FACIAL SURGERY

PLASTIC AND RECONSTRUCTIVE

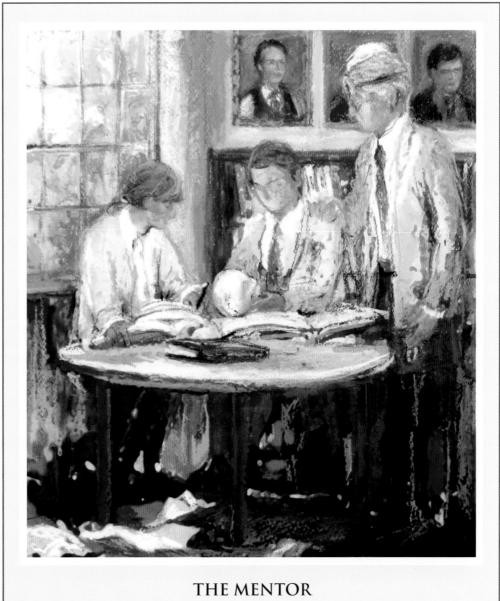

THE MENTOR

Artist: Jan Collins Selman, Selman Studio: *www.selmanstudio.com*
Mixed media, pastel and watercolor.

The mediocre teacher tells. The good teacher explains.
The superior teacher demonstrates. The great teacher inspires.
–William Arthur Ward (1921-1994)

FACIAL SURGERY

PLASTIC AND RECONSTRUCTIVE

Editors

MACK L. CHENEY, MD
Professor, Harvard Medical School;
Kletjian Chair and Director of Global Surgery,
Division of Facial Plastic and Reconstructive Surgery,
Massachusetts Eye and Ear Infirmary, Harvard Medical School,
Boston, Massachusetts

TESSA A. HADLOCK, MD
Director, Facial Plastic and Reconstructive Surgery
and Facial Nerve Center, Department of Otolaryngology,
Massachusetts Eye and Ear Infirmary, Harvard Medical School,
Boston, Massachusetts

With Illustrations By

ROBERT J. GALLA, MSI
TIFFANY SLAYBAUGH DAVANZO, MA, CMI
SARAH J. TAYLOR, MSMI

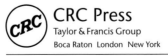

CRC Press
Taylor & Francis Group
Boca Raton London New York

CRC Press is an imprint of the
Taylor & Francis Group, an **informa** business

CRC Press
Taylor & Francis Group
6000 Broken Sound Parkway NW, Suite 300
Boca Raton, FL 33487-2742

Printed and bound in India by Replika Press Pvt. Ltd.

Printed on acid-free paper
Version Date: 20140721

International Standard Book Number-13: 978-1-4822-4091-7 (Pack - Book and Ebook)

Library of Congress Cataloging-in-Publication Data

Facial surgery : plastic and reconstructive / editors, Mack Cheney, Tessa
Hadlock ; with illustrations by Bob Galla, Tiffany Slaybaugh Davanzo, Sarah
J. Taylor.
   p. ; cm.
Preceded by: Facial surgery / [edited by] Mack L. Cheney. 1st ed. c1997.
Includes bibliographical references and index. Summary: "This landmark work covers the full range of aesthetic and reconstructive techniques in facial plastic surgery. Because of the coupling of aesthetics and function mandated by modern surgical standards, this book is organized by facial zone, rather than separated into aesthetic and reconstructive segments. The first six chapters highlight the basic principles of facial plastic and reconstructive surgery, including anatomy, proportions and beauty, visual documentation, and the principles of wound healing, aging, and flap design. Thereafter, sections are organized by facial zone or structure: the scalp and forehead, the eyelids and orbit, the nose, the ear, the bony facial skeleton, and the facial skin and soft tissue. Each section covers the range of aesthetic and reconstructive subjects relevant to the zone or structure in question. A separate section addresses conditions which affect multiple facial zones or tissues. The final section targets emerging trends and new directions in facial plastic and reconstructive surgery, designed to keep the reader both abreast of emerging technology, and intrigued and excited about the future possibilities for the specialty"--Provided by publisher.
ISBN 978-1-4822-4091-7 (hardback : alk. paper)
I. Cheney, Mack L. (Mack Lowell), 1955- , editor. II. Hadlock, Tessa A.,
editor.
[DNLM: 1. Face--surgery. 2. Reconstructive Surgical Procedures--methods.
WE 705]

RD523
617.5'2059--dc23   2014027822

Visit the Taylor & Francis Web site at
http://www.taylorandfrancis.com

and the CRC Press Web site at
http://www.crcpress.com

To Monty and Carmella for their prolonged and unwavering support—
with appreciation, admiration, and affection

Mack L. Cheney

■ ■ ■

This book is dedicated to the memories of Professor Farish Alston Jenkins, Jr.,
and Dr. William Wayne Montgomery, both the rarest of exceptional mentors

Of those to whom much is given, much is expected.
                              –John Fitzgerald Kennedy, 1961

Tessa A. Hadlock

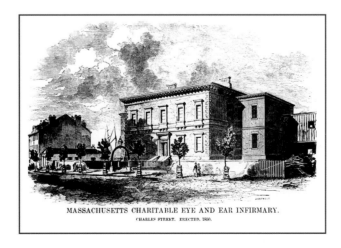

MASSACHUSETTS CHARITABLE EYE AND EAR INFIRMARY.
CHARLES STREET. ERECTED, 1850.

PUBLISHER Karen Berger

EDITORIAL COORDINATOR Megan Fennell

ASSISTANT EDITORS Heather Yocum, Ayse Eren

DIRECTOR OF EDITING Suzanne Wakefield

PROJECT EDITORS Hilary Hitchcock, Makalah Boyer

VICE PRESIDENT OF MANUFACTURING AND PRODUCTION Carolyn Reich

PRODUCTION Elaine Kitsis, Susan Trail, Madonna Gauding, Linda Maulin, Chris Lane

DIRECTOR OF GRAPHICS Brett Stone

GRAPHICS TECHNICIAN Ngoc-Thuy Khuu

DIRECTOR OF ILLUSTRATION Brenda Bunch

Contributors

PETER A. ADAMSON, MD, FRCSC, FACS
Professor and Head, Division of Facial Plastic
and Reconstructive Surgery, Department of
Otolaryngology-Head and Neck Surgery,
University of Toronto Faculty of Medicine,
Toronto, Canada

ROY AHN, ScD
Director of Research, Division of Global Health
and Human Rights, Department of Emergency
Medicine, Massachusetts General Hospital;
Instructor in Surgery, Harvard Medical School,
Boston, Massachusetts

DANIEL S. ALAM, MD
Section Head, Facial Plastic and Reconstructive
Surgery, Head and Neck Institute, Cleveland
Clinic; Associate Professor of Surgery, Case
Western Reserve, Lerner College of Medicine,
Cleveland, Ohio

MARCELO B. ANTUNES, MD
Private practice, Antunes Center for Facial
Plastic Surgery, Austin, Texas

BABAK AZIZZADEH, MD, FACS
Associate Clinical Professor, Department
of Surgery, David Geffen School of Medicine
of UCLA; Attending Surgeon, Department of
Surgery (Facial Plastic Surgery), Cedars-Sinai
Medical Center, Los Angeles, California

CAROLINE A. BANKS, MD
Clinical Fellow in Otology and Laryngology,
Department of Otology and Laryngology,
Massachusetts Eye and Ear Infirmary, Harvard
Medical School, Boston, Massachusetts

REGAN BERGMARK, MD
Resident, Department of Otology and Laryngology,
Massachusetts Eye and Ear Infirmary,
Harvard Medical School, Boston, Massachusetts

PRABHAT K. BHAMA, MD, MPH
Fellow, Department of Facial Plastic and
Reconstructive Surgery, Massachusetts Eye
and Ear Infirmary, Harvard Medical School,
Boston, Massachusetts

ELIZABETH A. BRADLEY, MD
Assistant Professor, Department of
Ophthalmology, Mayo Clinic, Rochester,
Minnesota

LORI A. BRIGHTMAN, MD, FAAD
Associate Adjunct Surgeon, Department of
Plastic Reconstructive Surgery, New York Eye
and Ear Infirmary, New York, New York

GARY C. BURGET, MD
Clinical Associate Professor, Section of Plastic
and Reconstructive Surgery, The University of
Chicago Pritzker School of Medicine; Attending
Surgeon, Department of Pediatric Plastic
Surgery, Lurie Children's Hospital, Chicago,
Illinois

THOMAS F. BURKE, MD, FACEP, FRSM
Chief, Division of Global Health and Human
Rights, Department of Emergency Medicine,
Massachusetts General Hospital; Assistant
Professor of Surgery, Harvard Medical School,
Boston, Massachusetts

MACK L. CHENEY, MD
Professor, Harvard Medical School; Kletjian
Chair and Director of Global Surgery, Division
of Facial Plastic and Reconstructive Surgery,
Massachusetts Eye and Ear Infirmary, Harvard
Medical School, Boston, Massachusetts

JOHN J. CHI, MD
Assistant Professor, Otolaryngology, Division
of Facial Plastic and Reconstructive Surgery,
Washington University School of Medicine,
St. Louis, Missouri

CAITLYN D. CLARK
Research Intern, Carolyn and Peter Lynch Center for Laser and Reconstructive Surgery, Massachusetts Eye and Ear Infirmary, Boston, Massachusetts

ROXANA COBO, MD
Coordinator, Service of Otolaryngology, Centro Medico Imbanaco, Cali, Colombia

MICHAEL S. COHEN, MD
Instructor, Department of Otology and Laryngology, Harvard Medical School, Boston, Massachusetts

DAWN K. DeCASTRO, MD
Clinical Instructor, Department of Oculoplastics and Reconstructive Surgery, Massachusetts Eye and Ear Infirmary, Boston, Massachusetts

JAIMIE DeROSA, MD, MS, FACS
DeRosa Facial Plastic Surgery, PC, Boston, Massachusetts

DANIEL DESCHLER, MD, FACS
Professor, Department of Otology and Laryngology, Harvard Medical School; Director, Division of Head and Neck Surgery, Department of Otolaryngology-Head and Neck Surgery, Massachusetts Eye and Ear Infirmary, Boston, Massachusetts

KEVIN S. EMERICK, MD
Assistant Professor, Department of Otology and Laryngology, Harvard Medical School, Boston, Massachusetts

AUDREY BAKER ERMAN, MD
Assistant Professor, Department of Otolaryngology, University of Arizona, Tucson, Arizona

CALLUM FARIS, MBBS, MRCS, FRCS
Consultant Otolaryngologist and Facial Plastic Reconstructive Surgeon, Department of Otolaryngology, Queen's Medical Centre, Nottingham, United Kingdom

PAUL E. FARMER, MD, PhD
Kolokotrones University Professor and Chair, Department of Global Health and Social Medicine, Harvard Medical School; Chief, Division of Global Health Equity, Brigham and Women's Hospital; Co-founder, Partners In Health, Boston, Massachusetts

BLAKE FAUSETT, MD, PhD
Department of Opthalmology and Visual Sciences, University of Michigan Kellogg Eye Center, Ann Arbor, Michigan

AARON FAY, MD
Assistant Professor, Department of Ophthalmology, Harvard Medical School, Boston, Massachusetts

JESSICA L. FEWKES, MD, FAAD
Assistant Professor, Department of Otology and Laryngology (Dermatology), Harvard Medical School, Boston, Massachusetts

SUZANNE K. FREITAG, MD
Assistant Professor, Harvard Medical School; Director, Ophthalmic Plastic Surgery Service, Department of Ophthalmology, Massachusetts Eye and Ear Infirmary, Boston, Massachusetts

RACHEL M. GILARDETTI
Researcher, Oral and Maxillofacial Surgery, Massachusetts General Hospital, Boston, Massachusetts

RICHARD GLIKLICH, MD
Leffenfeld Professor, Department of Otolaryngology, Massachusetts Eye and Ear Infirmary, Harvard Medical School, Boston, Massachusetts

GARRETT GRIFFIN, MD
Surgeon, Midwest Facial Plastic Surgery and Aesthetic Skincare, Woodbury, Minnesota

TESSA A. HADLOCK, MD
Director, Facial Plastic and Reconstructive Surgery and Facial Nerve Center, Department of Otolaryngology, Massachusetts Eye and Ear Infirmary, Harvard Medical School, Boston, Massachusetts

CHRISTOPHER J. HARTNICK, MD
Professor, Department of Pediatric
Otolaryngology, Massachusetts Eye and Ear
Infirmary, Boston, Massachusetts

RICHARD E. HAYDEN, MD
Professor and Chairman, Department of
Otolaryngology-Head and Neck Surgery,
Mayo Clinic Arizona, Phoenix, Arizona

MARC W. HERR, MD
Otolaryngologist, Brooke Army Medical
Center, San Antonio Military Medical Center,
Department of Otolaryngology-Head and Neck
Oncology/Microvascular Reconstruction, San
Antonio, Texas

MARC HALE HOHMAN, MD
Assistant Professor, Department of Surgery,
Uniformed Services University of the Health
Sciences, Bethesda, Maryland; Major, Medical
Corps, U.S. Army, Staff Plastic Surgeon, Madigan
Army Medical Center, Tacoma, Washington

ANTHONY D. HOLMES, MB, BS, FRACS
Clinical Professor, Department of Pediatrics,
University of Melbourne; Senior Plastic Surgeon,
Department of Plastic and Maxillofacial Surgery,
Royal Children's Hospital, Melbourne, Australia

BRITTANY E. HOWARD, MD
Resident, Department of Otolaryngology-
Head and Neck Surgery, Mayo Clinic Arizona,
Phoenix, Arizona

ADAM S. JACOBSON, MD
Attending Physician, Department of
Otolaryngology-Head and Neck Surgery,
Mount Sinai Beth Israel, New York, New York

CALVIN M. JOHNSON, JR., MD
Clinical Associate Professor, Department of
Otolaryngology-Head and Neck Surgery,
Tulane University School of Medicine,
New Orleans, Louisiana

ROBERT M. KELLMAN, MD
Professor and Chair, Department of
Otolaryngology and Communication Sciences,
SUNY Upstate Medical University, Syracuse,
New York

ELIAS KHOURY, MD, FRCS
Department of Otolaryngology, Charing Cross
Hospital, London, United Kingdom

ALYN J. KIM, MD
Physician, Department of Otolaryngology/
Head and Neck Surgery, Long Beach Memorial
Hospital and Miller Children's Hospital, Long
Beach, California

DAVID C. KIM, MD
Plastic Surgeon, Department of Plastic and Oral
Surgery, Boston Children's Hospital, Harvard
Medical School, Boston, Massachusetts

JENNIFER KIM, MD
Associate Professor, Department of
Otolaryngology, University of Michigan Health
System, Ann Arbor, Michigan

ANDREW J. KLEINBERGER, MD
Clinical Instructor, Department of
Otolaryngology-Head and Neck Surgery,
Boston University School of Medicine, Boston,
Massachusetts

CODY A. KOCH, MD, PHD
Physician, Koch Facial Plastic Surgery and Spa,
West Des Moines, Iowa

WAYNE F. LARRABEE, JR., MD, FACS
Department of Otolaryngology-Head and Neck
Surgery, University of Washington, Seattle,
Washington

NAHYOUNG GRACE LEE, MD
Instructor, Department of Ophthalmology,
Harvard Medical School; Ophthalmic Plastic and
Reconstructive Surgery, Massachusetts Eye and
Ear Infirmary, Boston, Massachusetts

PETER LIACOURAS, PHD
Director of Services, 3D Medical Applications
Center, Department of Radiology, Walter Reed
National Military Medical Center, Bethesda,
Maryland

ALICE C. LIN, MD
Chief of Microvascular and Robotic Surgery,
Department of Otolaryngology-Head and Neck
Surgery, SUNY Downstate Medical Center,
Brooklyn, New York

ROBIN W. LINDSAY, MD
Assistant Professor, Department of Otology and
Laryngology, Harvard Medical School; Surgeon-
Facial Plastic and Reconstruction, Department
of Otolaryngology, Massachusetts Eye and Ear
Infirmary, Boston, Massachusetts

RALPH MAGRITZ, MD
Visiting Professor, Ear, Nose, and Throat-Head
and Neck Surgery, Regensburg University,
Regensburg; Surgeon, Ear, Nose, and Throat,
Department of Head and Neck Surgery, Prosper
Hospital, Recklinghausen, Germany

RYAN M. MANZ, MD
Facial Plastic Surgery, Department of
Otolaryngology-Head and Neck Surgery,
Gunderson Health System, La Crosse, Wisconsin

VARTAN A. MARDIROSSIAN, MD
Assistant Professor, Department of
Otolaryngology, Florida Atlantic University,
Boca Raton, Florida; Jacobson and Mardirossian
Plastic Surgery Center for Excellence, Jupiter,
Florida

JOHN G. MEARA, MD, DMD, MBA
Associate Professor, Department of Surgery;
Global Health and Social Medicine, Harvard
Medical School; Plastic Surgeon-in-Chief,
Department of Plastic and Oral Surgery, Boston
Children's Hospital, Boston, Massachusetts

SARAL MEHRA, MD, MBA
Assistant Professor of Surgery (Otolaryngology),
Head and Neck Cancer and Reconstructive
Surgery, Yale University School of Medicine,
New Haven, Connecticut

GUSTAVO MIERY, MD
Assistant Professor, Department of Plastic
Surgery, Universidad el Bosque, Bogota, DC,
Colombia

ALI MOKHTARZADEH, MD
Department of Ophthalmology and Visual
Neurosciences, University of Minnesota,
Minneapolis, Minnesota

JEFFREY MOYER, MD, FACS
Associate Professor and Chief, Facial Plastic
and Reconstructive Surgery, Department of
Otolaryngology-Head and Neck Surgery,
University of Michigan, Ann Arbor, Michigan

CHRISTINE NELSON, MD, FACS
Bartley R. Frueh and Frueh Family Professor
in Eye Plastics and Orbital Surgery; Professor,
Ophthalmology and Visual Sciences, Depart-
ment of Ophthalmology, Kellogg Eye Center,
University of Michigan, Ann Arbor, Michigan

TERESA M. O, M.ARCH, MD
Co-director, Facial Nerve Center, Department
of Otolaryngology-Head and Neck Surgery,
Vascular Birthmark Institute of New York,
Lenox Hill and Manhattan Eye, Ear, and Throat
Hospitals, New York, New York

JON-PAUL PEPPER, MD
Assistant Professor, Department of
Otolaryngology-Head and Neck Surgery,
Keck School of Medicine of the University of
Southern California, Los Angeles, California

VITO C. QUATELA, MD, FACS
Clinical Associate Professor, Department
of Otolaryngology, University of Rochester,
Rochester, New York

ALICIA M. QUESNEL, MD
Instructor, Department of Otology and
Laryngology, Harvard Medical School;
Department of Otolaryngology, Massachusetts
Eye and Ear Infirmary, Boston, Massachusetts

KAVITHA K. REDDY, MD
Director of Dermatologic Surgery, Department
of Dermatology, Boston University School of
Medicine, Boston, Massachusetts

CAROLYN R. ROGERS, MD
Clinical Instructor of Surgery, Department of
Plastic and Oral Surgery, Boston Children's
Hospital, Boston, Massachusetts

DEREK J. ROGERS, MD
Clinical Fellow, Department of Pediatric
Otolaryngology, Massachusetts Eye and Ear
Infirmary, Boston, Massachusetts

HESHAM SALEH, MD, FRCS (ORL-HNS)
Honorary Senior Lecturer, Department of
Otolaryngology, Imperial College; Consultant
Rhinologist/Facial Plastic Surgeon, Department
of Otolaryngology, Charing Cross and Royal
Brompton Hospitals, London, United Kingdom

NADIA SHAIKH, MS
Student, University of Massachusetts Medical
School, Worcester, Massachusetts

JEFFREY H. SPIEGEL, MD, FACS
Professor and Chief, Division of Facial Plastic
and Reconstructive Surgery, Department of
Otolaryngology-Head and Neck Surgery,
Boston University School of Medicine, Boston,
Massachusetts

MICHAEL SULLIVAN, MD
Plastic Surgeon, The Sullivan Centre, Columbus,
Ohio

CATHRYN A. SUNDBACK, ScD
Assistant Professor in Surgery, Co-director of
the Laboratory of Tissue Engineering and Organ
Fabrication, Center for Regenerative Medicine,
Department of Surgery, Massachusetts General
Hospital, Boston, Massachusetts

OON TIAN TAN, MD, PHD
Director, Carolyn and Peter Lynch Center for
Laser and Reconstructive Surgery, Massachusetts
Eye and Ear Infirmary, Boston, Massachusetts

DEAN M. TORIUMI, MD
Professor, Department of Otolaryngology-
Head and Neck Surgery, University of Illinois at
Chicago, Chicago, Illinois

PATRICK TRÉVIDIC, MD
Head, Department of Surgery, Hôpital Sainte-
Anne, Paris, France

MARIA J. TROULIS, DDS, MSc
Associate Professor, Department of Oral and
Maxillofacial Surgery, Massachusetts General
Hospital, Harvard School of Dental Medicine,
Boston, Massachusetts

JASON P. ULM, MD
Assistant Professor of Surgery, Department
of Plastic and Reconstructive Surgery, Medical
University of South Carolina, Charleston, South
Carolina; Craniofacial Fellow, Department
of Plastic and Reconstructive Surgery,
Massachusetts General Hospital, Harvard
Medical School, Boston, Massachusetts

MARK L. URKEN, MD, FACS
Professor, Department of Otolaryngology,
Icahn School of Medicine at Mount Sinai;
Medical Director, Thane Foundation,
New York, New York

JOSEPH P. VACANTI, MD
John Homans Professor of Surgery, Harvard
Medical School, Boston, Massachusetts; Chief,
Department of Pediatric Surgery, Massachusetts
General Hospital; Surgeon-in-Chief,
Massachusetts General Hospital for Children;
Co-director, Center for Regenerative Medicine,
Massachusetts General Hospital; Director,
Laboratory for Tissue Engineering and Organ
Fabrication, Massachusetts General Hospital;
Chief, Pediatric Transplantation, Department
of Surgery, Massachusetts General Hospital,
Boston, Massachusetts

MARK VARVARES, MD, FACS
Donald and Marlene Jerome Endowed Chair,
Department of Otolaryngology-Head and Neck
Surgery; Director, St. Louis University Cancer
Center, Department of Otolaryngology-Head
and Neck Surgery, St. Louis University, St. Louis,
Missouri

HADÉ VUYK, MD, PHD
Facial Plastic Reconstructive Surgery Clinics,
Vleuten, The Netherlands

THOMAS J. WALKER, MD
Fellow, Facial Plastic and Reconstructive Surgery,
Department of Otolaryngology-Head and
Neck Surgery, University of Illinois at Chicago,
Chicago, Illinois

**MILTON WANER, MB, BCH (WITS),
FCS(SA), MD**
Co-director, Vascular Birthmark Institute of
New York, Department of Otolaryngology-Head
and Neck Surgery, Lenox Hill and Manhattan
Eye, Ear, and Throat Hospitals, New York,
New York

BRIAN J.F. WONG, MD, PHD, FACS
Professor and Vice-Chairman, Department
of Otolaryngology-Head and Neck Surgery,
Department of Biomedical Engineering,
Department of Surgery, and The Beckman
Laser Institute and Medical Clinic, University of
California, Irvine, Irvine, California

WENDY WILLIAMS, JD
Associate Director, Office of Global Surgery and
Health, Massachusetts Eye and Ear Infirmary,
Boston, Massachusetts

MICHAEL J. YAREMCHUK, MD
Professor, Department of Surgery, Harvard
Medical School; Chief of Craniofacial Surgery,
Department of Plastic Surgery, Massachusetts
General Hospital, Boston, Massachusetts

YEDEH YING, DMD
Clinical Fellow, Department of Oral and
Maxillofacial Surgery, Massachusetts General
Hospital, Boston, Massachusetts

Preface

A movement to create a subspecialty within otolaryngology/head and neck surgery began four decades ago, driven by the recognized need to focus aesthetic and reconstructive procedures in the head and neck toward a select group of individuals with specialized training. This concept has now fully matured in the United States as facial plastic and reconstructive surgery. The emergence of the distinct field of facial plastic and reconstructive surgery has likewise found solid footing in Europe, Central and South America, and Australasia and continues to resonate with surgeons across the globe; the field has entered an exciting new phase of global connectivity. The lines between and among specialties have blurred in positive and productive ways, and our modern understanding of the relationship between form and function has continued to evolve.

We have crafted this textbook to reflect these important trends. Authors from disparate specialties, including facial plastic and reconstructive surgery, oculoplastic surgery, plastic surgery, oral and maxillofacial surgery, dermatology, and others, have been brought together to produce a body of work that is intended to represent the best of cross-specialty collaboration and cross-continent communication.

This book arose from a precursor text of the same name, published in 1997. Like many works of that era, the original book represented an institutional approach to the field of facial plastic and reconstructive surgery. The contributing authors were practicing at or had received training at the Massachusetts Eye and Ear Infirmary and thus had been heavily influenced by the historic figures from this institution: Dr. Varaztad Kazanjian, Dr. Edgar Holmes, Dr. Aram Roopenian, Dr. Richard Webster, and Dr. William Montgomery. The current text is intended to capture a broader scope of intellectual energy and surgical creativity that globalization of our field and cross-specialty collaborations have fostered, while simultaneously preserving important elements of the historic work at The Infirmary and Harvard Medical School.

Throughout the chapters, historical perspective is deliberately emphasized to highlight the importance of thought leaders that have come before us. The current generation of surgeons owes much to past leaders, who forged the concept that form and function lie along an important continuum. Surgeons concentrating on aesthetic issues of the nose, ear, periocular region, and face must now have a thorough understanding of the ways in which aesthetic surgical manipulation can either enhance or impair function. Likewise, head and neck reconstructive surgeons must give intensive consideration to aesthetic outcomes when planning and executing complex reconstructive procedures.

Driven by the coupling of aesthetics and function mandated by modern surgical standards, this book is organized by facial zone, rather than separated into "aesthetic" and "reconstructive" segments. The first six chapters highlight the basic principles of facial plastic and reconstructive surgery, including anatomy, proportions and beauty, visual documentation, and the principles of wound healing, aging, and flap design. Thereafter, sections are organized by facial zone or structure: the scalp and forehead, the eyelids and orbit, the nose, the ear, the bony facial skeleton, and the facial skin and soft tissue. Each section covers the range of aesthetic and reconstructive subjects relevant to the zone or structure in question. A separate section addresses conditions which affect multiple facial zones or tissues. The final section targets emerging trends and new directions in facial plastic and reconstructive surgery, designed to keep the reader both abreast of emerging technology and intrigued and excited about the future possibilities for our specialty.

The book is accompanied by an e-book version, allowing access wherever the surgeon may be, and a wealth of operative videos. In addition, we include a pilot educational feature, modeled after modern Internet-based open access global teaching programs, which emphasizes learning through a coupling of both visual and oral teaching. This unique experiment, which we term "Medflix," is presented in the form of video-teaching supplements that accompany chapters on Anatomy, Facial Aging, Acute Auricular Injuries, Local Flaps for Auricular Reconstruction, Microtia, Mandibular Fractures, Facial Paralysis, Evaluating Patient Outcomes, and Tissue Engineering. These educational supplements are intended to appeal to both visual and auditory learners and those who prefer to watch, rather than read, a chapter.

Our hope is that residents, fellows, and mature surgeons across disciplines will gain valuable knowledge from the content presented herein.

Any project undertaken by two people is by necessity a complex melding of styles and strengths, involving fluid and occasionally lively interchange, whose aim is to produce a final product that integrates the ideas of both participants into a common vision. It is our sincere hope that this unified vision is reflected in the pages of this book.

Mack L. Cheney
Tessa A. Hadlock

Not to know what happened before one was born is always to be a child.
–Marcus Tullius Cicero (46 BC)

Acknowledgments

The interface of disciplines is where progress is made.
—Joseph E. Murray, MD (1919-2012)
Professor of Plastic Surgery,
Harvard Medical School, 1990 Nobel Laureate,
Physiology or Medicine

This project represents the collective efforts of many authors, illustrators, editorial staff members, and administrators. Particular acknowledgment goes to several key individuals who provided major support in the early, middle, and late phases of the book. First and foremost, Dr. Joseph Nadol, Chairman Emeritus of the Department of Otolaryngology at the Massachusetts Eye and Ear Infirmary, served as a champion of the project from its conception and generously permitted the use of extensive departmental resources, including the services of Robert Galla and Suzanne Day. Dr. Bradley Welling carried enthusiastic support for the project into his tenure at The Infirmary, for which we are extremely grateful.

Karen Berger at Quality Medical Publishing really made this book happen. From our first conversation, we shared a collective vision for what a useful, versatile, and handsome textbook should look like, and how it could be organized and designed. It was a wonderful union of philosophies that has now spanned three years. The entire QMP staff have been extraordinarily responsive and have helped us keep to a reasonable timeline, and for that we are certainly indebted. Sue Hodgson of Taylor & Francis Group demonstrated an amazing ability to jump into the project midway, and has truly helped us get over the finish line with enthusiasm. She has helped us to produce a book of which we can all be proud.

A book comes down to the contributors, and we owe profound gratitude to those who took time out of their busy lives to thoughtfully compose chapters at stages of their careers where the novelty of composing a chapter has completely worn off. A special thanks to the most senior authors, Drs. Burget, Cobo, Hayden, Holmes, Kellman, Larrabee, Quatela, Sullivan, Tan, Toriumi, Troulis, Urken, Varvares, Vuyk, and Waner, whose contributions are all the more valuable given the perspective with which they were composed.

An enormous acknowledgment must be made to our fellows, Drs. Prabhat Bhama and Caroline Banks, who not only made important writing contributions to six of the chapters, but who also spent countless hours pouring over details of artwork, page layouts, text, and video. They not only kept the project on track, but also provided a gentle, positive, and encouraging spirit when our editorial tempers ran short. Wendy Williams picked up the administrative torch at The Infirmary, and through her efforts the project was able to be completed in an efficient timeframe.

Projects such as this book require enormous commitments of time, effort, and energy. We would like to acknowledge the support of our families in generously sacrificing time together for the type of commitment such a project entails.

Contents

VOLUME

PART I ▪ GENERAL PRINCIPLES

VOLUME

Section V ▪ Bony Facial Skeleton

Section VI ▪ Facial Skin and Soft Tissue

PART III ▪ CONDITIONS AFFECTING MULTIPLE FACIAL ZONES OR TISSUES

Part IV ▪ Emerging Trends and New Directions in Facial Plastic Surgery

Facial Surgery

Plastic and Reconstructive

28

Nasoethmoid Complex, Frontal Sinus, and Skull Base Fractures

Robert M. Kellman

Trauma to the area of the root of the nose frequently results in fractures of the thin bones that lie deep to the nasal root. The concept of the nasoethmoid complex fracture, or nasoorbital ethmoid fracture, evolved from recognition of the characteristic way in which the bones of the ethmoid sinuses and medial orbits collapse in response to high-impact injury directed at the nasal root. The thin bones of the ethmoid sinuses and medial orbits give way, allowing the nasal bone to telescope posteriorly. Stranc[1,2] described this as the *ethmoid crush;* ultimately the name has changed variably to *nasoethmoid complex* (NEC) or *nasoorbitoethmoid* (NOE) fracture to more closely reflect the structures involved. Early treatment favored closed management of these injuries, with lead plates positioned over the lateral nasal bones, secured in place using percutaneously placed transnasal wires. It became apparent that this approach produced suboptimal outcomes, and routine open/direct repair has since become prevalent.

Fractures of the NEC, the frontal sinuses, and the anterior skull base present unique challenges to the craniomaxillofacial surgeon because of difficulties with surgical access for repair and controversies relating to the management of the frontal sinus cavities. These fractures are also associated with cerebrospinal fluid (CSF) leaks, and disagreements exist regarding their management. Furthermore, repair of NOE fractures requires access to and repair of the medial canthal ligaments, which represents a significant technical challenge. Failure to recognize an injury to this area may lead to deforming telecanthus, which may be very difficult to repair secondarily. A thorough understanding of proper NOE, frontal sinus, and skull base fracture management is essential for those charged with the care of these injuries.

ANATOMY, EPIDEMIOLOGY, AND CLASSIFICATION

The nasal bones project anteriorly from the frontal processes of the maxillae and attach superiorly to the very solid bone of the glabella, a portion of the frontal bone (Fig. 28-1).

The frontal bone is thick in this lower area, becoming thinner over the paired frontal sinuses. The supraorbital rims are likewise thick and solid and form ridges that extend inferiorly a variable distance over the globes. Posterior to the nasal bones, the maxilla contributes to the anterior lacrimal crest, and the lacrimal bones house and protect the lacrimal sacs behind the anterior lacrimal crests, providing a posterior crest to complete the lacrimal fossae.

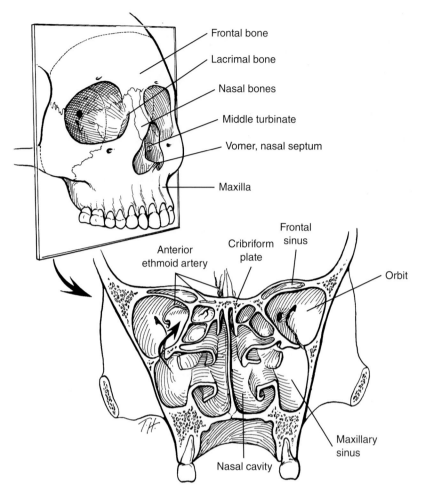

Frontal bone

Lacrimal bone

Nasal bones

Middle turbinate

Vomer, nasal septum

Maxilla

Anterior ethmoid artery

Cribriform plate

Frontal sinus

Orbit

Maxillary sinus

Nasal cavity

Fig. 28-1   Bony anatomy of the nasoorbitoethmoid complex.

In this zone, the medial canthal ligaments—formed by medial extensions of the orbicularis oculi muscles—split into anterior and posterior components and attach to the anterior and posterior lacrimal crests, respectively (see Chapter 11, Fig. 11-2). There are also superior extensions of the tendons, which secure the medial canthi superiorly and prevent inferior displacement. Behind the lacrimal bone, the very thin lamina papyracea (aptly named for its "paper thin" structure) separates the orbital contents from the ethmoid sinuses. Posteriorly, the optic nerves traverse through a foramen surrounded by the extremely thick and protective bone of the lesser wing of the sphenoid.

Because of their prominent position and relative thinness compared with the bones posterior to and surrounding them, the nasal bones are the most commonly fractured facial bones. The thicker bones of the glabella and frontal area require much more force to fracture and therefore are fractured less frequently. Frontal fractures are usually the result of high impact trauma, such as that seen in motor vehicle accidents involving unrestrained occupants, high-force assaults—typically with weapons rather than fists, falls, and industrial accidents.

The NEC/NOE fracture is usually the result of a direct high-energy impact to the nasal root/glabellar region. This impact results in "telescoping" of the solid nasal root posteriorly into the ethmoids and orbits, with associated disruption of the thin laminae of the medial orbits (Fig. 28-2).

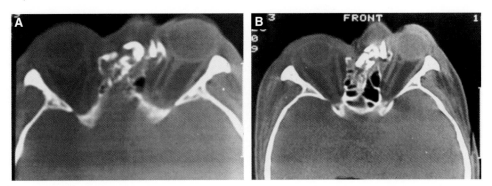

Fig. 28-2   Nasoethmoid complex fracture. **A,** Axial CT section shows marked comminution of the nasal bones, anterior ethmoid sinuses, and cribriform plate area with marked telescoping. Note displacement of the nasal bones and medial wall of the orbit laterally with encroachment on the medial rectus muscle and globe on the left. **B,** Axial CT section (at a slightly higher level than **A**) shows the comminution, telescoping, and displacement of fragments into both orbits, predominantly on the left.

Displacement/fracture of the maxillary and lacrimal components of the medial orbital area results in loss of fixation of the medial canthal ligaments. The lacrimal collecting system in the medial anterior orbit is affected. The collecting canaliculi are located in the medial upper and lower lids, and they join medially to form a common canaliculus that drains into the lacrimal sac, which resides between the anterior and posterior lacrimal crests in the medial orbital wall. The lacrimal sac drains into the nasolacrimal duct, which drains inferiorly into the nose, lateral to the inferior turbinate.

Fractures often involve the supraorbital rims and extend into the frontal sinuses. The supraorbital rims provide transit for the supraorbital and supratrochlear nerves and vessels, which pass through the rims along a notch or a foramen to innervate and vascularize the frontal area and scalp, and are thus at risk from injury or from surgical approaches to repair.

The frontal sinuses are mucosally lined bony cavities located completely within the frontal bones. They drain through openings (complete ducts in about 15% of cases) located medially and posteriorly within the sinuses, opening most frequently into the frontal recess of the anterior ethmoid sinuses.

Considering the significant force required to fracture the thick frontal/glabellar bone, it is noteworthy that injuries to the eyes and optic nerves are relatively infrequent. It has been theorized that the frontal sinuses within the frontal bones may provide a survival advantage by serving as a "crumple zone" to protect the brain from direct frontal trauma, and similarly, the collapse of the NEC with telescoping of the nasal root into the ethmoid sinuses—rather than into the orbit and posteriorly into the optic canals—might serve to protect the globes and optic nerves.[3,4]

The anterior skull base is composed of the sturdy bones of the orbital roofs laterally and the thinner roofs of the ethmoid sinuses and the cribriform plates medially (see Fig. 28-1).

Numerous classification systems have been proposed in attempts to characterize both frontal sinus and NOE fractures. The easiest and most useful way to classify frontal sinus fractures is by anatomic location: anterior wall, posterior wall, and floor, and by involvement of the frontal sinus outflow tract (FSOT). A

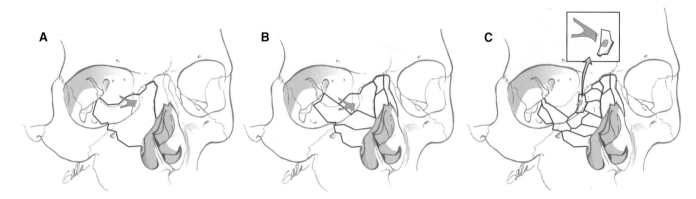

Fig. 28-3 **A,** Type I NOE fracture. **B,** Type II NOE fracture. **C,** Type III NOE fracture.

particularly useful classification of NOE/NEC was developed by Markowitz and Manson,[5] with type I (Fig. 28-3, *A*) involving a solid central fragment still attached to the medial canthal ligament, type II (Fig. 28-3, *B*) with comminution of the central fragment with the ligament still attached, and type III (Fig. 28-3, *C*) with severe comminution of the central fragment and disruption of the medial canthal ligament.

There is no well-defined classification for anterior skull base fractures that guides the approach to repair. Important issues to be considered with anterior skull base fractures include displacement, defect, CSF leak, and brain herniation. It is difficult to comprehensively describe these features using a simple classification system because current systems are generally radiologically based, and current radiologic assessments are often inadequate for assessing these critical clinical/anatomic uncertainties.

PATIENT EDUCATION AND PREOPERATIVE PLANNING

The key to preoperative planning is adequate assessment of the injury. Since fractures in this area may traverse the skull base, careful assessment for CSF rhinorrhea is mandatory. If any orbital bones have been fractured, an ophthalmology consultation is indicated, and any vision-threatening situation should guide the planned surgery. The status of the medial canthal attachments must be evaluated by manipulation to assess adequacy of their fixation. Extraocular movements must be evaluated and epiphora documented, because it may indicate injury of the lacrimal collecting system. A full cranial nerve examination should also be documented.

Risks of fracture repair include residual deformity, blindness, diplopia, persistent CSF leak, meningitis, epiphora, and cranial nerve deficits. Catastrophic risks are rare but must be mentioned.

INDICATIONS, LIMITATIONS, AND TECHNIQUES

For frontal sinus trauma, indications for exploration and intervention (and choice of intervention) remain more controversial than other areas of facial trauma and are considered based on anatomic location.

Frontal sinus fractures can be divided anatomically into anterior wall, posterior wall, and floor. Many fractures will traverse more than one site, and management will depend on each area injured.

ANTERIOR WALL

Isolated anterior wall fractures will not traverse the duct (that is, the FSOT) of the frontal sinus. Fractures may result in displacement of the anterior wall, which can create a cosmetic deformity; repair is designed to prevent deformity (Fig. 28-4).

Unfortunately, soft tissue swelling may mask the deformity. Repair of pure anterior wall fractures generally requires wide exposure (through the coronal approach) and is indicated for severely displaced frac-

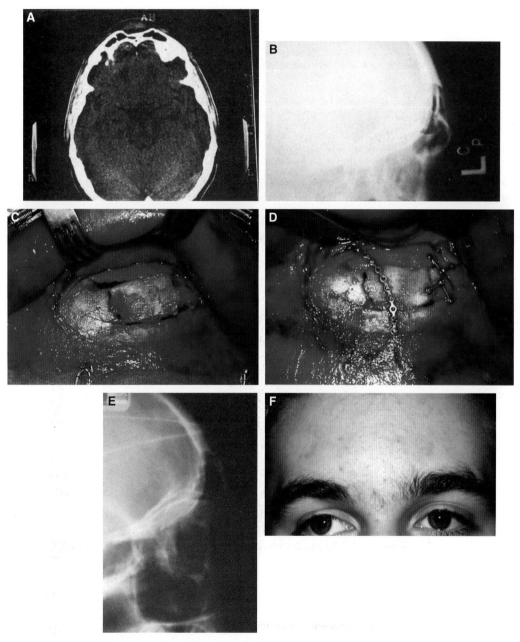

Fig. 28-4   **A,** CT scan of anterior frontal sinus fracture. **B,** Lateral radiograph of frontal sinus fracture. **C,** Coronal exploration. **D,** Repositioning of anterior fragments with miniplate fixation. **E,** Restoration of anterior frontal sinus wall. **F,** Result 6 months postoperatively.

tures. For mildly displaced fractures, either repair or observation is acceptable. If a deformity becomes apparent after several weeks, a camouflage approach using an implant/graft placed over the defect (outside of the sinuses) may be performed.

When the supraorbital rim is involved in anterior wall fractures, the floor of the frontal sinus will be injured as well. Fractures through the floor of the sinus have a high likelihood of injury of the FSOT. Involvement of the outflow tract changes the fracture from a cosmetic injury to an injury that has the potential to affect sinus function. Strong evidence suggests that obstruction of the FSOT will lead to complications that often require secondary surgery, and increase the risk of high morbidity infectious complications.[6,7] The conclusion from the traditional literature has been to obliterate or cranialize the frontal sinus when FSOT injury is found.[7-12] However, in the endoscopic age, some early evidence suggests that even in the presence of an FSOT injury, close observation with anatomic repair as needed may allow early discovery of impending sinus complications, which may be managed using endoscopic transnasal approaches to the frontal sinuses.[13]

Involvement of the posterior wall of the frontal sinus requires careful assessment and management. Donald and Bernstein[8] have popularized the cranialization procedure for posterior wall fractures associated with significant disruption of the bone. Both cranialization and obliteration have been shown to decrease the risks of complications and secondary surgical procedures in patients with posterior wall and FSOT injuries.[7] When the fracture extends posteriorly along the roof of the ethmoid and/or cribriform plate, the risk of meningitis is increased, and a management strategy should be considered.

Techniques

Repair of anterior wall frontal sinus fractures is typically performed using 1 to 1.5 mm plates and screws to minimize visibility of the hardware through the skin, through either an existing laceration, or through a bicoronal approach.

Obliteration of the frontal sinuses requires complete removal of all sinus mucosa. This requires drilling of the walls of the sinus until all potential invaginations of mucosa are completely exenterated, otherwise mucosa may regenerate and result in mucocele formation. Openings into the ethmoids/nose must be completely sealed with fascia or bone. The sinus cavity is then filled with the obliteration material of choice, preferably autogenous cancellous bone or fat.

When cranialization is selected, the posterior walls of the sinuses are removed completely. Mucosa is completely exenterated from the remaining sinus areas, including drilling. It is imperative that any communication with the ethmoid/nasal cavities be occluded. This should be embellished with a well-vascularized pericranial flap whenever possible, to assure separation between the sterile brain/dural space and the contaminated sinus/nasal area.

The approach to the ethmoid roof and cribriform area depends on the severity of the injury. If it is extensive, the subcranial approach (described later) provides broad exposure and access for dependable repair with a pericranial flap. For more limited injuries, endoscopic exploration and repair will allow proper assessment of ethmoid roof and cribriform injuries with access for repair of small defects.

Repair of NOE/NEC fractures involves two main goals: (1) repositioning of the medial canthal ligaments, and (2) restoration of nasal dorsal height. Failure to achieve these two important objectives will result in a significant cosmetic deformity that is difficult to repair secondarily. Inadequate medialization of the medial canthal ligament results in *telecanthus*, a term that refers to the appearance of hypertelorism although the eyes (orbits) themselves are not actually too far apart (it has also, therefore, been referred to as *pseudohypertelorism*) (Fig. 28-5).

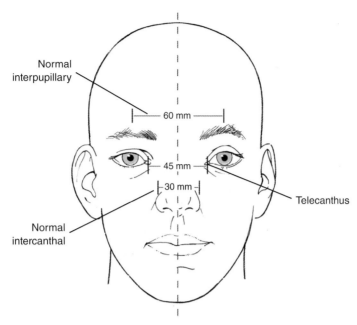

Fig. 28-5   Inadequate medialization of the medial canthal ligament.

The medial canthal ligament secures the medial canthus in position, and when it is released, the canthus becomes laterally, inferiorly, and anteriorly malpositioned. Correction of this sequela requires repositioning the medial canthal ligament medially, superiorly, and posteriorly. In type I fractures, the ligament remains attached to a substantial segment of bone, so that repositioning the bone and rigidly fixing it in place effectively repositions the ligament (see Fig. 28-3).

In type II fractures, although the ligament is still attached to a bony fragment, it is typically too small and unstable to be held in place with bone fixation alone (see Fig. 28-3, *B*). These injuries require some form of medial stabilization of the ligament, generally transnasally to the contralateral side. For type II fractures, there are two options: (1) to pass a wire/stitch through the small fragment and/or ligament and fix it in place, or (2) to disarticulate the ligament from the bone fragment and convert it to a type III injury (see Fig. 28-3, *C*).

A type III fracture involves complete separation of the ligament from the bone, usually caused by disruption of the medial attachment. When the ligament is free, it can be grasped with a suture (either wire or permanent suture) and fixed in proper anatomic position. Fixation of the medial canthal attachment (type II or III) can be accomplished ipsilaterally to a plate or contralaterally (more typical) behind the nasal bone, either to the contralateral medial canthal ligament or to a plate or bone at the superomedial frontoorbital junction. It is important to be sure that the ligament has been properly secured medially, superiorly, and posteriorly to avoid late deformity. The nasal dorsal height must be reestablished using bone grafts, if necessary, to avoid loss of nasal dorsal height and likely development of epicanthal folds.

CSF leaks should be assessed even if they stop spontaneously. Once a leak is recognized, it indicates a communication between the subdural space and the outside environment. If it stops, it could be caused by the development of a dural seal (which is indeed the goal of repair), or it could indicate that a hole has been plugged with brain, which leads to an encephalocele, leaving the patient at long-term risk of developing meningitis. If open surgery is planned, the area of the leak can be directly visualized and assessed and then repaired if indicated. If open surgery is not otherwise indicated, the site of the defect should be identified on CT and then visualized endoscopically, typically under anesthesia, particularly since it may require entry into one of the paranasal sinuses. Once the site of the leak is visualized, the need for repair may be assessed and endoscopic repair may be accomplished if indicated.

When the anterior skull base and posterior frontal sinus are fractured along with an NOE/NEC fracture, removal of the nasal/glabella complex allows the surgeon full access to the anterior skull base for visualization and repair. This subcranial approach, introduced by Raveh,[14] is a logical choice in severe trauma because much of the approach is completed by the fracture itself. The medial canthal ligaments are repaired directly by repositioning them medially and superiorly and fixating them to the contralateral frontal bone (called *centripetal suspension* by Raveh). Proper posterior positioning is assured by displacing the fixation wire/suture posteriorly when replacing the nasal dorsum (or with a bone graft).

ADJUNCTIVE PROCEDURES

Some advocate lumbar drainage as an initial step in management of CSF rhinorrhea. However, others recommend this approach only after assuring that a safe potential seal is present, after assessment and even initial repair of the defect.

Evaluation and consideration for possible cannulation of the lacrimal collecting system should be considered when indicated. Traditionally, cannulation was commonly performed in NOE fractures because nasolacrimal duct injuries are relatively common. However, many patients with minor duct injury develop long-term epiphora; thus it is reasonable to observe most of these patients and to reserve operative intervention only if epiphora develops or fails to resolve.

Controversy exists as to whether a percutaneous transnasal bolster should be applied after NOE repair to ensure maximal medialization of the overlying skin. However, bolstering can damage already traumatized skin, so this approach is not universally advocated. An alternative approach involves placing a secure case over the nasal dorsum with firm medial positioning, taking care not to devascularize the skin.

Management of posttraumatic sinus disease, particularly frontal sinus disease, is essential and may be performed using modern endoscopic sinus surgery techniques.

Intraoperative CT scanning guidance should be considered.[15] In most institutions, postoperative CT scans are performed in the days after surgery. Because the threshold for revision of a suboptimally reduced fracture is often high, the use of intraoperative scanning allows the surgeon to obtain a real-time assessment and an opportunity to reposition suboptimally repaired fractures before leaving the operating room.

POSTOPERATIVE CARE

Careful, frequent neurologic and visual assessments should be performed during the initial postoperative period. Developing and/or progressive visual loss can indicate the presence of an orbital hematoma that may require decompression. Neurologic checks are also essential to assure recognition of an intracranial hematoma or tension pneumocephalus. Elevating the head of the bed decreases postoperative swelling. The nasal tissues should be kept moist with nasal saline, although if a suspicious rhinorrhea exists, introduction of nasal saline may obscure evaluation for CSF leakage.

COMPLICATIONS

Complications include ocular and periocular injuries, which could lead to visual loss, diplopia, and globe malposition (enophthalmos, exophthalmos, or hypophthalmos). Failure to adequately stabilize the medial canthal ligaments leads to telecanthus/pseudohypertelorism. Failure to adequately restore nasal dorsal height can result in the development of epicanthal folds, which are notoriously difficult to repair. Damage to the lacrimal system results in epiphora. Persistent CSF rhinorrhea requires closure of the defect through which the leak is occurring. Closure requires precise localization of the defect, followed by open or endoscopic repair; most defects can be handled endoscopically. Chronic sinusitis, including delayed development of mucocele/mucopyocele, may occur. Many of these can be managed endoscopically, particularly now that the frontal sinus can be widely accessed using the Draf III (endoscopic Lothrop) procedure. In a patient who has had prior surgery, maneuvering may be more difficult, necessitating an open approach.

Coronal incisions can lead to hair loss and widened scars. Hair transplants will graft well into scar tissue, so alopecic areas may be addressed with subsequent hair transplantation. Forehead and scalp numbness may arise from damage to supraorbital/supratrochlear nerves, and loss of brow elevation may result from damage to the temporal branches of the facial nerve.

KEY POINTS

- NOE/NEC fractures represent a telescoping fracture pattern and posterior displacement of the glabella.
- Recognize NOE/NEC fractures through meticulous physical examination and CT scanning.
- Proper repositioning of medial canthal ligaments both posteriorly and superiorly is necessary to avoid telecanthus.
- Restoration of nasal dorsal height is essential, even when bone grafting is required, to avoid long-term deformity and epicanthal folding.
- Proper management of frontal sinus fractures requires classifying the injury by anterior table, posterior table, ductal involvement, and addressing each zone.
- It is critical to assess and manage CSF leaks, even those that appear to cease spontaneously.

REFERENCES

1. Stranc MF. The pattern of lacrimal injuries in naso-ethmoid fractures. Br J Plast Surg 23:339-346, 1970.
2. Stranc MF. Primary treatment of naso-ethmoid injuries with increased intercanthal distance. British J Plast Surg 23:8-25, 1970.
    The author explains the development of the current understanding of the nature of the nasoethmoid complex and the importance of proper fixation from a historical perspective.
3. Kellman RM. Maxillofacial trauma. In Flint PW, Haughey BH, Lund VJ, et al, eds. Cummings Otolaryngology Head and Neck Surgery, vol 1, ed 5. St Louis: Elsevier, 2010.
4. Kellman RM, Schmidt C. The paranasal sinuses as a protective crumple zone for the orbit. Laryngoscope 119:1682-1690, 2009.
5. Markowitz BL, Manson PN, Sargent L, et al. Management of the medial canthal tendon in nasoethmoid orbital fractures: the importance of the central fragment in classification and treatment. Plast Reconstr Surg 87:843-853, 1991.
    This reference includes the most current and relevant classification scheme for describing and planning the treatment of NEC/NOE fractures. It is a must-read for all surgeons managing craniomaxillofacial trauma.

6. Hybels RL, Newman MH. Posterior table fractures of the frontal sinus: I. An experimental study. Laryngoscope 87:171-179, 1977.

7. Rodriguez ED, Stanwix MG, Nam AJ, et al. Twenty-six-year experience treating frontal sinus fractures: a novel algorithm based on anatomical fracture pattern and failure of conventional techniques. Plast Reconstr Surg 122:1850-1866, 2008.

 Although it spans a long time period, this retrospective study includes the largest series of frontal fractures from a single institution. It is well analyzed and informative. A careful read is required to gain a full understanding of the findings and their implications.

8. Donald PJ, Bernstein L. Compound frontal sinus injuries with intracranial penetration. Laryngoscope 88:225-232, 1978.

9. Stanley RB, Becker TS. Injuries of the nasofrontal orifices in frontal sinus fractures. Laryngoscope 97:728-731, 1987.

10. Stanley RB. Management of frontal sinus fractures: a review of 33 cases. J Oral Maxillofac Surg 57:380-381, 1999.

11. Bell RB, Dierks EJ, Brar P, et al. A protocol for the management of frontal sinus fractures emphasizing sinus preservation. J Oral Maxillofac Surg 65:825-839, 2007.

12. Rohrich RJ, Hollier LH. Management of frontal sinus fractures: changing concepts. Clin Plast Surg 19:219-232, 1992.

13. Smith TL, Han JK, Loehrl TA, et al. Endoscopic management of the frontal recess in frontal sinus fractures: a shift in the paradigm? Laryngoscope 112:784-790, 2002.

14. Raveh J, Vuillemin T, Sutter F. Subcranial management of 395 combined frontobasal-midface fractures. Arch Otolaryngol Head Neck Surg 114:1114-1122, 1988.

15. Stanley RB Jr. Use of intraoperative computed tomography during repair of orbitozygomatic fractures. Arch Facial Plast Surg 1:19-24, 1999.

Midface Fractures

Jason P. Ulm ▪ *Michael J. Yaremchuk*

Midfacial fractures have been common among facial injuries across the ages, and descriptions of surgical approaches to their management are found in medical literature beginning in the latter half of the eighteenth century, with Wiseman's *Chirurgical Treatise*.[1] By the 1900s, when general anesthesia was in widespread use, myriad descriptions of surgical approaches to midfacial fractures began to emerge, including Lothrop's transantral approach to the maxilla[1] (Fig. 29-1) and Manwaring's towel-clip approach to fracture reduction.[1] Major pioneers in maxillofacial trauma included Varaztad Kazanjian, an Armenian dental surgeon who immigrated to the United States during the first World War; and John Converse, whose seminal works with Kazanjian described all kinds of external fixation devices (Fig. 29-2) and fracture

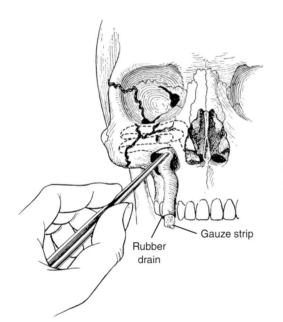
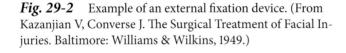

Fig. 29-1   Lothrop intraoral approach. (From Kazanjian V, Converse J. The Surgical Treatment of Facial Injuries. Baltimore: Williams & Wilkins, 1949.)

Fig. 29-2   Example of an external fixation device. (From Kazanjian V, Converse J. The Surgical Treatment of Facial Injuries. Baltimore: Williams & Wilkins, 1949.)

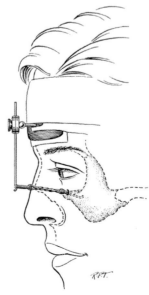

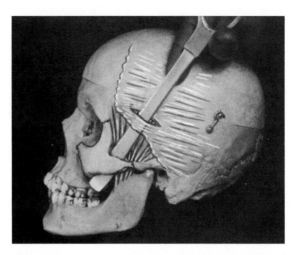

Fig. 29-3   Gillies' technique of a temporal incision to approach a zygomatic arch fracture. (From Gillies HD, Millard DR, eds. The Principles and Art of Plastic Surgery. Boston: Little Brown, 1957.)

management methods in *The Surgical Treatment of Facial Injuries.*[1] In the same era, Harold Gillies described a temporal incision technique for zygomatic arch repair (Fig. 29-3) in his landmark text *Plastic Surgery of the Face,*[2] which is still in common use today.

Although our understanding of the details and patterns of midfacial fractures has broadened with modern radiographic technology and our surgical tools have become more sophisticated, the fundamental goals of proper restoration of facial architecture remain identical to those of these pioneering and innovative facial surgeons of the past century.

ANATOMY

The midfacial skeleton is juxtaposed between the cranium superiorly and the mandible inferiorly. As the central component of the face, the midface is paramount in contributing to the topography of the cheeks, eyes, nose, and mouth.

Functionally, it houses the nasal cavity and paranasal sinuses, the orbits, and the occlusional elements of the maxilla. It also provides support and attachment for the muscles of mastication and those of facial expression.

Structurally, the maxilla is composed of a series of bony struts and buttresses. As the facial skeleton ages, the sinuses become more pneumatized and the bones become thinner in localized areas, contributing to the difference in fracture patterns seen in children and adults. The reinforced horizontal struts correspond to the supraorbital bar, the infraorbital rim and floor, the zygomatic arches, and the palatal shelf (Fig. 29-4).

The palatal strut provides the footing for the seven vertical pillars, or buttresses. The four anterior pillars consist of the paired lateral zygomaticomaxillary and the paired medial nasomaxillary buttresses. The posterior buttresses derive their name from their palatal orientation, their oblique posterior course,

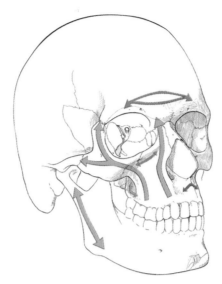

Fig. 29-4   Facial buttresses. The horizontal struts are depicted in blue. These include the supraorbital rim/bar, the infraorbital rim and orbital floor, the zygomatic arches, and the palatal shelf. The vertical buttress *(green arrows)* include the paired medial nasomaxillary, lateral zygomaticomaxillary, and the pterygomaxillary buttresses and the single nasal septum.

and the articulation with the sphenoid at the base of the skull. The paired parasagittal pterygoid (pterygomaxillarysphenoid) buttresses have thinner laminae near the palatal articulation (medial and lateral pterygoid plates), becoming more robust at the cranial end of the sphenoid. Fractures tend to occur in the thinner location, sparing the vital structures that pass through the superior sphenoid. The single sagittal nasal septum (vomerosphenoidalfrontal) buttress is the longest and often most overlooked of the seven buttresses. Unlike their anterior counterparts, direct exposure of the sagittal and parasagittal buttresses is often limited, and rigid fixation of these areas is not practical; the anterior buttress repair restores height and projection of the midface.

EPIDEMIOLOGIC FACTORS AND CLASSIFICATION

The causes of facial trauma vary across the globe. Cultural, socioeconomic, and environmental factors have an effect on the incidence and population most prone to these injuries. In the United States, motor vehicle collision and assault remain the predominant causes of adult facial trauma. Falls, sports injuries, industrial accidents, and gunshot wounds are the remaining sources.[3] Not surprisingly, most midfacial fractures are found in young men. The exception to this trend is midface fractures sustained by falls, which have a bimodal distribution, in infants and the elderly, with no predilection for either sex.[4] The pediatric facial skeleton is different from that of the adult, altering fracture distribution. In the United States, the most common fracture sites in children are the mandible and nasal bones, with midfacial fractures occurring less often.[4,5] In contrast, the adult population reports predominantly mandibular and midfacial fractures, including orbital, zygomaticomaxillary complex, LeFort, and nasoethmoid orbital.[3]

At the start of the twentieth century, René LeFort described predictable fracture levels of the midfacial skeleton (based on "lines of weakness") (Fig. 29-5).[6] The detail of enhanced CT imaging has demonstrated that more complex fracture patterns are typical today, often involving multiple fragments with different

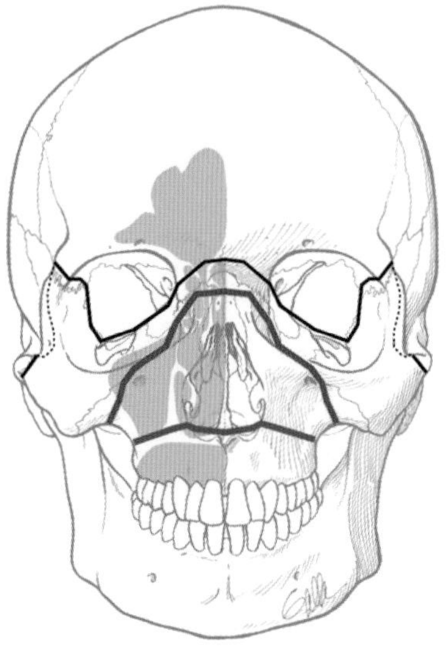

Fig. 29-5   LeFort fracture patterns. LeFort I *(green line)*. Maxillary alveolus: a transverse fracture pattern involving the lower maxilla, just superior to the tooth apices. The fracture extends from the nasal floor and piriform rims anteriorly to the posterior pterygomaxillary buttresses. LeFort II *(red line)*. Pyramidal shaped fracture pattern that separates the medial midface from the lateral midface and orbits. It extends in an oblique course from the posterior pterygomaxillary buttress across the lateral buttress (inferior to the zygomaticomaxillary junction) and anterior wall of the maxillary sinus (adjacent to infraorbital foramen) toward the nasofrontal suture. LeFort III *(black line)*. Craniofacial disjunction: a transverse fracture pattern that involve the zygomatic arch and the lateral orbital wall near the zygomaticofrontal suture, extending along the floor of the orbit to the medial orbital wall and the nasofrontal suture. In the midline it extends from the nasofrontal suture posteriorly through the ethmoid, vomer, and pterygoid plates, thus separating the face from the cranium.

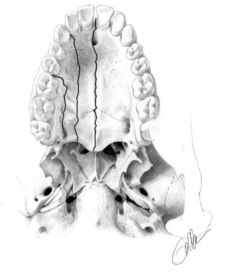

Fig. 29-6   Fracture patterns of the palate are typically paramedian or paralveolar. True sagittal fractures are rare.

levels of severity for each side. Nonetheless, LeFort's levels remain a relevant classification tool among various medical disciplines for the description of facial fractures.

When describing the fracture pattern of a complex injury, one should specify the *highest* level of LeFort fracture for *each side* of the face, adding any associated fractures (such as the frontal bone and mandible) when applicable.[7,8]

Sagittal fractures of the maxilla may occur either in isolation or in conjunction with LeFort injuries. These fractures typically traverse adjacent to the midline at the cuspid teeth, or more laterally at the maxillary tuberosity. The latter fracture leads to rotation and displacement of a dentoalveolar segment, causing maxillary widening, buccal crossbite, and malocclusion[9] (Fig. 29-6).

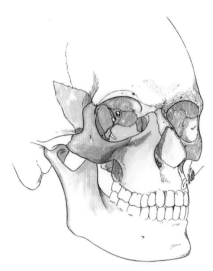

Fig. 29-7   The complex relationship between the zygoma *(pictured in red)* and the frontal, sphenoid, maxilla, and temporal bones is shown. The degree of energy transmitted will dictate the pattern of disruption at these articulations.

Zygomaticomaxillary Complex

The zygoma articulates with the frontal (ZF), sphenoid (ZS), maxilla (ZM), and temporal (ZT) bones (Fig. 29-7) to form the zygomaticomaxillary complex (ZMC). The amount of energy transmitted to the zygoma dictates the degree of disruption at these articulations. Manson et al classified injuries to the zygoma as *low, middle, and high-energy* injuries, depending on the force applied during impact. *Low-energy* fractures result in minimal or no bony displacement, with at least one articulation maintained, often the zygomaticofrontal suture.[7] These fractures occur approximately 18% of the time, and may not require stabilization after reduction.

Middle-energy fractures are most common (77%). These injuries yield complete disruption at all buttresses and lead to mild to moderate bony fragment displacement with varying degrees of comminution.

High-energy fractures are the least common (5%) and tend to occur with panfacial or LeFort injuries. These injuries nearly universally demonstrate comminution in the lateral orbit and lateral displacement and posterior segmentation of the zygomatic arch.

INDICATIONS AND LIMITATIONS

The primary goal of midfacial fracture repair is restoration of facial *height, width,* and *projection,* in addition to *occlusion.* Accomplishing this goal is facilitated through intricate knowledge of the skeletal infrastructure and its relationship with the soft tissue envelope. Zygoma fractures may lead to both functional and aesthetic disturbances. These disturbances include coronoid impingement, diplopia, infraorbital nerve anesthesia, and malar regression, enophthalmos, vertical dystopia, and altered shape of the palpebral fissure.

The following basic craniomaxillofacial principles and techniques are used: (1) adequate exposure and precise open reduction of all fractured segments, (2) rigid stabilization of fractured segments with the appropriate caliber plates and screws, (3) addressing skeletal defects with autologous bone grafts, and (4) reestablishment of soft tissue-skeletal relationship.

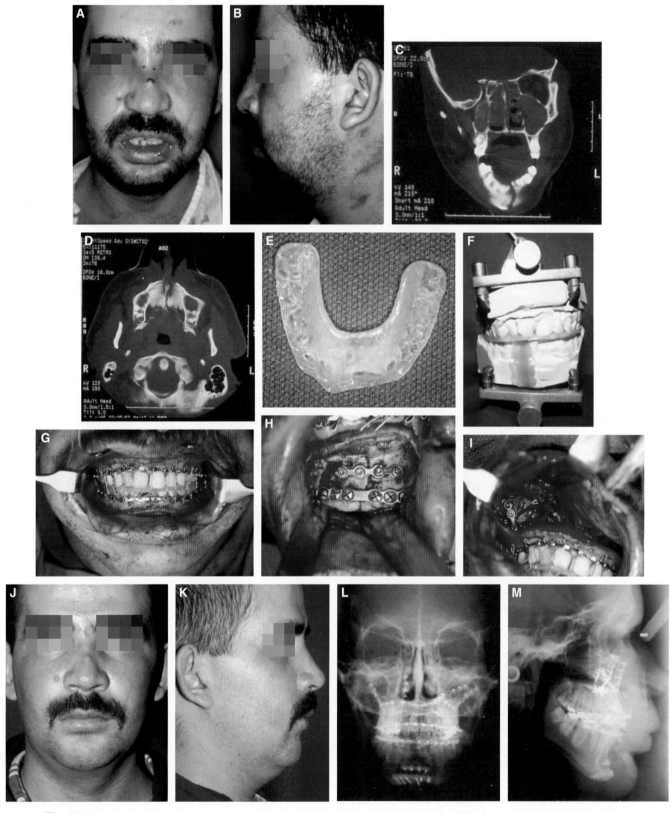

Fig. 29-8   **A-D,** This patient sustained bilateral LeFort II, sagittal palate, and mandibular symphyseal fractures from a fall. Preoperative photographs and CT scans show the degree of injury. **E** and **F,** The patient was placed in maxillomandibular fixation by making a mold from which a splint was fashioned to maintain proper occlusion. **G-I,** The bilateral, lateral, and medial buttresses were widely exposed and plated with 2.0 mm plates. The anterior maxillary wall was also plated to prevent soft tissue herniation into sinus. **J-M,** Postoperative images and radiographs demonstrate class I occlusion with good restoration of facial height, width, and projection.

Despite strict adherence to these principles, success of the reconstruction is sometimes limited by the degree and nature of the injury. Infection, scarring, and unpredictable bone resorption may contribute to undesirable sequelae. In severe cases, staged reconstruction is prudent. Extensive bone and soft tissue defects may require free tissue transfer to replace missing elements.

PATIENT EVALUATION AND PREOPERATIVE PLANNING

The initial patient evaluation includes appropriate triage and stabilization. Advanced trauma life support protocol is followed with preservation of the airway, C-spine stabilization, and thorough primary and secondary surveys. Telecanthus, periorbital ecchymosis (raccoon eyes), and blood within the external auditory meatus or nasopharynx indicate potential facial fractures. Malocclusion and midfacial mobility are characteristic of LeFort fractures. Malar depression, enophthalmos, trismus, and infraorbital nerve paresthesia suggest ZMC fractures.

Plain radiographs are of limited value in assessing facial trauma. Any patient with suspected facial fractures is best evaluated by fine-cut CT. Axial, coronal, and sagittal views help define the fracture patterns and the precise degree of displacement. Three-dimensional reconstructions of the scan are especially helpful in complex cases in which the skeletal components can be appreciated from multiple vantage points. Further, CT provides simultaneous evaluation of the relevant soft tissue structures within the orbit and cranial vault. Associated fractures and vascular injuries within the neck and cranial base can also be evaluated with this modality, which facilitates a complete, coherent, and systematic treatment and operative plan.

Preoperative photographs are necessary. Standard anterior and posterior, lateral, oblique, and basal views are done with adequate lighting and a dark background (see Chapter 3). Emergent operative treatment of midfacial fractures is rarely indicated. Facial fracture management is deferred until the patient is stabilized and other more critical injuries are treated. Significant nasopharyngeal hemorrhage is typically managed successfully with anterior and posterior nasal packing. In the rare circumstance that hemorrhage persists, angioembolization of the offending vessel may be performed by an interventional radiologist. Significant contamination and soft tissue destruction require urgent debridement and serial washouts.

The timing and treatment of midfacial fractures depends on the patient's other associated injuries, soft tissue edema, and coordination of involved services (such as neurosurgery, otolaryngology, oral and maxillofacial surgery, and plastic surgery). Occasionally, preoperative fabrication of oral splints is undertaken to delineate the occlusional relationship during surgery. Fig. 29-8 illustrates the utility of dental splinting in a complex panfacial fracture case.

TECHNIQUE

Maxillomandibular Fixation

Complex midfacial fractures, including bilateral LeFort fractures and unilateral fractures that involve a maxillary alveolar segment, require maxillomandibular fixation (MMF) to define the occlusional relationship and provide a reference for facial width and projection. If the mandible is not fractured, then MMF can be removed after rigid fixation of the midface is accomplished. Unless required for other reasons, a tracheostomy is avoided by using a nasotracheal tube or an oral endotracheal tube positioned behind the last molar. MMF is accomplished with either Erich arch bars, or four (or six) point screw fixation techniques with 24- or 26-gauge wire.

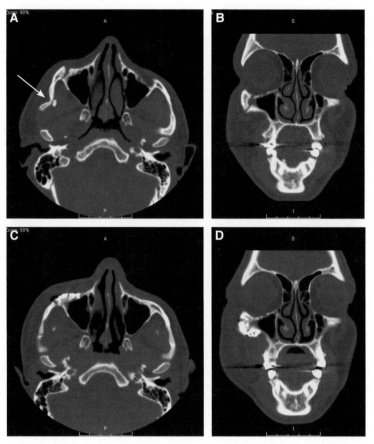

Fig. 29-9   **A** and **B,** Displaced ZMC fracture resulting in coronoid impingement. **C** and **D,** Postreduction scan, after an intraoral approach was used for plating of the zygomaxillary buttress.

APPROACHES

Access to midface fractures is achieved through four principal approaches: intraoral, periorbital, coronal, and Gillies. The surgical goals must align with the informed wishes of the patient, because the extent of the surgery can only be justified by the anticipated aesthetic result and degree of functional improvement.[10]

An intraoral approach through an upper gingivobuccal sulcus incision provides excellent access to the anterior maxilla and its four anterior buttresses (Fig. 29-9).

The superior maxilla, inferior orbital rim and floor, and medial zygoma are accessed through a periorbital approach. Of the lower eyelid approaches, the subciliary and subtarsal incisions have largely been supplanted by the transconjunctival approach in many practices, because it eliminates an additional skin incision, yields lower rates of ectropion, and can be extended medially (through transcaruncle), or laterally (through lateral canthotomy) for further orbital exposure. Occasionally, an existing lower eyelid laceration may provide sufficient access.

In elderly patients, a cutaneous incision made directly over the infraorbital rim at the junction of eyelid and cheek skin provides excellent exposure, an imperceptible scar, and is not likely to result in postoperative lid malposition.

Exposure of the superior and lateral orbital wall, including the ZF and ZS sutures, can be achieved through a lateral brow incision, an upper blepharoplasty incision, or a lateral extension of a lower eyelid approach.

For simple (isolated) zygomatic arch fractures, a Gillies approach provides remote access to the depressed segment. A 1.5 cm incision is made in the temporal scalp, approximately 4 cm superior and 2 cm anterior to the tragus. The deep temporal fascia is entered and a periosteal elevator is passed caudally between this layer and the underlying muscle. The arch is reduced laterally and position is confirmed with gentle palpation, comparing with the contralateral uninjured side. In complex cases, in which exposure of the zygomatic arch, lateral orbit, frontal and/or nasoethmoidal areas are required, the coronal incision is used.

After the appropriate incision is made, dissection proceeds in a subperiosteal plane until all fractures are exposed. Identification and preservation of the infraorbital nerve is ensured before reduction.

REDUCTION

All fractured areas are exposed before bony reduction is attempted; a methodical approach to reduction is applied based on CT imaging. In complex or bilateral LeFort fracture repair, placing the patient in MMF takes advantage of the uninjured mandible to define the occlusal relationship and provide a reference for facial width and projection. Repair begins at the most intact vertical buttress to restore facial height. Three-dimensional reduction of isolated ZMC segments can be accomplished using a Carroll-Girard screw. In LeFort III or ZMC fractures, accurate reduction is best confirmed along the lateral orbital wall at the zygomaticosphenoid articulation. A Gillies approach or intraoral reduction of the zygomatic arch is often sufficient, unless significant displacement or comminution warrants a coronal approach to permit plate stabilization.

PLATE AND SCREW SELECTION

Rigid fixation requires proper plate selection to ensure adequate stability while avoiding palpability through the overlying soft tissue. Lower midface fixation is achieved with miniplate systems (1.5 to 2.0 mm) using 4 to 6 mm screws, whereas the upper midface (ZF, infraorbital rim) requires microplates (1.0 to 1.3 mm) with 2 to 3 mm screws. After accurate reduction of all articulations is confirmed, the fractured buttresses are repaired, including the zygomaticofrontal sutures and the infraorbital rim, when needed. In general, plate design and shape is determined by the bony anatomy. The plates are bent and molded to the desired reduced position and applied with at least two screws placed on either side of the fracture line (Fig. 29-10). Autogenous bone grafts are incorporated into the repair when there are bone gaps greater than 5 mm.

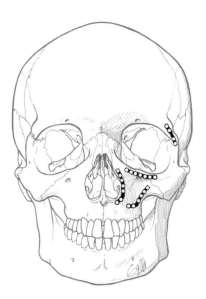

Fig. 29-10   Open reduction and internal fixation (ORIF) using plates and screws. Shown are typical plating options for a left-sided midface fracture. After adequate exposure and precise reduction, fractures are plated in a manner to restore the natural buttresses and struts of the facial skeleton.

PALATE

Palatal fractures are repaired using MMF and plating the involved maxillary segments and buttresses. Palatal fractures that occur in combination with both LeFort and mandible fractures pose a challenge in restoring facial width. Repair of these fractures is accomplished by using dental splints designed after impressions are made of both fractured dental arches and reconstructed through model surgery.

ADJUNCTIVE PROCEDURES

Soft tissue resuspension is necessary to avoid postoperative descent of the malar cheek mass and increased scleral show. This maneuver is performed at the time of closure, with reattachment of the malar fat pad to the infraorbital rim using permanent monofilament suture. A lateral canthopexy is also performed in cases of canthal disruption.[10]

SKELETAL AUGMENTATION

Inadequate skeletal reduction or untoward bone resorption can produce facial asymmetry and contour deformities. These sequelae can often be improved with skeletal augmentation. Anatomic porous polyethylene implants can be meticulously sculpted and rigidly fixed to the affected skeleton using an onlay technique. Alternatively, patient-specific implants can be manufactured to replicate the uninjured side, using computer-aided design and computer-aided manufacturing (CAD-CAM) technology. Postoperative occlusal issues may require orthodontic treatment.

POSTOPERATIVE CARE

Postoperative management includes efforts to ensure continued reduction through rigid stabilization, prevention of infection, and decreased edema (which can be accomplished through intermittent use of ice packs and head of bed elevation). Sinus precautions, decongestants, nasal saline spray, and a short course of antibiotics are administered. Vision is assessed in the recovery room, followed by a more complete eye exam in the early postoperative period. If MMF is continued postoperatively, the patient is placed on a pureed or soft diet. Close follow-up is required to monitor for signs of infection, malocclusion, and visual disturbances. Postoperative imaging is reserved for concerns of hardware malposition.

COMPLICATIONS

Complications from midfacial fractures and their repair are listed in Box 29-1. Malposition of the involved fragments can lead to alterations in facial width, height, projection, and occlusion. This complication may arise from unpredictable bone graft resorption, inadequate reduction, or failure of rigid stabilization. Inaccurate reduction of the zygoma can lead to a depressed malar eminence and increased orbital volume, resulting in enophthalmos and facial asymmetry. Postoperative diplopia should be evaluated by CT scanning to ensure that the extraocular muscles are not impinged. In most cases, the contusion and edema of the periorbital tissues will resolve over 3 to 6 months, resulting in improvement or resolution of the diplopia. Persistent cases should be referred to a strabismus specialist for evaluation.

Box 29-1   Complications of Midface Fractures and Repair

- Malocclusion
- Malposition
- Enophthalmos
- Diplopia
- Lower lid malposition
- Entropion
- Ectropion
- Trismus
- Infraorbital nerve injury
- CSF leak
- Infection
- Traumatic optic neuropathy

KEY POINTS

- The midfacial skeleton is composed of vertical buttresses and horizontal struts that house the orbits, nasal cavity, and sinuses, and provide attachment to facial musculature.
- Facial fractures are assessed best with thin-sliced computed topography using coronal, sagittal, and axial views, with three-dimensional reconstruction for complex cases.
- Fracture patterns are described specifying the *highest* level of LeFort fracture for *each* side of the face.
- Repair is directed at restoration of facial *height, width, projection,* and preinjury *occlusion,* while minimizing iatrogenic injury and alteration of the delicate soft tissue-skeletal relationship.
- Basic craniomaxillofacial principles are used: (1) adequate exposure and precise reduction of fractured segments, (2) stabilization with plates and screws, (3) reestablishment of soft tissue-skeletal relationship.
- MMF and/or dental splints are necessary to define facial width in fractures that involve the occlusional elements.
- Resuspension of the malar fat pad to infraorbital rim and lateral canthopexy are critical maneuvers to avoid postoperative cheek/lid malposition.

REFERENCES

1. Kazanjian V, Converse J. The Surgical Treatment of Facial Injuries. Baltimore: Williams & Wilkins, 1949.
2. Gillies H. Plastic Surgery of the Face. New York: Thieme-Stratton Corp, 1983.
3. Erdmann D, Follmar K, DeBruijn M, et al. A retrospective analysis of facial fracture etiologies. Ann Plas Surg 60:398-403, 2008.
4. Zimmerman CE, Troulis MJ, Kaban LB. Pediatric facial fractures: recent advances in prevention, diagnosis and management. Int J Oral Maxillofac Surg 34:823-833, 2005.
5. Imahara S, Hopper R, Wang J, et al. Patterns and outcomes of pediatric facial fractures in the United States: a survey of the National Trauma Data Bank. J Am Coll Surg 207:710-716, 2008.
6. LeFort R. Étude expérimentale sur les fractures de la mâchoire supérieur. Rev Chir Paris 23:208, 360, 479, 1901.
7. Manson P, Markowitz B, Mirvis S, et al. Toward CT-based facial fracture treatment. Plas Reconstr Surg 85:202-212, 1990.
   In addition to the traditional anatomic description of various facial fractures, the authors describe how additional classification of fracture pattern based on the degree of energy of the injury provides enhanced preoperative analysis. CT scans can thus be used to determine the degree and method of exposure and fixation required.

8. Manson P. Some thoughts on the classification and treatment of LeFort fractures. Ann Plas Surg 17:356-363, 1986.

9. Hendrickson M, Clark N, Manson PN, et al. Palatal fractures: classification, patterns, and treatment with rigid internal fixation. Plast Reconstr Surg 101:319-332, 1998.

10. Yaremchuk MJ, Kim WK. Soft tissue alterations with acute, extended open reduction and internal fixation of orbital fractures. J Craniofac Surg 3:134-140, 1992.

   The authors discuss and present data on common morbidities associated with the repair of orbital fractures. Diligent preoperative treatment planning for repair of facial fractures and meticulous technique and soft tissue repositioning during closure can minimize iatrogenic deformities.

30

Mandibular Fractures

Rachel M. Gilardetti ▪ Yedeh Ying ▪ Maria J. Troulis

The first known medical description of mandibular fractures was in the Edwin Smith *Surgical Papyrus* in the seventeenth century BC[1,2] (Fig. 30-1).[3] During the pre-Christian era, people were superstitious regarding mandibular fractures; many believed that death from such afflictions was inevitable. In the *Surgical Papyrus,* an Egyptian writes:

> One having a fracture in his mandible, over which a wound has been afflicted, thou will a fever gain from it. An ailment not to be treated.

Death usually followed, presumably caused by infection.[2,4]

Hippocrates' works established many of the principles of modern surgery. Today these principles are coupled with advances in equipment and technology to effectively treat mandibular fractures. Hippocrates invented a method for immobilizing a dislocated mandible intraorally by using gold or linen threads as wires, which were tied around teeth near the fracture site.[1,2] This intraoral fixation technique served as the foundation for mandibular fracture immobilization and represented a milestone on which subsequent mandibular surgeons have built modern strategies. Hippocrates also devised an extraoral immobilization technique, where Carthaginian leather strips were glued to the skin.[2]

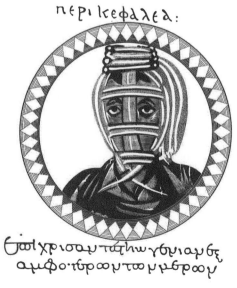

Fig. 30-1 First known depiction of a mandible fracture.

With the introduction and subsequent widespread use of gunpowder, facial gunshot wounds became commonplace, and complex facial fractures resulting from these wounds required various treatment approaches. The traditional method of simple ligatures around appropriate teeth was not effective in keeping the "extensively damaged" mandibular bone fragments in a strict, confined position. In 1779 Chopart and Desault invented a simple dental splint that contained an iron trough that settled over the occlusal surface of the mandibular teeth.[1,2] The iron trough was secured directly beneath the mandible with an external screw device, improving the immobilization of the bony segments for better healing.

In the nineteenth century a surge of innovation in mandibular fracture treatment resulted from the introduction of anesthesia, which transformed all surgical disciplines. In 1840 Baudens devised a novel internal fixation method using circumferential wiring to immobilize an oblique fracture.[1,2] Thomas Gunning's splint was the first customized intraoral dental device[1]; vulcanite was secured with screws onto the hard palate and mandible, then secured to an external head cap.[1,2] Gilmer and Salicetti are credited with first using intermaxillary fixation,[1] and Gilmer further described full arch bars on both the mandible and maxilla.[1,2]

The battlefield injuries that occurred during World Wars I and II involved extensive maxillofacial damage and forced surgeons to become more adept at managing these complex problems. Before these wars, mandibular fractures were treated either by approximate fixation (immobilization) with internal wiring or by external fixation with metal pins or custom-made cap splints.[2] During and after World War II, the concept of reduction and alignment of the bony fragments and rigid fixation began to develop. With the introduction of antibiotic therapy, direct fixation of bony fragments became more widespread because the risk of infection decreased. Numerous materials were used for rigid internal fixation: stainless steel Vitallium monocortical miniplates were introduced in the 1960s but were cumbersome to use because they lacked malleability.[2] In the early 1970s improved malleable stainless steel and titanium miniplates were introduced and continue to be popular internal fixation materials today.[5,6] Biodegradable polylactide plates have also been used for internal fixation of mandibular fractures; after healing, the plate biodegrades and no foreign body remains.[2,5,6]

ANATOMY

The mandible is the largest and strongest bone in the facial skeleton and serves many functions. The morphology of the lower third of the face is largely dictated by mandibular features. The mandible follows the ringbone rule, which states that if a fracture or dislocation is present in a ringbone, there is a high likelihood that another bony injury is present.[7] Two hemimandibles are fused at the midline, the symphysis. The body of the mandible is the horizontal parabola-shaped portion and has both external and internal cortical layers. The external cortical layer is stronger and is used as an anchoring surface for osteosynthesis plates and screws[5] (Fig. 30-2).

The mandibular canal is a concave path extending from the mandibular lingula to the mental foramen. When using internal fixation, the surgeon will find the mandibular canal an important anatomic reference because it houses the alveolar nerve bundle. Damage to the inferior alveolar nerve may result from treating fractures (during the insult, reduction, or fixation),[8] and dental malocclusion, another complication of poor fracture reduction, can result and may impair mastication.[1,5]

Mandibular fractures are affected by the force that the muscles attached to the mandible exert on the fragments. Understanding how the musculature affects fracture lines is critical to planning surgical treatment. The relationship between the orientation of the fracture line and the vector of muscle pull can result in a

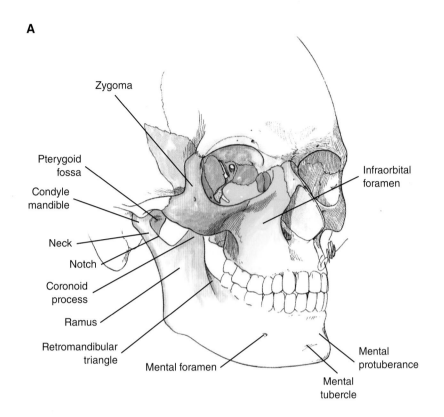

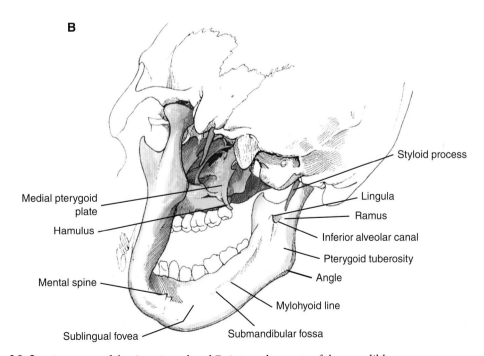

Fig. 30-2 Anatomy of the **A,** external and **B,** internal aspects of the mandible.

positive influence on the fracture line, aligning the fragments, or a negative influence, where muscle activity promotes malalignment. Fractures of the mandibular angle are especially vulnerable to forces exerted by overlying muscles. The masseter, temporalis, and medial pterygoid muscle can displace angle fractures unfavorably by positioning the proximal segment superiorly and medially[1] (Fig. 30-3).

However, these same muscles can minimize dislocation in horizontally and vertically favorable fractures by aiding in fracture stabilization and reduction[1] (Fig. 30-4).

In condylar fractures, the lateral pterygoid muscle can displace the condylar bone fragment in an anteromedial direction and result in condylar dislocation from the fossa.[7] The mylohyoid, geniohyoid, and anterior digastric muscle all have a tendency to displace a bilateral parasymphyseal fracture in a posteroinferior manner.[7]

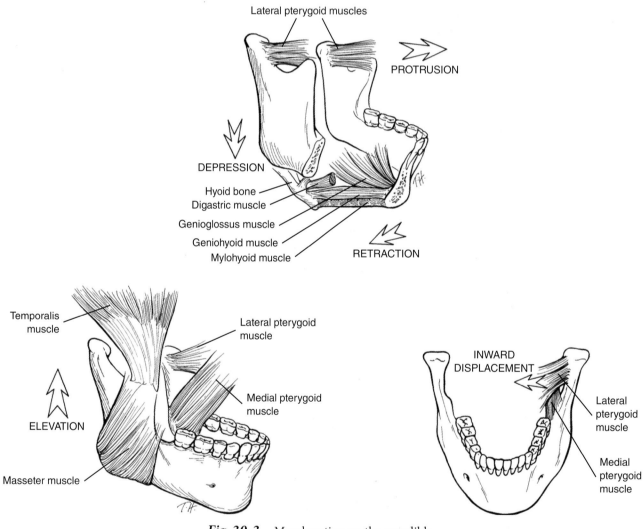

Fig. 30-3   Muscle action on the mandible.

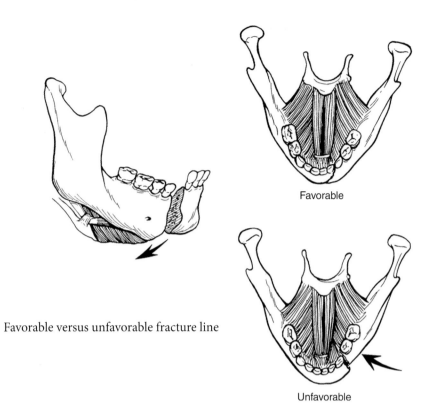

Fig. 30-4   Favorable versus unfavorable fracture line orientation.

Favorable

Unfavorable

EPIDEMIOLOGY

Epidemiologic data regarding facial fractures emerge most frequently from large urban trauma centers.[9-11] The cause and frequency of mandibular fractures vary by geographic location and mechanism of injury. Generally, injuries and deaths resulting from motor vehicle accidents occur with a higher incidence in rural areas than in urban areas,[11,12] whereas injuries caused by violent assaults are more common in urban settings.[6,12] It has been consistently reported that men sustain mandibular fractures more frequently than women, regardless of country or other demographic factors.[10,11,13-17]

The mandible is the second most commonly injured area of the maxillofacial skeleton (the nose is most commonly injured), accounting for 36% to 59% of all maxillofacial fractures,[16] which are far more common in teenagers and adults than in children. Unerupted dentition in children improves mandibular stability, and a thicker layer of adipose tissue protects the more flexible bones.[17,18] Although facial fractures are uncommon in young children, when they do occur, the mandible is the most common site for fracture. Falling, bicycle accidents, jungle gyms, and backseat vehicular accidents are among the most common causes of fractures in infants and children.[17-19]

LOCATION OF MANDIBULAR FRACTURES

The direction of the vector force and mechanics from the injury determine the site and pattern of mandibular fractures. Patient age and the presence of dentition also directly affect the fracture features. Mandibular fractures occur most often in areas where tensile strain is present. Within the mandible, the frequency of fracture locations has been described with ranges of 21% to 33% in the body, 29% to 36% in the condylar region, 20% to 23% in the mandibular angle, and 8% to 15% in the symphysis area.[7,15] More than 50% of mandibular fractures involve multiple sites.[15] This is important during the preliminary survey of the patient, and special attention should be paid to the cervical spine.

CLASSIFICATION

Although many classification systems exist for describing mandibular fractures, the most widely employed systems are based on either the anatomic location[3] (Fig. 30-5) or fracture pattern[15] (Table 30-1).

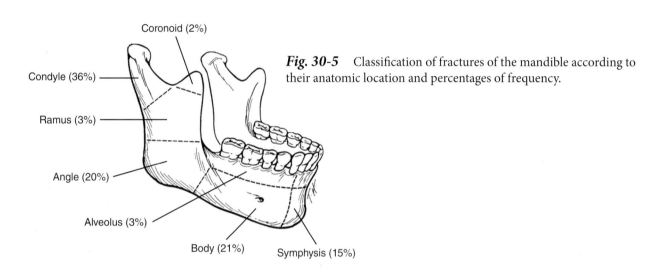

Fig. 30-5   Classification of fractures of the mandible according to their anatomic location and percentages of frequency.

Coronoid (2%)
Condyle (36%)
Ramus (3%)
Angle (20%)
Alveolus (3%)
Body (21%)
Symphysis (15%)

Table 30-1   Mandibular Fractures Based on Fracture Pattern

Fracture Name	Description
Simple	Single break that does not obstruct through the external environment; skin and mucosa and periodontal membrane are intact
Compound	Fracture obstructs through the external environment; skin or mucosa or periodontal membrane communicates with the bone break
Comminuted	Multiple fragmentation is produced
Greenstick	Incomplete loss of continuity of the bone; one cortex is broken, although the other cortex is bent
Complex or complicated	Structures adjacent to the bone (nerves, vessels, joints) are damaged
Telescoped or impacted	One bony segment is driven into the other
Indirect	Fracture arises at some distance from the contact force
Pathologic	Fracture occurs in a bone weakened by pathology (osteoporosis, cyst)
Displaced	Condylar segment movement in relation with movement at fracture site
Dislocated	Condylar head moves and thus no longer articulates with glenoid fossa

For fractures located at the mandibular angle and condyle, the direction of the fracture line dictates classification. At the angle, when viewing a fracture site in the horizontal plane, a favorable fracture is one in which the musculature resists upward forces on the proximal segment. When a fracture is viewed in the vertical plane, a favorable fracture indicates muscular resistance to medial pull on the proximal segment. Fractures with severe displacement are considered to have relatively unfavorable alignment, and those without displacement have relatively favorable alignment.

PATIENT EVALUATION AND PREOPERATIVE PLANNING

Per standard advanced trauma life support (ATLS) protocols, securing the airway is the highest priority after a maxillofacial trauma occurs. Endotracheal intubation or cricothyrotomy are performed when necessary to secure the airway. During history taking, it is helpful to understand the type and direction of the force that created the injury. Common symptoms reported by patients with mandibular fracture include pain, malocclusion, trismus, and sensory disturbance.

CLINICAL EVALUATION

The presence of any hematomas, lacerations, and swelling around the mandible should be noted. Lacerations under the chin are common in symphysis and subcondylar fractures.

An intraoral examination can reveal malocclusion, tooth injuries, and an impaired interincisal opening. The mandible should be palpated to inspect for loose teeth by placing the thumbs on the teeth and the fingers on the lower border of the mandible. Having the patient bite down lightly can reveal a malocclusion. If the patient is edentulous, dentures should be used if they are available; these can be helpful in setting landmarks and reducing the fracture (or stabilizing the fracture if wiring the dentures in).

RADIOGRAPHIC EVALUATION

Radiographic views in multiple perspectives are required to accurately assess the fracture site. A minimum of two views oriented in 90 degrees to one another are required for accurate radiographic assessment. A panoramic radiograph of the entire mandible, including the condyle, is the most informative view (Fig. 30-6). However, the patient is required to sit upright, which may be impossible in certain clinical situa-

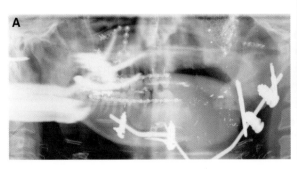 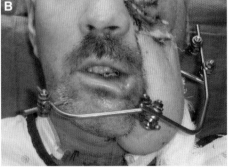

Fig. 30-6   External pin fixation in a complex fracture of the mandible. **A,** Panorex view demonstrating external fixator and internal plates. **B,** Photograph of device in place.

tions. For severely traumatized patients, lateral oblique views may be used. Lateral oblique radiography is also useful for diagnosing fractures in the ascending ramus, angle, alveolus, coronoid process, and posterior body. The Caldwell posteroanterior view can reveal fracture displacements of the ramus, angle, body, and symphysis. The reverse Towne radiograph is ideal for inspecting medial displacement of the condylar region, whereas an occlusal view can reveal anteroposterior displacement in the symphysis area. For condyle process fractures, CT scans of the temporomandibular joints should be performed. High-resolution CT scans are most thorough in the modern era for diagnosing the range of mandible fractures. CT scans are commonly obtained at urban centers and for the most part (except Panorex) replace plain films.

PREOPERATIVE PLANNING

The goals of mandibular reconstruction/repair are to obtain stable occlusion and reestablish full range of motion. The presence and condition of dentition are important factors that affect surgical treatment. The patient's occlusion is the cornerstone to the reestablishment of correct function; thus dentures are commonly used in an edentulous patient, where a critical landmark is unavailable during fracture reduction. Patients with atrophic mandibles pose a reconstructive challenge. Fractures in atrophic mandibles can be difficult to treat properly because there is a reduced cross-section, leading to less contact area between bone fragments and poorly vascularized, sclerotic bone.[8,20]

TECHNIQUE

Treatment of all mandibular fractures has two common goals: to return the patient to form and function (with particular focus on restoring the patient's occlusion) and to achieve osseous union. There are multiple methods to achieve these goals.

Closed reduction is both simple and safe and can satisfactorily treat the majority of mandible fractures. The technique involves direct or indirect interdental wiring, with or without arch bars, to produce maxillomandibular fixation (MMF). This fixation provides immobilization of the jaw for a specified period. Using 24- or 26-gauge wires, an arch bar is adapted to both the maxilla and mandible.[8] This immobilizes the fractured segments and fixes the jaw by using the patient's occlusion. The occlusion will then determine the anatomic reduction. If inadequate reduction is noted on postoperative imaging, a secondary technique for fixation should be considered.

EXTERNAL PIN FIXATION

In complex mandibular fractures, such as those acquired through gunshot wounds where the mandible is severely comminuted, an external fixator is considered if intermaxillary fixation is not possible (see Fig. 30-6). An open technique would jeopardize blood supply through the periosteum to the smaller bony fragments, resulting in an increased risk of infection and nonunion.[21] The technique is based on the principle of anchoring pins into the bone fragments to form a bridge to reconstruct the mandible. These pins are typically transcutaneous and allow reduction with minimal surgical exposure.

OPEN REDUCTION

Advances in rigid plate fixation have dramatically reduced and in some cases even eliminated the requirement for MMF, and this has become a predictable and reliable treatment option. Rigid internal fixation methods include interosseous wiring, lag screw technique, or plate fixation.

The lag screw technique, introduced in the 1970s by Brons and Boering,[20] delivers compressive forces to reduce the fracture. Fixation is performed by driving the screw head through both fragments of the fracture, engaging only the distal segments with the threads of the screw. This approach pinches the two fragments together by drawing the proximal bony fragment toward the distal fragment with pressure applied by the head of the lag screw. Lag screw reduction is limited to the chin region, given the anatomic location of the nerve bundle and accessibility of the fracture site (this requires a sagittal type fracture to allow for screw placement and bony reduction).

Plate fixation was first described by Michelet[22] and colleagues as placing plates along the physiologic tension zone of the mandible. This was later modified and refined by Champy et al.[23] Today open reduction and rigid internal fixation using titanium plating systems is common. The optimal technique depends on biting forces, the location of anatomic structures, and the amount of bone available (Figs. 30-7 and 30-8).

MINIMALLY INVASIVE TECHNIQUES: ENDOSCOPIC

Widespread interest in minimally invasive techniques across many surgical disciplines has prompted the development of minimally invasive techniques for mandible fracture repair. Decreased morbidity is achieved through minimizing the length of the extraoral incisions, and the technique has been shown to decrease the risk of facial nerve injury.[24] The approach involves a 1.5 cm incision to gain access to the lateral ramus.[25] An optical cavity is then created through subperiosteal dissection along the lateral aspect of the ramus. The endoscope is then passed into this cavity, permitting identification of the relevant anatomy such as the sigmoid notch, anterior and posterior ramus borders, and the fracture line. Fixation is then performed either transcutaneously with the assistance of a trocar in the preauricular region or directly through the access incision (Fig. 30-9).

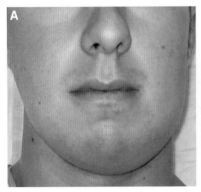
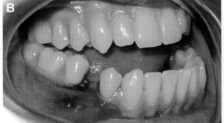
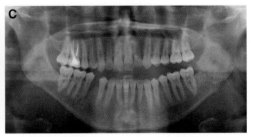

Fig. 30-7   **A** and **B,** This 20-year-old man had a sports injury to the chin and presented 1 day later complaining of a malocclusion and increasing pain. **C,** Frontal intraoral imaging showed premature occlusion of the right posterior teeth and significant widening between premolars with gingival laceration.

Continued

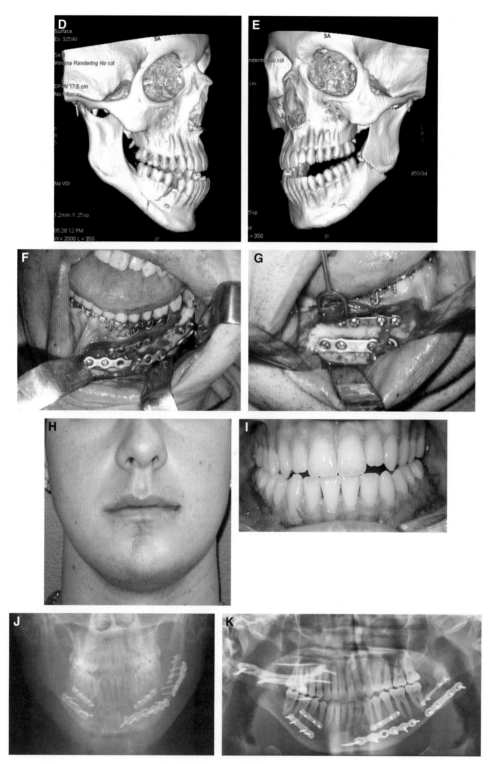

Fig. 30-7, cont'd   **D** and **E,** Three-dimensional reconstruction of CT imaging showing fractures through the right body, left body, and left angle. **F** and **G,** Intraoperative photos of rigid fixation at all three fracture sites. **H** and **I,** Postoperative photos. **J** and **K,** Postoperative radiographs.

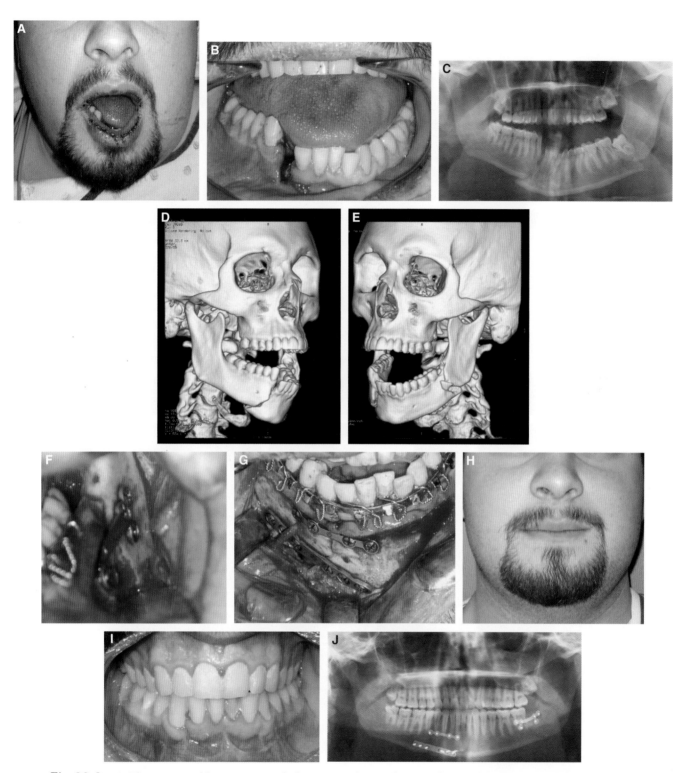

Fig. 30-8   **A,** This 21-year-old man presented after an assault complaining of pain, malocclusion, and difficulty swallowing. **B,** Intraoral photograph showing step-off between the right canine and lateral incisor. **C,** Panorex verifying the left angle and right parasymphysis fractures. **D** and **E,** Three-dimensional reconstruction of CT imaging showing displacement of the fractures. **F** and **G,** Intraoperative photographs of rigid fixation of the right parasymphysis fracture and miniplating of the left angle. **H** and **I,** Postoperative photos of plates and screws with good reduction and occlusion. **J,** Postoperative radiograph of the fixation.

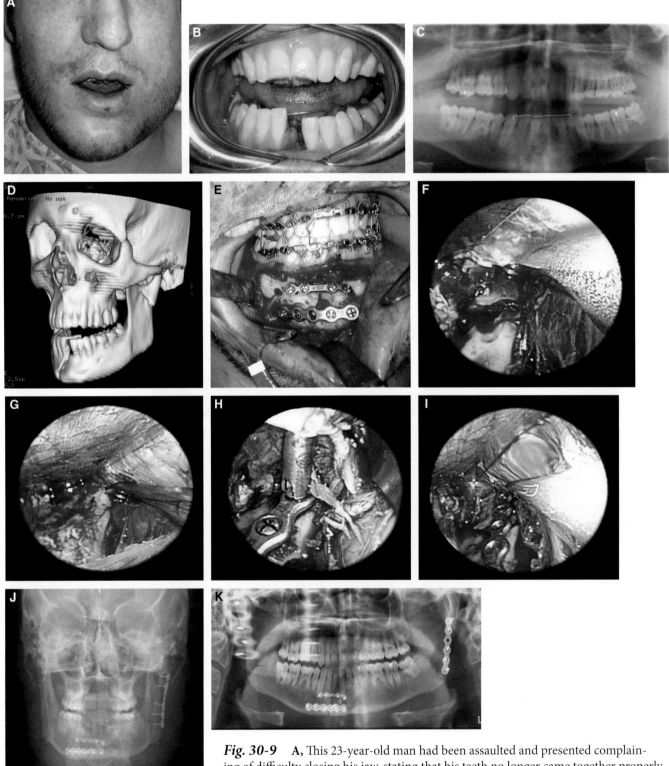

Fig. 30-9   **A,** This 23-year-old man had been assaulted and presented complaining of difficulty closing his jaw, stating that his teeth no longer came together properly. **B,** Step-off noted between the central incisors with a gingival laceration and inability to close his mouth. **C,** Preoperative radiograph and **D,** three-dimensional reconstruction showing displaced symphyseal and left subcondylar fractures. **E,** Intraoperative view of rigid fixation of the symphysis. **F,** Endoscopic photograph of the subcondylar fracture. **G-I,** Reduced fracture fixation technique with plates and screws. **J** and **K,** Plates and screws in place on postoperative radiographs.

POSTOPERATIVE CARE

Regardless of surgical technique, appropriate postoperative management is essential to the restoration of normal function. Patient compliance is critical to achieve this outcome. Meticulous attention to soft diet, oral hygiene, and physical therapy must be emphasized at all postoperative visits. When MMF is avoided, close follow-up is needed to ensure patient compliance; in this patient population early return to function may lead to less discipline with diet and oral hygiene, and thus increase the complication rate. The standard postoperative diet is a "non-chew" or blenderized diet. Significant masticatory forces during the initial postoperative phase increase the risk of nonunion.[26] If MMF is employed, the length of fixation varies depending on the fractures and can range from 2 to 8 weeks, depending on the fracture location, severity, comminution, and the patient's age, among other factors. During the time that MMF is in place, the fixation must remain tight and stable. If the occlusion is stable for 4 to 6 weeks, the patient may be released from MMF (depending on the injury) and be transitioned to guiding elastics to ensure a reproducible occlusion, or the arch bars can be removed.

COMPLICATIONS

Malunion typically occurs when basic principles of reduction, stabilization, and fixation have been violated and the bone has healed in a nonanatomic position, resulting in malocclusion.[27] This complication may also occur despite proper surgical technique and patient compliance. Correction of this complication usually requires added treatment.

Nonunion—defined as mobility in the segments after 4 to 8 weeks of treatment (during the period of transition from blenderized diet to open reduction and internal fixation)[10]—is rare, occurring in approximately 3% of patients.[28] Other causes of nonunion may be improper or inadequate fixation of the fractures, or osteomyelitis of the fracture. Reexploration, with debridement of the bone and proper reduction of bone fragments, is the usual management approach. Infections are the most common complication after open mandibular fracture repair. Several factors have been attributed to postoperative infection, including patient noncompliance with postoperative regimens, substance abuse such as smoking, gross contamination of the wound, and delay in treatment. Nerve injury is rare, and occurs when inadequate attention is paid to the course of the inferior alveolar nerve. Most commonly, injury to the nerve occurs as a result of the injury itself, rather than the surgical repair.[29]

KEY POINTS

- The primary aim of mandibular fracture repair is to restore function and preoperative occlusion.
- Fractures are typically caused by motor vehicle accidents or assaults.
- Advances in mandible plating systems have permitted the development of rigid internal fixation strategies through both intraoral and extraoral approaches.
- Mandible fractures are commonly multifocal.
- The most common mandible fracture sites are the body, condylar region, and mandibular angle.
- The mandibular canal is an important anatomic reference for fixation to avoid injury.
- Mandible-associated musculature influences displacement of fractures.
- Clinical examination permits accurate diagnosis of the type and classification of the fracture, even before imaging.

Continued

- Modern three-dimensional reformatted CT imaging provides high resolution and accurate diagnosis of mandible fractures.
- Reestablishing occlusion and functional movements are the goals of all mandibular reconstructive procedures.
- Closed reduction is the most traditional means of managing mandible fractures.
- Open reduction and internal fixation are necessary when closed reduction does not permit adequate reduction.
- Minimally invasive approaches and advances in endoscopy have resulted in the development of techniques that decrease the incidence of nerve injury and improve aesthetic outcomes.
- Patient compliance with diet and oral hygiene is critical postoperatively and should be reinforced at each postoperative visit.
- Complications include malunion, nonunion, infections, and nerve injury.

REFERENCES

1. Bahram R, Woodbury SC, Silverstein KE, et al. Mandibular fractures. In Fonseca RJ, Walker RV, Betts NJ, et al, eds. Oral and Maxillofacial Trauma, vol 1, ed 3. Philadelphia: Saunders-Elsevier, 2005.

   The chapter addressed classification of mandibular fractures and how such injuries can be vertically or horizontally displaced in favorable or unfavorable ways. The authors described how the masseter, temporal, and medial pterygoid can unfavorably displace angle fractures.

2. Mukerji R, Mukerji G, McGurk M. Mandibular fractures: historical perspective. Br J Oral Maxillofac Surg 44: 222-228, 2005.

3. Dingman R, Natvig P. The mandible. In Dingman R, Natvig P, eds. Surgery of Facial Fractures. Philadelphia: WB Saunders, 1964.

4. Breasted JH. Edwin Smith Surgical Papyrus. Facsimile and hieroglyphic transliteration with translation and commentary. Am J Orthod Oral Surg 30:399-504, 1944.

5. Gerlach KL, Erle A, Eckelt U, et al. Surgical management of mandibular, condylar neck, and atrophic mandible fractures. In Booth PW, Schendel SA, Hausamen JE, eds. Maxillofacial Surgery, vol 1, ed 2. London: Churchill Livingstone, 2007.

6. Oqundare BO, Bonnick A, Bayley N. Pattern of mandibular fractures in an urban major trauma center. J Oral Maxillofac Surg 61:713-718, 2003.

   This retrospective study evaluated mandibular fractures at an urban level I trauma center in Washington, DC. The analysis showed that 86% of the patients were men and that 79% of the mandibular fractures were caused by interpersonal violence.

7. Li K, Weber A, Cheney ML. Mandibular fractures. In Cheney ML, ed. Facial Surgery: Plastic and Reconstructive. Baltimore: Williams & Wilkins, 1997.

8. Erich JB, Austin LT. Traumatic Injuries of Facial Bones: An Atlas of Treatment. Philadelphia: WB Saunders, 1944.

9. Alvi A, Doherty T, Lewen G. Facial fractures and concomitant injuries in trauma patients. Laryngoscope 113:102-106, 2003.

10. Laski R, Ziccardi VB, Broder HL, et al. Facial trauma: a recurrent disease? The potential role of disease prevention. J Oral Maxillofac Surg 62:685-688, 2004.

11. Smith H, Peek-Asa C, Nesheim D, et al. Etiology, diagnosis, and characteristics of facial fracture at a Midwestern level I trauma center. J Trauma Nurs 19:57-65, 2012.

12. Peek-Asa C, Zwerling C, Stallones L. Acute traumatic injuries in rural populations. Am J Public Health 94:1689-1693, 2004.

13. Anyanechi CE, Saheeb BD. Mandibular sites prone to fracture: analysis of 174 cases in a Nigerian tertiary hospital. Ghana Medical J 45:111-114, 2011.

14. Bither S, Mahindra U, Halli R, et al. Incidence and pattern of mandibular fractures in rural population: a review of 324 patients at a tertiary hospital in Loni, Maharashtra, India. Dent Traumatol 24:468-470, 2008.

15. Chacon GE, Larsen PE. Principles of management of mandibular fractures. In Miloro M, ed. Peterson's Principles of Oral and Maxillofacial Surgery, vol 2, ed 2. Hamilton, ON, Canada: BC Decker, 2004.

> *The authors discussed the different types of mandibular fractures, how to evaluate such fractures, and the procedures most appropriate for treating each. The article also analyzed the epidemiology, preoperative planning, and postoperative planning for mandibular fractures.*

16. Sojat AJ, Meisami T, Sandor G, et al. The epidemiology of mandibular fractures treated at the Toronto General Hospital: a review of 246 cases. J Can Dent Assoc 67:640-644, 2001.

17. Zimmermann CE, Troulis MJ, Kaban LB. Pediatric facial fractures: recent advances in prevention, diagnosis and management. Int J Oral Maxillofac Surg 35:2-13, 2006.

18. Imahara SD, Hopper RA, Wang J, et al. Patterns and outcomes of pediatric facial fractures in the United States: a survey of the National Trauma Data Bank. J Am College Surg 207:710-716, 2008.

19. Lida S, Matsuya T. Pediatric maxillofacial fractures: their aetiological characters and fracture patterns. J Cranio-maxillofac Surg 30:237-241, 2002.

20. Brons A, Boering C. Fractures of the mandibular body treated by stable internal fixation: a preliminary report. J Oral Surg 28:407-415, 1970.

21. Converse JM. External fixation in fractures of the mandibular angle. J Bone Joint Surg 24:154-161, 1942.

22. Michelet FX, Deymes J, Dessus B. Osteosynthesis with miniaturized screwed plates in maxillo-facial surgery. J Maxillofac Surg 1:79-84, 1973.

23. Champy M, Lodde JP, Schmitt R, et al. Mandibular osteosynthesis by miniature screwed plates via a buccal approach. J Maxillofac Surg 6:14-21, 1978.

24. Ellis E, McFadden D, Simon P, et al. Surgical complications with open treatment of mandibular condylar process fractures. J Oral Maxillofac Surg 58:950-958, 2000.

25. Troulis MJ. Endoscopic open reduction and internal rigid fixation of subcondylar fractures. J Oral Maxillofac Surg 62:1269-1271, 2004.

26. Li Z, Zwang W, Li JB, et al. Abnormal union of mandibular fractures: a review of 84 cases. J Oral Maxillofac Surg 64:1225-1231, 2006.

27. Dodson TB, Perrott DH, Kaban LB, et al. Fixation of mandibular fractures: a comparative analysis of rigid internal fixation and standard fixation technique. J Oral Maxillofac Surg 48:362-366, 1990.

28. Mathog RH, Toma V, Clayman L, et al. Nonunion of the mandible: an analysis of contributing factors. J Oral Maxillofac Surg 58:746-752, 2000.

29. Tuovinen V, Nørholt SE, Sindet-Pedersen S, et al. A retrospective analysis of 279 patients with isolated mandibular fractures treated with titanium miniplates. J Oral Maxillofac Surg 52:931-935, 1994.

31

Implants and Skeletal Modifications

Vartan A. Mardirossian ▪ *Jeffrey H. Spiegel*

Facial surgeons may encounter clinical situations in which volume, normal adjacent tissue, and the appropriately matched tissue necessary for reconstruction of a defect are all inadequate. When adequate native tissue is not available, the surgeon may employ an "imported" material—either alloplastic or autologous—as a graft.

The characteristics of the missing tissue dictate the desired properties of any graft. The ideal graft exhibits properties that include no immune or carcinogenic effects, no inflammatory reaction, sufficiently similar properties to the missing or deficient tissue, ease of fabrication and sculpting, and complete biostability without breakdown in physical or chemical composition. In addition, practical considerations (including ease of availability, low cost, simplicity of sterilization, purity, low incidence of migration, predictable tissue ingrowth and regeneration, and limited potential for litigation) factor into the choice of implant best suited for consistent and favorable reconstruction. A wide and potentially confusing array of grafting and implantation materials is available to the reconstructive surgeon. In this chapter we review the most commonly used materials, with a focus on bone and cartilage graft integration. We will also discuss applications of implants and skeletal modifications to clinical practice.

Bone, cartilage, and a number of soft tissue (fascia, fat, dermis, muscle) implants, can be autografts (from the same patient), homografts/allografts (from same species), or xenografts (from a different species). In addition, there are synthetic tissue replacement materials, or *alloplasts,* and these are many and varied. Although use of autograft similar tissue is typically the best choice for reconstruction, sometimes alloplasts are the best available option for reconstruction. Generally, the use of autologous grafts is favored whenever possible and practical. A variety of bone, cartilage, and soft tissue autografts are usually available through concealed incisions and serve as satisfactory replacement tissues that incur no immunologic reactivity. Donor site morbidity is the most significant drawback of autologous tissues.

Skeletal modifications sometimes involve subtraction by contouring techniques, rather than the addition of grafting materials. These techniques are particularly relevant in gender transition surgery. The facial sites most commonly involved in bone contouring are the forehead and the mandible. Specifically, the supraorbital ridge, the angle of the mandible, the body of the mandible, and the chin may be contoured to change the appearance of the face. A full understanding of both grafting techniques and contouring techniques of existing bone permits the surgeon to perform a wide array of skeletal and soft tissue modifications.

The beginning of the twentieth century marked an increase in the use of synthetic materials in plastic and reconstructive surgery, before our modern understanding of complex immunologic mechanisms and reactions. The first implants were made of readily available materials, many of which proved to be either pathogenic or toxic. Since then, three generations of implants have evolved. The first generation of implants was designed to match the characteristics of the tissue they were intended to replace, with minimal or no immune response from the patient (that is, inert materials). Metallic implants were developed for this purpose, the first of which were composed of vanadium steel and introduced in the early 1900s for mandibular reconstruction plates.[1] Its use was complicated by mechanical failure, corrosion, and poor biocompatibility. The second generation of implants shifted the emphasis from bioinert to bioactive implants: both nonresorbable and resorbable polymers that promote implant-tissue integration. In the 1980s, bioactive glass composite implants and hydroxyapatite were extensively employed in head and neck reconstruction, but ultimately fell out of favor because of poor wear properties and the complication of long-term ruptures.[1] To circumvent the problems of nonbiodegradable materials, a move was initiated toward the development of biodegradable synthetic implants without long-term foreign material. Biodegradable plates made of polyglycolic acid would degrade over time, so the issue of stress shielding was resolved.[1] However, an ongoing problem was their adaptation and resistance to varying forces in the head and neck, which has ultimately limited their utility. The newest, third generation of implants includes different forms of synthetic absorbable and nonabsorbable scaffolds developed to allow seeding and multiplication of stem cells to generate new bone and cartilage[2-4] (see Chapter 50 for full discussion).

BONE GRAFTS

Bone grafts are used for the reconstruction of acquired or congenital defects and deficiencies of the bony skeleton. The two major types of bone, membranous and endochondral, may be used for bone grafts and are defined by their embryologic development (Fig. 31-1).

The physiologic and microanatomic differences between these types of bone, influence graft behavior and may dictate donor graft choice. All bones are derived from mesenchyme by two different processes, depending on anatomic location. The flat bones of the face, calvarium, and ribs develop by direct deposition of bone in areas of vascularized mesenchyme by the process of intramembranous ossification, and hence are called *membranous bones*. The long bones and the iliac crest develop from a cartilage precursor by the process of endochondral ossification, and are thus called *endochondral bones*.[5,6]

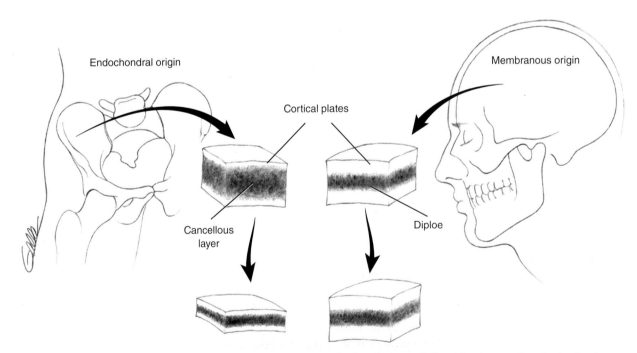

Fig. 31-1 Two major types of bone, membranous and endochondral, are defined by their embryologic development. The diagram illustrates that cancellous bone grafts are subject to significant volume loss over time, compared with volume maintenance of bone grafts of membranous origin. Diploe is a specialized cancellous layer found in short, flat, and irregular bones of membranous origin.

Membranous and endochondral bones are composed of a cortical outer layer and an inner cancellous region (in membranous bone, this is called *diploe*). Both components of bone, cortical and cancellous, may be used for bone grafts, either individually or together, depending on the requirements for reconstruction. Endochondral bone typically contains a greater proportion of cancellous bone than membranous bone does. The anatomic configuration of the cortical and cancellous components of bone has an influence on their healing as bone grafts. Cortical bone is characterized by a very dense or compact arrangement of both organic matrix and the predominantly hydroxyapatite inorganic mineral component. The cortical layer is traversed by microtubules (haversian canals) containing capillaries that connect with each other and with larger tubules called *nutritive canals*. Bone is deposited in concentric layers around the haversian canals to create a microscopic unit, the osteon.

Cancellous bone is composed of loosely woven trabeculae of organic and inorganic bone separated by large spaces filled with blood and marrow cells and osteoprogenitor (mesenchymal) cells. Cancellous bone does not contain haversian systems.

The most common source of bone graft is autologous, although bone allografts are derived from living or cadaver donors of the same species. These latter grafts generally elicit an immunologic response in the recipient and, like other allografts, carry a risk for the transfer of certain diseases. Bone allografts are occasionally employed in situations where the need for bone graft material exceeds the availability and practicality of autologous donor sites (such as with whole femur or humerus grafts) or where the morbidity of autograft bone harvest must be avoided. Purified rib and other types of bone are typically available from tissue banks as an allograft. Bone xenografts are derived from different species (usually bovine or porcine) and are infrequently used because of their immunogenicity and high rate of resorption.[7]

Autologous bone graft integration to the recipient site occurs through four processes: incorporation, osteoconduction, osteoinduction, and osteogenesis.

Incorporation is the process of adherence of the host tissues to the bone graft and the envelopment and admixture of necrotic and viable new bone. Incorporation requires immobilization of the bone graft, close contact of the surrounding soft tissues and bone to the bone graft, and a viable and well-vascularized recipient bed. The incorporation of cortical and cancellous bone is similar. Both are influenced by the age and the physiologic skeletal metabolism of the recipient, in addition to the proliferative activities of local and regional osteoprogenitor cells and the biochemical properties of the repair site.

Osteoconduction, or *creeping substitution,* is the predominant mechanism by which free, nonvascularized bone grafts "take." It is characterized by capillary and osteoprogenitor cellular ingrowth from the recipient bed into the bone graft, usually along the vascular channels and spaces previously occupied by the graft's cells. The bone graft essentially functions as a scaffold for cellular ingrowth and the deposition of new bone as the old bone is resorbed.[7]

Osteoinduction refers to the process by which local mesenchymal cells in contact with the matrix of the bone graft differentiate into osteoprogenitor cells and form new bone. This process is thought to be regulated by bone morphogenic protein (a component of the organic matrix) and specific enzymes and enzyme inhibitors.[7,8]

Osteogenesis refers to the formation of new bone by surviving cells within the bone graft. It is the predominant mechanism for new bone growth in vascularized bone grafts. Osteogenesis occurs to a much lesser extent in nonvascularized bone grafts and occurs especially poorly in cortical bone grafts where the density of the bone impairs early revascularization. Survival of graft surface cells and osteocytes is typically limited to a maximum depth of 0.3 mm.[7]

Healing of Nonvascularized Autologous Bone Grafts
Primary Stage

Nonvascularized bone grafts are especially useful to bridge gaps in otherwise healthy bone up to 6 cm in length. Their survival depends largely on immobilization and good vascularity of the recipient bed. Irradiated tissue is thus a contraindication for their placement. Whether cortical bone or cancellous bone is used is important because the mode, rate, and strength of the reparative process vary. The primary stage of autologous bone graft repair lasts for approximately 2 weeks and is similar in cortical and cancellous grafts. After transplantation the graft is encompassed briefly by a blood clot and a robust inflammatory reaction develops in the surrounding soft tissues. In the first week, the inflammatory reaction bathes the graft in a fluid exudate suspended in a lattice of scant, fibrous connective tissue. Capillary buds begin to proliferate around the graft. During the second week, the inflammatory reaction around the bone graft begins to subside, and fibrous granulation tissue and giant cells with osteoclastic activity dominate it. Within the bone graft, osteocytic autolysis proceeds to necrosis of the tissue within the haversian canals and marrow spaces. As the granulation response progresses, capillary buds infiltrate the graft through these anatomic portals and invading macrophages phagocytize the necrotic cellular debris. Coincident with the ingrowth of capillaries, primitive mesenchymal cells repopulate the now empty lacunae, haversian canals, and trabeculae.[9]

The primary stage of autologous bone graft repair lasts for approximately 2 weeks and is similar in cortical and cancellous grafts. After the primary stage of bone graft repair, cortical and cancellous bone grafts diverge with respect to their rate, mechanism, and completeness of repair.

Cancellous Bone Grafts

After the primary period of repair, cancellous bone grafts are usually completely revascularized, because of the larger channels available for capillary penetration and the facilitated access of phagocytes and osteoclasts. The rate of revascularization and repair of cancellous bone is related to its density (the number of trabeculae). Although the primary method of revascularization is thought to occur by capillary ingrowth as described earlier, under certain circumstances revascularization of cancellous bone may occur within several hours of transplantation by the process of inosculation (end-to-end alignment of the transplant and recipient vessels). In general, capillary penetration of the cancellous bone graft occurs within 4 days and is complete by 2 to 4 weeks.

As the vascular integration of a cancellous bone graft proceeds, the primitive mesenchymal cells that have repopulated the edges of the vacant trabeculae of the graft differentiate into osteogenic cells and then into osteoblasts that deposit a layer of osteoid (appositional bone formation) that eventually surrounds and seals the underlying core of devitalized bone graft. In time, new bone with a structure similar to that of the old bone graft replaces the entire cancellous bone graft. The marrow spaces of the renovated cancellous bone graft eventually refill with hematopoietic marrow cells.[10,11]

Because the mechanical strength of a cancellous bone graft is not affected appreciably by necrotic bony surfaces, this process tends to increase the mechanical strength and radiodensity of the graft. Over time, as the necrotic bone is resorbed gradually, the mechanical strength of a cancellous bone graft returns to normal.

Cortical Bone Grafts

The secondary repair and vascular integration of a cortical bone graft occurs through the preexisting haversian canals, starting first at the periphery and then proceeding to the interior of the graft. Because these channels are smaller and more widely dispersed than the vascular spaces of cancellous bone, the rate of revascularization and repair in a cortical bone graft decreases substantially. Generally, the capillary penetration of a cortical bone graft does not occur until the sixth day, and complete vascular integration takes 1 to 2 months.[12,13]

Capillary ingrowth into a cortical bone graft is facilitated by increased osteoclastic activity, which results in resorption and widening of the haversian canals. By the fourth week, the osteoclastic activity of the periphery of the graft and its interior is quantitatively equivalent. The increased osteoclastic activity in a cortical bone graft persists for more than a year after grafting. Although this osteoclastic activity is increased, it is primarily directed toward widening of the haversian canals with very little resorption of the remaining interstitial bone. After the haversian canals are widened to an appropriate size, the osteoclastic activity ceases. Mesenchymal cells then line the canals, differentiate into osteoblasts, and begin to form new appositional bone approximately 12 weeks after grafting. The new bone effectively seals the necrotic bone from further osteoclastic activity. The result is an admixture of new and necrotic bone that persists over time. The proportion of viable new bone to necrotic bone in cortical bone grafts increases up to 6 months after transplantation and remains unchanged thereafter.

Because a cortical bone graft is repaired initially by osteoclastic activity, the mechanical strength of the graft decreases as a direct function of the graft's porosity.[14] These grafts are approximately 40% to 50% weaker than normal bone at 6 weeks to 6 months after transplantation. As new bone is formed to create a permanent admixture of new and necrotic bone in a cortical bone graft, its mechanical strength and radiodensity gradually increase over time and are nearly normal 1 to 2 years after transplantation. As with other bone grafts, the stress loading imparted on the remodeled graft affects its strength.

LOCAL WOUND FACTORS IN BONE GRAFT REPAIR

The appearance of osteocytes, osteoblasts, and osteoclasts in and around the graft site characterizes the integration of cortical and cancellous bone grafts. These cells exert their respective activities on the repair process, which differs according to the type of graft. The observation of these cells in the bone soon after grafting suggests that some osteogenic elements survive the transplantation process. It is thought that the production of new bone cells resides in a primitive mesenchymal or osteoprogenitor cell. The periosteum, endosteum, intracortical elements, and marrow elements represent the four main sources from which surviving osteoprogenitor cells in the bone graft may be derived. Endosteal lining cells and marrow stroma together are responsible for the production of more than half of the new bone in the graft.[7] The source for the remaining new bone is the population of recipient site osteoprogenitor cells.

The stimulus for osteoprogenitor cells to differentiate into bone repair cells is thought to be the result of their contact with substances released from the necrotizing bone and marrow tissue within the graft. In endochondral bone induction, the recipient site mesenchymal cells that produce type II collagen serve as the progenitors of chondroblasts. These cells lay down a cartilage precursor that induces the attachment of osteoprogenitor cells and ultimately leads to new bone formation. In membranous bone grafts, the target cell for bone morphogenic protein is the perivascular connective tissue cell, or *pericyte,* in the recipient bed. The membranous bone graft provides a supplementary supply of marrow, mesenchymal cells, and a requisite structural framework on which new bone formation may occur.

COMMON SOURCES OF NONVASCULARIZED BONE AUTOGRAFTS
Iliac Bone Grafts

The ilium is an excellent source of cortical, cancellous, or combined cortical-cancellous bone grafts. It is the most commonly used donor site for nonvascularized autologous bone graft material, and is also a common source for vascularized bone grafting material.[15] Iliac bone has a tough, dense, cortical layer that lends itself well to the reconstruction of high-stress areas such as the long bones and hand. Its dense cortical component facilitates rigid fixation. These desirable qualities are offset by the relative rigidity and brittleness of the cortical component, which makes shaping and bending difficult. The inner table of the ilium is preferred as a donor site, because the outer cortex has more muscular attachments and thus increased morbidity associated with its harvest. A large volume of cortical and cancellous bone can be harvested from the ilium. The iliac crest is especially applicable in situations requiring a large amount of cancellous "filler" bone in reconstructions such as in the treatment of bony nonunions, alveolar cleft defects, and arthrodeses. In children, the iliac crest is covered by a cartilaginous apophysis that must be preserved for normal growth and development of the ilium. The primary disadvantage of the iliac crest donor site is its postoperative morbidity, which is related to the amount of bone harvested. Patients frequently report prolonged pain and may require crutches for a period of time to support ambulation. Injury to the lateral femoral cutaneous nerve during bone graft harvest, must be avoided which would result in significant postopertive pain.

Rib Grafts

Autologous rib grafts are cortico-cancellous membranous bone grafts that are used primarily in the reconstruction of cranial defects and as onlay bone grafts of the facial skeleton to correct acquired and congenital deformities. Rib grafts are soft and flexible, particularly in younger patients, and therefore are not desirable for the reconstruction of defects subjected to high stresses. A unique quality of the rib is that both bone and cartilage can be harvested in the same field. Rib grafts provide a relatively large volume of bone graft material for facial reconstruction. If the rib periosteal envelope is left in situ at the donor site, the rib will regenerate in both children and adults; however, the "take" of a rib graft is enhanced if its periosteum is left intact on the graft.

The primary disadvantage of rib grafts is their resorption when used as onlay grafts.[16] This is perhaps a result of the greater cancellous component of rib as compared with calvarial bone. The harvest of a rib graft carries the risk of pneumothorax and postoperative atelectasis caused by splinting. Split-rib grafts provide an excellent material for cranioplasty, and when compared with alloplastic materials, the incidence of infection is reduced with their use.[17]

Calvarial Bone Grafts

The calvarium is composed of membranous bone with a large cortical component represented by the inner and outer tables. The cancellous component of calvarial bone is the diploe, which varies in thickness and is poorly developed in children. Calvarial bone can be used as a source of bone graft material for a wide variety of reconstructive challenges in the facial skeleton.

Because of its dense cortical plates, minimal secondary resorption is expected. Because of its proximity to the face, and ease of inclusion into one operating field, the calvarium is a preferred donor site for bone grafts to the face and calvarium. Usually it is harvested as a split graft to preserve the inner table of cortical bone for protection of the brain and meninges. A popular site for harvest is the superior temporal line near the vertex, where the bone is thick and provides the opportunity to harvest a significant amount of bone while avoiding entry into the extradural space. When large amounts of bone are required for reconstruction, the calvarium is harvested as a full-thickness graft and then split into its inner and outer tables, with one of the tables returned to the donor defect. Split calvarial bone grafts are excellent as onlay, inlay, or bridging grafts of the facial skeleton and calvarium because they retain their volume better than endochondral bone grafts. In children, split calvarial bone is flexible and can be easily contoured. In adults, calvarial bone becomes rigid and brittle and does not lend itself well to bending. As with other bone grafts possessing a cortical component, calvarial bone grafts can be rigidly fixed with wires, plates and screws, or pins. In older children and adults, the well-developed diploe can be harvested as a cancellous bone graft for closure of alveolar clefts and smaller spaces in the facial skeleton. Specifically in the case of nasal onlay grafting it can provide nearly complete dorsal nasal reconstruction for saddle nose deformity and commonly provides good tip support without the need for a columellar strut (Fig. 31-2).

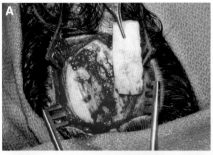
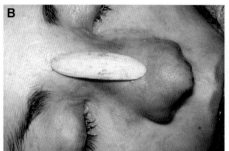
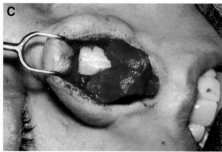

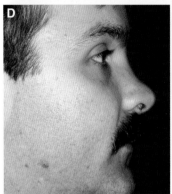
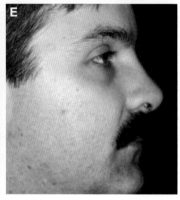

Fig. 31-2   Repair of saddle nose deformity. **A,** Calvarial bone graft harvest. **B,** Positioning of the graft. **C,** Placement of the graft. **D,** Preoperative profile view of saddle nose deformity. **E,** Final appearance months postoperatively. No columellar strut was necessary to achieve this long-term result.

Bone Allografts

The use of bone allografts for reconstruction is appealing from many perspectives. Their use obviates donor site morbidity, the additional operative time required for graft harvest, and there are no practical limitations on the quantity of graft material available for reconstruction. The shortcomings of bone allografts lie principally in the immunogenicity resulting from the genetic disparity between the host and recipient and the adverse effects that the host immune response has on graft incorporation and healing.[18]

Immunogenicity in bone allografts is derived primarily from the cells of the graft and, to a lesser extent, the organic matrix. Freezing removes the antibody response but has little effect on cell-mediated immunity. Freeze-drying of the bone graft decreases both types of immune response but will not completely eliminate these mechanisms of immunologic response.[19,20]

The host response to bone allografts is similar to that of other tissue allografts and varies from complete acceptance and repair of the graft to frank rejection based on the level of genetic disparity between the graft and host. In most cases, the host response to bone allografts falls somewhere between these two extremes, with variable levels of creeping substitution and resorption occurring simultaneously.[21]

The primary phase of healing in a bone allograft is similar to bone autografts with the formulation of an inflammatory granulation tissue response. A secondary osteogenic response may be initiated by the host 4 to 6 weeks after bone transplantation and persists until final healing is concluded.

Bone allografts generally progress to a satisfactory result, although their healing rate may be substantially delayed. Union of the graft to the host bone occurs gradually, by calluses formed both periosteally and endosteally. The replacement of necrotic bone by creeping substitution of new bone to create the typical admixture of new and necrotic bone (as seen in bone autografts) is limited or absent in bone allografts. This absence of creeping substitution, in combination with selective resorption of the graft, substantially reduces the graft's ability to withstand stress, and results in an increased incidence of fractures. Periosteal new bone formation around the bone allograft serves as the interface for attachment of soft tissues, but is tenuous when compared to bone autografts.

Demineralized freeze-dried bone allografts have been shown experimentally to retain the capacity for bone induction and may well find future application in the clinical arena.[22] However, their lack of strength after demineralization limits their utility as bone substitutes to counteract stress loads. Because of the superiority of autologous bone for graft material and the variable immunogenicity elicited by allografts, cadaveric bone grafts have a limited role.

CARTILAGE

Cartilage grafts are especially well suited to augmentation of the facial skeleton because of their resistance to remodeling and resorption. Cartilage is composed of three primary elements: chondrocytes, matrix, and bound water. Chondrocytes produce both type II collagen and proteoglycan matrix, two elements essential for maintaining the viability of cartilage. Chondrocytes are derived from mesenchymal cells containing chondrogenic DNA, which stimulates their differentiation. Mesenchymal cells, myoblasts, and fibroblasts containing the chondrogenic DNA also may be stimulated to differentiate into chondrocytes and form cartilage in the presence of bone morphogenic protein. Chondrocytes reside in lacunae within the cartilage matrix and under normal circumstances are not replaced during the life of the cartilage.[18]

The bound water in cartilage matrix facilitates the diffusion of nutrients because cartilage has no blood vessels and derives its entire nutritive support from the surrounding perichondrium or synovium. The compressive and tensile forces acting on cartilage in its normal environment cause migration and shifting of the water layers, which promote the diffusion of nutrients throughout the matrix. This diffusion is thought to be a primary mechanism in cartilage nutrition. Immobilization of cartilage (as occurs in cartilage grafting) results in thinning or resorption, which may be a direct consequence of impaired nutrition.[23]

Three types of cartilage are found in the human body. Hyaline cartilage is the lining cartilage of joints, the thoracic costal cartilage, the supporting cartilage of the tracheobronchial tree, and the nasal septum. As a graft, this cartilage is uniquely suited to resist compressive and expansive forces. Elastic cartilage has an abundance of elastin in its matrix and is found in the nasal tip, the external ear, and in the corniculate cartilage of the larynx. Its flexibility and shape memory as a scaffold allow for repeated deformation with return to its original shape. Fibrocartilage is composed of a predominantly fibrous matrix and is found in the intervertebral disks and in tendon attachments to bone. Fibrocartilage is tough and resilient and is capable of withstanding prolonged comprehensive and tensile stresses.

HEALING AND REPAIR OF AUTOLOGOUS CARTILAGE GRAFTS

Most cartilage grafts employed for reconstruction are autologous and are clearly superior to allografts and xenografts. The success of transplantation of an autologous cartilage graft can be defined in terms of the ultimate survival of the graft and the degree to which its structure and volume are maintained. In an autologous cartilage graft, this maintenance depends on the viability of its chondrocytes, which are necessary for maintaining the collagen/proteoglycan matrix. Unlike bone, cartilage does not heal by "creeping substitution" and normally does not become vascularized. New cells from the recipient bed do not replace chondrocytes in a cartilage graft. Therefore survival of the chondrocytes within the graft depends on the diffusion of nutrients from the surrounding soft tissues, and this is related to the condition of the recipient bed (that is, well vascularized versus scarred or irradiated), the adequacy of local mechanical forces in promoting the diffusion and distribution of nutrients, and the size of the graft.

Clinical experience with autologous cartilage grafts has been characterized by variable rates of resorption, depending on the type of cartilage used as a graft, how the graft is prepared before implantation, and where it is implanted. For example, hyaline cartilage resists vascular invasion if it is kept in an environment that allows motion such as bending and compression. If rib cartilage is transferred to a relatively immobile site (such as the nose), vascular invasion and partial resorption occurs. Cartilage grafts placed beneath the periosteum undergo more resorption and ossification than those placed above the periosteum. This may relate to pressure forces and immobilization of the graft in a subperiosteal pocket, both of which are thought to impair graft nutrition. Ear cartilage, which is elastic and subjected to similar external forces as nasal cartilage, demonstrates less resorption when transferred as a graft to the nose.[22,24] As with bone grafts, allograft cartilage is an alternative and may be indicated when autologous cartilage is unavailable or in insufficient supply.

SOURCES OF CARTILAGE
Nasal Septum

The hyaline cartilage found in the nasal septum is well suited for reconstruction. Its donor site morbidity is low, it is easily obtainable by experienced nasal surgeons through a standard septoplasty, and it is readily sculpted to reproduce even subtle contours. This is particularly useful when the quadrangular cartilage is used for nasal tip grafts. Other common uses for septal cartilage include nasal dorsal augmentation, spreader grafts and batten grafts in nasal reconstruction and rhinoplasty (Fig. 31-3), laryngotracheal interposition grafts (Fig. 31-4), and for orbital floor repair. Nasal septal cartilage has a low resorption rate and has shown up to 95% survival after 20 years.[25,26]

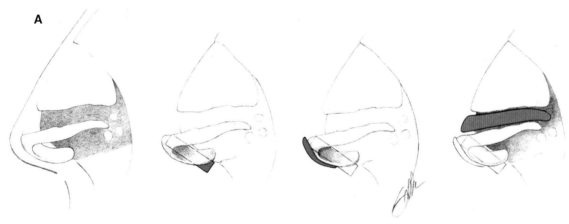

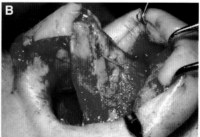

Fig. 31-3   **A,** Columellar strut, tip graft, and batten grafts fashioned from septal cartilage. **B,** Intraoperative photograph of batten graft placement.

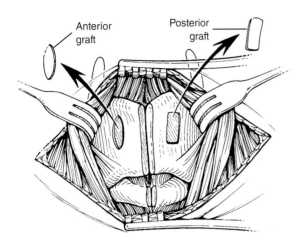

Fig. 31-4   Harvest of thyroid cartilage grafts for anterior and posterior cricoid expansion grafts.

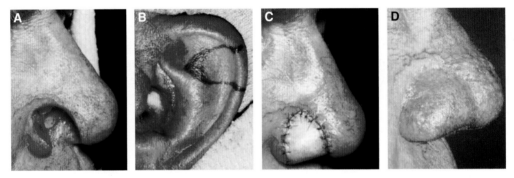

Fig. 31-5   **A,** Full thickness alar defect measuring 1.5 cm. **B,** Composite auricular graft donor site. **C,** Composite graft sutured into position. **D,** Result after 6 months.

Auricular Cartilage

Auricular cartilage is often useful when septal cartilage is unavailable or when a more pliable and resilient graft is desired. The cymba conchae and cavum conchae can be harvested as cartilage/perichondrial grafts with minimal auricular deformity. A portion of the helical rim (up to 1.5 cm) may be taken as a cartilage or skin and cartilage composite graft creating no obvious deformation of the ear (Fig. 31-5). The cartilage may be used for nasal or lower eyelid reconstruction (Fig. 31-6), and composite grafts are well suited for nasal alar repair (see Fig. 33-5) or contralateral ear reconstruction. Conchal cartilage may also be used for reconstruction of nasal defects, particularly of the lateral crus of the lower lateral cartilage (Fig. 31-6).

Costal Cartilage

Rib cartilage is an excellent source when large volumes of cartilage are necessary. It provides superior strength yet inferior pliability, and displays a tendency to warp when compared to hyaline cartilage. The donor site involves a subcostal scar and potential for intraoperative pneumothorax and postoperative splinting. Rib grafts are used to make auricular frameworks in microtia repair where the contralateral cartilage forms a natural curve that helps mimic the contour of the ear. Rib is commonly used for laryngotracheal reconstruction, nasal reconstruction, facial augmentation, and total auricular reconstruction (Fig. 31-7).

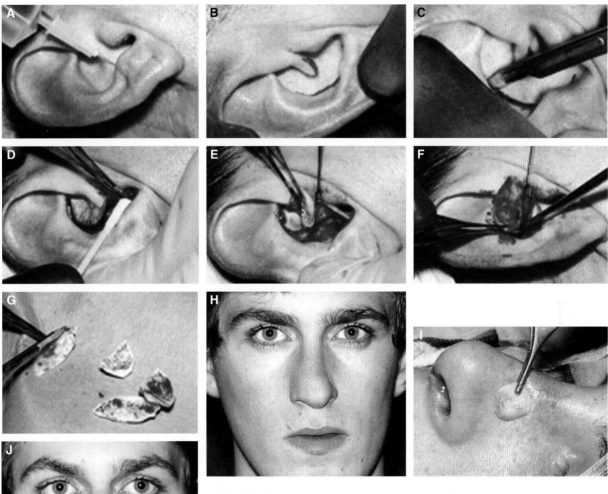

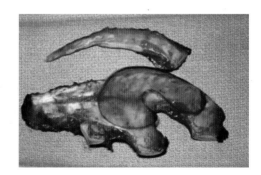

Fig. 31-6   Harvesting conchal cartilage graft from concha cavum and cymba. **A,** Infiltration of local anesthetic with vasoconstrictor. **B,** Outlined region of concha showing proposed harvest. **C,** Incision. **D,** Elevation of the skin using blunt dissection. **E,** Retraction of the skin with scleral hook with an emphasis on maintaining the root of the helix. **F,** Medial elevation of cartilage. **G,** Carving of grafts on back table. **H-J,** Clinical photographs of a case in which conchal cartilage addresses a nasal deformity.

Fig. 31-7   Example of stock costal cartilage harvest for microtia repair.

Allografts

Cadaveric cartilage is occasionally used as a grafting material. Irradiation, chemical treatment, lyophilization, and freezing of the cartilage decreases the risk of immunogenicity and disease transmission risk, while preserving the viability of the graft.[27] Allograft cartilage exhibits higher resorption rates than autologous cartilage. The method of preservation and site of implantation affect the amount of cartilage that survives. These grafts may be used for any of the common reconstructions that require strength and pliability, although autologous grafting material is more desirable.

ALLOPLASTIC MATERIALS

Numerous alloplastic materials have been used in clinical practice to repair tissue, replace structural elements, augment tissue, stabilize fractures, and bond other materials to tissue, among other applications. The success of implanted alloplastic materials has paralleled the growth in knowledge regarding the optimal physical/chemical composition of biomaterials, their fabrication, and their ability to decrease their reactivity in a biologic environment.[27]

All implanted alloplastic materials behave as foreign bodies, eliciting local inflammatory cellular responses. Biocompatibility is a requisite for successful incorporation and retention of an alloplast. Biocompatibility is directly related to the durability of the material and its mechanical, physicochemical, and electrochemical properties. Of key importance are the surface characteristics of the biomaterial and the events that occur at the tissue-biomaterial interface.[27]

The chemical composition of the alloplast largely determines the inflammatory reaction generated by its presence. Those materials that most closely mimic the elements occurring in organic materials (carbon and calcium) are less immunogenic.[28] Thus the closely matching valence structure of silicone, titanium, and hydroxyapatite make them excellent implants from a biochemical perspective.

The durability of an alloplastic material is often equated with its degree of inertness, but alloplasts may eventually undergo degradation. This process occurs by mechanical and physical events intrinsic to the material itself (such as fatigue) and by the processes of hydrolysis, phagocytosis, and lysis generated by the local cellular milieu. Important concerns regarding degradation include undesirable local, regional, and systemic side effects elicited by the microfragmentation of alloplasts in a biologic environment, and events that may lead to toxic side effects in the host. Particles smaller than 60 μm in diameter may be ingested by circulating macrophages. Often without the ability to lyse the particle, the macrophage itself is disrupted, releasing potent mediators of inflammation. This becomes a vicious cycle of ongoing inflammation around the implant.

The site of implantation plays a major role in determining biocompatibility. Proplast (Novomed, Houston, TX) is an example of an implant that the physician may encounter but is not commonly available for clinical use. Proplast implants are composed of either polytetrafluoroethylene (PTFE) and graphite or PTFE and aluminum oxide, and are generally well tolerated; however, they fail at a high rate when used under the mechanical stress of the mandibular joint, which causes them to sheer and produce microfragmentation.[29]

Beyond the degree of inertness, many other factors intrinsic to an alloplast have been found to affect the immediate cellular environment, including the size and shape of the material and its surface configuration, porosity, and composition. All of these components have an influence on the preferential affinity and adhesiveness of cells to the surface of a biomaterial and define its biocompatibility.

Clinical experience has shown that retention of an alloplastic material is enhanced by its placement deep in tissues, which diffuses the impact of any mechanical or physical disharmony between the material and the surrounding soft tissues. A thin soft tissue covering predisposes an alloplast to exposure by the simple mechanism of trauma caused by daily contact of the overlying tissue with the environment. Tissue responses to biomaterials have been studied primarily in the context of surface-mediated, cellular inflammatory reactions generated by native host tissues surrounding implants, which vary according to implantation site. This surface-mediated cellular response depends on cellular adherence, which influences (and is influenced by) the type of protein that initially adsorbed to the surface of the alloplast. Activation of complement on the alloplast surface is thought to be an important step in the pathway to macrophage adhesion and activation, and, in turn, plays a pivotal role in modulation of the cellular inflammatory response. The inflammatory cellular reaction to an alloplast decreases over time, thus a highly biocompatible alloplast ceases to provide a stimulus for continued inflammatory response. A chronic foreign-body response persists to a variable degree around the biocompatible implant, and the intensity of this reaction is thought to relate to the efficiency of cellular adherence and the physical and chemical stability of the implant. Thus an implanted, biocompatible alloplast material eventually becomes invested by a layer of fibrous tissue and assumes a steady state with its biologic environment.

Because tissue adherence to an alloplast is considered a major factor in its retention in the human body, methods to improve tissue adherence have evolved as important components of the design and manufacturing process. Alloplasts with pore sizes of 30 to 50 μm or greater allow fibrous tissue ingrowth to provide firm anchorage of the material to the surrounding soft tissues. Specific polymers have been fabricated with these favorable pore sizes for augmentation of the facial skeleton (for example, malar and chin implants), and for repairing fascial defects of the abdominal wall. Alloplast porosity may also serve to promote osteogenic conduction in implanted ceramic when invasion of the implant by the "creeping substitution" of osteoprogenitor cells is a defined goal. One disadvantage of implant porosity is the alteration of the physical characteristics of the alloplast, such as strength and flexibility. A second disadvantage is that extensive tissue ingrowth can limit ease of implant removal.

Surface texturing has been shown to increase soft tissue adhesion and elicit favorable foreign-body-type morphologic changes in the macrophages and foreign-body giant cells in contact with the implant (increased cytoplasmic-to-nuclear ratio).[30] The mechanisms by which surface texture initiates these cellular changes are not completely understood.

Textured materials are composed of surface spikes. It has been proposed that the radius of the curvature of the spike tip could change the surface energy of cells next to the implant sufficiently to affect the type, rate of adsorption, and conformation of adsorbed proteins, which may then induce morphologic changes in the cells reacting to the implant. Different cellular reactions to a biomaterial can be induced by altering the height and width of surface micropillars (that is, changing the size and shape of the surface texture spike).

The rough surface produced by surface texturing may cause chronic trauma to the surrounding soft tissues and has been shown to cause malignant changes in cells adjacent to implanted biomaterials in rodents; but thus far this has not been observed in humans.

Although texturing and porosity have been shown to improve tissue adherence to an implant, these surface characteristics may also promote bacterial colonization, which can result in extrusion of the implant. The preferential affinity of the implant surface to bacteria or eukaryotic cells is thus an important determinant of outcome.

Specific Implant Materials
Silicone

Silicone is a generic term for a family of polymers derived from the element silicon [Si^{14}]. As an implantable biomaterial, it is most commonly used in the form of the dimethylsiloxane polymer, which is a large molecule of repetitive units containing silicone, oxygen, and methane. The extent of polymerization determines its viscosity and hence its physical state: liquid, gel, or solid. Silicone polymers are easily contaminated with heavy metals, low-chain-length polymers, and other impurities during the manufacturing process, and their refinement requires specialized filtration and sterilization. Only medical-grade silicone is approved for implantation in the human body.[31]

Numerous implants of complex shapes and volumes can be custom fabricated by varying the viscosity of silicone to simulate the differing physical and mechanical properties of soft tissues and bone (that is, liquid, viscous gel, and solid). The rubbery consistency and flexibility of high-viscosity silicone make it particularly suited as an onlay material for the augmentation of tissues. This type of silicone is also used for fabricating inflatable saline-filled mammary implants. The availability of liquid and viscous gel silicones for human implantation has been hindered at times because of concerns over their potential for migration and toxicity in tissues, and a presumed but unproven association with human adjuvant disease.

The surface of most implantable silicones is smooth, which diminishes tissue adherence and may play a role in implant extrusion, especially if the implant is placed near the skin surface (for example, in the nose and ear). Silicone cannot at present be rendered porous in such a way as to improve its incorporation in tissues without substantially altering its physical characteristics. Texturing of the implant's surface has been introduced as a method to enhance tissue adherence and to modify the fibrous capsule that forms around the implant.

Although silicones are considered to be biologically inert, they do evoke an inflammatory response in humans. The degree of inflammatory response (especially injectable forms) varies widely among individuals. Medical-grade silicones are widely used in medicine for lubricating disposable syringes and needles and as coatings for suture materials. It is estimated that an insulin-dependent patient with diabetes injects 2 to 5 ml of medical-grade silicone into his or her body each year from the needles and syringes used for insulin injection.

Although antibodies to medical-grade silicone have never been demonstrated, the particulation of silicone implants has been associated with conditions such as silicone synovitis and siliconoma. In both conditions, the presence of silicone in the tissues elicits a granulomatous foreign-body reaction that appears to be related to the size of the silicone particle (Fig. 31-8). In silicone synovitis, fragmentation of silicone joint-replacement implants (particularly in the wrist and basilar joint of the thumb) is followed by migration of the particles into adjacent synovial spaces and bone. The foreign-body reaction produces synovitis, with attendant destruction of joint spaces and tendons and inflammatory resorption of bone.

Siliconomas (or silicone granulomas) are characterized by the formulation of granulomatous reactions around particles of liquid silicone. Most cases have been associated with the injection of nonmedical-grade liquid silicone or liquid silicone that has been tainted with other substances to provoke a more vigorous inflammatory response, thus inducing fibrous encapsulation that minimizes migration. Siliconomas may occur at the sites of liquid silicone injection in the skin or subcutaneous tissues, at sites of particle migration, or internally in the major organs, such as the liver, spleen, and kidneys. Silicone granulomas are characterized clinically by the appearance of firm, erythematous, ill-defined masses in the skin and subcutaneous tissues. Of interest, these siliconomas can occur seemingly at any time after placement, even 30 years after injection. In advanced stages, the skin may assume a peau d'orange quality, with associated tenderness. Removal of injected silicone is often requested, but not readily achievable as it often necessitates

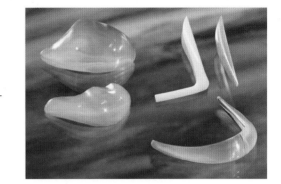

Fig. 31-8   Solid silicone implants come in many configurations and represent an excellent option for aesthetic augmentation of the malar area and chin. (Courtesy of Implantech.)

en-bloc resection of the silicone with a large amount of normal tissue, typically in anatomically delicate areas such as the cheeks or the lips.

In reconstructive surgery, silicone implants are used primarily for augmentation of the bony skeleton. When silicone implants are placed subperiosteally for augmentation of the bony skeleton (such as the chin or zygoma), bone resorption beneath the implant occurs routinely, presumably because of the effects of pressure and foreign-body reaction. Less bony resorption follows placement of the implant superficial to the periosteum. Deformation of the calvarial vault and bony thorax has also been observed beneath tissue expanders and silicone implants placed in these areas.[22]

The stability of a silicone implant in tissue resides primarily in fibrous encapsulation of the implant, which varies among individuals. For solid silicone implants, this does not pose a significant problem. In gel-filled or saline-filled silicone implants used for soft tissue or breast augmentation, the quality of the reconstruction depends on the softness of the implant in its tissue environment, which corresponds to the degree of fibrous encapsulation and contraction.

Solid silicone implants come in many configurations and represent an excellent option for aesthetic augmentation of the malar area and chin (Fig. 31-8). These implants are easy to place and require less tissue dissection for pocket creation than that required for more rigid materials. In addition, screw fixation is not required or desired, because compression of the implant around the screw could result in a palpable abnormality on the face. Facial implants can be sculpted from a block of solid silicone, but prefabricated shapes can be used in most applications and have the advantage of tapering to a very thin edge, which prevents the patient from identifying the edge of the implant or feeling a step-off deformity.

Tapered soft solid silicone tubes are also available as lip implants (PermaLip, SurgiSil, Inc.). These implants are easily placed and removed, although keeping the implants centered appropriately until they heal may be challenging for surgeons new to this procedure.

Silicone malar augmentation is most readily performed through an intraoral approach. A small sublabial incision is made and a subperiosteal dissection is executed from lateral to the infraorbital nerve to the malar eminence and continued over the zygomatic arch. This subperiosteal pocket should be very close in size to the dimensions of the implant so that a tight fixation is achieved (Fig. 31-9). The implant is placed into the pocket and the sublabial incision is closed. Fixation of the implant to the dermis with a temporary transcutaneous suture may be helpful at times, particularly in revision cases. Great care is necessary to ensure that the implant is not folded on itself and that the heights are symmetrical.

Chin augmentation is routinely performed with silicone implants, and a number of different configurations are available, depending on the area of deficiency and the aesthetic goals. For example, some implants augment primarily in the anterior vector, but others add a lateral augmentation. Implants are typically placed

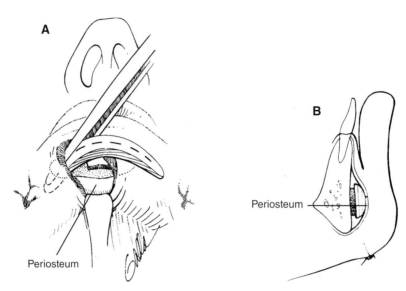

Fig. 31-9 **A** and **B,** Subperiosteal pocket size in relationship to the implant's dimensions to achieve a tight fixation.

through a small sublabial intraoral pocket. Critics of this technique argue that infection rates are higher and that the implant rides too high on the chin when using this approach, although in practice these are not common complications. Alternatively, a submental incision approach can be chosen, but this technique results in a potentially unsightly external scar. As with many surgical procedures, individual surgeon comfort and experience is likely the best predictor of outcome.

Methylmethacrylate

Methylmethacrylate, or *acrylic,* is the polymerized ester of acrylic acid, $CH_2 = CHCOOH$, or an ester of methacrylic acid, $CH_2 = (CH_3)COOH$. In its cured, polymerized state, methylmethacrylate is a rigid, porous, translucent material with low specific gravity. The material does not conduct electricity and is not carcinogenic, and can be shaped by burring and drilled for wiring or screw fixating. A great advantage of methylmethacrylate is that it can be prepared intraoperatively and molded in situ before hardening to achieve a desired contour or shape. Powdered granules of polymerized methacrylate polymer are mixed with a liquid monomer; the material is then placed in situ and shaped until it hardens (approximately 7 minutes). Final curing takes an additional 7 minutes. The polymerized monomer bonds to form an acrylic composite. An exothermic reaction generating temperatures up to 100° C ensues as the material polymerizes, and this sterilizes the alloplast. The heat generated by the curing of methylmethacrylate is sufficient to kill cells; therefore the surrounding tissues must be cooled by irrigation until the polymerization process is complete. Cold curing of methylmethacrylate by this technique has been shown experimentally to limit heat buildup in the immediately adjacent tissues to 68° C, which peaks 5 to 6 minutes after mixing.[32]

Allergic systemic reactions, hypotension, and cardiac arrest have been reported with the use of methylmethacrylate, although these phenomena are primarily a result of escape and absorption of monomers during the curing process.[33] Once the material has polymerized and the monomer becomes bonded, no further toxicity is seen, although approximately 4% of the monomer remains unbonded in the final acrylic composite. Toxic reactions to methylmethacrylate are associated with the use of large volumes of polymer when put in extensive direct contact with soft tissue and bone during orthopedic procedures; these reactions have rarely been encountered in head and neck reconstruction.

The reactivity of methylmethacrylate in tissues is slightly higher than that observed for silicone polymers but is still considered relatively mild. A typical foreign-body reaction develops after implantation, which

Table 31-1   Table of Alloplasts

Material	Product/Trade Names	Advantages	Disadvantages
Silicone	Silastic Silicone gel Bioplastique	Multiple forms Inert Removable	Controversial Contains impurities if not medical grade Bioplastique not FDA approved Public distrust May extrude on nasal dorsum Microfragmentation under stress loads
Titanium	Craniofacial plates	Strong, low profile	Expensive
Gold	Eyelid weights	Inert Removable	Often palpable Eyelid contour distortion
Calcium phosphate (hydroxyapatite [HA])	Ceramic HA Dense HA (solid or granular) Porous HA (coral) Nonceramic HA (cement)	Good tissue ingrowth Strong after integration Biocompatible	Need 3-6 month immobility for bony ingrowth Difficult to shape (brittle)
Polytetrafluoroethylene (PTFE)	Teflon	Injectable	Granuloma formation Migrates Not recommended for vocal cord augmentation
PTFE + graphite PTFE + aluminum oxide Expanded PTFE	Proplast I Proplast II Gore-Tex	Good for skeletal augmentation Well tolerated Shapeable for natural contour Easily removable Strong Excellent soft tissue correlate	Subject to microfragmentation if placed in areas of stress
Polyethylene (high density)	Plastipore Medpor	Carvable Good soft tissue ingrowth (125-250 μm pores)	Difficult to remove Should not be placed in regions of stress
Polymide mesh	Supramid	Good tissue ingrowth Shapeable	May contract
Polyester mesh	Mersilene Dacron	Good tissue ingrowth Shapeable Good for skeletal augmentation (such as genioplasty)	Difficult to remove

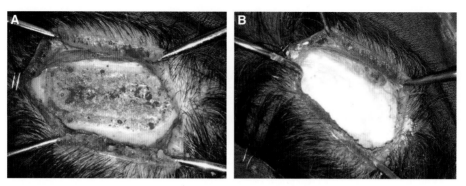

Fig. 31-10   **A** and **B**, Calvarial bone graft defect being repaired with methylmethacrylate.

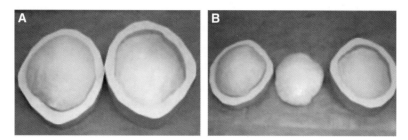

Fig. 31-11   **A**, Prefabricated mold. **B**, Methylmethacrylate implant made from a prefabricated mold.

appears to be related to the size of the polymethylmethacrylate particles on the implant surface. The inflammatory reaction eventually abates as the implant becomes enveloped by fibrous tissue. Adherence of the soft tissues to the implant surface occurs mostly at the points of surface irregularity, because its pore size is insufficient for cellular ingrowth.

Methylmethacrylate has been used extensively in orthopedic surgery as a cement to stabilize joint replacement prostheses in bone. In these situations, new bone formation occurs adjacent to the fibrous capsule enveloping the cement and enhances its mechanical fixation to the bone.

In head and neck surgery, methylmethacrylate implants have been used primarily for the reconstruction of cranial defects. The advantages of methylmethacrylate for this purpose reside in its low morbidity and its ability to be shaped and contoured intraoperatively. As calvarial patch materials, the acrylics work well because of the immobility and relatively low stresses intrinsic to this environment (Fig. 31-10). Occasionally the methylmethacrylate implant loosens, causing erosion of the overlying soft tissues, which leads to exposure and/or infection. In these situations, the implant must be removed and the defect repaired—either with autologous bone or with acrylic—if the reconstruction is performed after the wound has completely healed and the soft tissue covering is adequate. Other reported disadvantages of methylmethacrylate include seroma, persistent burning sensations in the area of placement caused by residual free monomer, and difficulty keeping the surface of the implant smooth when molding it to match the normal cranial contours.

Methylmethacrylate has also been used in three-dimensional printers for the creation of custom craniofacial implants.[34] A fine-cut CT scan determines the precise dimensions for a custom implant. This material is then fabricated using a three-dimensional printer and the resulting implant is sterilized and packaged for delivery to the physician (Fig. 31-11).[34] These custom implants can be a useful means by which to obtain the necessary hard tissue replacement.

Calcium Phosphate Ceramics

The use of calcium phosphate ceramics in reconstructive surgery has grown considerably over the past 15 years because of their high biocompatibility and desirable qualities as bone substitutes in reconstructive surgery. These materials are composed of crystals of compounded calcium phosphate that are found in nature or produced synthetically. This family of compounds is biologically inert, nontoxic, and, in pure form, does not elicit inflammatory or foreign-body responses. Calcium phosphate ceramics can become bonded to viable adjacent bone, and depending on their porosity and structure, can serve as osteogenic conductors (osteoconductive or osteophytic) of new bone formation. This osteoconductive property is dependent on rigid fixation of the material to bone; mobility results in fibrous encapsulation. The major disadvantages of these ceramics are their brittleness and susceptibility to breakage when exposed to inherent stresses. This brittleness makes shaping of the materials before implantation somewhat complicated, although with extreme care they can be sawed, burred, or drilled. Two types of calcium phosphate ceramics are commonly used in reconstructive surgery: hydroxyapatite and tricalcium phosphate.

Hydroxyapatite

Hydroxyapatite is a calcium phosphate ceramic that represents the major mineral component of bone. It is found in nature, as the mineral skeleton of porous coral, which has a morphologic structural configuration and porosity (500 to 600 μm) analogous to human bone.[19] Hydroxyapatite can be manufactured as porous coralline hydroxyapatite, block form, and granular hydroxyapatite. This material can be processed to remove its organic component and leave a pure hydroxyapatite replica of the coral skeleton. In its unimplanted state, this ceramic is weaker than cancellous bone in humans. After implantation as an onlay or inlay graft in long bones, its large pore size allows tissue ingrowth and osteogenesis to occur by the conductive process. Its ultimate strength in vivo is in the orientation of its channels in relation to the applied forces. This material develops an average mechanical strength three times greater than cancellous bone 6 months after implantation because of the overlay of new bone (representing approximately 30% of the new tissue ingrowth, with the remainder composed of fibrovascular tissue). The success of this material in promoting new bone formation is related to its rigid stabilization and close approximation to viable bone. It forms a very tight bond with adjacent bone by a natural cementing mechanism. Up to one third of the porous hydroxyapatite implant may be absorbed over time, although this does not appear to weaken the implant appreciably if the deposition of new lamellar bone occurs. Of some concern is the fact that only 30% of available interstices of the porous hydroxyapatite implant eventually become filled with new bone.[35,36]

Porous coralline hydroxyapatite has been employed successfully as a bone substitute in orthognathic surgery (as a filler material after tooth extraction or in mandibular advancements) and as an onlay material for chin and malar augmentation. If the material becomes exposed, the soft tissues do not heal over it, which results in the need for partial or complete removal. The use of porous hydroxyapatite has produced encouraging results in experimental clinical trials for the grafting of short segmental defects in long bones. As a replacement for calvarial bone, its incorporation is incomplete, although new methods of impregnating this substance with osteogenesis-inducing factors (such as bone morphogenetic protein) are currently being investigated. When compared with onlay bone grafts, porous hydroxyapatite demonstrates less absorption and better maintenance of volume and contour. The major concern with this material is its variable and incomplete filling with new bone.

Hydroxyapatite can be manufactured to create synthetic ceramics of varying density and porosity. Dense, nonporous hydroxyapatite in block form does not allow cellular infiltration, but instead becomes encapsulated, similar to other nonporous biomaterials. In this form, the implant has had limited use as an onlay graft for augmentation of the facial skeleton. Dense hydroxyapatite is hard and brittle and is prone to fracture when subjected to load-bearing stresses. To obviate these shortcomings, the material has been converted to a particulate form that when implanted adjacent to bone becomes invaded by reparative bone and fibrous tissues, thereby improving its viscoelastic properties. The tissue response to hydroxyapatite particles appears to be influenced by the shape of the particles, with smooth particles showing less inflammation than sharp particles. Granular hydroxyapatite has been employed successfully for alveolar ridge augmentation and as a filler substance for dental extractions. This material has also been bonded to tooth implants and provides reliable rigid fixation of the tooth substitute to alveolar bone.

Hydroxyapatite is also available as an injectable particulate mixed with a water-based gel. This material can be used as a soft tissue volume enhancer of moderate duration (typically 9 to 15 months), but is preferred in deeper and immobile tissue locations. For example, injectable hydroxyapatite is useful to augment the malar eminences but is not recommended in the lips. It has also been used as a means to augment the nasal dorsum.

Polytetrafluoroethylene

Although no longer readily available, Proplast is a composite of Teflon fluorocarbon polymer (polytetrafluoroethylene [PTFE]) and black vitreous carbon fibers (Proplast I) or white aluminum oxide fibers (Proplast II) that surgeons may encounter in patients who underwent implantation when Proplast was on the market. The addition of vitreous carbon or aluminum oxide to Teflon makes it wettable in tissues and therefore promotes protein adsorption and tissue adherence and ingrowth. Proplast is highly porous (70% by volume), with pore sizes ranging from 70 to 500 μm, which is sufficiently large to allow fibrovascular tissue ingrowth for firm anchorage of the implant in tissues.

Although their biologic activities were similar, the two types of Proplast differed in their physical properties. Proplast I is black and has a soft spongy consistency, whereas Proplast II is white and is harder (although it deforms and compresses more when subjected to equal pressures). Both materials could be burred or cut with scissors or a knife (although Proplast I lent itself more easily to shaping because of its softness). Because of its black color, Proplast I could be seen through areas covered by thin skin, such as the nasal dorsum, and therefore was less desirable for placement in these areas.

Proplast was used extensively for augmentation of the chin, malar region, nasal dorsum, and bony calvarium. Its primary advantages were its stability and compatibility in tissues, and the firm anchorage achieved by fibrous tissue ingrowth. Proplast implants in the chin have a higher rate of infection and displacement (7.4%) than do implants in other areas of the face.[37] The amount of long-term soft tissue augmentation achieved with this material is approximately 50% of the original result obtained at surgery, and this appears to remain stable beyond the first year. Although infection infrequently complicated its use, many surgeons advocated the instillation of antibiotic solutions directly into the Proplast implant by means of a needle and syringe, irrigation of the implant pocket with antibiotic solution, and prophylactic systemic antibiotics. As with other alloplasts that are placed subperiosteally, Proplast has been shown to cause bone resorption, presumably because of a pressure effect.

Other PTFE-based products include Gore-Tex and Teflon. Teflon is no longer recommended as an injectable filler for vocal cord augmentation. Frequent migration and occasional granulomas (notoriously difficult to treat) can be avoided by performing medialization procedures through a thyroid cartilage window using Silastic blocks or Gore-Tex. Both of these products can be easily removed.

Gore-Tex is modified PTFE (ePTFE) and has been used extensively for more than 20 years as a variety of implants with good tolerance in more than one million patients. It is approved by the FDA for soft tissue augmentation and numerous studies illustrate its utility in nasal and facial skeletal augmentation, cheiloplasty, static facial suspensions, thyroplasty, and to fill deep rhytids by inserting it into the subcutaneous tissue.[38-42] The flexibility and compressibility of Gore-Tex make it an attractive soft tissue substitute, and its resistance to tensile forces make it a good material for suspensions, sutures, and hernia repairs. Gore-Tex has a micropore (0.5 to 30 μm) design that allows for some tissue ingrowth. The implant is eventually surrounded by a thin fibrous capsule that helps prevent migration. Removal of the implant may be difficult, and if infected or exposed it must be completely removed. Gore-Tex is available in 1, 2, and 4 mm sheets, as carvable blocks, and as suture material. The site of implantation is only restricted by depth; Gore-Tex should not be placed immediately below the dermis, especially in highly mobile areas such as the lips or nasolabial folds, although its use in these locations has been described.

ePTFE has been available and used in a number of forms for lip augmentation. This includes strips and tubes, once known under the trade name Softform. These materials are not recommended for lip augmentation because the ePTFE tubes appear to stiffen over time, likely representing tightening of the fibrous capsule and eventually become palpable or deforming.

Porous polyethylene is available under the trade name Medpor. This material permits fibrovascular ingrowth and can easily be cut and shaped in the operating room. Available in a number of prefabricated shapes and sizes, these implants have commonly been used for reconstruction of temporal defects, although cheek, chin, mandible, nasal, orbital, auricular, and other reconstruction applications are available.

SKELETAL CONTOURING

Contouring of the facial bones can give the face a more attractive shape. It has been shown that an oval and nonprotruding supraorbital ridge with a nonprotruding glabellar ridge is a characteristic of the feminine face and accentuates the shape and luminosity of the eyes.[43] This change, in turn, leads to a far more attractive facial appearance. Mandible contouring, on the other hand, brings softer and more feminine features to the lower face. Additionally, in some individuals the malar eminences may be overly developed; these patients commonly request reduction in malar size.

FOREHEAD CONTOURING

The eyes, the eyebrows, and the forehead are the most important areas in determining sex and likely facial attractiveness. Bony contouring of the forehead is capable of transforming the appearance of the forehead from masculine to feminine, and from unattractive to attractive. Masculine foreheads usually have a prominent supraorbital ridge, often referred to as *frontal bossing*. The frontal bone is readily accessed through a coronal or pretrichial approach. The bone is contoured once the coronal flap is elevated in the subperiosteal plane. Simply burring the bone to reduce its appearance is rarely possible. If the anterior table of the frontal sinus is thick enough, then the forehead shape can be changed in this fashion without affecting the sinus anatomy. This, however, is a rather rare finding. Usually during the process of setback the anterior table of the frontal sinus has to be removed, remodeled ex vivo, and then replaced with the help of rigid fixation. During this process no frontal mucosa is removed and the anterior frontal table is stabilized with titanium plates and screws. The empty linear spaces created as a result of the anterior table repositioning are filled with the bone pate obtained during the contouring of the frontal bone. Additionally, the lateral eyebrows and the area of the nasion may be contoured to create a harmonious continuity with the new oval shape of the forehead. These forehead cranioplasty techniques permit significant changes in facial appearance (Fig. 31-12).

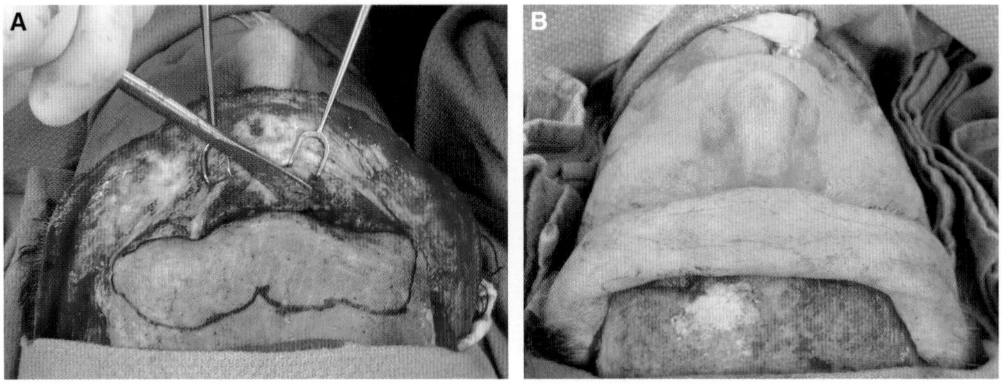

Fig. 31-12   **A** and **B,** Cranioplasty techniques.

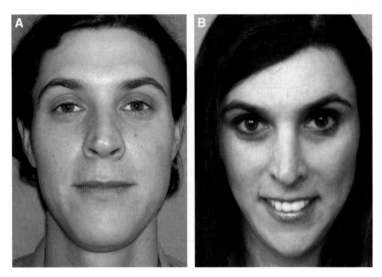

Fig. 31-13   Skeletal augmentation and modification. **A,** Preoperative view of patient. **B,** Postoperative view after facial feminization procedures. Note the mandible contouring.

MANDIBLE CONTOURING

Men who are considered attractive often have square chins and wide mandibles, whereas women tend to have a narrower, tapered, delicate shape to the mandible. When the wrong mandible shape is present for an individual's sex, the resulting appearance can be disturbing. Women with strong jaws may be considered unattractive, and men may request mandible enhancement, commonly with onlay of mandible angle implants or chin augmentation. Mandible contouring involves partial or complete removal of the cortical bone of the angle and the body, and modification of the chin. After subperiosteal dissection is performed through a sublabial approach, the areas of prominent bone are shaped with a surgical rasp, drill, or microsaw, curving down from back to front to achieve a well-rounded contour (Fig. 31-13).

Once the bone and muscle have been contoured, the wound is closed with dissolving sutures. Genioplasty typically requires an anterior sublabial incision and division of the mentalis muscle with a cuff to allow correct reapproximation.

Genioplasty can be performed to slide the inferior border of the mandible at the symphysis forward to augment the chin. The sliding genioplasty was originally performed through an extraoral approach but is

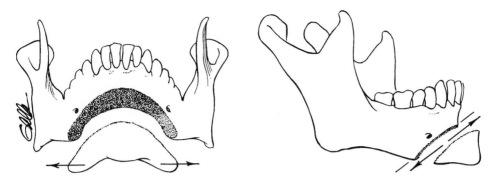

Fig. 31-14   The genial segment can be moved in all directions. In conjunction with selective bone reduction or grafting at the osteotomy site, correction of a variety of chin deformities can be achieved.

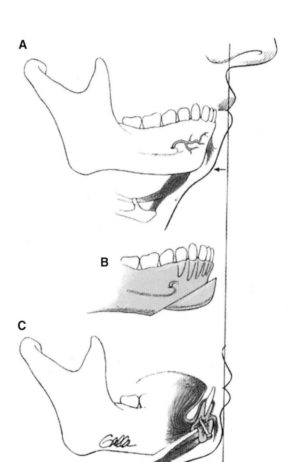

Fig. 31-15   **A-C,** The advancement of the genial segment creates an anterior pull on the suprahyoid musculature. This results in improvement of the neckline contour.

now commonly done through an intraoral incision to correct microgenia. The major advantage of sliding genioplasty over augmentation mentoplasty is the avoidance of alloplastic material. It is of paramount importance to use precision when performing the osteotomies and applying rigid fixation. The genial segment should be mobile in all directions, permitting correction of various chin deformities (Fig. 31-14). Sliding genioplasty can also improve the contour of the neckline (Figs. 31-15 and 31-16).

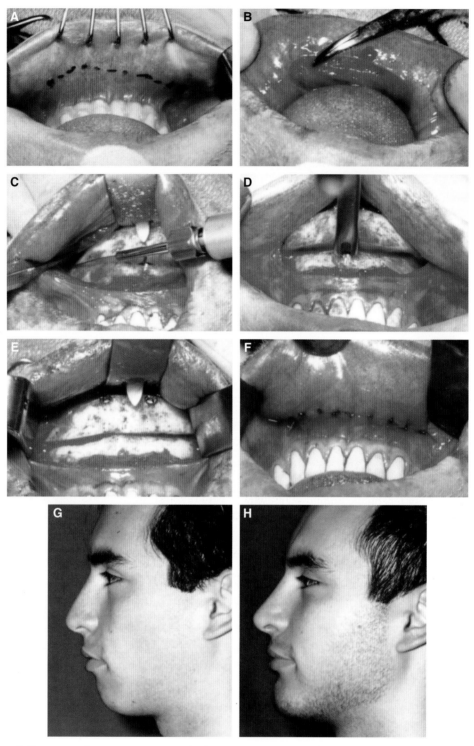

Fig. 31-16 Sliding genioplasty. **A,** Incision marked at 15 mm anterior to the depth of the vestibule. **B,** Incision made just through the mucosa; the hemostat points to a terminal branch of the mental nerve. **C,** Osteotomy made with a reciprocating saw under copious irrigation. The saw should be a minimum of 5 mm below the mental foramina to prevent injury of the inferior alveolar nerves. **D,** The genial segment being advanced with a bone clamp. **E,** The genial segment is fixed with two screws. To ensure stability, it is important for the screws to engage the outer cortex of the genial segment and the inner cortex of the mandible. **F,** Two-layer, soft tissue closure completed. The closure of the periosteum and mentalis muscle is important to prevent postoperative chin ptosis. **G,** Preoperative view showing insufficient chin projection. **H,** Postoperative view showing improved chin position.

CONCLUSION

Skeletal augmentation and modification require knowledge of alloplastic materials and their properties, and a good understanding of bone healing and reconstruction techniques. However, the results of these modifications can be dramatic. The adage that "beauty is only skin deep" lacks accuracy, since it is often the skeletal structure that more closely correlates with perceptions of attractiveness.

Future developments in skeletal modifications will likely involve the creation of ex vivo autografts through tissue engineering and ultimately the differentiation of stem cells into custom replacement tissues.

KEY POINTS

- Various grafting and implant materials have been introduced since the beginning of the twentieth century.
- After the primary stage of bone graft repair, cortical and cancellous bone grafts diverge with respect to their rate, mechanism, and completeness of repair.
- Iliac bone, rib, calvarial bone, and bone allografts are currently in clinical use.
- Cartilage grafts are especially adapted to augmentation of the facial skeleton because of their resistance to remodeling and resorption.
- Clinical experience with autologous cartilage grafts has been characterized by variable rates of resorption, depending on the type of cartilage used as a graft, how the graft is prepared before implantation, and where it is implanted.
- Septal, auricular, and costal grafts and allografts are the currently employed cartilage grafting sources. Alloplastic materials include silicone, methylmethacrylate, ceramics, hydroxyapatite, and polytetrafluoroethylene.
- The success of implanted alloplastic materials has paralleled the growth in knowledge of the physical and chemical composition of biomaterials, their fabrication, and their reactivity in a biologic environment.
- Skeletal contouring is most commonly employed for the frontal bone and mandible.
- Contouring of the facial bones can give the face a more attractive shape.
- Oval and nonprotruding supraorbital ridges with a nonprotruding glabellar ridge are characteristic of the feminine face, and accentuate the shape and luminosity of the eyes.

REFERENCES

1. Papel ID. Facial plastic and reconstructive surgery, ed 3. New York: Thieme, 2009.
2. Jimi E, Hirata S, Osawa K, et al. The current and future therapies of bone regeneration to repair bone defects. Int J Dent 2012:148261, 2012.
3. Smith JO, Sengers BG, Aarvold A, et al. Tantalum trabecular metal—addition of human skeletal cells to enhance bone implant interface strength and clinical application. J Tissue Eng Regen Med 8:304-313, 2014.
4. Boeckel DG, Shinkai RS, Grossi ML, et al. Cell culture-based tissue engineering as an alternative to bone grafts in implant dentistry: a literature review. J Oral Implantol 38 Spec No:538-545, 2012.
5. Smith JD, Abramson M. Membranous versus endochondral bone grafts. Arch Otolaryngol 99:203-205, 1974.

6. Zins JE, Whitaker LA. Membranous versus endochondral bone: implications for craniofacial reconstruction. Plast Reconstr Surg 72:778-785, 1983.

> *Based on observations in humans that suggested improved membranous bone graft take, an experimental study was undertaken in 15 rabbits and 7 monkeys to evaluate the differences between membranous and endochondral bone grafts. The study confirmed the increased resorption of endochondral bone grafts when compared with membranous grafts, and substantiated clinical impressions that cranial donor sites are preferable for craniofacial recipient areas when clinically feasible.*

7. Burchardt H. Biology of bone transplantation. Orthop Clin North Am 18:187-196, 1987.
8. Huggins CB. The formation of bone under the influence of epithelium of the urinary tract. Clin Orthop Relat Res 59:7-19, 1968.
9. Peer LA. Fate of autogenous human bone grafts. Br J Plast Surg 3:233-243, 1951.
10. Ostrup LT, Fredrickson JM. Distant transfer of a free, living bone graft by microvascular anastomoses. An experimental study. Plast Reconstr Surg 54:274-285, 1974.
11. Puckett CL, Hurvitz JS, Metzler MH, et al. Bone formation by revascularized periosteal and bone grafts, compared with traditional bone grafts. Plast Reconstr Surg 64:361-365, 1979.
12. Burchardt H. The biology of bone graft repair. Clin Orthop Relat Res 174:28-42, 1983.
13. Pinholt EM, Solheim E, Talsnes O, et al. Revascularization of calvarial, mandibular, tibial, and iliac bone grafts in rats. Ann Plast Surg 33:193-197, 1994.
14. Lieberman JR, Friedlaender GE. Bone Regeneration and Repair: Biology and Clinical Applications. Totowa, NJ: Humana Press, 2005.
15. Ebraheim NA, Elgafy H, Xu R. Bone-graft harvesting from iliac and fibular donor sites: techniques and complications. J Am Acad Orthop Surg 9:210-218, 2001.
16. Phillips JH, Rahn BA. Fixation effects on membranous and endochondral onlay bone graft revascularization and bone deposition. Plast Reconstr Surg 85:891-897, 1990.
17. Jandial R, McCormick P, Black PM. Core Techniques in Operative Neurosurgery. Philadelphia: Elsevier, 2011.
18. Elves MW. Newer knowledge of the immunology of bone and cartilage. Clin Orthop Relat Res 120:232-259, 1976.
19. Friedlaender GE, Strong DM, Sell KW. Studies on the antigenicity of bone. I. Freeze-dried and deep-frozen bone allografts in rabbits. J Bone Joint Surg Am 58:854-858, 1976.

> *Immune responses directed against osteochondral allograft-associated immunogens have been demonstrated in a variety of animal models and, to a more limited degree, in human recipients. The most extensively studied—and presumably most potent source of sensitization—are cell-surface transplantations found on the heterogeneous cell types ubiquitous to skeletal tissues.*

20. Friedlaender GE. Immune responses to osteochondral allografts. Current knowledge and future directions. Clin Orthop Relat Res 174:58-68, 1983.
21. Holmstrand K, Longacre JJ, Destefano GA. Biophysical studies of split-rib grafts in the repair of defects of the cranium. Preliminary results of experimental studies in Rhesus monkeys. Plast Reconstr Surg Transplant Bull 26:286-300, 1960.
22. Brown BL, Kern EB, Neel HB III. Transplantation of fresh allografts (homografts) of crushed and uncrushed cartilage and bone: a 1-year analysis in rabbits. Laryngoscope 90:1521-1533, 1980.
23. Donald PJ. Cartilage grafting in facial reconstruction with special consideration of irradiated grafts. Laryngoscope 96:786-807, 1986.

> *The author reports an experiment undertaken to investigate the physiology of irradiated cartilage grafts after prolonged implantation on the facial skeleton of sheep and dogs. Many of the grafts acquired chondrocytes from the host and produced new proteoglycan matrices in addition to undergoing some degree of ossification. A comparison is made with the clinical situation in humans.*

24. Mankin HJ, Doppelt S, Tomford W. Clinical experience with allograft implantation. The first ten years. Clin Orthop Relat Res 174:69-86, 1983.
25. González-Sixto B, Pérez-Bustillo A, Samaniego E, et al. Cartilage graft in the reconstruction of the pinna of the ear. Actas Dermosifiliogr 104:633-634, 2013.
26. Sheen JH, Sheen AP. Aesthetic Rhinoplasty. St Louis: CV Mosby, 1978.
27. Rubin LR. Biomaterials in Reconstructive Surgery. St Louis: CV Mosby, 1983.

28. Costantino PD, Friedman CD. Soft-tissue augmentation and replacement in the head and neck. General considerations. Otolaryngol Clin North Am 27:1-12, 1994.

   The information in this monograph helps integrate reconstructive options so that autologous tissues are used whenever possible and synthetic materials are appropriately selected and applied when necessary.

29. Valentine JD, Reiman BE, Beuttenmuller EA, et al. Light and electron microscopic evaluation of Proplast II TMJ disc implants. J Oral Maxillofac Surg 47:689-696, 1989.

30. Stanford CM. Surface modification of biomedical and dental implants and the processes of inflammation, wound healing and bone formation. Int J Mol Sci 11:354-369, 2010.

31. McGrath MH, Burkhardt BR. The safety and efficacy of breast implants for augmentation mammaplasty. Plast Reconstr Surg 74:550-560, 1984.

32. Jefferiss CD, Lee AJ, Ling RS. Thermal aspects of self-curing polymethylmethacrylate. J Bone Joint Surg Br 57:511-518, 1975.

33. Gosavi SS, Gosavi SY, Alla RK. Local and systemic effects of unpolymerised monomers. Dent Res J (Isfahan) 7:82-87, 2010.

34. Kim BJ, Hong KS, Park KJ, et al. Customized cranioplasty implants using three-dimensional printers and polymethyl-methacrylate casting. J Korean Neurosurg Soc 52:541-546, 2012.

35. Wolford LM, Wardrop RW, Hartog JM. Coralline porous hydroxylapatite as a bone graft substitute in orthognathic surgery. J Oral Maxillofac Surg 45:1034-1042, 1987.

36. el Deeb M, Holmes RE. Tissue response to facial contour augmentation with dense and porous hydroxylapatite in rhesus monkeys. J Oral Maxillofac Surg 47:1282-1289, 1989.

37. Terino EO, Flowers RS. The Art of Alloplastic Facial Contouring. St Louis: Mosby–Year Book, 2000.

38. Wang TD. Gore-Tex nasal augmentation: a 26-year perspective. Arch Facial Plast Surg 13:129-130, 2011.

39. Redbord KP, Hanke CW. Expanded polytetrafluoroethylene implants for soft-tissue augmentation: 5-year follow-up and literature review. Dermatol Surg 34:735-743; discussion 744, 2008.

40. Constantinides M, Galli SK, Miller PJ. Complications of static facial suspensions with expanded polytetrafluoroethylene (ePTFE). Laryngoscope 111:2114-2121, 2001.

41. Suehiro A, Hirano S, Kishimoto Y, et al. Comparative study of vocal outcomes with silicone versus Gore-Tex thyroplasty. Ann Otol Rhinol Laryngol 118:405-408, 2009.

42. Krauss MC. Recent advances in soft tissue augmentation. Semin Cutan Med Surg 18:119-128, 1999.

43. Spiegel JH. Facial determinants of female gender and feminizing forehead cranioplasty. Laryngoscope 121:250-261, 2011.

   Feminization of the forehead through cranioplasty is safe and has a significant impact in determining the gender of the patient. The strong association between femininity and attractiveness can now be attributed more specifically to the upper third of the face and the interplay of the glabellar prominence of the forehead and the shape and position of the hairline and eyebrows. These results have strong implications for a paradigm shift in the method of facial analysis used to select aesthetic procedures and illuminate the process by which femininity and attractiveness are interpreted in faces.

32

Free Tissue for Reconstruction of the Bony Facial Skeleton

Saral Mehra ▪ *Adam S. Jacobson* ▪ *Mark L. Urken*

Defects of the facial skeleton can have a profound effect on a patient's ability to eat, speak, and integrate into society. A variety of pathologic processes can result in defects in the facial skeleton, ranging from benign and malignant neoplasms to trauma, congenital deformities, systemic diseases, and side effects of treatment plan (that is, medications and radiation). Historically, reconstruction of the facial skeleton was extremely difficult and was plagued by major complications and poor aesthetic and functional results.[1-4] Advances in surgical techniques and surgical instruments have greatly enhanced our ability to reconstruct defects of the facial skeleton, permitting surgeons to refocus their efforts from simply trying to restore form, to optimizing function (such as speaking, masticating, and swallowing) and aesthetic outcomes for these patients.

In the 1970s a number of pedicled osteomyocutaneous flaps were described for facial reconstruction, including the pectoralis major muscle with rib, the sternocleidomastoid muscle with clavicle, the trapezius muscle with scapula, and the temporalis muscle with calvarial bone. Shortcomings of these techniques were that (1) they did not address the needs of the entire facial skeleton, (2) the vascular supply to the bone was not reliable, (3) there was limited versatility with respect to the soft tissue component of these flaps, and (4) prosthetic rehabilitation was suboptimal.[5-7]

In the 1980s, alloplasts, including gap-bridging metallic reconstruction plates, became popular, but these often resulted in intraoral and extraoral exposure of the hardware, plate fracture, instability of the retaining screws, and infection in the overlying soft tissue. These complications were especially common when postoperative radiotherapy was administered.[8-12]

The introduction of free tissue transfer using microvascular surgical techniques revolutionized the reconstruction of the facial skeleton in terms of reproducibility, function, versatility, and aesthetic outcomes. During the period between 1979 and 1989, the iliac crest/internal oblique,[13,14] the scapular osteocutaneous free flap,[15] radius osteocutaneous flap,[16] and the fibular free flap[17] were sequentially introduced into the literature for reconstruction of the facial skeleton and associated soft tissue. These procedures led to marked improvements in reconstruction of the facial skeleton, as well-vascularized flaps resisted infection caused by salivary contamination and incorporated versatile bone and soft tissue components that were customizable.

Widespread interest in surgical midface reconstruction emerged later, in the late 1990s and the early 2000s, likely because palatomaxillary pathology is less common, and because of the simplicity and suitability of palatal obturators. Before the widespread use of free vascularized bone for the reconstruction of palatomaxillary defects, many reconstructive options were described, such as (1) local flaps, including buccal mucosa, buccal fat, tongue, palatal mucosa, and nasolabial skin, (2) regional flaps, such as forehead, temporalis, temporoparietal fascia, deltopectoral, pectoralis major, and submental flaps, and (3) free soft tissue flaps. Although these techniques were variably able to achieve separation of the oral and sinonasal cavities, none of these techniques restored bone to the midface. The lack of bony skeletal reconstruction meant that prosthodontic rehabilitation was difficult, if not impossible, leaving patients with poor aesthetic and functional outcomes.

A number of authors have attempted to compare prosthetic obturation with free flap reconstruction for palatomaxillary defects.[18-20] The advantages of transferring free bone and soft tissue include the ability of these tissues to withstand the detrimental effects of oral flora, saliva, and adjuvant radiotherapy. In addition, with the introduction of vascularized bone, the osteogenic potential is retained and permits formation of a union with native bone, vastly improving the bone's ability to accept dental implants to achieve complete rehabilitation of the oral cavity and to withstand the forces of functional mastication.[21] Finally, with success rates of free tissue transfer ranging from 90% to 99%, the perceived risks of flap failure are greatly reduced compared with several decades ago.[22-24]

ANATOMY OF THE FACIAL SKELETON

For a detailed discussion of bony facial anatomy, see Chapter 1. Briefly, the facial skeleton is composed of the primary bones (mandible, maxilla, frontal bone, nasal bones, and zygoma) and the vomer, lacrimal, orbital, ethmoid, and sphenoid bones.

The mandible is composed of a fused left and right half with multiple segments, including the condyle, coronoid process, ramus, angle, body, and parasymphysis (Fig. 32-1). In addition, the inferior alveolar neurovascular bundle courses through the ramus and body of the mandible. The inferior alveolar nerve supplies sensation to the chin and lower lip through the mental nerve.

The paired right and left maxillae and their bony attachments represent more complex anatomy (Fig. 32-2). The maxilla provides structural support between the skull base and the occlusal surface, opposes the forces of mastication from the mandible, anchors the upper dentition, separates the oral from nasal cavities, supports the globe, and supports the muscles of facial expression.[25]

From a functional and anatomic viewpoint, the main considerations are the vertical buttresses (nasomaxillary, zygomaticomaxillary, and pterygomaxillary buttresses) that support the vertical forces of mastication, provide a stable occlusal surface to oppose the mandible, and allow for an even distribution of forces across the skull base.[26] The four processes (zygomatic, alveolar, palatine, and frontal) are critical for support and projection of the midface and the separation of the oral cavity from the sinonasal cavity. In addition to the maxilla, the orbital floor and orbital rim provide orbital support and frontal projection and are important considerations in midfacial reconstruction. Finally, the nasolacrimal apparatus is an important consideration in resection and reconstruction of the palatomaxillary complex.

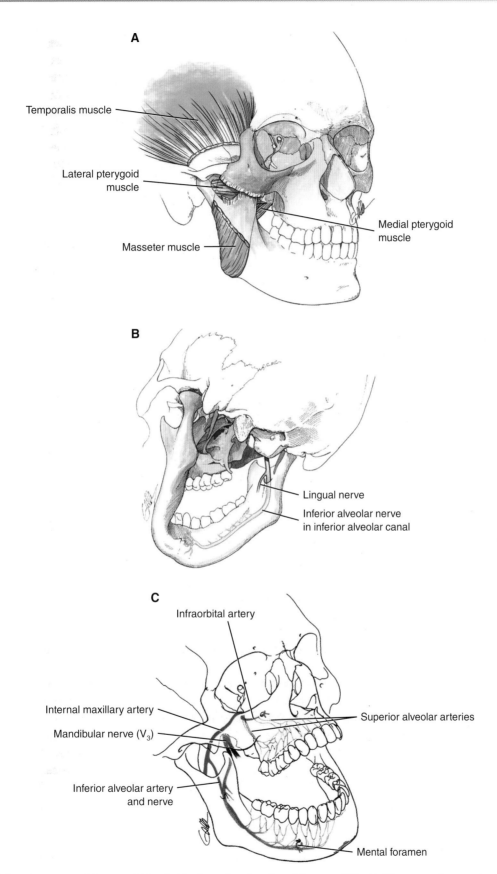

Fig. 32-1   Anatomy of the mandible. **A,** The bony landmarks of the mandible. **B,** The muscular attachments of the mandible. **C,** The inferior alveolar nerve running through the inferior alveolar canal.

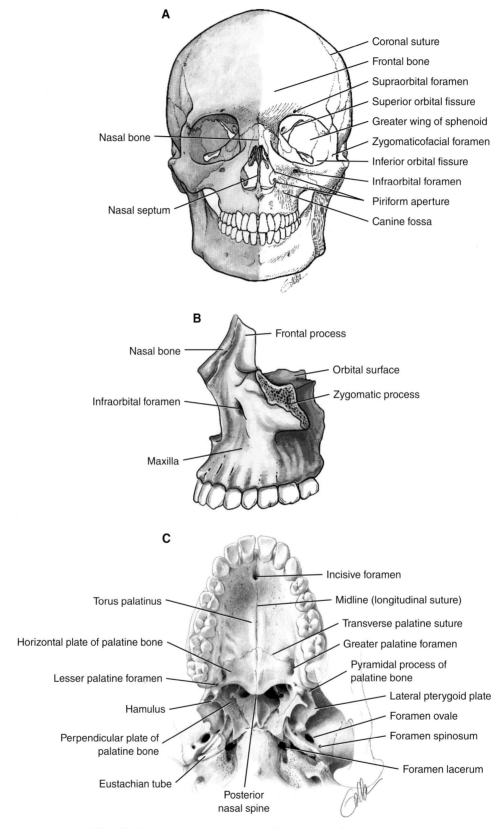

Fig. 32-2   Anatomy of the **A,** midface, **B,** maxilla, and **C,** palate.

INDICATIONS AND PATIENT EVALUATION

The most common indication for free tissue transfer for reconstruction of the bony facial skeleton is after tumor extirpation of a malignant or benign neoplasm, typically squamous cell carcinoma. In addition, free tissue transfer is commonly used for reconstruction after a segmental mandibulectomy for advanced osteoradionecrosis.[27] Benign odontogenic and nonodontogenic neoplasms may also require resection and reconstruction of the facial skeleton. Congenital anomalies such as destructive high flow vascular malformations, severe facial clefting, and clinically significant facial microsomia are additional indications for reconstruction using free tissue. Finally, severe trauma may necessitate free tissue for optimal cosmetic and functional outcome.

Factors to consider in determining the appropriate reconstructive option for each patient include patient, surgeon, tumor, and defect factors, as shown in Box 32-1.

Regarding patient factors, age alone need not be a major consideration; rather, performance status, patient preference, and severity of comorbid conditions should be guiding factors in deciding on the use of free tissue transfer in the elderly.[28,29]

When free tissue is being considered for malignancy or an aggressive benign pathologic condition, tumor factors must be taken into account, including the stage of disease, the biology of the disease, and the need to monitor for disease recurrence. In addition, prior therapy is a major consideration in choosing free tissue transfer. For malignant pathology, reconstructive matters are best discussed in the context of a multidisciplinary head and neck cancer team.[30]

The surgeon's familiarity with the various donor sites and availability of appropriate postoperative monitoring are key components in deciding on the optimal reconstructive approach. In addition, a critical appraisal of the defect must be performed using a classification system that accounts for bone and soft tissue requirements.

The goals of reconstruction of the facial skeleton are to restore form and facial symmetry, maintain a safe and comfortable airway, separate cranial from sinonasal contents, support the globe, restore dentition to maintain occlusal relationships, improve the patient's ability to eat in public, and to make intelligible speech possible.[31]

Box 32-1   Goals When Using Free Tissue for Oromandibular Reconstruction

- Establish mandibular continuity and contour by way of osseous union of bone segments.
- Establish a normal condylar position and normal occlusion.
- Establish height of the neomandible in the tooth-bearing segment that achieves a reasonable match to the native mandible to facilitate dental restoration and ultimately normal masticatory function.
- Preserve normal mandibular motion in relation to opening aperture and chewing stroke.
- Restore opposing dentition in all four quadrants to facilitate functional mastication.
- Place dental implants primarily for rapid dental rehabilitation.
- Restore normal lower lip height to achieve labial competence.
- Restore oral competence.
- Restore sensation to the lips and oral soft tissues.
- Restore and maintain maximal tongue mobility.

> **Box 32-2   Goals When Using Free Tissue for Midface Reconstruction**
>
> • Provide surgical closure of the oral cavity and eliminate the need for a palatal obturator.
> • Separate the sinonasal cavity from the anterior cranial fossa if a craniofacial resection is performed.
> • Provide support for the globe with appropriate vertical position and orbital volume to achieve symmetry of the upper third of the face.
> • Restore the maxillary buttresses to withstand the vertical forces of mastication.
> • Restore functional dentition.
> • Prevent epiphora through restoration of the patency of the nasolacrimal duct.
> • Achieve symmetry in the projection of the upper and middle third of the face.
> • Restore facial skin with both color-matched and texture-matched skin.
> • Restore facial mimetic motion or static suspension where impaired.
>
> Data from Urken ML, Okay DJ. Reconstruction of palatomaxillary defects. In Urken ML, ed. Multidisciplinary Head and Neck Reconstruction: A Defect-Oriented Approach. Philadelphia: Lippincott Williams & Wilkins, 2010.

Midfacial reconstruction should be considered separately from oromandibular reconstruction for several reasons. First, the midface is nonmobile and thus does not shift with movement. Second, the prognosis for near-complete functional recovery is excellent for palatomaxillary defects, because the tongue is rarely involved. Third, small defects in the palate may be effectively reconstructed with soft tissue flaps alone, but segmental defects of the mandible are not amenable to these flaps alone for optimal functional recovery. In addition, palatomaxillary defects affect oral function only when the pterygoid plates are involved, or when significant muscle loss is present. In palatomaxillary restoration, obturators can achieve two of the main goals of reconstruction: separation of the oral and sinonasal cavity and restoration of dentition. However, a prosthesis cannot achieve the main goals of oromandibular reconstruction,[32] as outlined in Boxes 32-1 and 32-2.

DEFECT CLASSIFICATION

A classification system is important for communication, comparison of end results, and selection of appropriate reconstructive options. A number of classification systems have been developed for oromandibular[33-36] and palatomaxillary defect analysis.[25,26,37-48]

Oromandibular Defect Classification

Several classification systems have been described for segmental mandible defects, as shown in Table 32-1. For mandible defects we use a classification scheme based on the parts of the mandible (Fig. 32-3). The letters C, R, B, and S indicate a defect in the condyle (C), ramus (R), body (B), and symphysis (S).[34,49] The superscript M is applied to indicate a marginal mandibular resection.

For central defects the superscript H is applied when a hemisymphyseal defect is present; this distinction is made because of the functional disturbance created by detaching a greater portion of the suprahyoid and tongue musculature, especially bilaterally. Moreover, it is more difficult to contour the bone when the entire symphysis must be reconstructed.

For lateral defects, the classification system takes into account the functional impact that occurs when the condyle and ramus are resected. Successful reconstruction of the condyle has a significant effect on the

Table 32-1   The Most Common Segmental Mandible Defects

Authors of Classification System	Description
Jewer et al, 1988	H C L This system denotes defects that involve lateral defects of any length plus the condyle *(H)*, or lateral defects of any length that do not include the condyle *(L)*, and central defects that include the two canines and four incisors *(C)*.
Urken et al, 1991	C R B S Superscripts $^{h, m}$ The letters *C, R, B,* and *S* indicate a defect in the condyle, ramus, body, and symphyseal (between the two canine teeth) region, respectively. The superscript ^{h} denotes a hemisymphyseal defect, and the superscript ^{m} denotes a marginal mandibular defect. The soft tissue component of the oromandibular defect is added, as shown in Fig. 32-3.
Boyd et al, 1993	H C L Subscripts $_{o, m, s}$ This is a modification of Jewer's system, and adds the epithelial component of the defect as $_o$ (neither skin nor mucosal component), $_m$ (mucosa), and $_s$ (skin).

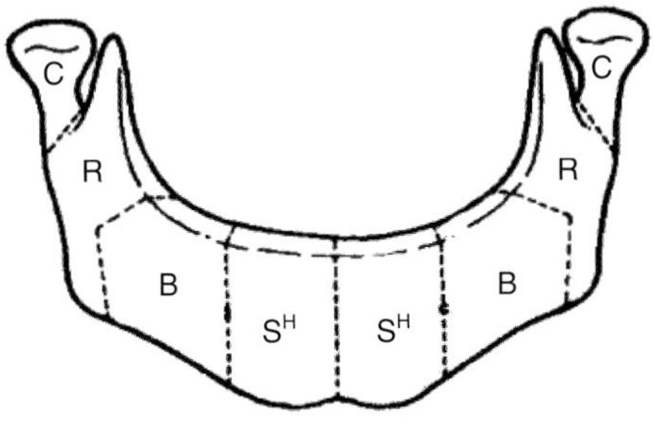

DEFECT	ABBREVIATION*
BONE	
Condyle	C
Ramus	R
Body	B
Symphysis	
Total	S
Hemi	S^H

*For marginal resection, add superscript ^{M}.

DEFECT	ABBREVIATION*
MUCOSA	
Labial	L
Buccal	B
Soft palate	
Hemi	SP^H
Total	SP^T
Floor of mouth	
Anterior	FOM^A
Lateral	FOM^L
Pharynx	
Lateral	PH^L
Posterior	PH^P
TONGUE	
Mobile	
1/4 1/2 3/4	$T^M_{1/4}$ $T^M_{1/2}$ $T^M_{3/4}$
Nonfunctional	T^M_{NF}
Tongue base	
1/4 1/2 3/4	$T^B_{1/4}$ $T^B_{1/2}$ $T^B_{3/4}$
Nonfunctional	T^B_{NF}
Total glossectomy	TG

DEFECT	ABBREVIATION*
CUTANEOUS DEFECT	
Cheek	C^C
Neck	C^N
Mentum	C^M
Lips	C^L
Upper	$C^{UL}_{1/4}$ $C^{UL}_{1/2}$ $C^{UL}_{3/4}$ C^{UL}_T
Lower	$C^{LL}_{1/4}$ $C^{LL}_{1/2}$ $C^{LL}_{3/4}$ C^{LL}_T
NEUROLOGIC DEFECT	
Mental	N_M
Inferior alveolar	N_{IA}
Lingual	N_L
Hypoglossal	N_H
Facial	N_F

*For bilateral nerve defect, add superscript ^{B}.

Fig. 32-3   Classification of mandibular defects. The letters *C, R, B,* and *S* indicate the defect of the condyle, ramus, body, and symphysis, respectively. The superscript ^{H} is used to indicate a hemisymphyseal defect. The superscript ^{M} denotes a marginal resection in that specific part of the mandible. In addition, the associated soft tissue and neurologic defect should be part of a complete oromandibular defect classification because of the important effect they have on functional outcome.[49]

Table 32-2 Criteria Required for a Universal Description of Maxillectomy Defects

Criterion	Outcome
Dental status	Teeth absent or present (right posterior, right anterior, left anterior, left posterior)*
Oroantral/nasal communication status	Absent or present
Contiguous structure involvement	Soft palate, lip, cheek, nose, orbital contents, zygoma, pterygoid process, or none
Superior-inferior extent	Anterior base of skull level, orbital level, nasal/sinus level, palatal level, or alveolar level
Anterior-posterior extent	Right anterior, left anterior, right posterior, or left posterior regions
Medial-lateral extent	Isolated, unilateral, bilateral defects

Bidra AS, Jacob RF, Taylor TD. Classification of maxillectomy defects: a systematic review and criteria necessary for a universal description. J Prosthet Dent 107:261-270, 2012.
*Posterior teeth include all premolars and molars.

Table 32-3 The Most Commonly Used Maxillary and Midface Defect Classification Systems

Authors of Classification System	Description
Brown and Shaw, 2010	Vertical Class I II III IV V VI Horizontal Class a b c d This system, a modification of the original from 10 years earlier, includes a vertical component that varies based on the height of the defect where class V and VI are suprastructure defects and the horizontal class describes the amount of palate and alveolar ridge sacrificed.
Yamamoto et al, 2004	Category I Category II Category III This system focuses on the importance of the three maxillary buttresses (zygomaticomaxillary, pterygomaxillary, and nasomaxillary) and their role in maxillectomy defects. Each category has different vertical buttresses that are ablated and must be reconstructed to restore midfacial form and function.
Okay and Urken et al, 2001	Class I (a,b) Class II (a,b) Class III Class IV Superscript [f, z, s, o] This system combines oncologic, reconstructive, and prosthodontic considerations and is based on defect location, size, and specific teeth available for optimal obturator retention. It also describes the vertical component of the defect and associated soft tissue requirements for reconstruction.
Cordeiro and Santamaria, 2000	Type 1 Type 2 Type 3 (a,b) Type 4 This system uses the concept of the maxilla as a hexahedron in which the roof supports the globe, the medial wall is the lateral nasal wall, the floor forms the anterior portion of the hard palate and alveolus, and the other walls contribute to the sinuses. The classification is based on the number and location of the missing walls in the maxillectomy defect.

function of the mandible during mastication. The rationale for subdividing body and ramus defects is that there is significant functional impairment when the masticator muscle sling is completely disrupted. When the entire angle is removed, the defect is classified as a ramus defect *(R)* and reflects an almost complete disruption of the masticator sling.

Because long-term studies have shown that the functional and aesthetic results of reconstruction of the facial skeleton correlate more with the extent of the soft tissue defect and subsequent reconstruction than with the extent of the bony defect, we developed a more inclusive classification system for oromandibular defects that takes into account soft tissue and neurologic defects.[50] The complete oromandibular classification system is shown in Fig. 32-3.

PALATOMAXILLARY DEFECT CLASSIFICATION SYSTEM

For palatomaxillary defects, Bidra et al[51] performed a systematic review of 14 different maxillectomy and midfacial defect classification systems. They used the acronym *DOC-SAM* to identify six criteria necessary for a universal description of maxillectomy defects (the first letters of the first column in Table 32-2 define the acronym). A summary of the most commonly used maxillary and midface defect classification schemes is presented in Table 32-3, with the Okay and Urken classification scheme presented in detail in Fig. 32-4.

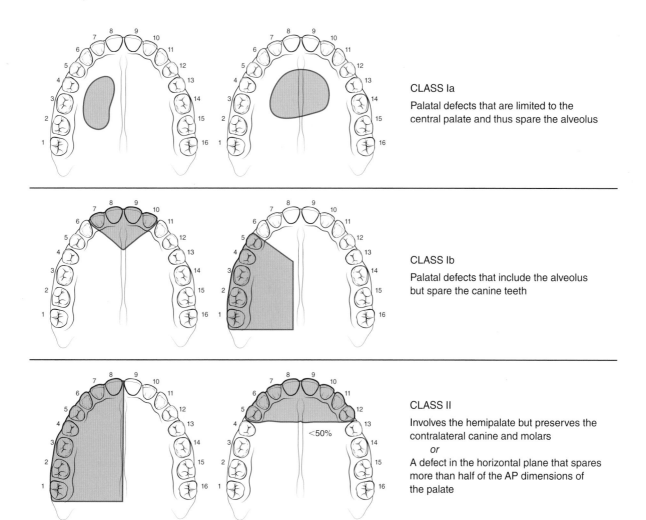

CLASS Ia

Palatal defects that are limited to the central palate and thus spare the alveolus

CLASS Ib

Palatal defects that include the alveolus but spare the canine teeth

CLASS II

Involves the hemipalate but preserves the contralateral canine and molars
or
A defect in the horizontal plane that spares more than half of the AP dimensions of the palate

Fig. 32-4   Okay and Urken classification of palatomaxillary defects.

Continued

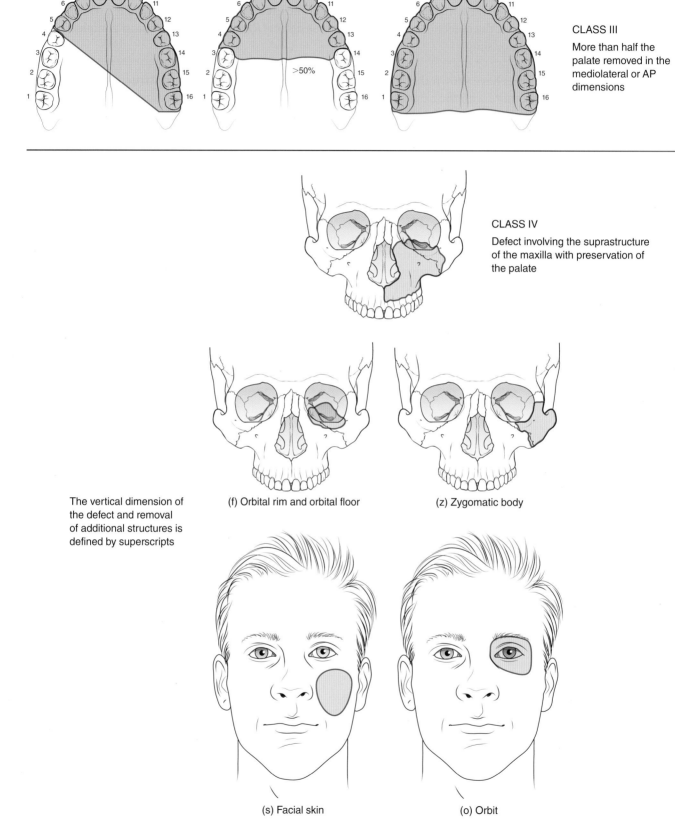

CLASS III

More than half the palate removed in the mediolateral or AP dimensions

CLASS IV

Defect involving the suprastructure of the maxilla with preservation of the palate

The vertical dimension of the defect and removal of additional structures is defined by superscripts

(f) Orbital rim and orbital floor

(z) Zygomatic body

(s) Facial skin

(o) Orbit

Fig. 32-4, cont'd   Okay and Urken classification of palatomaxillary defects.

PREOPERATIVE PLANNING

After careful consideration of the planned defect characteristics, extensive preoperative planning must ensue, with particular attention to which donor site is ideal for the composite reconstruction. In addition to defect characteristics, the surgeon must have an understanding of patient and disease factors to provide the optimal reconstruction.

When tumor or trauma causes distortion of the outer mandibular cortex it prevents accurate precontouring of the reconstruction plate. In this situation, optimal functional and aesthetic outcome can be achieved in one of three ways: (1) using an external fixator to maintain position of the remaining native mandibular bone before excision, (2) using stock mandibular plates based on average mandible sizes, or (3) using computer-generated models to create a model after virtual tumor removal with a precontoured reconstruction plate. An example of the use of computer planning for the preoperatively anatomically distorted mandible is shown in Fig. 32-5.

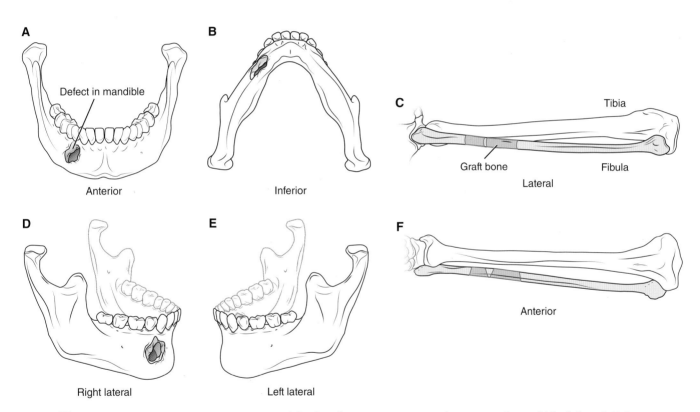

Fig. 32-5   Virtual surgical planning is used for free flap reconstruction of a segmental mandible defect. **A-F,** Preoperative tumor or trauma.

Continued

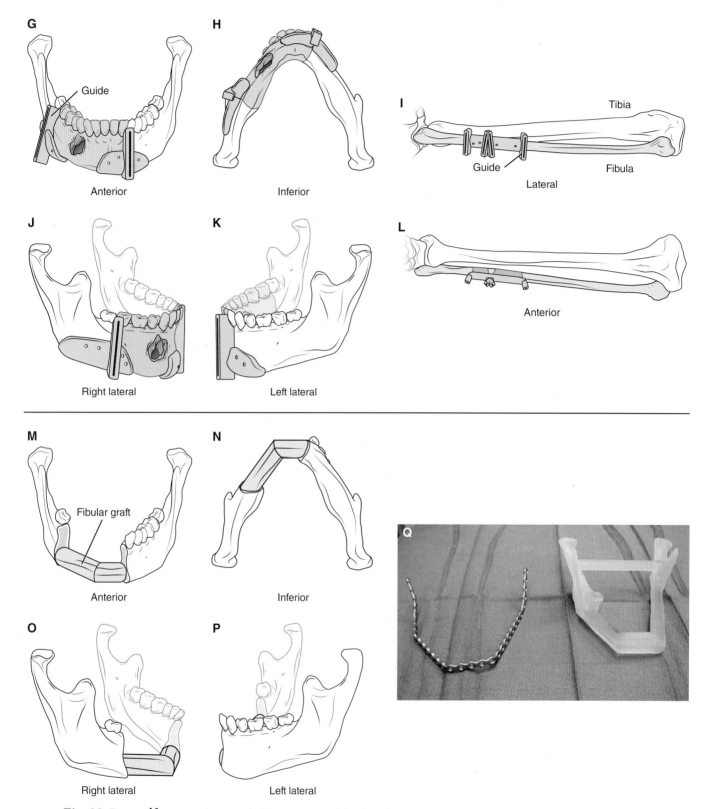

Fig. 32-5, cont'd   Virtual surgical planning is used for free flap reconstruction of a segmental mandible defect. **G-L,** External factors. **M-P,** Stock mandibular plates. **Q,** Computer-generated precontoured reconstruction plate.

Overview of Donor Sites

A number of donor sites have been described for the purpose of reconstruction of the facial skeleton, including the ilium, fibula, scapula, humerus, ulna, tibia, rib, and metatarsus.[52-55] The optimal donor site varies for each defect and depends on a critical analysis of the soft tissue and bone requirements of the deficit. The three main donor sites used in contemporary reconstruction of the facial skeleton are the scapula, iliac crest, and fibula.

The radial forearm flap may also be used, although the potential for fracture of the radius and the paucity of bone that can be reliably transferred makes it a poor osteocutaneous flap. As a soft tissue flap it continues to play an important supportive role in facial reconstruction because of its large, thin, pliable soft tissue component.[56,57] Soft tissue free flaps such as the rectus abdominis and anterolateral thigh, with or without nonvascularized bone grafts, have also been used extensively for midface defects, because they have reliable skin paddles with a large volume of soft tissue to obliterate dead space[44,58] (Fig. 32-6) (Table 32-4).

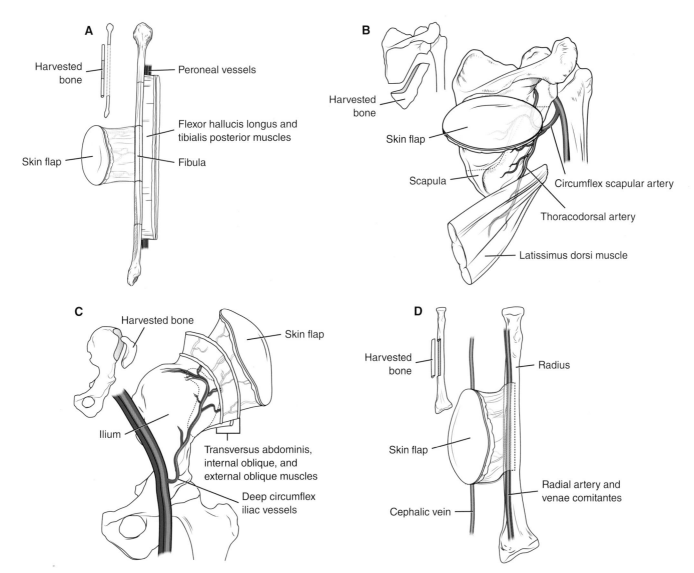

Fig. 32-6   The most common osteocutaneous flaps used in free tissue reconstruction of the facial skeleton. **A,** Fibula. **B,** Subscapularis system. **C,** Iliac crest. **D,** Radial forearm.

Table 32-4   Donor Sites Used in Free Tissue Reconstruction of the Facial Skeleton

Donor Site	Advantages	Disadvantages	Donor Site Considerations	Osseointegration/ Dental Implants	Tissue Type	Anatomy
Fibula	Readily osteomized for contouring because of rich periosteal blood supply Up to 25 cm of bone available Long vascular pedicle	Limited soft tissue for large composite defects Limited alveolar height Limited mobility of skin relative to bone because of short cutaneous perforators	Potential weakness of extension and flexion of great toe Contraindicated with atherosclerotic disease of the lower extremity Skin graft often required	++	B++ M− S+	A Peroneal V Peroneal N Lateral sural cutaneous
Scapula (subscapularis system)	Very versatile with multiple bone and soft tissue segments Allows early ambulation Intermediate length vascular pedicle	Intraoperative positioning limits two-team approach	Decreased range of motion of the shoulder (short term) Primary closure usually possible	+	B+ M++ S++	A Circumflex scapular A Angular artery A Thoracodorsal artery perforators N None
Iliac crest (DCIA system)	Bone height comparable to that of native mandible Can restore vertical component of midface defects Excellent bone stock for implantation Large muscular paddle available	Short vascular pedicle Very limited soft tissue mobility in relation to bone	Hernia formation Delayed ambulation Risk of gait difficulty	++	B++ M++ S++	A Ascending branches of deep circumflex iliac artery V Ascending branches of deep circumflex iliac artery N None
Radial forearm	Pliable skin with minimal soft tissue Multiple skin islands possible Long, large, consistent vascular pedicle	Poor monocortical bone stock	Risk of radial bone fracture Skin graft typically required	−	B− M S++	A Radial V Venae comitantes and cephalic N Medial and lateral antebrachial cutaneous

B, Bone; *DCIA*, deep circumflex iliac artery; *M*, muscle; *S*, skin.

FIBULAR FREE FLAP

The fibular free flap, based on the peroneal artery and its two venae comitantes, has become the dominant flap for oromandibular reconstruction and many midface reconstructions. Preoperative assessment of the circulation to the foot is critical when the fibula donor site is being considered. Although physical examination of pulses and skin changes that are indicative of vascular disease is important, objective tests such as the ankle-to-arm index, color flow Doppler, CT angiogram, and MR angiogram have been advocated as noninvasive tests to evaluate the safety of harvesting a fibular flap (Fig. 32-7). More detailed vascular imaging provides information regarding not only the integrity of three-vessel runoff to the foot, but also the presence and severity of atherosclerosis.

In deciding which fibula to harvest, the surgeon must determine both the ideal orientation of the skin paddle and the location of the pedicle relative to available donor vessels. As a general rule, harvesting a contralateral fibula will place the skin paddle intraorally and the pedicle oriented toward the ipsilateral side of the neck. In some cases, the skin paddle can be mobile enough to place intraorally or extraorally; this is facilitated by a lengthy perforator and/or by isolating the perforator on a small cuff of fascia. Even when the pedicle is planned for the contralateral neck, the generous length of the pedicle can permit anastomosis to recipient vessels in the ipsilateral neck (Fig. 32-8).

Finally, if the fibula is selected, one must consider that the height of the transferred bone is approximately one fourth of the height of the dentate mandible, which can affect lip position and oral competence. The size mismatch can be overcome in a number of ways, as shown in Fig. 32-9, including adding additional nonvascularized bone, "double-barreling" the flap with an osteotomy, insetting the fibula above the inferior border of the native mandible, and prosthetic correction using implants. Preoperative consultation with an oral and maxillofacial prosthodontist is critically important in assessing the status of the remaining teeth and the options for dental rehabilitation in the reconstructed segment. Although this extent of planning is ideal, in reality, many technical decisions must be made intraoperatively depending on flap type, vessel length, and defect characteristics.

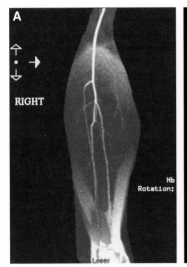 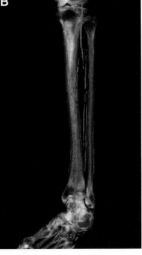

Fig. 32-7 **A,** MR angiogram of the right lower extremity showing normal three vessel runoff. **B,** CT arteriogram of the right lower extremity showing a high takeoff of the anterior tibial artery, with normal three-vessel runoff with mild calcific atherosclerotic changes noted at the distal tibial/peroneal trunk.

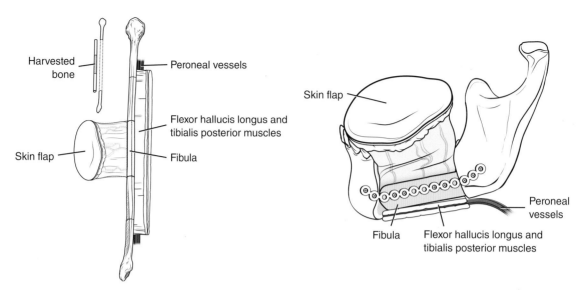

Fig. 32-8   Skin and vessel orientation in a fibula free flap. For oromandibular reconstruction, a contralateral fibula will have the skin paddle intraorally and the pedicle on the ipsilateral side. This can change, depending on the mobility of the skin paddle relative to the bone, as dictated by the perforators and the location of the recipient vessels.

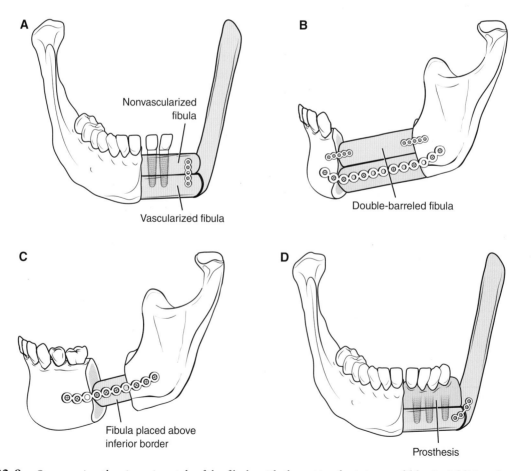

Fig. 32-9   Overcoming the size mismatch of the fibula with the native dentate mandible. **A,** Additional nonvascularized bone added. **B,** "Double-barreled" vascularized fibula. **C,** Placing the fibula above the inferior border. **D,** Using prosthesis to "correct" height discrepancy.

Scapular Free Flap (Subscapular System of Flaps)

Although limited by the difficulty in performing a two-team approach, the scapular flap based on the subscapular vascular system is an excellent choice for large composite defects because it provides three-dimensional mobility of its soft tissue components and availability of a broad sheet of latissimus dorsi muscle (Fig. 32-10). In addition, this flap is an excellent choice for patients with known peripheral vascular disease because the donor vessels are rarely involved by atherosclerotic vascular disease. In addition, the recovery from the harvest of a composite flap based on the subscapular system of flaps does not interfere with the patient's ability to ambulate postoperatively. However, although dental restoration is possible in some cases, the thickness and height of the lateral border of the scapula make this less likely than with a fibula or iliac crest. Preoperative consultation should include a discussion of these factors. Use of the subscapular system of flaps and inclusion of the scapular tip through the angular artery can improve the possibility of dental restoration.[15,59]

Because donor site morbidity is minimal, the main consideration in choosing which scapula to harvest is patient positioning as it relates to the extirpative surgery; therefore the ipsilateral scapula is typically used. If possible, the nondominant shoulder is selected.

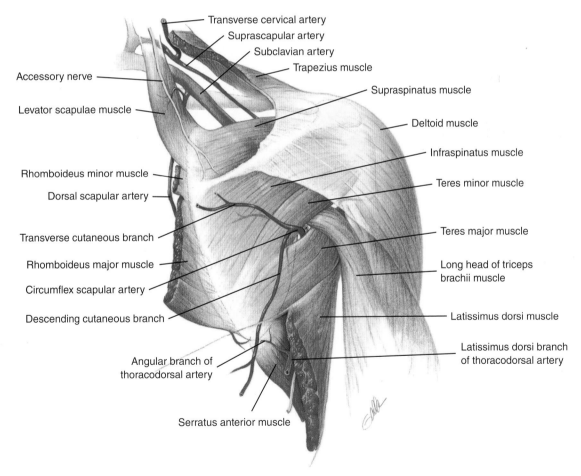

Fig. 32-10   The subscapular artery is shown passing through the triangular space and dividing into transverse and descending branches. Note the angular branch from the thoracodorsal artery that supplies the bone of the angle of the scapula.

Iliac Crest/Internal Oblique Free Flap (DCIA System)

Historically, the iliac crest free flap based on the deep circumflex iliac artery (DCIA) and vein was the approach of choice for bony reconstruction (Fig. 32-11). Although it is still used in select cases because it has excellent bone stock and enables the transfer of a large amount of muscle, its current use is limited because of donor site morbidity and the availability of other flaps. Like the scapular free flap, the iliac crest donor vessels are compromised by atherosclerotic vascular disease much less frequently than the peroneal system of the fibular free flap. However, this flap is not suited for patients who are likely to become debilitated by the harvest, who have a history of surgical procedures to the ipsilateral hip or abdomen, or who have a small atrophic mandible.

The determination of which iliac bone to harvest requires careful planning with consideration of whether the skin paddle or internal oblique muscle will reconstruct the intraoral defect, how the natural contour of the pelvis can simulate the natural shape of the mandible, whether the iliac crest or cut surface of the iliac bone will create the neoalveolus, and on which side of the neck the recipient vessels are located.

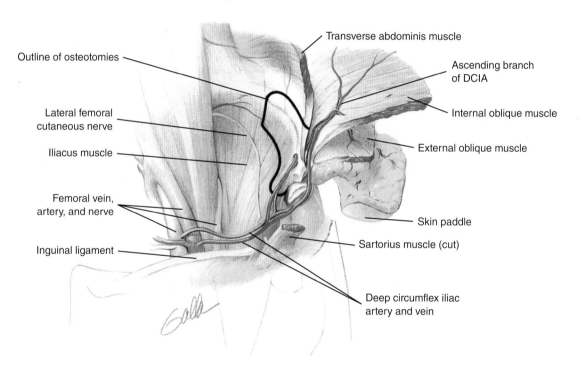

Fig. 32-11 The blood supply to the iliac crest and internal oblique osteomyocutaneous flap. The deep circumflex iliac artery (DCIA) gives off the ascending branch that is an axial blood supply to the internal oblique muscle. The DCIA continues on the medial aspect of the iliac crest to supply the iliac bone and sends cutaneous perforators to supply the skin laterally.

Radial Forearm Free Flap

The radial forearm osteofasciocutaneous free flap, based on the radial artery, venae comitantes, and cephalic vein, has fallen out of favor for reconstruction of the facial skeleton because of the poor monocortical bone stock and risk of fracture of the radius (Fig. 32-12). If this flap is used for bony reconstruction, one must be aware of the potential complications, including radial bone fracture, which leads to decreased grip and pinch strength, decreased sensation to the hand, and poor donor site cosmesis.[60-63] If used as a bony free flap, it is reasonable to obtain orthopedic surgical consultation for placement of a stress shielding plate to prophylactically strengthen the radial bone after harvest.[64] In a recent series of 34 patients who underwent radial bone harvest with placement of a 3.5 mm plate, there were no cases of radial bone fracture and no cases of persistent plate exposure.[60]

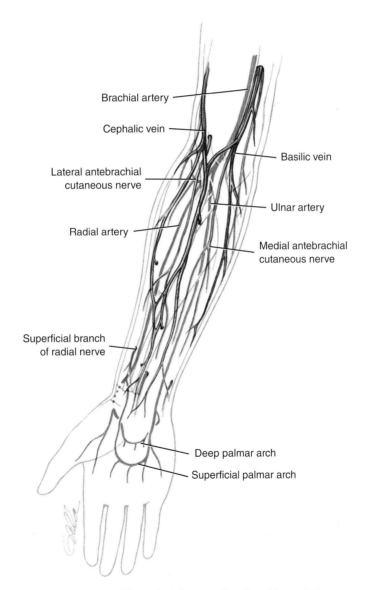

Fig. 32-12   The neurovascular anatomy of the radial forearm free flap. The radial artery supplies inflow. Outflow is through the cutaneous veins of the forearm (usually the cephalic vein) and/or the venae comitantes of the radial artery. The lateral antebrachial cutaneous nerve provides the primary sensory innervation to the region.

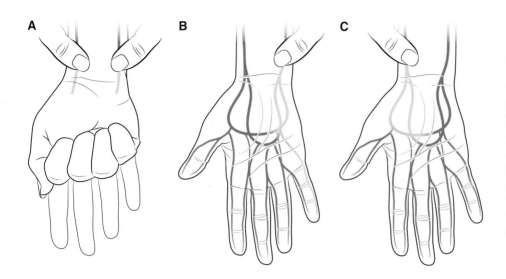

Fig. 32-13   The Allen test. **A,** The blood supply to the hand is through the radial artery and ulnar artery, with communication between the two through the superficial and deep palmar arches. **B** and **C,** Before a radial forearm free flap is harvested, the Allen test is performed to assess the status of the arch and limit the risk of hand ischemia with sacrifice of the radial artery.

The nondominant arm is typically chosen as the donor site, and an Allen test is performed on the hand to determine if the ulnar artery provides sufficient collateral circulation to the hand through vascular communications with the palmar arch (Fig. 32-13). Although an ulnar transposition flap has been described for closure of small soft tissue defects,[65] usually a split-thickness skin graft placed over intact paratenon of the flexor tendons is required for coverage. The arm is splinted for 7 days to immobilize the skin graft and prevent shearing forces from tendon movement that may lead to poor take of the graft.

OPERATIVE TECHNIQUES

Oromandibular Reconstruction

Primary reconstruction of a segmental mandible defect is important because the scarring and fibrosis that occur if reconstruction is delayed make it difficult to restore the natural mandible position. This effect is compounded by postoperative radiation. With contemporary surveillance imaging and frozen section analysis, primary reconstruction can overcome the perceived oncologic disadvantages of tumor bed monitoring and risk of residual disease. Furthermore, the addition of well-vascularized tissue improves the safety of adjuvant radiation and chemotherapy, and immediate reconstruction contributes to the patient's psychological well-being after potentially disfiguring surgery.

Considerations in Choice of Donor Site

In the past, the iliac crest free flap was the major donor site used for oromandibular reconstruction. The fibular free flap is currently the most commonly used flap for oromandibular reconstruction, with up to 70% to 90% of cases in some contemporary large consecutive series.[66,67] Up to 25 cm of bone is available that can be osteotomized multiple times and it provides excellent bone stock for dental implantation. The scapula is reserved for a select group of patients when the iliac crest and fibula are suboptimal. Although the likelihood of dental rehabilitation is lower with the scapular free flap, it has a number of distinct advantages and is used in cases of extensive soft tissue defects, older age, and preexisting gait disturbance.

The radial forearm osteocutaneous free flap has an extremely limited role in oromandibular reconstruction because of the potential for complications and poor bone stock. Some authors advocate its use for small lateral mandible defects that do not require osteotomies, will not receive dental implants, and require a large intraoral mucosal lining.[60,68-70] In rare cases, implants can be placed into the native mandible lateral to the radial bone to permit dental rehabilitation.[71]

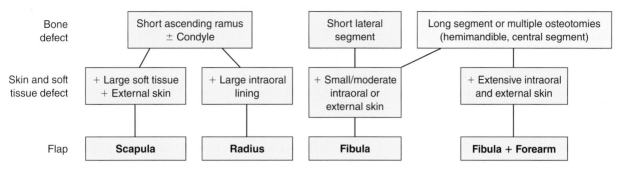

Fig. 32-14   Cordeiro and Disa algorithm for oromandibular reconstruction techniques. This algorithm does not take patient factors into account and does not consider the iliac crest free flap. (From Cordeiro PG, Disa J, Hidalgo DA, et al. Reconstruction of the mandible with osseous free flaps: a 10-year experience with 150 consecutive patients. Plast Reconstr Surg 104:1314-1320, 1999.)

The optimal donor site for oromandibular reconstruction can be determined based on a number of considerations, including patient and defect (bone and soft tissue) factors; one such algorithm is shown in Fig. 32-14.[72] Although algorithms provide useful guidelines considering defect factors, they may not take into account patient factors and may not consider all options (for example, in this algorithm the iliac crest free flap, which is an excellent choice in select oromandibular defects, is omitted). A discussion of donor site based on the location of the bony defect is presented later in this chapter.

Condyle and Ramus

The main goals of reconstructing defects involving the condyle and ramus are to maintain near normal range of motion during functional mandibular excursion and to prevent malocclusion, trismus, difficulty with mastication, and loss of mandibular height.[72] A discussion of temporomandibular joint reconstruction is provided later in this chapter. The fibular free flap is the preferred flap for correcting defects in this region, although the iliac crest, scapular, and even radial forearm can be used in certain cases.

Horizontal Segment

Reconstruction of horizontal segment defects of the mandible must take into account both the projection of the lower face and the ability to provide a platform for dental rehabilitation. All three flaps are suitable; the best choice will be determined by patient and defect-related factors.

Symphysis

In reconstruction of defects of the symphysis, one of the significant concerns related to the bone inset is to avoid overprojection of the neomandible, which would affect appearance and functional dental rehabilitation. In the normal native mandible, the alveolus is located more lingually than the inferior border of the mandible; therefore placing straight bone directly at the level of the inferior border will result in superior overprojection. Orientation of dental implants placed into an overprojected neomandible will result in significant rehabilitative challenges for the prosthodontist. If the scapular flap is chosen, it is advisable to harvest a wider piece of bone to appropriately increase height and support the lower lip, but because the blade of scapula is very thin it may be difficult to support dental rehabilitation. It is advisable to preserve the angular artery when making osteotomies in the scapular free flap, particularly if the tip of the scapula will play an important role in the final reconstruction.

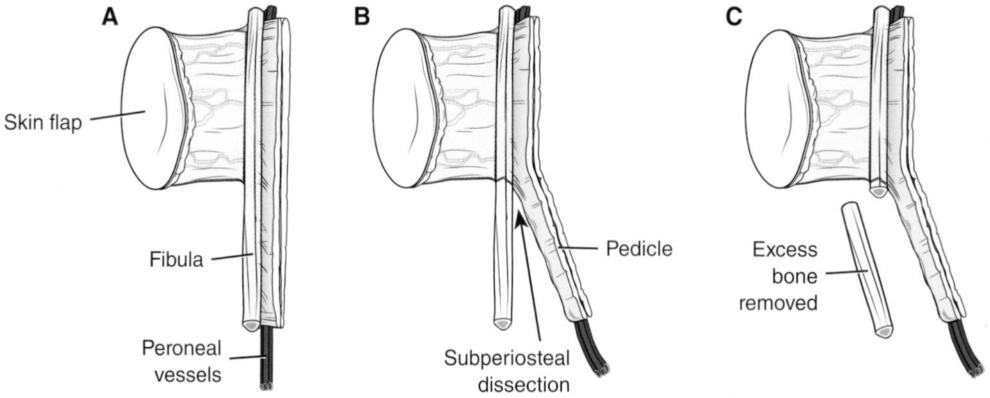

Fig. 32-15   Lengthening the vascular pedicle of the fibular free flap. **A,** The flap is harvested. **B,** The pedicle is lengthened by a subperiosteal dissection to the point of bone needed for the reconstruction. **C,** The excess bone is cut with a reciprocating saw.

Flap Contouring and Inset

Before the segmental resection is performed it is important to apply rigid internal fixation hardware (such as a 2.4 mm locking reconstruction plate [LRP]) along the inferior border of the mandible to maintain the position of the proximal and distal segments and to preserve the natural jawline. The preferred internal fixation hardware is an LRP secured with bicortical screws to the proximal and distal mandibular segments, and designed to prevent mobility and nonunion of the interposed bone flap. Either an external fixator or preoperative computer models can be used to achieve symmetry and a good functional outcome when it is not possible to modify a plate to mirror the natural contour of the outer mandibular cortex (such as in cases of extensive trauma, distortion of the natural mandible contour, or malignancy extending to or through the periosteum of the outer cortex).

When the fibular free flap is used, the pedicle may be lengthened and excess bone discarded by subperiosteal dissection; the excess bone is discarded by using a reciprocating saw and kept on the back table in case a nonvascularized bone graft is necessary (Fig. 32-15).

Next, the bone graft is contoured and inset, as shown in Fig. 32-16. The graft is placed within the defect in the native mandible with the pedicle on the lingual aspect of the neomandible. Wedge-shaped osteotomies are performed in the bone graft to achieve a contour that matches that of the plate. Great care must be taken not to injure the underlying vascular pedicle. The minimum length of each segment should be approximately 2 to 3 cm to decrease the likelihood of devascularizing the individual segments, which are each maintained in position by monocortical drilling and placement of a 26-gauge wire between each fibular segment. After the bone is contoured and secured under the reconstruction bar, the minimum number of monocortical locking screws that will ensure stability are placed into the bone flap to secure it to the plate. Minimizing the number of the screws placed into the neomandible preserves the opportunity to strategically place dental implants. With use of an LRP, maxillomandibular fixation is not necessary.

PALATOMAXILLARY AND MIDFACE RECONSTRUCTION
Considerations in Choice of Donor Site

Although mandibular reconstruction using the fibular free flap has become standard, a single most popular reconstructive method has not emerged for palatomaxillary or midface reconstruction. The numerous and somewhat disjointed defect classification systems and reconstructive algorithms have precluded the

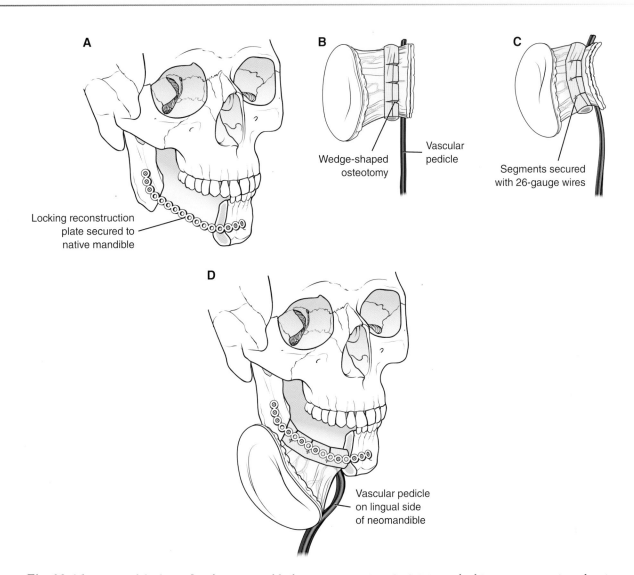

A, Locking reconstruction plate secured to native mandible

B, Wedge-shaped osteotomy   Vascular pedicle

C, Segments secured with 26-gauge wires

D, Vascular pedicle on lingual side of neomandible

Fig. 32-16   Inset of the bone flap for oromandibular reconstruction. **A,** A 2.4 mm locking reconstruction plate is secured into place with three or four bicortical locking screws on each side of the native mandible. **B,** After flap harvest, wedge-shaped osteotomies are made to match the contour of the plate. Care is taken not to disturb the underlying vascular pedicle. **C,** The individual segments are maintained in position using 26-gauge wires through monocortical drill holes. **D,** The bone flap is then placed between the native mandible, deep to the reconstruction bar, with the pedicle on the lingual surface of the neomandible; the minimum number of monocortical locking screws that are needed to ensure stability are placed into the bone flap to secure it to the plate.

development of a standardized approach and technique for palatomaxillary and midface reconstruction. However, most agree that in considering reconstruction of the midface, one must first address the bony defect, followed by assessment and addressing of the associated soft tissue deficit (including the skin, soft palate, buccal lining, and nasal lining). Individualized treatment of aesthetically and functionally critical structures such as the oral commissure, nasal airway, and eyelids must be developed and executed.[68] Combinations of microvascular free tissue transfer, local flaps, and maxillofacial prostheses will likely achieve a better overall result than a single technique alone. Guidelines for palatomaxillary reconstruction based on the Okay classification system are presented in Fig. 32-17, and Fig. 32-18 provides a generalized algorithm for reconstruction of midface and maxillary defects.

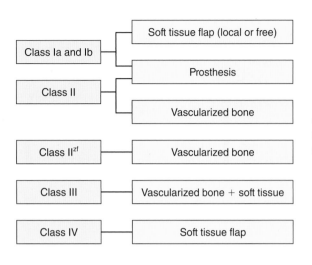

Fig. 32-17   A systematic approach to maxillary and midface reconstruction based on the Okay and Urken defect classification.

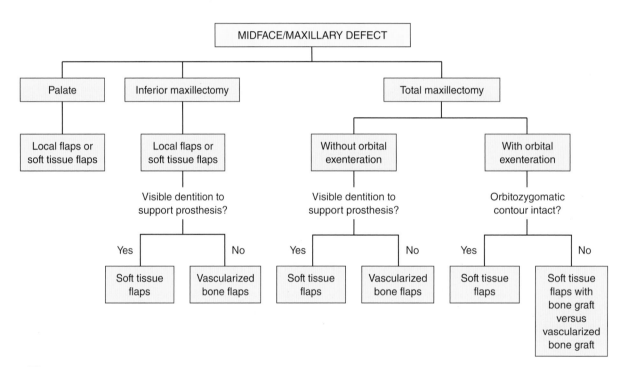

Fig. 32-18   Generalized algorithm for midface and maxillary defects independent of any classification system.

These guidelines do not specify which flap to use, since this requires a thorough evaluation of various patient and defect characteristics. The fibular, scapular, and iliac crest free flaps can all be effective, as shown in Fig. 32-19.

The osteocutaneous radial forearm free flap is reserved for only a select few palatomaxillary defects, including bony defects limited to the anterior maxillary arch with a significant soft tissue palatal defect. One important consideration is that prosthetic rehabilitation of the palatomaxillary defect provides functional dentition and separation of the oral cavity from the sinonasal cavities. It is essential that the introduction of a regional or free flap into a defect in the palate not interfere with the ability to achieve those goals, and that it enhance the patient's functional result over what can be achieved with a prosthesis.

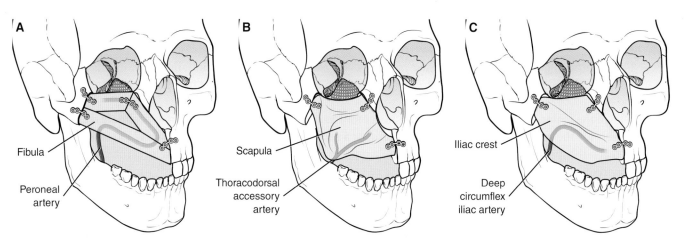

Fig. 32-19   Use of various donor sites for reconstruction of class III defects of the maxilla with involvement of the floor of the orbit and/or body of the zygoma. **A,** Fibula. **B,** Scapula tip/latissimus dorsi. **C,** Iliac crest/internal oblique.

Okay and Urken Class I Defects

For limited defects of the hard palate (class Ia and Ib), either an obturator or a soft tissue flap such as a palatal island pedicled flap or radial forearm free flap is useful to restore function. The exception is the class Ib defect of the premaxilla, which is best restored with vascularized bone.

Okay and Urken Class II Defects

For class II defects, patients either undergo rehabilitation with an obturator, if the remaining bone and dental support is adequate for retention, or a vascularized bone–containing free flap to serve as a suitable platform for dental rehabilitation.

Okay and Urken Class III Defects

For class III defects, or those that include the floor of the orbit or body of the zygoma (f and z defects), a vascularized bone–containing composite free flap is the optimal reconstructive technique because prosthetic obturators cannot provide adequate support for the orbit and midface without becoming too bulky. The specific flap selected will depend on a number of factors, but the iliac crest/internal oblique composite flap is the preferred option. This flap permits the transfer of vascularized bone that has sufficient caliber to permit support of the globe and replication of the inferior orbital rim, while permitting dental implants to be integrated into the neopalate.

The fibular free flap is ideal for palatomaxillary defects limited to the infrastructure because of the flap's long vascular pedicle and ability to undergo extensive contouring with closing wedge osteotomies. The bone is fixed using titanium miniplates at the two midfacial vertical buttresses (see Fig. 32-19). The skin of the fibular flap can be used to reline the neoalveolus and separate the oral cavity from above; however, when the skin paddle is too thick or the defect too large, a second thin, pliable, bivalved soft tissue flap may be required to achieve the reconstructive goals.

Okay and Urken Class IV Defects

Class IV defects consist of suprastructure defects in which the alveolus is intact, and a soft tissue flap (such as the temporoparietal fascia flap, radial forearm free flap, rectus abdominis free flap, or anterolateral thigh free flap) with a titanium implant for orbital floor support is usually sufficient to restore form.

Flap Contouring and Inset

Flap contouring is achieved in a similar fashion as for mandible reconstruction; however, in this setting reconstruction plates are not used. The key steps in flap contouring are shown in Fig. 32-20.

One of the major challenges in free tissue transfer for the midface is in the selection of appropriate recipient vessels for the microvascular anastomoses because a minimum pedicle distance of 10 to 12 cm is required to reach the ipsilateral neck.[73] Although usually not a problem for the fibular or radial forearm, other flaps may require pedicle lengthening with the use of vein grafts or arteriovenous loops.[74,75] The pedicle is then passed through a subcutaneous or submucosal tunnel to the cervical vessels.

Alternatively, using the superficial temporal artery and vein may obviate the need for lengthy pedicles. The drawbacks of using these vessels are that they (1) are often resected, (2) have increased susceptibility to vasospasm, (3) tortuous, (4) are of limited caliber, and (5) place the facial nerve at risk. However, a number of recent reports have shown a high success rate using this vascular system and suggest these vessels are a safe and reliable vessel option for defects of the upper face and scalp.[76-78]

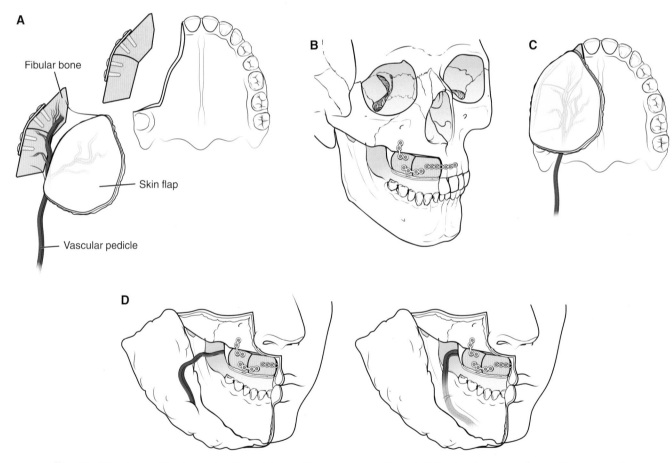

Fig. 32-20   Inset of the bone flap for palatomaxillary reconstruction. **A,** Osteotomies are performed to contour the flap to fit the required defect and recreate the natural maxillary alveolus contour. The vascular pedicle placed on the palatal side of the bone with monocortical miniplates to achieve fixation of each segment. **B,** The flap is then secured with miniplates anteriorly to the remaining alveolus, in the midline, and posteriorly at the level of the body of the zygoma. **C,** The soft tissue component of the flap is brought into place. **D,** The vascular pedicle is passed into the neck either through the cheek in a subcutaneous plane or through a submucosal plane along the body of the mandible.

Adjunct Procedures in Palatomaxillary Reconstruction

Depending on the requirements of the defect and reconstruction, additional procedures may be considered to address postoperative functional problems.[30] For example, a coronoidectomy is often performed on the ipsilateral side to prevent impingement of the coronoid process of the mandible with the posterior edge of the flap, which would result in trismus and potential compromise of the vascular pedicle. In addition, nasal trumpets are sometimes left in place for 2 weeks to stent and maintain a nasal airway during recovery and to prevent nasal stenosis. When the medial canthus and lacrimal sac have been disrupted by the resection, a medial canthopexy and dacryocystorhinostomy are performed. Finally, the cheek flap must be resuspended to prevent ptosis of the cheek and excessive pull on the lower lid.

SPECIAL TECHNIQUES AND CONSIDERATIONS

TEMPOROMANDIBULAR JOINT RECONSTRUCTION

In some cases of trauma or disease, mandible resection may extend to include the condyle and temporomandibular joint (TMJ). The goals of reconstruction in this case are to maintain TMJ range of motion to prevent malocclusion, trismus, loss of posterior mandible height, and difficulty with speech and mastication. There are a number of options for TMJ reconstruction as shown in Fig. 32-21. Excellent functional outcomes have been achieved by shaping the end of a vascularized bone graft into a neocondyle and securing it into the glenoid fossa to prevent drift. Interposition of soft tissue into the joint space is performed at the same time to prevent a bony union if the cartilaginous disc has been removed.[79,80]

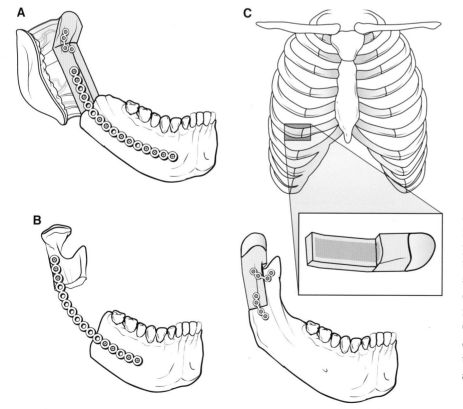

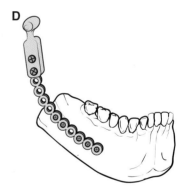

Fig. 32-21   Four methods of temporomandibular joint reconstruction. **A,** The preferred method is shaping the end of the vascularized bone graft to resemble a condyle. **B,** Replacement of a resected condyle after frozen section analysis of marrow space in cases of malignancy. **C,** Use of an autologous graft (such as costochondral bone or cartilage) shaped to resemble a condyle. **D,** Implantation of a prosthetic condyle.

Reimplantation of the resected condyle has been shown to result in similar postoperative functional outcomes as in patients with undisturbed condyles.[53] Nonvascularized autologous grafts are subject to resorption, fracture, and late complications, especially in the face of postoperative radiation. Finally, alloplastic materials such as titanium implants are not approved for permanent TMJ reconstruction, and may cause erosion of the glenoid fossa and migration into the middle cranial fossa.[81]

DOUBLE-BARRELED FIBULAR FLAPS

In patients who are not candidates for prosthetic dental restoration, restoring the height of the anterior mandible is important to provide support for the lower lip and to facilitate the reestablishment of oral competence. The technique of creating a double-barreled fibula involves performing an ostectomy while guarding the vascular pedicle and preserving the continuity of the periosteum. This helps to achieve immediate oral competence and allows for more successful dental implantation by reducing the crown to root ratio[82] (Fig. 32-22). This is not relevant, however, in patients with atrophic native mandibles.

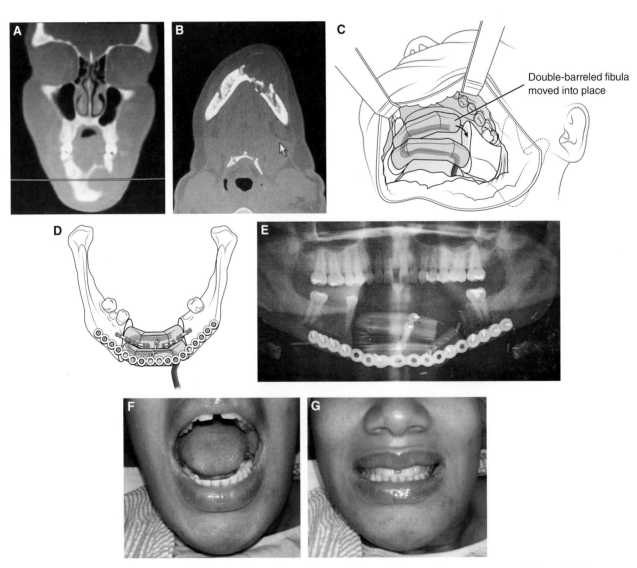

Fig. 32-22 The double-barreled fibula free flap. This technique helps achieve oral competence and allows for immediate dental implantation with good outcome.

Double Flaps for Facial Reconstruction

Double flaps should be considered in a number of cases, including (1) reconstruction of massive soft tissue defect with intricate three-dimensional requirements, (2) reconstruction of the total lower lip and symphysis, (3) reconstruction of the mandible in conjunction with a half to three quarters of the tongue, and (4) when there is nonviability of a critical portion of the soft tissue component of a composite free flap.[21,83-85] In oromandibular reconstruction one major advantage is the ability to use a vascularized bone-containing free flap to provide optimal bone reconstruction and a separate sensate soft tissue flap to reline the oral cavity and oropharynx.

Sandwich Flaps

A double flap is not ideal for situations in which standard osteocutaneous flaps for maxillary reconstruction are too bulky and/or a significant amount of mucosal lining is required for nasal and oral defects. Instead, the radial forearm osteocutaneous "sandwich" flap has been described.[86] When used for bilateral subtotal maxillectomy defects requiring restoration of the maxillary arch in addition to significant intraoral and nasal lining, the bone is osteotomized and contoured to recreate the maxillary arch. The large skin island is folded around the bone, as in a sandwich, and used to replace both the palatal and nasal lining (Fig. 32-23).

Sensate Flaps

A sensate flap involves harvesting a sensory nerve along with the vascular pedicle and coapting it to a donor sensory nerve in the head and neck region. An example of this approach is the sensate radial forearm free flap, with coaptation of the lateral antebrachial cutaneous nerve to the lingual nerve. Sensory recovery after oromandibular and palatomaxillary reconstruction may play a role in improving functional outcomes after facial reconstruction. Although some sensory recovery occurs in nonsensate flaps through neuronal ingrowth, it has been shown to be significantly improved and targeted when sensate flaps are used.[87-89] Further study is required to assess the functional impact of sensate flaps.

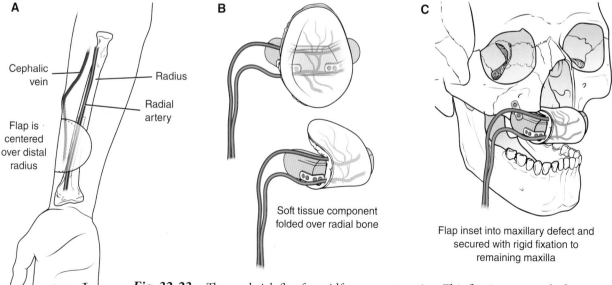

A

Cephalic vein

Radius

Radial artery

Flap is centered over distal radius

B

Soft tissue component folded over radial bone

C

Flap inset into maxillary defect and secured with rigid fixation to remaining maxilla

Fig. 32-23   The sandwich flap for midface reconstruction. This flap is composed of an osteofasciocutaneous radial forearm free flap and can be used instead of a double flap when there is a defect of the maxillary arch and large, thin, pliable soft tissue is required for oral and nasal lining in a midface defect.

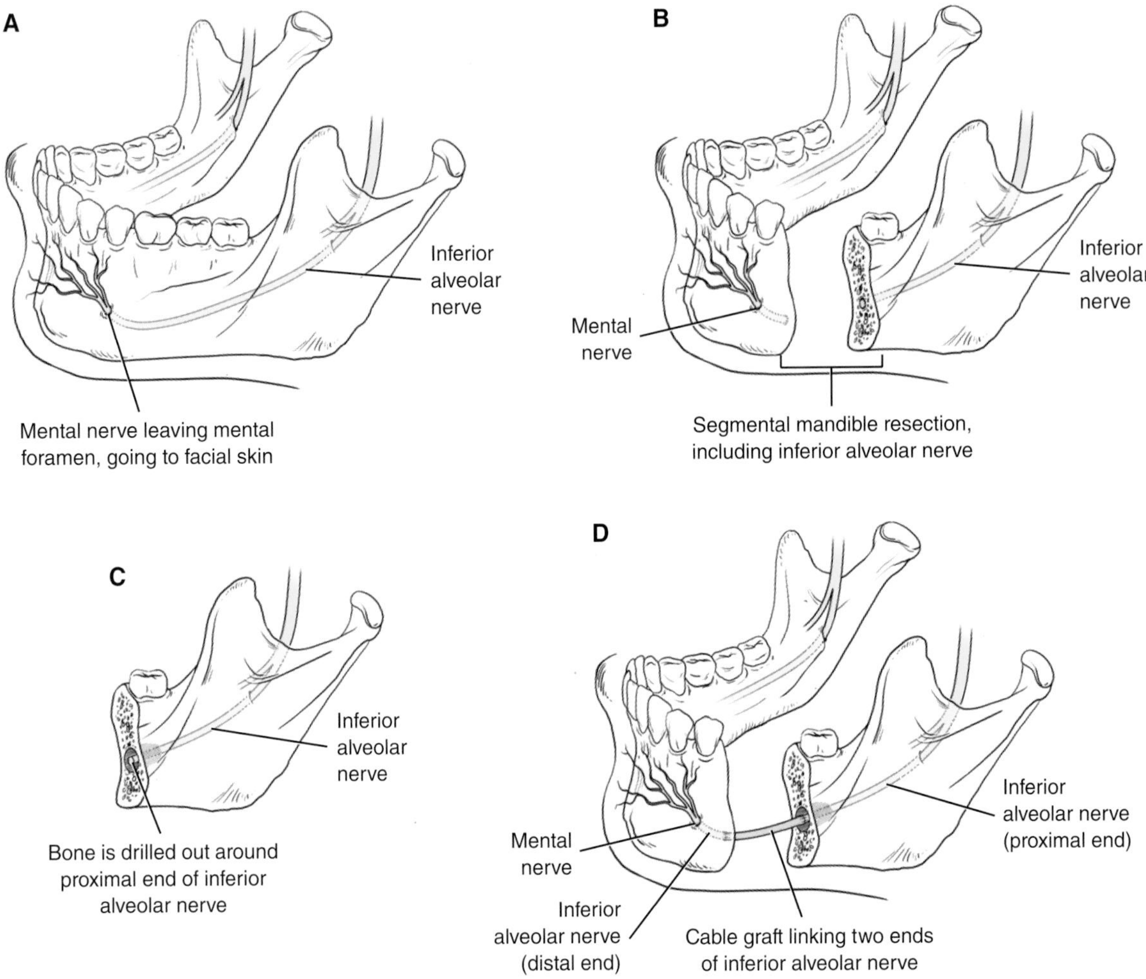

Fig. 32-24   Interposition nerve graft. A cable nerve graft between the proximal end of the inferior alveolar nerve to the mental nerve as it enters the facial skin can restore sensation to the lower lip region.

INTERPOSITION NERVE GRAFTS

In a segmental mandibulectomy, the inferior alveolar nerve is divided within the mandible. This deficit leads to a loss of sensation of the lower lip and chin. In these cases, the use of a nerve graft to connect the proximal stump of the inferior alveolar nerve to the mental nerve as it enters the skin can restore sensation.[34,90] The lateral femoral cutaneous, sural, or greater auricular nerves may be used as cable grafts (Fig. 32-24).

DENTAL REHABILITATION

Dental rehabilitation is integral to complete functional and cosmetic rehabilitation of the facial skeleton, including restoration of mastication, facial aesthetics, and support for the lower lip to maintain oral competence. The use of vascularized bone grafts has facilitated primary placement of endosteal implants.

The advantages of primary implantation include rapid dental rehabilitation with reduced surgical procedures, and in the case of malignancy in which postoperative radiation will be given, it permits approximately 3 months of integration before the onset of radiation damage to the bone. Considerations in primary endosteal implants include (1) patient motivation, (2) available bone stock, (3) radiation status of the palate or mandible, (4) adequate tongue function for manipulating the food bolus between the upper and lower occlusal surfaces, and (5) the financial resources to complete fabrication of the dental prosthesis.[21]

Ideally, planning for implantation begins before resection and should be part of the reconstructive plan. Patient factors to be considered include good oral hygiene, reasonable interincisal opening, and a favorable prognosis for survival and swallowing function. In a review of 728 fixtures in 183 patients with malignancy, there was an overall success rate of 95% for implant stability, including 88% for those who had postoperative radiation.[91]

Pediatric Mandible and Midface Reconstruction

Free tissue transfer for reconstruction of the facial skeleton is exceedingly uncommon in the pediatric patient. In contrast to adults, tumors requiring extensive bony resections in the pediatric population are typically benign or sarcomatous in nature. Other indications include congenital bony deformities, trauma, and vascular malformations.

Many of the techniques and principles in facial skeletal reconstruction described in this chapter can be applied to the pediatric population. The pediatric patient is growing, however, so there are specific goals in reconstructing the facial skeleton in this population; these include (1) preserving or restoring maxillomandibular relations to promote normal craniofacial development, (2) reducing deformity and morbidity of the facial skeleton in the growing child, and (3) avoiding secondary problems with growth at the site of flap harvest.[92]

Because long-term data and large case series are unavailable in the pediatric population, two unresolved questions regarding free tissue reconstruction of the pediatric facial skeleton are (1) the long-term growth potential of reconstructed mandibles in children and the need for further corrective surgeries after skeletal maturity has been reached, and (2) the impact of donor site morbidity resulting from flap harvest.

Mandible growth occurs through epiphyseal proliferation and bone remodeling. Some studies have shown fibular growth in the implanted mandible, with a number of case series measuring facial symmetry at 1 to 4 years postoperatively.[93-95] However, other reports suggest that the fibula does not grow concomitantly with the child, and that additional flaps and/or orthognathic surgery (such as sagittal split osteotomies or distraction osteogenesis) may be indicated to maintain facial symmetry in the long term as patients reach skeletal maturity.[96,97] Long-term studies with radiographic and cephalometric data are still required to resolve this issue. The removal of fixation hardware as early as possible in the postoperative period is thought to help facilitate growth.

There is concern about the impact of bone harvest on function and physical development of a child. There is discrepancy among studies regarding the impact on the donor site. Although some studies support minor disturbances, including great toe flexion contractures and valgus deformity after fibular bone harvest,[95] most contemporary studies show that scapular and fibular graft harvests in the pediatric population have very little morbidity if standard harvesting techniques are used. There is limited evidence for physical development abnormalities at the donor sites.[94,97,98]

POSTOPERATIVE CARE

There is considerable variation across the country and the world in the routine postoperative management of free flap patients. Many practices are based on departmental or personal preferences rather than evidence.[99-100] Issues to consider are the routine use of tracheotomy for airway management, monitoring in intensive care units, length of sedation time, ventilation, vasoactive or cardioactive drugs, active versus

Table 32-5   Mechanism of Action and Considerations of Anticoagulation After Free Tissue Transfer

	Mechanism of Action	**Considerations**
Aspirin	Antiplatelet action by inhibiting thromboxane, but not prostacyclin	Has been shown to reduce the rate of graft occlusion in a range of vascular procedures if given preoperatively or within 24 hours of surgery Retrospective studies have shown no difference in bleeding complication or flap failure between groups using aspirin and groups using no anticoagulation[106]
Heparin	Inhibits thrombin and, subsequently, inhibits thrombin-induced activation of factor V and factor VIII	Not routinely used in free tissue transfer because systemic heparin can result in significant bleeding complications
Dextran	Interferes with the formation of fibrin networks, increases the degradation of fibrin, decreases von Willebrand's factor and factor VII, and expands intravascular volume	Animal studies have shown better immediate postoperative vessel patency with use of dextran infusion[107] Associated with a number of complications, including anaphylactoid reactions, volume overload, renal damage, and acute respiratory distress syndrome A prospective trial showed no improvement in flap outcome with the use of dextran[108]

passive drainage, anticoagulation regimens[44,53,101-108] (Table 32-5), methods and frequency of flap monitoring, and time to restart an oral diet. Unfortunately, until a national database is developed to assess different types of postoperative care on outcomes and compare units, there is no robust data to support any particular regimen, and the decisions are best left up to policies and procedures within each reconstructive unit.

After discharge from the hospital, patients are often referred for physical therapy, jaw opening exercises, tongue exercises, and swallowing therapy to help with functional outcome. A number of patients will require flap modification, including removal of mandibular reconstructive plates 12 to 18 months after surgery to prevent exposure through the external skin, flap debulking, or removal of a monitoring paddle. Dental rehabilitation that includes implant placement must be performed with a carefully considered timing to permit strategic schedules of intervention relative to radiotherapy. Patients are also followed for aesthetic and functional outcomes as described in the next section.

RESULTS AND FUNCTIONAL OUTCOMES

Although there is little doubt that the advent of free tissue transfer has transformed surgical outcomes for head and neck cancer patients, with surgical oncologists able to perform more aggressive resections and give additional adjuvant therapy, a continued focus on function and aesthetics is still necessary. With the maturation of free tissue transfer techniques, aesthetic and functional outcomes are being analyzed and the importance of studying quality of life in cancer patients is increasingly being recognized.[101] Retrospective studies have shown excellent functional and aesthetic outcomes in free tissue transfer.[102]

In a 10-year follow-up study of patients with oromandibular defects reconstructed with free tissue transfer, results were found to be stable over time with 75% of patients demonstrating good to excellent aesthetic results and all patients maintaining excellent volume in the grafted bone.[53] In addition, 85% of patients had easily intelligible speech, 70% were tolerating a regular diet, and 60% had good form and function with implants or dentures. Of note, those with suboptimal speech had partial glossectomy, which supports the statement that management of the tongue is the most important functional factor in a patient's postoperative quality of life.[103]

For maxillectomy and midfacial defects, Cordeiro and Santamaria[44] evaluated 50 patients who underwent a variety of midface reconstructions, analyzed the functional and aesthetic outcomes, and found satisfactory results. The following parameters were evaluated:
1. *Speech:* Normal, near normal, intelligible, unintelligible
2. *Diet:* Unrestricted, soft, liquid
3. *Eye globe position and function:* Vertical dystopia, enophthalmos, visual disturbance, ectropion
4. *Oral competence:* Ability to retain intraoral liquids, presence of drooling, need for tube feeding
5. *Aesthetic result:* Facial symmetry, malar prominence, cheek contour, scars, eyelid position

Most of the available functional outcome data are retrospective in nature. In a prospective study, Seikaly et al[104] looked at functional outcomes at various times after mandibulectomy with fibular free flap reconstruction and found relative stability between preoperative and postoperative speech and swallowing outcomes. Additional studies have highlighted the importance of the soft tissue component in optimizing functional outcomes of facial skeletal reconstruction.[105] Ideally, multiinstitutional studies to evaluate functional outcomes, including quality of life parameters such as those shown in Fig. 32-25, will be designed and will serve as a guide as we strive for sound oncologic surgery in conjunction with the enhanced restoration of form and function.

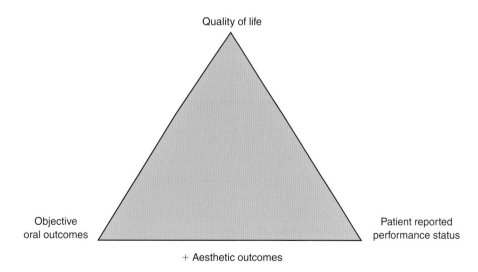

Fig. 32-25   The functional outcomes triangle for free flap reconstruction. A combination of objective, patient reported, and validated quality of life surveys compared across institutions are necessary to identify surgical factors related to improved patient outcomes after free tissue transfer for reconstruction of the facial skeleton.

Key Points

- The goals of reconstruction of the facial skeleton are to restore form and facial symmetry, maintain a safe and comfortable airway, separate cranial from sinonasal contents, support the globe, restore dentition to maintain occlusal relationships, improve the patient's ability to eat in public, and restore intelligible speech.
- Patient, surgeon, tumor, and defect factors are all important considerations in determining the most appropriate reconstruction for a particular patient.
- The three main donor sites used in contemporary reconstruction of the facial skeleton with vascularized bone are the scapula, iliac crest, and fibula. The radial forearm osteocutaneous flap can also be used.
- Preoperative consultation with an oral and maxillofacial prosthodontist is important to assess the status of the remaining teeth and the options for dental rehabilitation in the reconstructed segment. Dental rehabilitation that includes implant placement must be performed with carefully considered timing to permit strategic schedules of intervention relative to radiotherapy.
- Prosthetic rehabilitation of the palatomaxillary defect provides functional dentition and separation of the oral cavity from the sinonasal cavities. The introduction of a regional or free flap into a defect in the palate must not interfere with attaining those goals and must enhance the patient's functional result over what can be achieved with a prosthesis.
- Long-term studies with radiographic and cephalometric data are still required on the topic of pediatric mandible growth after free tissue reconstruction.
- With the maturation of free tissue transfer techniques, aesthetic and functional outcomes are being analyzed, and the importance of studying quality of life in cancer patients is increasingly being recognized.

REFERENCES

1. Lawson W, Loscalzo LJ, Baek SM, et al. Experience with immediate and delayed mandibular reconstruction. Laryngoscope 92:5-10, 1982.
2. Shpitzer T, Neligan PC, Gullane P, et al. The free iliac crest and fibula flaps in vascularized oromandibular reconstruction: comparison and long-term evaluation. Head Neck 21:639-647, 1999.
3. August M, Tompach P, Chang Y, et al. Factors influence the long-term outcomes of mandibular reconstruction. J Oral Maxillofac Surg 58:731-737, 2000.
4. Urken ML, Buchbinder D, Weinberg H, et al. Functional evaluation following microvascular oromandibular reconstruction of the oral cancer patient: a comparative study of reconstructed and non-reconstructed patients. Laryngoscope 101:935-950, 1991.
5. Conley J. Use of composite flaps containing bone for major repairs in the head and neck. Plast Reconstr Surg 49:522-526, 1972.
6. Panje W, Cutting C. Trapezius osteomyocutaneous island flap for reconstruction of the anterior floor of the mouth and the mandible. Head Neck Surg 3:66-71, 1980.
7. Cuono CB, Aruyan S. Immediate reconstruction of a composite mandibular defect with a regional osteomusculocutaneous flap. Plast Reconstr Surg 65:477-484, 1980.
8. Klotch DW, Prein J. Mandibular reconstruction using AO plates. AM J Surg 154:384-388, 1987.
9. Vuillemin T, Raveh J, Sutter F. Mandibular reconstruction with the titanium hollow screw reconstruction plate (THORP) system: evaluation of 62 cases. Plast Reconstr Surg 82:804-814, 1988.
10. Stoll P, Wachter R. AO reconstruction plate systems for the repair of mandibular defects 3-DBRP versus THORP-system. J Carniomaxillofac Surg 20:40-45, 1992.
11. Spencer KR, Sizeland A, Taylor GI, et al. The use of titanium mandibular reconstruction plates in patients with oral cancer. Int J Oral Maxillofac Surg 28:288-290, 1999.
12. Gullane PJ. Primary mandibular reconstruction: analysis of 64 cases and evaluation of interface radiation dosimetry on bridging plates. Laryngoscope 101:1-50, 1991.

13. Taylor GI, Townsend P, Corlett R. Superiority of the deep circumflex iliac vessels as the supply for free groin flaps. Plast Reconstr Surg 64:595-604, 1979.

14. Sanders R, Mayou BJ. A new vascularized bone graft transferred by microvascular anastomosis as a free flap. Br J Surg 66:787-788, 1979.

15. Swartz WM, Banis JC, Newton ED, et al. The osteocutaneous scapular flap for mandibular and maxillary reconstruction. Plast Reconstr Surg 77:530-545, 1986.

    This cadaveric and clinical study is the seminal article that describes the scapula free flap and its use in reconstruction of facial defects of the facial skeleton. The advantage this tissue has over previous reconstructive methods is the ability to have multiple cutaneous panels on a separate vascular pedicle from the bone, thereby allowing for improvement in three-dimensional spatial relationships for the most complex facial skeleton and soft tissue reconstructive needs.

16. Soutar DS, Scheker LR, Tanner NS, et al. The radial forearm flap: a versatile method for intra-oral reconstruction. Br J Plast Surg 36:1-8, 1983.

17. Hidalgo DA. Fibula free flap: A new method of mandible reconstruction. Plast Reconstr Surg 84:71-79, 1989.

18. Rogers SN, Lowe D, McNally D, et al. Health-related quality of life after maxillectomy: a comparison between prosthetic obturation and free flap. J Oral Maxillofac Surg 61:174-181, 2003.

19. Genden EM, Okay D, Stepp MT, et al. Comparison of functional and quality of life outcomes in patients with and without palatomaxillary reconstruction: a preliminary report. Arch Otolaryngol Head Neck Surg 129:775-780, 2003.

20. Moreno MA, Skoracki RJ, Hanna EY, et al. Microvascular free flap reconstruction versus palatal obturation for maxillectomy defects. Head Neck 32:860-868, 2010.

21. Urken ML, Buchbinder D, Constantino PD, et al. Oromandibular reconstruction using microvascular composite flaps: report of 210 cases. Arch Otolaryngol Head Neck Surg 124:46-55, 1998.

22. Gerressen M, Pastaschek CI, Riediger D, et al. Microsurgical free flap reconstructions of head and neck region in 406 cases: a 13-year experience. J Oral Maxillofac Surg 71:628-635, 2013.

23. Suh JD, Sercarz JA, Abemayor E, et al. Analysis of outcome and complications in 400 cases of microvascular head and neck reconstruction. Arch Otolaryngol Head Neck Surg 130:962-966, 2004.

24. Wong CH, Wei FC. Microsurgical free flap in head and neck reconstruction. Head Neck 32:1236-1245, 2010.

25. Futran ND, Mendez E. Developments in reconstruction of midface and maxilla. Lancet Oncol 7:249-258, 2006.

26. Yamamoto Y, Kawashima K, Sugihara T, et al. Surgical management of maxillectomy defects based on the concept of buttress reconstruction. Head Neck 26:247-256, 2004.

27. Baumann DP, Yu P, Hanasono MM, et al. Free flap reconstruction of osteoradionecrosis of the mandible: a 10-year review and defect classification. Head Neck 33:800-807, 2011.

28. Ferrari S, Copelli C, Bianchi B, et al. Free flaps in elderly patients: outcomes and complications in head and neck reconstruction after oncological resection. J Craniomaxillofac Surg 41:167-171, 2013.

29. Shaari CM, Buchbinder D, Costantino PD, et al. Complications of microvascular head and neck surgery in the elderly. Arch Otolaryngol Head Neck Surg 124:407-411, 1998.

30. Urken ML, Buchbinder D, Okay D. Functional palatomaxillary reconstruction. Oper Tech Otolaryngol Head Neck Surg 16:36-39, 2005.

31. Bak M, Jacobson AS, Buchbinder D, et al. Contemporary reconstruction of the mandible. Oral Oncology 46:71-76, 2010.

32. Urken ML, Okay DJ. Reconstruction of palatomaxillary defects. In Urken ML, ed. Multidisciplinary Head and Neck Reconstruction: A Defect-Oriented Approach. Philadelphia: Lippincott Williams & Wilkins, 2010.

33. Jewer DD, Bod JB, Maktelow RT, et al. Orofacial and mandibular reconstruction with the iliac crest free flap: a review of 60 cases and a new method of classification. Plast Reconstr Surg 84:391-403, 1989.

34. Urken ML, Weinberg H, Vickery C, et al. Oromandibular reconstruction using microvascular composite free flaps. Report of 71 cases and a new classification scheme for bony, soft tissue, and neurologic defects. Arch Otolaryngol Head Neck Surg 117:733-744, 1991.

35. Boyd JB, Gullane PJ, Rotstein LE, et al. Classification of mandibular defects. Plast Reconstr Surg 92:1266-1275, 1993.

36. David D, Tan E, Katsaros J, et al. Mandibular reconstruction with vascularized iliac crest: a 10 year experience. Plast Reconstr Surg 82:792-801, 1998.

37. Aramany MA. Basic principles of obturator design for partially edentulous patients. Part I: classification. J Prosthet Dent 40:554-557, 1978.

38. Wells MD, Luce EA. Reconstruction of midfacial defects after surgical resection of malignancies. Clin Plast Surg 22:79-89, 1995.

39. Spiro RH, Strong EW, Shah JP. Maxillectomy and its classification. Head Neck 19:309-314, 1997.

40. Umino S, Masuda G, Ono S, et al. Speech intelligibility following maxillectomy with and without a prosthesis: an analysis of 54 cases. J Oral Rehabil 25:153-158, 1998.

41. Davison SP, Sherris DA, Meland NB. An algorithm for maxillectomy defect recontruction. Laryngoscope 108:215-219, 1998.

42. Brown JS, Rogers SN, McNally DN, et al. A modified classification for the maxillectomy defect. Head Neck 22:17-26, 2000.

43. Triana RJ, Uglesic B, Virag M, et al. Microvascular free flap reconstructive options in patients with partial and total maxillectomy defects. Arch Facial Plast Surg 2:91-101, 2000.

44. Cordeiro PG, Santamaria E. A classification system and algorithm for reconstruction of maxillectomy and midfacial defects. Plast Reconstr Surg 105:2331-2346, 2000.

45. Okay DJ, Genden E, Buchbinder D, et al. Prosthodontic guidelines for surgical reconstruction of the maxilla: a classification system of defects. J Prosthet Dent 86:352-363, 2001.

46. Carrillo JF, Guemes A, Ramirez-Ortega MC, et al. Prognostic factors in maxillary sinus and nasal cavity carcinoma. Eur J Surg Oncol 31:1206-1212, 2005.

47. Rodriguez ED, Martin M, Bluebond-Langner R, et al. Microsurgical reconstruction of posttraumatic high-energy maxillary defects: establishing the effectiveness of early reconstruction. Plast Reconstr Surg 120(7 Suppl 2):103S-117S, 2007.

48. Brown JS, Shaw RJ. Reconstruction of the maxilla and midface: introducing a new classification. Lancet Oncol 11:1001-1008, 2010.

49. Buchbinder D, Okay DJ, Urken ML. Oromandibular reconstruction. In Urken ML, ed. Multidisciplinary Head and Neck Reconstruction: A Defect-Oriented Approach. Philadelphia: Lippincott Williams & Wilkins, 2010.

50. Hidalgo DA, Pusic AL. Free-flap mandibular reconstruction: a 10-year follow-up study. Plast Reconstr Surg 110:438-449, 2002.

51. Bidra AS, Jacob RF, Taylor TD. Classification of maxillectomy defects: a systematic review and criteria necessary for a universal description. J Prosthet Dent 107:261-270, 2012.

   This article summarizes various maxillectomy/midfacial defect classification systems and identifies six criteria that an ideal classification system should include to satisfy both prosthodontic and surgical needs. The six criteria identified in this systematic review for a universal description of a maxillectomy defect are (1) dental status, (2) oroantral/nasal communication status, (3) soft palate and other contiguous structure involvement, (4) superoinferior extent, (5) anteroposterior extent, and (6) mediolateral extent of the defect. The authors conclude that a criteria-based description appears more objective and amenable for universal use than a classification-based description. However, the Okay and Urken classification, with the modifications previously published and presented in this chapter, does indeed address all six aspects.

52. Duncan MJ, Manktelow RT, Zuker RM, et al. Mandibular reconstruction in the radiated patient: the role of osteocutaneous free tissue transfers. Plast Reconstr Surg 76:829-840, 1985.

53. Netscher D, Alford EL, Wigoda P, et al. Free composite myo-osseous flap with serratus anterior and rib: indications in head and neck reconstruction. Head Neck 20:106-112, 1998.

54. Lovie MJ, Duncan GM, Glasson DW. The ulnar artery forearm free flap. Br J Plast Surg 37:486-492, 1984.

55. Testelin S. History of microsurgical reconstruction of the mandible. Ann Chir Plast Esthet 37:241-245, 1992.

56. Zenn MR, Hidalgo DA, Cordeiro PG, et al. Current role of the radial forearm free flap in mandibular reconstruction. Plast Reconstr Surg 99:1012-1017, 1997.

57. Villaret DB, Futran NA. The indications and outcomes in the use of osteocutaneous radial forearm free flap. Head Neck 25:475-481, 2003.

58. Bianchi B, Bertolini F, Ferrari S, et al. Maxillary reconstruction using rectus abdominus free flap and bone grafts. Br J Oral Maxillofac Surg 44:526-530, 2006.

59. Coleman JJ III, Sultan MR. The bipedicled osteocutaneous scapula flap: a new subscapular system free flap. Plast Reconstr Surg 87:682-692, 1991.

60. Bardsley AF, Soutar DS, Elliot D, et al. Reducing morbidity in the radial forearm flap donor site. Plast Reconstr Surg 86:287-294, 1990.

61. Smith AA, Bowen CV, Rabczak T, et al. Donor site deficit of the osteocutaneous radial forearm flap. Ann Plast Surg 32:372-376, 1994.

62. Swanson E, Boud JB, Manktelow RT. The radial forearm flap: reconstructive applications and donor-site defects in 35 consecutive patients. Plast Reconstr Surg 85:258-266, 1990.

63. Inglefield CJ, Kolhe PS. Fracture of the radial forearm osteocutaneous donor site. Ann Plast Surg 33:638-643, 1993.

64. Nunez VA, Pike J, Avery C, et al. Prophylactic plating of the donor site of osteocutaneous radial forearm flaps. Br J Oral Maxillofac Surg 37:210-212, 1997.

65. Jaquet Y, Enepekides DJ, Torgerson C, et al. Radial forearm free flap donor site morbidity: ulnar-based transposition flap vs split-thickness skin graft. Arch Otolaryngol Head Neck Surg 138:38-43, 2012.

66. Cordeiro PG, Disa J, Hidalgo DA, et al. Reconstruction of the mandible with osseous free flaps: a 10-year experience with 150 consecutive patients. Plast Reconstr Surg 104:1314-1320, 1999.

67. Chang D, Oh HK, Robb GL, et al. Management of advanced mandibular osteoradionecrosis with free flap reconstruction. Head Neck 23:830-835, 2001.

68. Santamaria E, Cordeiro PG. Reconstruction of maxillectomy and midfacial defects with free tissue transfer. J Surg Oncol 94:522-531, 2006.

69. Cordeiro PG, Santamaria E, Disa JJ. Mandible reconstruction. In Shah JP, ed. Cancer of the Head and Neck. Hamilton, ON, Canada: BC Decker, 2001.

70. Boyd JB. Mandible reconstruction with the radial forearm flap. Oper Tech Plast Reconstr Surg 3:241-247, 1996.

71. Foster RD, Anthony JP, Singer MI, et al. Microsurgical reconstruction of the midface. Arch Surg 131:960-966, 1996.

72. Disa JJ, Cordeiro PG. Mandible reconstruction with microvascular surgery. Semin Surg Oncol 19:226-234, 2000.

73. Cordeiro PG, Disa JJ. Challenges in midface reconstruction. Semin Surg Oncol 19:218-225, 2000.

74. Vogt PM, Steinau HU, Spies M, et al. Outcome of simultaneous and staged microvascular free tissue transfer connected to arteriovenous loops in areas lacking recipient vessels. Plast Reconstr Surg 120:1568-1575, 2007.

75. Cavadas PC. Arteriovenous vascular loops in free flap reconstruction of the extremities. Plast Reconstr Surg 121:514-520, 2008.

76. Chia HL, Wong CH, Tan BK, et al. An algorithm for recipient vessel selection in microsurgical head and neck reconstruction. J Reconstr Microsurg 27:47-56, 2011.

77. Shimizu F, Lin MP, Ellabban M, et al. Superficial temporal vessels as a reserve recipient site for microvascular head and neck reconstruction in vessel-depleted neck. Ann Plast Surg 62:134-138, 2009.

78. Hansen SL, Foster RD, Dosanjh AS, et al. Superficial temporal artery and vein as recipient vessels for facial and scalp microsurgical reconstruction. Plast Reconstr Surg 120:1879-1884, 2007.

79. Khariwala SS, Chan J, Blackwell KE, et al. Temporomandibular joint reconstruction using a vascularized bone graft with Alloderm. J Reconstr Microsurg 23:25-30, 2007.

80. Wax MK, Winslow CP, Hansen J, et al. A retrospective analysis of temporomandibular joint reconstruction with free fibula microvascular flap. Laryngoscope 110:977-981, 2000.

81. Shenaq SM, Klebuc MJ. TMJ reconstruction during vascularized bone graft transfer to the mandible. Microsurgery 15:299-304, 1994.

82. Chang YM, Wallace CG, Tsai CY, et al. Dental implant outcome after primary implantation into double-barreled fibula osteoseptocutaneous free flap-reconstructed mandible. Plast Reconstr Surg 128:1220-1228, 2011.

83. Wei, FC, Demirkan F, Chen HC, et al. Double free flaps in reconstruction of extensive composite mandibular defects in head and neck cancer. Plast Reconstr Surg 103:39-47, 1999.

84. Bianchi B, Ferrari S, Poli T, et al. Oromandibular reconstruction with simultaneous free flaps: experience on 10 cases. Acta Otorhinolaryngol Ital 23:281-290, 2003.

85. Wei FC, Yazar S, Lin CH, et al. Double free flaps in head and neck reconstruction. Clin Plast Surg 32:303-308, 2005.

86. Cordeiro PG, Bacilious N, Schantz S, et al. The radial forearm osteocutaneous "sandwich" free flap for reconstruction of the bilateral subtotal maxillectomy defect. Ann Plast Surg 40:397-402, 1998.

87. Kim JH, Rho YS, Ahn HY, et al. Comparison of sensory recovery and morphologic change between sensate and nonsensate flaps in oral cavity and oropharyngeal reconstruction. Head Neck 30:1099-1104, 2008.

88. Urken ML. Targeted sensory restoration to the upper aerodigestive tract with physiologic implications. Head Neck 26:287-293, 2004.

89. Urken ML, Weinberg H, Vickery C, et al. The combined sensate radial forearm and iliac crest free flaps for reconstruction of significant glossectomy-mandibulectomy defects. Laryngoscope 102:543-558, 1992.

90. Chang YM, Rodriguez ED, Chu YM, et al. Inferior alveolar nerve reconstruction with interpositional sural nerve graft: a sensible addition to one-stage mandibular reconstruction. J Plast Reconstr Aesthet Surg 65:757-762, 2012.

91. Samouhi PB. Rehabilitation of oral cancer patients with dental implants. Curr Opin Otolaryngol Head Neck Surg 8:305-313, 2000.

92. Futran ND, Okay DJ, Urken ML. Pediatric mandibular and maxillary reconstruction. In Urken ML, ed. Multidisciplinary Head and Neck Reconstruction: A Defect-Oriented Approach. Philadelphia: Lippincott Williams & Wilkins, 2010.

93. Olvera-Caballero C. Mandibular reconstruction in children. Microsurgery 20:158-161, 2000.

94. Genden EM, Buchbinder D, Chaplin JM, et al. Reconstruction of the pediatric maxilla and mandible. Arch Otolaryngol Head Neck Surg 126:293-300, 2000.

95. Crosby MA, Martin JW, Robb GL, et al. Pediatric mandibular reconstruction using a vascularized fibula flap. Head Neck 30:311-319, 2008.

96. Phillips JH, Rechner B, Tompson BD. Mandibular growth following reconstruction using a free fibula graft in the pediatric facial skeleton. Plast Reconstr Surg 116:419-424, 2005.

97. Guo L, Ferraro NF, Padwa BL, et al. Vascularized fibular graft for pediatric mandibular reconstruction. Plast Reconstr Surg 121:2095-2105, 2008.

98. Iconomou TG, Zuker RM, Phillips JH. Mandibular reconstruction in children using the vascularized fibula. J Reconstr Microsurg 15:83-90, 1999.

99. Marsh M, Elliott S, Anand R, et al. Early postoperative care for free flap head & neck reconstructive surgery—a national survey of practice. Br J Oral Maxillofac Surg 47:182-185, 2009.

100. Spiegel JH, Polat JK. Microvascular flap reconstruction by otolaryngologists: prevalence, postoperative care, and monitoring techniques. Laryngoscope 117:485-490, 2007.

101. Morton RP. Toward comprehensive multidisciplinary care for head and neck cancer patients: quality of life versus survival. Otolaryngol Head Neck Surg 147:404-406, 2012.

102. Shpitzer T, Neligan PC, Gullane PJ, et al. Oromandibular reconstruction with the fibular free flap. Analysis of 50 consecutive flaps. Arch Otolaryngol Head Neck Surg 123:939-944, 1997.

103. Urken ML, Moscoso JF, Lawson W, et al. A systematic approach to functional reconstruction of the oral cavity following partial and total glossectomy. Arch Otolaryngol Head Neck Surg 120:589-601, 1994.

104. Seikaly H, Maharaj M, Rieger J, et al. Functional outcomes after primary mandibular resection and reconstruction with the fibular free flap. J Otolaryngol 34:25-28, 2005.

   This study is among the first to prospectively examine functional outcomes in a cohort of patients who had undergone free flap reconstruction of the facial skeleton. This type of study is necessary to continuously improve on outcomes in free flap reconstruction. The cohort of patients had oral cavity cancer and had undergone mandibulectomy with primary fibular free flap reconstruction for the facial skeleton. There was a particular emphasis on longitudinal comparison of the preoperative function with that in postoperative and postradiotherapy periods. Speech and swallowing data were gathered, including analysis for speech intelligibility and modified barium swallows for problems with various phases of swallowing at various treatment time points. The authors found no significant difference across any of the evaluation times for single-word or sentence intelligibility, and the swallowing data showed no instances of posttreatment aspiration or laryngeal penetration. There were also no significant differences in any of the swallowing parameters across treatment times.

105. Wagner JD, Coleman JJ III, Weisberger E, et al. Predictive factors for functional recovery after free tissue transfer oromandibular reconstruction. Am J Surg 176:430-435, 1998.

106. Lighthall JG, Cain R, Ghanem TA, et al. Effect of postoperative aspirin on outcomes in microvascular free tissue transfer surgery. Otolaryngol Head Neck Surg 148:40-46, 2013.

107. Wolfort SF, Angel MF, Knight KR, et al. The beneficial effect of dextran on anastomotic patency and flap survival in a strongly thrombogenic model. J Reconstr Microsurg 8:375-378, 1992.

108. Disa JJ, Polvora VP, Pusic AL, et al. Dextran-related complications in head and neck microsurgery: do the benefits outweigh the risks? A prospective randomized analysis. Plast Reconstr Surg 112:1534-1539, 2003.

33

Soft Tissue Injuries of the Face

Tessa A. Hadlock ▪ *Mack L. Cheney*

The face defines an individual's window to the world. It conveys individual beauty, unique identity, and emotion, transmits nonverbal communication, and is vital for myriad critical human functions, among them speaking and eating. The face occupies a vulnerable position on the body, since it is rarely covered and is prone to soft tissue injury from virtually any modality. Most common mechanisms of facial injury include motor vehicle accidents and falls, although sports injuries, violence, and abuse are also substantial contributors to soft tissue injury.[1-4]

Soft tissue injuries of the face require special attention because of their dual impact on function and aesthetics. Any injury to the face elicits a strong emotional response from the patient because of the potential for permanent scarring and disfigurement. Although in certain cultures facial scarring is thought to represent beauty, strength, and honor, in general the significant negative psychological aspect of acute facial injury must be deeply appreciated; systematic and timely repair of the traumatized tissues of the face will minimize the likelihood of long-term sequelae.[5-7]

GENERAL PRINCIPLES

WOUND ASSESSMENT

Soft tissue injuries of the face are unique in that they may involve skin, hair-bearing facial areas, subcutaneous tissues, glands, ducts, nerve branches, vessels, muscles, and even the underlying bony skeleton. Each of these structures must be carefully considered as a facial injury is assessed.

After adequate stabilization and evaluation of the patient, including airway assessment and control of bleeding, and through bony and vascular evaluation with CT scanning if indicated, assessment of the extent of soft tissue injury may be performed. A complete history regarding the circumstances and mechanism of injury is important, along with meticulous inspection of the wound to determine the possible presence of foreign bodies, traumatic tattooing, and special risks of infection. Physical examination must also involve meticulous attention to facial nerve function, facial muscle function, facial sensation, eyelid function, lacrimal system continuity, parotid duct continuity, and potential vascular trauma. Wound cultures may be taken when relevant. Proper documentation of findings is essential before any injury is manipulated, to avoid disagreement regarding the onset of any facial movement or function deficits after repair.

Free margins must be individually assessed for direct involvement or for their proximity to the zone of injury, given the risk of distortion during repair (Fig. 33-1). These areas, including the eyelid margin, the vermilion border of the lip, the alar margin, and the helical margin of the ear, offer little or no resistance to soft tissue forces at the closure line.

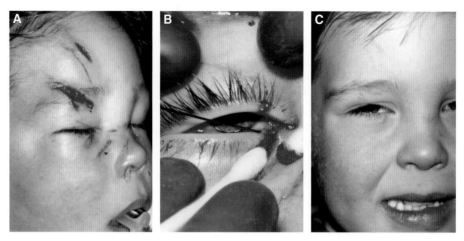

Fig. 33-1 Dog bite injury of the scalp and free margin of the lower eyelid in a child. **A,** Initial presentation. **B,** Lacrimal exploration shows injury of the lacrimal apparatus in association with free margin laceration of the lower eyelid. Meticulous reconstruction and stenting of the lacrimal system ensures proper realignment of this free margin structure. **C,** Result at 3 months postoperatively.

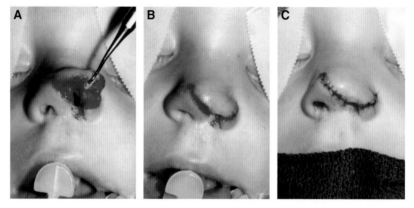

Fig. 33-2 Traumatic laceration of the nose with involvement of the nasal alar free margin. **A,** Acute injury. **B,** Repositioning of the soft tissue avulsion injury. **C,** Reapproximation of free margins with careful attention to the free margin of the alar structures.

When not meticulously realigned and protected from the contractile forces of healing, soft tissue distortion of these margins is common, and secondary revision of these areas may prove difficult or impossible (Fig. 33-2).

Photographic documentation of the injury is essential; a complete record of the extent of injury is necessary not only for the early postoperative management, but also as a reference for future revisional surgery. It is also not uncommon for these injuries to lead to litigation, and photographs may be extremely valuable in clarifying the extent and location of the injury.

Prevention of infection is of paramount importance. A recent review of management strategies following soft tissue injury to the face provides support for routine antibiotic prophylaxis to prevent bacterial infection.[8] Tetanus prophylaxis must also be universally considered. Guidelines for tetanus immunoprophylaxis,

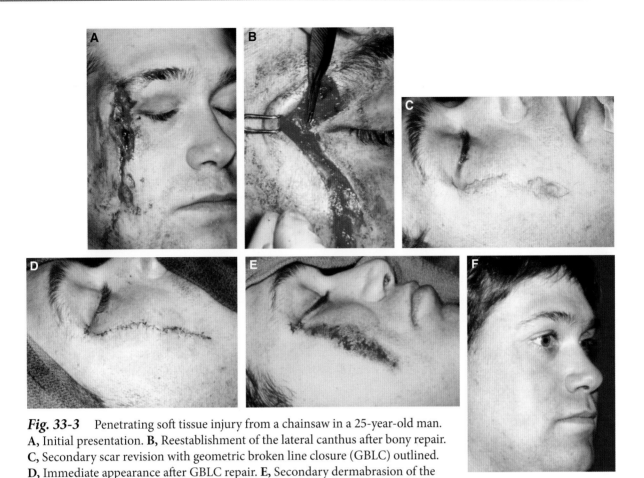

Fig. 33-3   Penetrating soft tissue injury from a chainsaw in a 25-year-old man.
A, Initial presentation. **B,** Reestablishment of the lateral canthus after bony repair.
C, Secondary scar revision with geometric broken line closure (GBLC) outlined.
D, Immediate appearance after GBLC repair. **E,** Secondary dermabrasion of the
scar after 6 weeks. **F,** Final result 1 year after injury.

established by the American College of Surgeons Committee on Trauma, must be adhered to.[9] When there
is concern for herpes simplex reactivation, as in patients who are prone to cold sore outbreaks, antiviral
drugs may decrease the risk of a herpetic outbreak.[10]

If immediate repair of the soft tissue injury is warranted, either local, regional, or general anesthesia is
administered, depending on the clinical circumstances. The repair begins by a close examination of the
wound for any evidence of a foreign body and to make a careful determination of the need for debridement of nonvital tissue. The wound should be scrubbed with an antiseptic solution and irrigated with a
sterile bacitracin solution. Wounds in which significant contamination has occurred may require forceful
irrigation with a 19-gauge catheter.

The length of time from initial injury to treatment is important; the risk of soft tissue infection increases
with the time lapse between injury and proposed repair. However, the head and neck regions have an advantage compared with other parts of the body because of their generous vascular supply, and wounds
in this region may be closed primarily even 12 to 24 hours after the initial injury. In highly contaminated
soft tissue injuries, delayed closure may be the best option. When soft tissue injuries accompany osseous
fractures, repairing the underlying bony injury before completing the soft tissue repair is the standard
procedure (Fig. 33-3).

SPECIFIC TYPES OF INJURY AND MANAGEMENT

ABRASIONS

Abrasions are superficial injuries involving the epidermis and dermis, and they normally heal with local wound care measures. However, failure to carefully remove any foreign material from the dermal layer may result in traumatic tattooing of the soft tissue. This problem can be avoided by vigorous soft tissue cleansing; solvents such as acetone are occasionally necessary to remove grease or oil. After careful wound evaluation and debridement, the abrasion is managed best by application of a topical antibiotic ointment to minimize desiccation and crusting and to optimize rapid reepithelialization. Traumatic tattooing, when it does arise, may be treated secondarily with combination laser therapies, microincision techniques, and camouflaging makeup.[11,12]

BURNS

Although the head and neck compose only 9% of total body surface area, they are a common site for burn injury, and burns of the face, scalp, and neck have a profound long-term impact on an individual's health-related quality of life.[7] Burn injuries can be divided into full-thickness and partial-thickness defects. First-degree burns are limited to the epidermis and cause pain, erythema, and minimal associated tissue loss. These injuries typically heal within 5 to 10 days. Second-degree or deep partial-thickness burns penetrate the dermis and damage the adnexa. These wounds produce severe pain but retain the ability to regenerate epithelium. Second-degree burns usually require 10 to 30 days for complete healing. Third-degree or full-thickness burns result in irreversible damage to the deep dermis of the skin. The area is typically insensate from loss of sensory end-organs. This injury results in secondary scarring and requires a prolonged period of healing, with the possible need for secondary skin grafting.

Initial assessment and treatment of patients who have sustained head and neck burns must include an adequate assessment of the airway. It is not uncommon for patients who have facial burns to have accompanying mucosal injury to the upper and lower respiratory tract. An early tracheostomy may be necessary, although conservative management with intubation for up to 10 days may be appropriate.

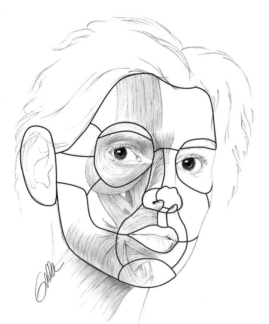

Fig. 33-4   The aesthetic subunits of the face.

The treatment of third-degree head and neck burns should begin with cleaning and debridement of necrotic tissue. Prophylaxis against herpes simplex virus reactivation is indicated.[10] Early excision of burned areas and grafting are currently the treatments of choice. In planning large skin grafts to the face, the concept of *aesthetic units* is an important guide in optimizing outcome (Fig. 33-4). Large grafts that encompass a full aesthetic unit often result in a more satisfactory cosmetic outcome than smaller grafts whose borders do not correspond to aesthetic subunit borders.

Secondary scar contracture, resulting in loss of range of motion, may be minimized by daily passive range of motion exercises and the use of conforming splints. Preserving good range of motion is of particular importance in the neck and along the margin of the mandible.[13] Tissue expanders are sometimes employed in facial burn injuries, because their use will provide a more exact tissue match for the burned area than skin grafts do, and expansion provides enough surface area to adhere to total, rather than partial, facial subunit replacement principles.[14]

LACERATIONS

Lacerations result from sharp injuries to the facial skin and underlying soft tissue. A classification schema that describes laceration injuries by depth, pattern, and associated injury was proposed by Lee et al[15] under the hypothesis that systematic evaluation will lead to more codified treatment algorithms. The depth of penetration should be carefully explored in the acute setting. Specific examination of ductal and neural branch injury must be undertaken so that microsurgical repair of any violated duct or nerve may be executed (see Penetrating Injuries for discussion of management of these injuries). After careful exploration and management of any injury to these structures, the wound should be closed using a multilayered technique. Particular attention should be given to any free margins that may be violated by the laceration.

AVULSION LACERATIONS

In avulsion lacerations, a component of the soft tissue has been elevated as a result of trauma. This type of injury can result in a trapdoor defect, with an avulsed flap of tissue. Trapdoor defects heal in an unpredictable fashion and may produce a pattern of lymphatic and venous obstruction that predispose the area to secondary contour deformities. Several measures in the acute period may be used to minimize the likelihood of this unfavorable sequela. Careful soft tissue handling techniques and meticulous trimming of the margins to viable bleeding edges both encourage proper flattening of the avulsed segment, and a pressure dressing improves the long-term result. Frodel et al[16] described a series of facial avulsion injuries with venous congestion successfully managed with medicinal leech therapy.

Autologous fat transfer has been advocated by some to manage contour deformities associated with facial avulsion injuries, although the application of this technique to the trauma patient must be modified somewhat from that used in the aging face population.[17]

COMPLETE AVULSION INJURIES

It is not uncommon for facial trauma to result in loss of segments of soft tissue. Small areas may be closed by using undermining techniques with primary closure. When primary closure is not possible, other options may be used in the acute setting, including split-thickness skin grafts or local flaps, or the wound can be allowed to heal by secondary intention. After an appropriate period of healing, secondary defects may be managed using delayed soft tissue techniques. However, if free margins are involved, soft tissue coverage with grafts or flaps should be employed as a primary modality, since their use minimizes the likelihood of permanent distortion of these important landmarks (Fig. 33-5).

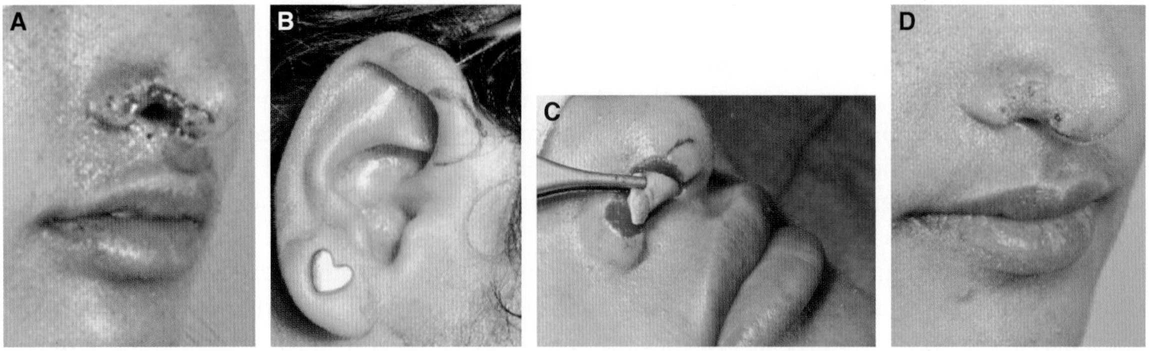

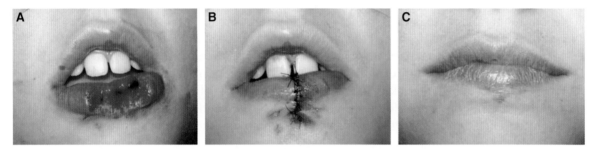

Fig. 33-5   Dog bite injury to the alar margin in an 18-year-old female. No fragment was available for reattachment. **A,** Initial presentation. **B,** Outline of a composite graft to be taken from the right helical root. **C,** Composite graft placed into the defect. **D,** Completed repair, showing preservation of the free alar margin.

Fig. 33-6   **A,** Dog bite injury to the lower lip with extensive tissue loss of the lower lip structures. **B,** Primary closure using advancement mucosal techniques, followed by appropriate antibiotic coverage. **C,** Result 6 months postoperatively.

Animal and Human Bites

Dog bites account for approximately 80% of the animal bites seen in emergency departments. Children are particularly susceptible to these injuries, and the midfacial area is most commonly affected.[18] Animal bite wounds are typically polymicrobial; alpha-hemolytic streptococci and *Staphylococcus aureus* are the most common contaminating aerobes. Frequently found anaerobic organisms include *Bacteroides* and *Fusobacterium.* For management of an animal bite to the face, the surgeon should employ basic surgical principles, including liberal irrigation and meticulous primary closure (Fig. 33-6). If the bite is more than 12 hours old, it may be advantageous to delay primary closure for 4 to 7 days. Broad-spectrum antibiotic coverage is recommended in this setting. If the bite results in a complete avulsion injury, a composite graft may be required to properly address the defect and prevent free margin distortion (see Fig. 33-5).

Human bites yield a higher incidence of soft tissue infection. In contrast to animal bites, which tend to be located in the central aspect of the face, the lips and auricles are common sites for human bite injuries. The most common organisms cultured from human bite injuries are alpha-hemolytic *Staphyloccocus* and *Bacteroides.* If the wound is managed in the acute phase, it is best to attempt primary closure. However, if there has been a delay longer than 12 hours in the repair, secondary closure using delay techniques is advisable. Broad-spectrum antibiotic coverage is recommended as well as topical antibiotic ointment. Human bites involving cartilaginous structures of the face are managed best with parenteral antibiotics and require multistep reconstructive interventions (see Chapters 23 and 24).

Penetrating Injuries

Penetrating wounds to the face may harbor elusive but devastating injuries, including traumatic arteriovenous fistulas, duct transection, and neural injury. Penetrating injuries commonly result from detonation of improvised explosive devices (IED) in war zones and during terrorist activity. These pose a high risk of airway compromise and vascular injury and require evaluation at a level I trauma center based on the risk of life-threatening damage.[19]

In a stable patient in whom the airway has been managed and vascular injury either ruled out or treated, any penetrating injury in the midface must be assessed for parotid duct and lacrimal duct continuity. Parotid duct lacerations, if unrepaired, result in a persistent parotid duct fistula or sialocele. When identified, parotid duct injuries require repair in the operating room under microscopic guidance. The lacerated edges of the duct should be anastomosed using microsurgical techniques over a stent (Fig. 33-7).

Penetrating soft tissue injuries of the head and neck commonly involve peripheral cranial nerves, including facial nerve injuries (Fig. 33-8). Early and aggressive exploration of these wounds, with identification and repair of the proximal and distal nerve stumps under microscopic magnification, promotes the likelihood of satisfactory recovery of facial movement.

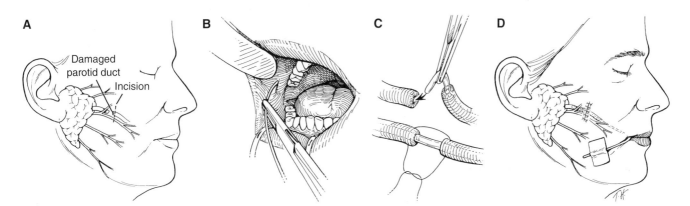

Fig. 33-7   **A,** Laceration overlying the parotid duct. **B,** To identify the distal segment of the parotid duct, the orifice is stented with Silastic tubing. **C,** Silastic tubing is threaded through the distal duct and is used as a stent to provide continuity between the lacerated segments of the duct. The duct should be reapproximated with 9-0 nylon. **D,** The Silastic stent is draped through the duct to the oral commissure and left in position for 2 to 3 weeks.

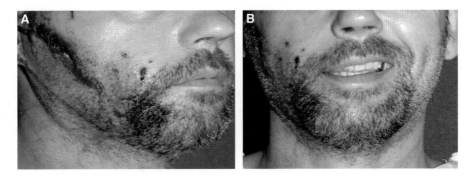

Fig. 33-8   This 40-year-old man sustained a penetrating injury to the right cheek when a grinding wheel shattered and a fragment was lodged against the main trunk of his right facial nerve. **A,** Initial presentation. **B,** Patient smiling, with nasolabial fold effacement and lack of oral commissure movement.

Continued

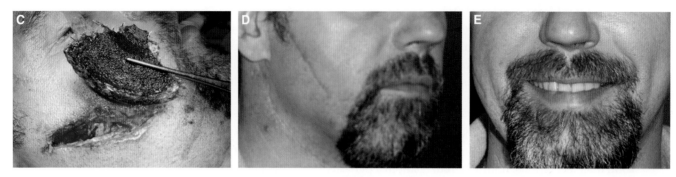

Fig. 33-8, cont'd   **C,** Intraoperative photograph of a fragment of grinding wheel removed through the laceration. The facial nerve was contused but not severed. **D,** Scar appearance after 4 months. **E,** The patient gained return of normal facial nerve function.

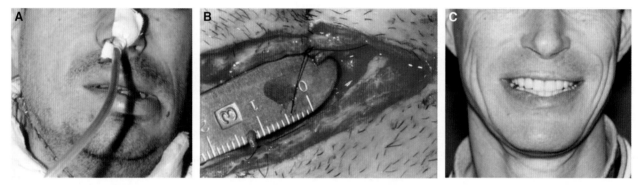

Fig. 33-9   **A,** Laceration of the upper neck from a knife wound, resulting in a defect of the marginal mandibular nerve. Note the lack of depressor action of the right lower lip. **B,** Lacerated ends of the marginal nerve are identified and stimulated. The nerve margins are freshened and reapproximated with 10-0 nylon suture. **C,** Return of lip depressor function after 6 months.

In many cases the damaged nerve may be repaired by simple mobilization of the nerve divisions and reapproximation with microsurgical techniques (Fig. 33-9). Occasionally a cable graft is required if the injury has resulted in significant tissue loss. The discontinuous nerve endings should be judiciously debrided at both the proximal and distal stumps to eliminate any devitalized tissue and freshen the proximal stump for axonal sprouting. Sometimes the distal stump of the nerve is easier to identify based on the retention of stimulability for up to 72 hours after transection; however, the proximal stump cannot be found even under microsurgical magnification.

In cases involving the facial nerve, the main trunk of the nerve is identified using standard landmarks, and an anterograde dissection toward the open wound is executed until the transected edge is identified

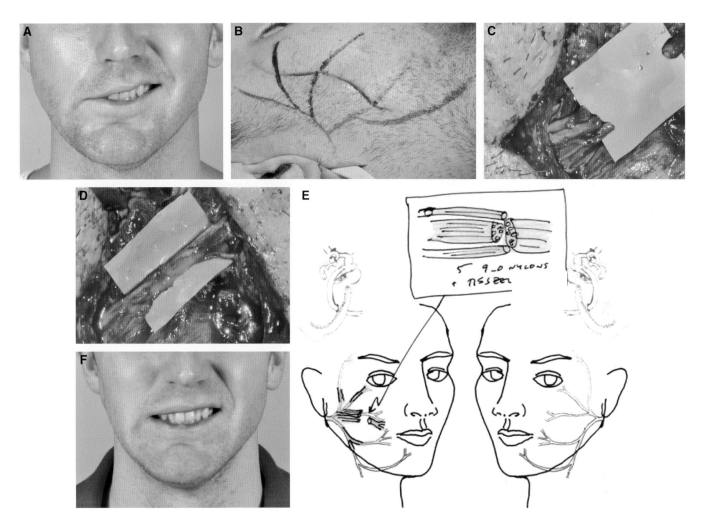

Fig. 33-10   Extensive facial laceration from a stab injury. **A,** Patient smiling with right facial weakness. **B,** The expected location of the facial nerve branches are drawn in purple. **C,** Severed ends of the facial nerve. **D,** Microsurgical repair. **E,** Operative drawing depicting the operative details. **F,** Final result with the patient smiling 6 months postoperatively.

so that neural coaptation to the distal stump can take place (Fig. 33-10). Soft tissue repair is accomplished after the peripheral nerve has been adequately recoapted.

Blunt Trauma

Blunt trauma may result from falls, motor vehicle accidents, blows to the face with a blunt object, and from recreational activities such as sports, paintball, and other target-oriented events.[2-4,20] Contusions manifest with swelling and ecchymosis and occasionally significant hematoma formation. In general, once bony and other structural injuries are ruled out or managed, conservative contusion management with topical application of ice to decrease edema is adequate treatment. However, hematomas, when identified, require

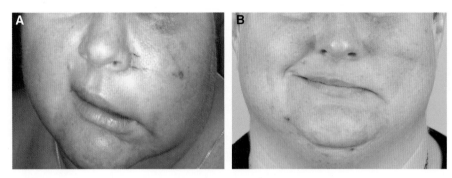

Fig. 33-11   A blunt trauma injury with facial muscle disinsertion. **A,** The patient is seen several days after a fall in which he struck a coffee table with his left cheek. Note the ecchymosis and facial weakness. No skin broach occurred. **B,** Five months later, with appreciable facial weakness corresponding to zygomaticus major disinsertion.

immediate drainage. If not evacuated, these collections can lead to abscess formation, excessive stretching of the facial soft tissue and musculature, and may even lead to disinsertion of the muscles from their attachments (Fig. 33-11). Pigmentary changes and secondary subcutaneous atrophy are not uncommon in these types of wounds, and cases of posttraumatic lipoma formation have been described.[21]

GUNSHOT WOUNDS

Gunshot wounds to the head and neck area require careful evaluation and management of the airway, vascular structures, and soft tissue. It is not uncommon for associated bony defects to be incurred from gunshot wounds. CT scanning is the imaging modality of choice for comprehensive assessment. Airway compromise is the most immediate threat to life and is always addressed emergently. After the airway is stabilized, if necessary, vascular injuries are best managed with angiography and embolization for control, and the soft tissue component may be managed conservatively, without immediate repair.[22] Both entry and exit wounds should be carefully evaluated; the exit wounds often produce significant tissue destruction and may require acute debridement. A recent study of wartime facial blast injuries supports the concept of aggressive debridement back to bleeding tissue. A switch from the standard practice of conservative debridement to aggressive debridement with primary closure resulted in a tenfold decline in the wound infection rate.[23]

Traumatic tattoos that result from gunshot wounds may be treated with laser therapy. However, for wounds incurred at close range, cases have been described in which laser heat ignited the powder fragments, triggering microexplosions of the powder and additional soft tissue trauma.[24] Therefore caution must be exercised when dealing with close-range wounds with retained gunpowder tattooing.

POSTOPERATIVE CONSIDERATIONS

Soft tissue injuries require careful attention in the acute setting but also require meticulous postoperative care and follow-up to optimize outcome. The wound should be monitored closely in the early phase of healing to determine whether any early intervention may minimize scar contracture and/or hypertrophic scarring. Local flaps and grafts may be necessary to maximize the long-term outcome. In addition, local steroid injections may prevent hypertrophic scarring in specific situations, such as in a highly mobile facial zone like the lip, or in a patient known to form keloids. Facial scars mature over a 12- to 18-month period, and then may require further management with delayed techniques (see Chapter 34).

Key Points

- The psychological impact of facial scarring and its effect on an individual's quality of life is substantial.
- Soft tissue injuries of the face may involve skin, hair-bearing structures, subcutaneous tissues, ducts, nerves, vessels, and the underlying bone.
- After airway stabilization and control of bleeding, meticulous assessment of facial muscle function, sensation, and parotid and lacrimal duct function must be performed and documented.
- Infection is avoided by prophylactic administration of antibiotics, prevention of herpes simplex reactivation, tetanus prophylaxis, and debridement of devitalized tissue.
- Free margin alignment is critical to the aesthetic outcome.
- Facial burns are best treated using a facial subunit concept to replace entire units with grafts or tissue expansion.
- Avulsion injuries may develop lymphatic and venous congestion.
- Gunshot wounds and penetrating trauma may cause traumatic vascular injury, which is best treated with angiography and embolization.

REFERENCES

1. Fasola AO, Obiechina AE, Arotiba JT. Soft tissue injuries of the face: a 10 year review. Afr J Med Sci 29:59-62, 2000.
2. Deits J, Yard EE, Collins CL, et al. Patients with ice hockey injuries presenting to US emergency departments, 1990-2006. J Athl Train 45:467-474, 2010.
3. Crow RW. Diagnosis and management of sports-related injuries to the face. Dent Clin North Am 35:719-732, 1991.
4. McGregor JC. Soft tissue facial injuries in sport (excluding the eye). J R Coll Surg Edinb 39:76-82, 1994.
5. Mammen L, Norton SA. Facial scarification and tattooing on Santa Catalina Island (Solomon Islands). Cutis 60:197-198, 1997.
6. Levine E, Degutis L, Pruzinsky T, et al. Quality of life and facial trauma: psychological and body image effects. Ann Plast Surg 54:502-510, 2005.
7. Warner P, Stubbs TK, Kagan RJ, et al. The effect of facial burns on health outcomes in children aged 5 to 18 years. J Trauma Acute Care Surg 73(3 Suppl 2):S189-S196, 2012.
8. Abubaker AO. Use of prophylactic antibiotics in preventing infection of traumatic injuries. Dent Clin North Am 53:707-715, 2009.
9. Hetzler DC, Hilsinger RL. The otolaryngologist and tetanus. Otolaryngol Head Neck Surg 95:511-515, 1986.
10. Haik J, Weissman O, Stavrou D, et al. Is prophylactic acyclovir treatment warranted for prevention of herpes simplex virus infections in facial burns? A review of the literature. J Burn Care Res 32:358-362, 2011.
11. Sun B, Guan WW. Treating traumatic tattoo by micro-incision. Chin Med J (Engl) 113:670-671, 2000.
12. Martins A, Trindade F, Leite L. Facial scars after a road accident—combined treatment with pulsed dye laser and Q-switched Nd-YAG laser. J Cosmet Dermatol 7:227-229, 2008.
13. Gonzales-Ulloa M. Reconstruction of the face covering by means of selective skin in regional aesthetic units. Br J Plast Surg 9:212-221, 1956.
    Strong introduction to the concept of regional subunits in the face.
14. Khalatbari B, Bakhshaeekia A. Ten-year experience in face and neck unit reconstruction using tissue expanders. Burns 39:522-527, 2013.
15. Lee RH, Gamble WB, Robertson B, et al. The MCFONTZL classification system for soft tissue injuries to the face. Plast Reconstr Surg 103:1150-1157, 1999.
16. Frodel JL, Barth P, Wagner J. Salvage of partial facial soft tissue avulsions with medicinal leeches. Otolaryngol Head Neck Surg 131:934-939, 2004.

17. Lam SM. Fat transfer for the management of soft tissue trauma: the do's and the don'ts. Facial Plast Surg 26:488-493, 2010.

18. Horswell BB, Chahine CJ. Dog bites of the face, head and neck in children. W V Med J 107:24-27, 2011.

19. Maier H, Tisch M, Lorenz KJ, et al. [Penetrating injuries in the face and neck region. Diagnosis and treatment] HNO 59:765-782, 2011.

20. Sbicca JA, Hatch RL. Target lesions and other paintball injuries. J Am Board Fam Med 25:124-127, 2012.

21. Aust MC, Spies M, Kall S, et al. Lipomas after blunt soft tissue trauma: are they real? Analysis of 31 cases. Br J Dermatol 157:92-99, 2007.

22. McLean JN, Moore CE, Yellin SA. Gunshot wounds to the face—acute management. Facial Plast Surg 21:191-198, 2005.

Review of the English language literature regarding gunshot wounds and their acute management.

23. Shvyrkov MB, Yanushevich OO. Facial gunshot wound debridement: debridement of facial soft tissue gunshot wounds. J Craniomaxillofac Surg 4:e8-e16, 2013.

24. Fusade T, Toubel G, Grognard C, et al. Treatment of gunpowder traumatic tattoo by Q-switched Nd:YAG laser: an unusual adverse effect. Dermatol Surg 26:1057-1059, 2000.

34

Scar Revision

Callum Faris ▪ *Hadé Vuyk*

Scars cannot be completely eliminated with current approaches, but revision, irregularization, resurfacing, and repositioning strategies have led to dramatic improvements in aesthetic outcomes for scarring. The word *scar* is derived from the Latin *eschara,* which means "scab." The *Oxford Dictionary* defines a scar as "a mark left on the skin or within body tissue where a wound, burn, or sore has not healed completely and fibrous connective tissue has developed." A scar results from damage to the skin that involves the mid and deeper dermis. Wounds injuring only the epithelium and superficial dermis tend to heal without long-term scarring.

A crude form of dermabrasion to treat prominent scars existed in the early twentieth century,[1] but was popularized by Kurtin in the 1950s.[2] The origins of Z-plasty are less clear, with Horner being credited with describing the first Z-shaped incision incorporating the use of a single transposition flap in 1837.[3]

Double Z designs emerged later, with McCurdy's description in 1898[4]; however, it was not until 1904 that Berger described what we would consider a Z-plasty in the modern era.[5] Borges composed a landmark text in 1959, which is considered the basis of modern scar revision; it included a case of a W-plasty.[6] The geometric broken line was added by Webster in 1969.[7] Neumann was the first to describe the modern use of tissue expansion in reconstruction in the 1950s,[8] followed by the introduction of the CO_2 laser in the 1960s by Kumar Patel of Bell Laboratories. It was 40 years later (after refinements in laser technologies) that Manstein[9] developed fractional photothermolysis in 2004.

WOUND HEALING

There are three main phases to wound healing: inflammatory, proliferative, and remodeling/maturation[10] (see Chapter 4 for a comprehensive discussion).

In the remodeling phase, success depends on a balance of synthesis and lysis.[11] Aberrations in this phase of collagen formation result in abnormal healing. A deficiency will result in prolonged healing and poor scar tensile strength (such as in malnutrition). Conversely, an excess of collagen results in hypertrophic scarring (with the scar limited to the wound area) or keloid formation (with the scar extending beyond wound edge; Fig. 34-1). Ordinarily, neovascularization will progressively fade, and the accompanying erythema will resolve. The final state of healing is achieved after approximately 1 year. A scar will ultimately reach 80% of the tensile strength of normal skin.[12]

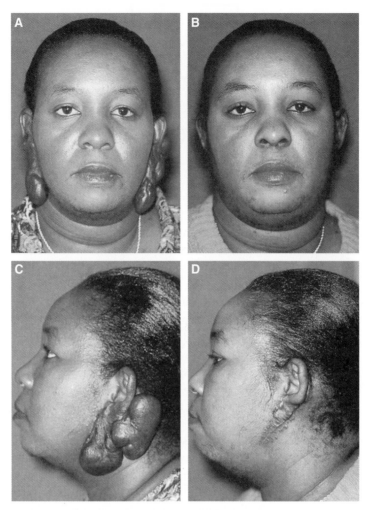

Fig. 34-1   This patient had large keloids of the auricle that had been excised four previous times. She underwent preoperative preparation with Kenalog-40, excision, and low-dose radiation of 500 rads in the postoperative period.

PATHOGENESIS OF POOR SCAR FORMATION

There are several common factors that lead to poor wound healing and scar formation: tissue infection, inflammation, ischemia, foreign bodies, and traumatic tissue handling.[13] These unfavorable wound bed factors exacerbate the degree of injury by maintaining the wound in the proliferation second stage and stopping progression to the third stage of matrix remodeling scar formation. These factors increase the risk of scar contracture or hypertrophic scarring.

Orientation and geometry factors can also lead to poor scar formation. Poor scar orientation or geometry can lead to poor lymphatic drainage and edema. Curved circular scars can lead to pin-cushioning, and failure to anticipate potential deformities arising from scar contracture across concave or mobile surfaces also predisposes to disfigurement. The overall length and geometry of the laceration can lead to poor scar formation, even if the wound itself has healed optimally. Traumatic wounds, especially from blunt or crush injuries, often involve diffuse surrounding areas of soft tissue destruction that result in poor scarring. Mobile areas of the face are at higher risk for scars. Most of these factors are beyond the surgeon's control.

Table 34-1   Characteristics of Scars

	Age	Risk Factors	Symptoms	Color	Size	Natural History
Immature scar	Any age	Not applicable	Not applicable	Red raised	Within confines of wound	Spontaneous resolution
Hypertrophic	Young	Tension, infection	Pruritic, painful	Red raised	Within confines of wound	Spontaneous resolution; may be prolonged and require treatment
Keloid	Peak <30	FH, higher Fitzpatrick skin types V and VI Genetic AD	Pruritic, burning, painful	Red raised	Extends beyond wound borders	Rarely resolves spontaneously

Data from Panuncialman J, Falanga V. The science of wound bed preparation. Clin Plast Surg 34:621-632, 2007.
FH, Family history; *AD,* autosomal dominant.

ABERRATIONS OF NORMAL SCAR FORMATION: FIBROPROLIFERATIVE LESIONS

Hypertrophic scarring and keloid formation result from aberrations of the normal wound-healing process. Both phenomena result from an increase in collagen synthesis, deposition, and accumulation, but their exact pathogenesis is not well understood. Historically, the two processes have been classified separately, although they are caused by similar pathobiologic processes (Table 34-1). There are many situations in which a scar has elements of both keloid and hypertrophic scarring.[14] It has been suggested that a continuum exists between the two conditions.[15] In the early stages of scar development, it may be difficult to distinguish a hypertrophic scar from a potential keloid. Key differences are that after several months a keloid scar will continue to extend beyond the original site of injury and become irritable, and its surface tends to round and become smoother.[16]

Hypertrophic scars arise most frequently from excessive tension across the wound, and are red, pruritic, and often painful. They are limited to the confines of the wound, and rarely exhibit more than 4 mm of elevation from the skin surface. A hypertrophic scar will usually flatten gradually, although the process may take months to more than a year. Histologically, hypertrophic scars demonstrate fibrillary collagen bundles parallel to the skin surface with an absence of elastin. Myofibroblasts are present with normal fibroblasts and mast cells, which gives rise to pruritus.

Keloid scarring is far more common in patients with higher Fitzpatrick skin types and occurs in up to 16% of Afro-Caribbean patients. There are varying reports of autosomal and autosomal dominant patterns of inheritance.[17,18] In susceptible individuals, keloids tend to occur in particular areas, including the shoulder, sternum, and earlobe, often after minor injury.[19] The hallmark of keloid scarring is invasion; the advancing edge of the fibroproliferative lesion extends beyond the boundaries of the wound. Histologically, the lesion has thickened eosinophilic collagen bands, often with an absence of elastin. Keloids are highly vascular, with few myofibroblasts and atypical fibroblasts (enlarged nuclei) and mast cells.[20]

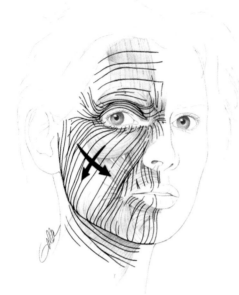

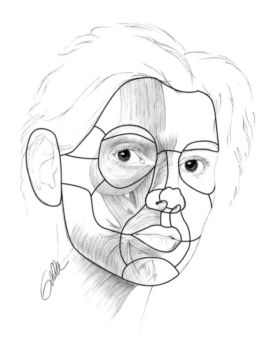

Fig. 34-2   Facial RSTLs. These lines roughly conform to the observed facial rhytids that occur with facial aging. The lines of maximal extension always fall perpendicular to the RSTLs.

Fig. 34-3   Facial subunits.

CHARACTERISTICS OF AN IDEAL SCAR

Scars cannot be eliminated but may be improved with proper manipulation and care. The ideal scar should be thin, level, and placed within the relaxed skin tension lines (RSTLs) (Fig. 34-2) or borders of anatomic subunits (Fig. 34-3). Care should be taken to not disturb facial landmarks.[21] Under certain circumstances it is appropriate to intentionally deviate from these principles to increase scar camouflage. Understanding how to apply scar management principles, and when it is appropriate to deviate from them, is somewhat of an art, and represents an interesting challenge for a facial reconstructive surgeon.

OPTIMIZING A SCAR

Basic wound management, including proper tissue handling and suture techniques, cannot be overemphasized. Prevention of poor scar formation is uniformly preferable to scar revision. Surgical strategies of paramount importance include meticulous technique, gentle handling of tissue, sharp anatomical dissection, meticulous hemostasis, removal of necrotic tissue, obliteration of dead space, orientation along RSTLs, and minimization of wound closure tension. Wound closure should be performed under aseptic

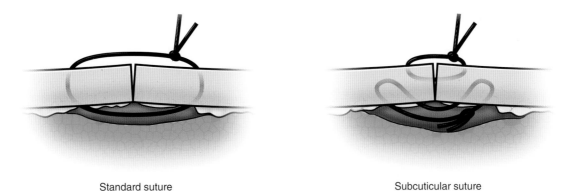

Standard suture   Subcuticular suture

Fig. 34-4   Comparison between standard and subcuticular everting sutures. Subcuticular everting sutures are preferred to attain more favorable eversion.

conditions with sharp dissection and gentle handling of tissue to minimize further tissue trauma. In traumatic wounds, cleansing the wound appropriately with copious normal saline is paramount. Debriding devitalized tissue and reducing foreign body contamination help to eliminate factors that predispose to poor wound healing. Surgical wound edges should be freshened to make them linear, with the blade held perpendicular or beveled outward to promote skin eversion, thus decreasing the likelihood of a depressed scar. A balance must be struck between debridement of questionable tissue and the creation of an excessive tissue defect requiring adjunctive techniques to achieve a tension-free closure. In all cases, atraumatic undermining should be performed in the immediate subdermal plane (leaving at least 1 to 2 mm fat on the undersurface) to reduce tension on the wound edges and to permit skin eversion. The surgeon should approximate the dermis with absorbable sutures, using a subcuticular buried everting technique with vertical mattress sutures, which greatly promotes wound eversion (Fig. 34-4).

A recent meta-analysis of randomized, controlled trials that compared the cosmetic outcomes and complications of traumatic lacerations and surgical incisions closed with absorbable sutures versus nonabsorbable sutures failed to demonstrate a clear benefit of nonabsorbable sutures over absorbable sutures.[22] The aim is to achieve tension-free skin closure with everted wound edges and minimal iatrogenic skin trauma. The presence of any dead space below the wound must be obliterated to reduce the likelihood of seroma formation, which frequently results in excessive fibrosis and scar retraction.

Several incision planning variables promote ideal scar formation. For best results, incisions should be placed in the RSTLs, which are perpendicular to the lines of maximal extensibility and muscles of facial expression. Placement of incisions in these lines maximally reduces tension across the wound, which in turn minimizes scar widening in the postoperative phase. Since rhytids tend to follow the RSTLs, linear incisions along these lines may be camouflaged within natural rhytids.

Tissue deficiency, either cutaneous or deep, is one of the most common reasons for poor wound healing and poor scar formation. Tissue deficiency will lead to excess tension across the wound and result in increased risk of hypertrophic and widened scar formation. In cases in which cutaneous tissue loss results from tumor excision or trauma, a surgeon generally must decide to (1) close the wound primarily with increased tension over the wound edges and risk hypertrophic scarring, (2) recruit more tissue from adjacent tissue reservoirs through skin flap movement or tissue expansion, or (3) allow the area to heal by secondary intention. Although this latter strategy can produce good cosmetic outcomes in concave areas on the face, it rarely produces optimal results in scars greater than 2 cm.[23]

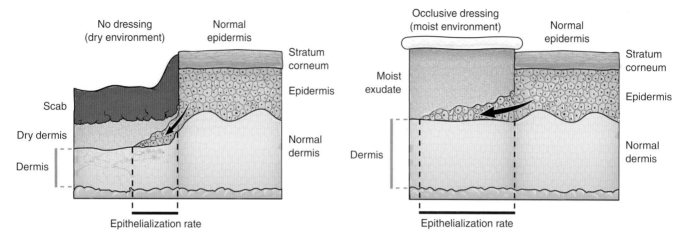

Fig. 34-5   Wound bed environment factors. Keeping the wound bed moist encourages reepithelialization and helps prevent depressed scar formation.

Table 34-2   Dressings and Their Characteristics

Dressing Type/Material	Moisture Vapor Transmission Rate	Properties/Use
Polyurethane film	300-800	No absorptive capacity Not for infected wounds Not for heavily exudative wounds
Absorptive wound fillers (calcium alginate)	800-5000	Highly absorptive Hemostatic
Gauze	1200	Heavily exudative wounds

Data from Panuncialman J, Falanga V. The science of wound bed preparation. Clin Plast Surg 34:621-632, 2007.

WOUND BED FACTORS

The aim of wound management is to create optimal conditions for reepithelialization. Studies have shown that a moist wound bed will increase the rate of epithelialization by up to 100%.[24] If wound moisture is not maintained, the wound bed will dry and scab. The epithelium will migrate beneath the scab, with loss of dermis increasing the risk of poor scar formation and a depressed scar[25,26] (Fig. 34-5).

Occlusive or semiocclusive dressings are helpful in increasing wound bed moisture; however, excess moisture can present a problem in heavily exudative wounds. In such wounds, exudate must be wicked away by the dressing to prevent wound maceration, seroma, and infection. Ideal wound bed conditions are maintained by matching the dressing to the degree of exudate being produced.[27] Dressings that maintain a moist wound environment are described as being moisture retentive. This property is measured by the moisture vapor transmission rate (MVTR). A dressing is moisture retentive when its MVTR is less than 840 g/m^2/24 hr. The MVTR is therefore a guide for prescribing dressings, depending on whether one wants to create a moist healing environment or whether the primary goal is control of heavy exudate[28] (Table 34-2).

ADJUNCT MEASURES TO PREVENT POOR SCAR FORMATION

SILICONE GEL

A Cochrane review showed only weak evidence for the benefits of using silicone gel sheeting as prevention for abnormal scarring in high-risk individuals.[29] More recent animal studies suggest that silicone dressings do have some positive effects on wound healing.[30]

The most widely accepted mechanism for the success of gel sheeting in prevention of abnormal scarring is the increase in hydration of the wound, which is caused by occlusion.[31] The use of silicone gel sheeting should begin soon after surgical closure, after the incision has fully epithelialized. It must be applied for at least 12 hours a day with twice-daily washing, for a minimum of 6 months and up to 2 years.[32]

BOTULINUM TOXIN

Decreased wound tension is advantageous and results in improved scar cosmesis. Overall wound tension is a product of static and dynamic tension across the wound. Static tension results from stretching tissue to overcome tissue deficiency during wound closure and does not vary after skin closure. Dynamic tension results from the action of mimetic facial muscles during facial expression, which increases tension across the wound. If chemodenervation is used at the time of wound closure, dynamic tension may be eliminated and cosmesis improved in the immobilized scar. This manipulation has improved scar outcome in animal models and in one randomized controlled trial studying the effects of botulinum toxin in traumatic forehead lacerations or elective excisions of forehead masses.[33,34]

PREVENTION OF ABNORMAL SCARRING

Factors that reduce the risk of abnormal healing and poor scar formation[12,32,33,35,36] are listed in Box 34-1.

Box 34-1   Prevention of Abnormal Scarring

- Avoid excessive movements that stretch the wound.
- Avoid direct stretching of the wound.
- Use taping and consider gel sheeting.
- Keep the wound clean by irrigation and the use of antibacterial lotions.
- Remove sutures in a timely fashion.
- Consider using botulinum toxin to immobilize the tissue.

TREATMENT OF ESTABLISHED KELOID AND HYPERTROPHIC SCARRING

Various treatments are available for both keloids and hypertrophic scars. The treatments for hypertrophic scarring include silicone sheeting, corticosteroid injection, pressure therapy, excisional techniques, and radiotherapy. The treatment of keloid scars involves similar therapies, but generally requires combinations of these strategies. A recent meta-analysis of 70 studies using single and combined modality therapy showed that overall there was a mean improvement of 60% following any intervention.[37] Several authors have suggested treatment algorithms for keloids and hypertrophic scars.[32,35,36] However, no uniform, widely accepted consensus exists for treatment.

EXCISION

Simple excision of hypertrophic scars without addressing the underlying causative factor often leads to recurrence. Simple excision of keloid scars has resulted in recurrence rates of 45% to 100%.[19,32] Intralesional excision of a hypertrophic scar has been shown by one investigator to lead to a higher rate of improvement, 77% versus 25%.[38] Conversely, for surgical management of keloids, Tan et al evaluated margin status (complete versus incomplete excision) and have quoted recurrence rates of 25% to 80% compared with 10% to 35% when the leading edge was included in the specimen.[39]

For hypertrophic scarring, some authors[35] have recommended tension-releasing techniques such as Z-plasty or W-plasty. However, if hypertrophic scarring recurs after the use of such tension-releasing techniques, a visually inferior scar may result. Therefore alternative nonsurgical techniques (such as corticosteroid, silicone, or pulsed dye laser) may be more appropriate for linear hypertrophic scarring.

Attempts to reduce inflammation and aberrant healing should be pursued in both keloids and hypertrophic scars. The use of minimally reactive sutures such as monofilament Monocryl for deep sutures and Prolene for skin are appropriate.

CORTICOSTEROID THERAPY

The effectiveness of corticosteroids in the treatment of hypertrophic and keloid scarring is thought to be a consequence of reduction of the inflammatory response, and of diminished collagen synthesis through inhibition of fibroblast proliferation. A general consensus is that injected triamcinolone is efficacious as first-line therapy for the treatment of keloids, and as second-line therapy for the treatment of hypertrophic scars (after silicone sheeting).[32] Some keloid and hypertrophic scars respond well to monotherapy with intralesional steroids (recurrence rates are 9% to 50%).[32,40] Side effects that are associated with steroid use include telangiectasia, hypopigmentation, and atrophy; these occur in over 50% of cases.[41,42] Results may be improved when corticosteroids are combined with other therapies, such as surgery.[36,43,44] Other positive effects of steroid combination therapies are a reduction in the necessary steroid dose, which can improve the side effect profile.[41,45]

FLUOROURACIL

Fluorouracil (5-FU) inhibits fibroblastic activity and reduces transforming growth factor beta (TGF-β), an important cytokine in abnormal scarring. It is an established treatment for keloid and hypertrophic scarring and is often used in conjunction with other modalities. It has a low side effect profile that includes minor erythema and pigmentation changes, and is generally well tolerated. Its use involves the cumbersome precautions of cytostatic therapy and difficulties in patient education and consent for use in a benign condition.

Intralesional 5-FU as a monotherapy has been shown in a small study to have equivalent effectiveness to intralesional corticosteroid or pulsed dye laser, or a combination of 5-FU and intralesional corticosteroid.[41] More promising outcomes have been shown for combination therapy with 5-FU with other modalities; combination therapy with 5-FU and corticosteroids (or 5-FU with corticosteroids and pulsed dye laser) is effective and appears synergistic.[45,46] A trial of surgical excision with adjuvant 5-FU outperformed surgery with silicone sheeting by 75%, compared with 43% for keloid-free recurrence.[47]

Despite the data reported in various studies, an optimal modality for keloids and hypertrophic scarring has not yet been identified. Combinations of established therapies and emerging therapies seem the most likely future direction for reducing recurrence rate while also reducing treatment morbidity.

HISTORY AND PATIENT ANALYSIS

The importance of a thorough history cannot be overstated, including details of the original trauma or surgery and any prior treatment and unsuccessful attempts at scar revision. Patient factors such as medications (for example, Accutane, anticoagulants, and immunosuppressive agents), diabetes, and smoking may adversely affect further revisions.

SCAR ANALYSIS

It must be determined whether a scar is at an early, evolving stage or whether it is mature. The surgeon must systematically assess what it is about the scar that is unsightly, bearing in mind that the ideal scar should be thin, level with no contour deformity or step-off, and within the RSTLs or borders of anatomic subunits.[21] The patient should be asked whether the scar causes pain or pruritus or limits function or normal social functioning. Working methodically through these characteristics can help to systematize an approach to scar revision (Table 34-3).

Table 34-3   Prevention of Abnormal Scarring

	Ideal	Nonideal
Timing	Early (some improvement still possible)	Late (likely chronic)
Color	Normal pigment match	Erythematous
Width	Narrow	Wide, >1-2 mm
Contour	Flush	Depressed, raised
Length	Short	Long linear scar, complex scar (stellate)
Alopecia	Not present	Associated hair loss
Orientation to RSTLs or BOAS	Scar parallel to RSTLs or in BOAS	Scar not parallel to RSTLs or outside BOAS
Tissue deficiency superficial	Not present	Yes
Tissue deficiency deep	Not present	Yes
Distortion of landmark through scar contracture or misalignment	Not present	Contracture, distortion, notching

BOAS, Border of the aesthetic subunit; *RSTLs,* relaxed skin tension lines.

Table 34-4   Scar Scoring Systems

	Patient and Observer Scar Assessment Scale (POSAS)	Vancouver Scar Scale (VSS)
Vascularity	1-10	0-3
Pigmentation	1-10	0-3
Pliability	1-10	0-3
Height/relief	1-10	0-3
Thickness	1-10	–
Painful (P)	1-10	–
Itching (P)	1-10	–
Color (P)	1-10	–
Stiffness (P)	1-10	–
Thickness (P)	1-10	–
Irregular (P)	1-10	–

Data from Draaijers LJ, Tempelman FR, Botman YA, et al. The Patient and Observer Scar Assessment Scale: a reliable and feasible tool for scar evaluation. Plast Reconstr Surg 113:1960-1965; discussion 1966-1967, 2004; and Sullivan T, Smith J, Kermode J, et al. Rating the burn scar. J Burn Care Rehabil 11:256-260, 1990.
(P) denotes score graded by patient.

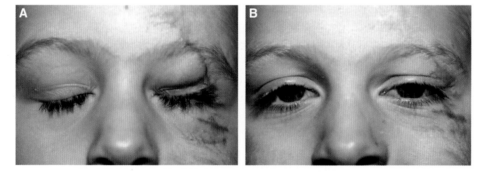

Fig. 34-6   Scar response to simple massage and observation. **A,** An early scar with tethering of the anterior and/or middle lamella scarring resulting in a degree of lagophthalmos. **B,** A conservative approach was undertaken with manual upper eyelid massage, and the tethering resolved over the next 2 months.

There are various scoring systems that are used in grading scars. Two common scales are the Patient and Observer Scar Assessment Scale (POSAS) and the Vancouver Scar Scale (VSS).[48,49] The scale was originally designed for burn scars and encompasses limited characteristics[48,49] (Table 34-4). POSAS is the more comprehensive scale.[48] This scale is most frequently employed and is recommended because it takes into account the most important aspect of scar analysis, the patient's perspective.[50]

Timing

Ideally, 1 year should pass before scar revision is contemplated. Simple observation results in a more pleasing outcome for even quite unaesthetic immature scars (Fig. 34-6). There are, however, some indications for early intervention. If gross distortion of an anatomical landmark is causing functional issues or severe cosmetic deformity that prevents normal social functioning, earlier intervention is warranted. Other examples include lower eyelid cicatricial ectropion causing ocular irritation, and lip tethering causing oral incompetence.

Color

A scar should have a good pigment match to the tissues surrounding it. However, as the scar progresses through the healing phase from an immature scar, it will change in color from more erythematous to more normally pigmented. In mature scars, hyperpigmentation is more common in Fitzpatrick skin types that are higher than IV, but may occur in lower skin types if there is excessive sun exposure in the first 6 months after injury.

Persistent erythema during the earlier phases of wound healing may indicate infection, whereas erythema that is present in the mature phases suggests an abnormality of wound remodeling, such as hypertrophic scarring or keloid formation. It is often difficult to predict whether an immature scar (one that has erythema and is raised and itchy) will resolve or develop into a hypertrophic scar. If erythema persists beyond 1 month (especially if present with pruritus and pain), the risk of true hypertrophy increases, and therapeutic intervention should be considered (such as corticosteroid injections, silicone sheeting, or pulsed dye laser therapy).[32]

Width

Wide scars result from excessive tension across the wound, or a wound that has healed by secondary intention. This scar characteristic should alert the surgeon to tissue deficiency or poor surgical technique applied in the primary operation. Nonsurgical techniques are not suited to decreasing the width of these scars. It is essential to assess the vectors of tension across the wound, orientation to the RSTLs, and local tissue reservoirs that can be recruited by undermining and skin mobilization without distortion of landmarks. In addition, during surgical revision, correct approximation of the dermis with long-term absorbable sutures such as PDS is essential to prevent recurrence. The use of a subcuticular buried everting technique or vertical mattress sutures (see Fig. 34-4) will achieve this aim. A tension-free, everted skin closure with minimal iatrogenic skin trauma is the goal.

A hypertrophic scar, such as a vertical sternal scar, that is poorly oriented to RSTLs will not respond well to simple fusiform excision and primary closure without recruitment of excess tissue to decrease wound tension. Employment of this incorrect approach will lead to recurrence of the hypertrophic scarring, often with poorer results; employing reorientation techniques such as geometric broken line closure or W-plasty of the scar to the RSTLs without recruitment of excess tissue can lead to obvious recurrence in a more noticeable pattern such as the geometric broken line closure or W-plasty. If local skin mobilization is not sufficient, the surgeon must consider using local flaps or tissue expansion.[51]

Table 34-5   Height-Discrepant Scar Deformities

Type of Deformity	Cause	Suggested Treatment
Step-off	May be a result of incorrect alignment at closure or a true mismatch in tissue thickness from tissue loss	Dermabrasion, CO_2 laser, reexcision
Pin-cushioning	Any curved incision with centripetal contracture	Subcutaneous thinning and Z-plasty
Hypertrophic/keloid	Thinned epidermis with thickened fibrous tissue present, either confined to boundaries of scar or progressing beyond boundaries	Multimodality treatment

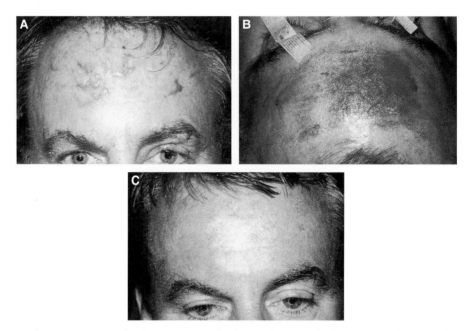

Fig. 34-7   **A,** This man was involved in a motor vehicle accident in which he struck the windshield, sustaining multiple lacerations and abrasions of the forehead. **B,** Dermabrasion with a wire brush was used 3 months after the accident to reduce the irregularity of the forehead. **C,** Result 6 months after dermabrasion.

Contour

A scar may be flush, elevated, or depressed. In an elevated scar, a distinction is made between types of elevation, because the treatment will depend on the etiologic factors (Table 34-5).

Small step-offs are treated effectively with dermabrasion or CO_2 laser therapy to eliminate contour deformity (Fig. 34-7). Larger step-offs require excision and repeat closure with correct alignment of tissues, including subcutaneous fat, dermis, and epidermis. For a true tissue thickness mismatch, dermal fillers, dermal grafts, or a soft tissue flap or implant may help to produce correct alignment. Pin-cushioning responds well to steroid injections and/or invasive techniques, such as subcutaneous tissue excision in combination with peripheral Z-plasties.

A scar may be depressed as a result of tethering of the dermis to the underlying fascia. In atrophic scars, excess wound tension over an unsupported wound can lead to scar widening, with thinning of the dermis and epidermis. Tethered scars require release of the fibrous bands from the fascia to the dermis, using minimally invasive techniques such as subcision (with a hypodermic needle) or formal scar excision and formal undermining, with or without dermal/subcutaneous grafts. Wide atrophic scars often require excisional techniques, accompanied by measures to address underlying wound tension through tissue mobilization, the use of RSTLs, or both.

LENGTH

Long linear scars are not aesthetically acceptable on the face. Longer scars on the forehead and neck may be appropriately subtle if they are oriented into the RSTLs. For example, a direct brow-lift scar, when performed in the presence of preexisting rhytids, may mimic a horizontal rhytid. Long scars malpositioned to the RSTLs are not aesthetic and often require reorientation and irregularization for camouflage. Irregularization techniques (multiple Z-plasties, W-plasties, and geometric broken line closures) do increase overall length, but increase camouflage because of their irregular nature. In scar irregularization, each of the limbs should be less than 10 mm in a Z-plasty, and range from 4 to 6 mm in W-plasty and geometric broken line closure.[52]

Assessment of the facial subunits and RSTLs in relation to the scar is essential. Facial units are defined by forehead, temple, cheek, periorbital, scalp, and nose. All of these units contain subunits, with the exception of the cheek. Both the aesthetic subunit principle and RSTLs can contribute to plan development in scar revision. They use different principles, and hence may dictate disparate revision approaches. The surgeon must assess on an individualized basis which is the more appropriate principle to employ to camouflage the scar.

FACIAL SUBUNITS

The basis for the aesthetic facial subunit principle is that the contour of the face differs between zones (see Fig. 34-3). These contour differences are primarily a result of underlying bony/cartilaginous skeletal features, although varying skin thickness also contributes to the differences. This combination produces a series of gently flowing convex hills and concave valleys.[53] The transition in shape from convex to concave creates changes in light reflection and shadowing, producing transition zones. These zones can be defined as the borders of aesthetic subunits (see Fig. 34-3). The transition zones between facial units and subunits are used to hide incisions and scars. Excision of the scar and advancement of the remaining tissue to the boundaries of the borders of the aesthetic subunits result in a less conspicuous scar. Alternatively, a whole subunit can be replaced. For example, the whole affected ala or nasal tip may be reconstructed as a single unit.

The role of RSTLs in incisions and scar formation is somewhat different from the borders of aesthetic subunits and are by definition perpendicular to lines of maximal extensibility and muscles of facial expression. If incisions are placed in these lines, this maximally reduces the tension across the wound, which has the effect of minimizing scar widening in the postoperative phase.[54] A secondary beneficial effect of placing an incision in the RSTLs is that rhytids tend to follow these lines. Therefore linear scars oriented along the RSTLs can be camouflaged as rhytids. This orientation can have a powerful camouflaging effect, depending on the presence or absence of preexisting rhytids.

TISSUE DEFICIENCY

If a tissue deficiency is identified (Table 34-6) and is limited to the skin layer, the excess tension during wound healing may result in a widened, hypertrophic, atrophic-depressed scar associated with alopecia in hair-bearing areas. If there is an underlying tissue deficiency (from depressed fractures or tissue loss from traumatic wounds), a depressed complex scar frequently develops, with an associated contour deformity or concavity that may extend to the surrounding area. For optimal scar revision in these complex situations (Box 34-2), one must replace tissue with similar tissue, recruiting excess tissues through local flaps, tissue expansion, and regional flaps.

If a contour deformity results from a deep tissue deficiency, one must assess the bony and/or fascial/fat deficiency that contributes to the contour deformity. Corrective osteotomies should be considered where bony deformity exists. Implants, fascial flaps, dermal grafts, and lipofilling are also effective masking techniques for significant contour defects for which one wishes to avoid osteotomies. In thorough scar analysis, all of these factors must be carefully considered and a systematic characterization of the scar undertaken.

Table 34-6   Common Scar Deformities

Scar Type	Appearance
Immature	Red, raised
Hypertrophic	Red, painful, raised
Poor color match	Hypopigmented/hyperpigmented
Depressed	Indented
Raised	Step-off, irregular
Poorly oriented	Off RSTLs or not in BOAS
Irregular	Stellate
Tissue deficiency cutaneous	Increased wound tension, webbing, hypertrophic scarring, possible contour deformity
Tissue deficiency deep	Contour deformity
Distortion of landmark	Alar stenosis, brow elevation, ectropion, lagophthalmos, lip eversion

---

Box 34-2   Goals of Scar Revision of Increasing Complexity

- Improve color of scar
- Smooth out contour deformity of raised scar
- Eliminate depressed scar
- Make scar narrower
- Reorient scar to RSTL or BOAS
- Break up long linear scar
- Correct cutaneous tissue deficiency
- Replace entire subunit with flap and reorientation of scars into BOAS
- Correct deep tissue deficiency
- Correct facial landmark distortion

COUNSELING REALISTIC EXPECTATIONS

Scars cannot be removed completely; they may be relocated or camouflaged by reorientation or other techniques. The most difficult cases lie at each end of the spectrum. On one end, complex traumatic wounds present requirements for simultaneous correction of cutaneous tissue deficiency, facial landmark distortion, and deep tissue deficiency, and can be difficult to improve. At the other end, a simple but lengthy linear scar on the cheek of a young, attractive patient with high aesthetic demands may be equally challenging in terms of patient satisfaction. Managing patient expectations is essential, especially if small gains are the expected outcome.

TYPES OF INVASIVE SURGICAL TECHNIQUES

The common scar revision techniques include fusiform excision, serial excision, tissue expansion, Z-plasty, W-plasty, graft placement, and reconstruction with a graft/flap.

Indications for fusiform excision with linear closure include the following:
- Wide scar in a relaxed skin tension line
- Scar not well oriented to RSTLs (less than 30 degrees)
- Depressed scar
- Poor scar color[3]

Fusiform revision is ideal for wide scars that are well oriented to the RSTLs. A scar should be considered for fusiform excision and primary closure in the RSTL if the scar is less than 30 degrees off the lines. The internal angles of the fusiform excision should be less than 30 degrees to avoid standing cutaneous vector deformities on closure. If the fusiform excision is planned to extend beyond a subunit border, an M-plasty should be performed to avoid this violation. When scars that are increasingly divergent from the RSTLs are treated with fusiform excision, an increase both in scar length and in discarding healthy tissue results (Fig. 34-8). Therefore scars more than 30 degrees divergent from the RSTLs should be reoriented using alternative techniques to avoid excessive tissue loss and unnecessary lengthening.[3,21]

Fig. 34-9 illustrates an example of a depressed mature scar, with a step-off. The scar is well oriented in the RSTLs; it is also short and wide. It most likely resulted from poor surgical technique during primary surgery. The poor aesthetic result is accentuated because it resides within a convex subunit. There is no notching or distortion of the alar margin. The main issue in this circumstance is scar depression and step-

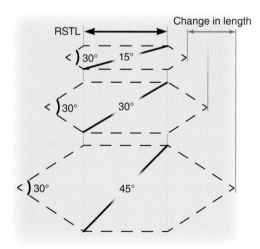

Fig. 34-8   For the same length scar, as it becomes more divergent from the RSTLs, fusiform excision and primary closure results in increased tissue loss and a longer linear scar.

off. Scar reorientation is not required, because the scar lies in the RSTLs and is not of sufficient length to require techniques such as W-plasty or geometric broken line closure to camouflage it. Scar excision and primary closure with correct surgical technique will produce the optimal scar in this instance. Excess skin eversion (overcorrection) is the goal, because a depressed scar is far more difficult to address than a raised scar, postoperatively. Any residual raised scar is managed by shave scar excision of the raised portion of the scar under local anesthetic (Fig. 34-9).

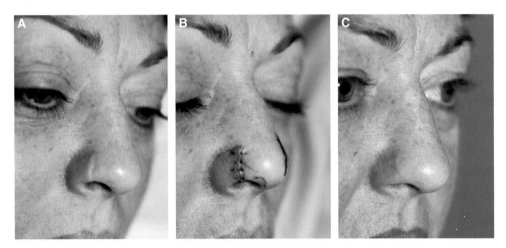

Fig. 34-9   Management of a depressed scar in the RSTLs. **A,** Preoperative view. Note the scar has a short length. **B,** Simple excision and undermining with primary closure. **C,** One year postoperatively, a good result is shown, with the scar well placed in the RSTLs.

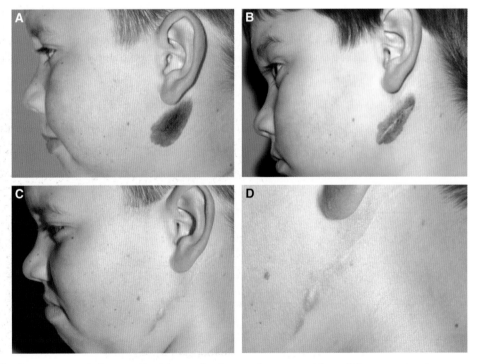

Fig. 34-10   Large congenital nevus. Excision and primary closure would result in excess tension across the wound because of high skin tension and poor laxity in pediatric skin. **A,** Preoperative view. **B,** After the first stage of excision and closure in the RSTLs. **C,** Result 6 months after the second and final stage of serial excision. **D,** Closeup view reveals some hypertrophic scarring inferiorly, which was treated conservatively.

SERIAL EXCISION

Serial excision is a staged excision technique. It can be used on any scar or diseased area when two criteria are met. It must be (1) amenable to fusiform excision and primary closure, and (2) the resulting tissue deficiency must preclude closure without distortion of nearby structures, or introduce unacceptable tension across the wound.

Serial excision involves sequential partial excision of the scar or cutaneous inequality, with wide undermining and closure of the wound with acceptable tension across the wound, with no distortion of anatomical landmarks (Fig. 34-10). The number of procedures required depends on the elasticity of the surrounding skin and the size of the scar or area being excised. Serial excision relies mainly on biologic tissue creep, an inherent biomechanical property of skin (see Chapter 4).

TISSUE EXPANSION

Tissue expansion is similar to serial partial excision in that it takes advantage of skin's ability to respond dynamically to mechanical forces and to increase with time (see Figs. 4-9 through 4-12).

In cases in which a deficiency exists, adjacent tissue is the most appropriate match for similar dimension, texture, and color. Adjacent tissue is therefore generally the first choice as a tissue reservoir, which can be recruited by appropriate undermining and local flaps. However, alternatives must be sought in cases in which a defect is large, or only small tissue reservoirs exist. Regional flaps, tissue expansion, and free tissue transfer are all options. Tissue expansion is an extremely useful technique when the size of the defect surpasses the ability of large flaps to produce sufficient tissue to close the defect.

Tissue expansion involves placement of a silicone expander, which is ultimately inflated by percutaneous injection of saline solution through a remote port. The implant is expanded every 1 to 2 weeks, using aseptic technique. Overly aggressive inflation causes persistent blanching of skin and intractable pain. Self-expanding osmotic silicone expanders (Fig. 34-11) represent a newer technology, requiring fewer hospital

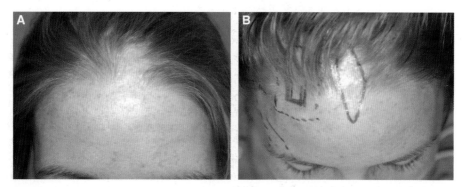

Fig. 34-11   Wide scar crossing from forehead facial unit onto the scalp subunit. **A,** Closeup view of the defect. **B,** The midline diamond marking shows the area of tissue to be excised. Remote insertion of a tissue expander is through an incision on the side of the scalp in the vicinity of the ear (not visible). Placement of a rectangular self-inflating implant in an adjacent tissue is outlined.

Continued

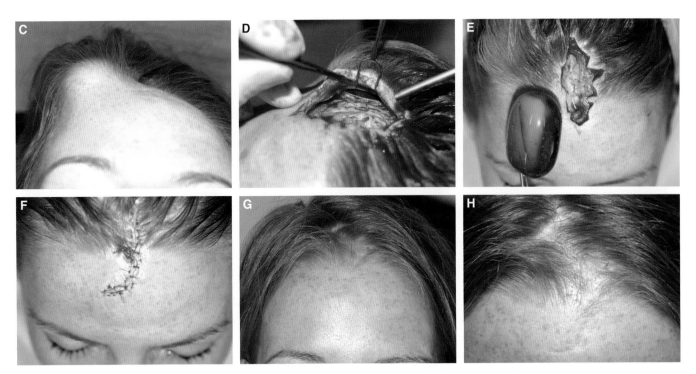

Fig. 34-11, cont'd   **C,** Note that even a small defect requires excessive width measured over the implant after expansion; usually an attempt is made to generate three times the amount of required tissue. **D,** The scar is excised in a geometric broken line pattern skirting the defect to aim camouflage and interpose hair-bearing tissue at the normal hairline/forehead transition. **E,** The tissue expander is removed. **F,** Horizontal advancement with attention to avoid excess tension and limit damage to the hair follicles. The scar is irregularized and interrupted as hair is moved over the previous scarred area. **G,** Postoperative result after 6 months, with reconstitution of frontal hairline. There is still some alopecia related to the expansion. **H,** Postoperative view 1 year later.

visits and, given the more gradual expansion, causing less discomfort. This approach offers a new exciting horizon with tissue expansion and may become the preferred method for tissue expansion.[55]

Rapid intraoperative expansion is an alternative which produces a small amount of immediate tissue lengthening to aid tension-free closure. Rapid intraoperative tissue expansion uses the plastic region of the stress/strain curve. It allows the surgeon to use mechanical creep to increase length immediately intraoperatively to aid closure. Two or three cycles of expansion and disinflation with subsequent release are undertaken intraoperatively. The tissue is rapidly expanded beyond its elastic limit while pallor and blanching are carefully monitored for 3 minutes. This technique has the advantage of producing rapid expansion without the need for further surgical stages and the delay required with standard tissue expansion. With this method, 1 to 2 cm of expansion can be gained to facilitate primary closure.

When using tissue expansion, the surgeon must determine the volume of the expander, the shape of the expander, and the proposed incision placement for insertion of the expander. One must also select the layer for insertion, the location of the port, and choose both the frequency of injection and the amount of filling with each stage. The volume required can be estimated by the widest portion of the defect *(x)*. The amount of expansion required for sufficient advancement is 2.0 to 2.5*x* for the width of the dome for linear areas, and 2.5 to 3*x* for curved areas to account for the increased tissue requirements. Incision placement

Table 34-7   Scar Irregularization Techniques Summary

	Lengthening	Tissue Loss	Camouflage	Complexity
Z-plasty	+++	−	+	+
W-plasty	+	++	++	++
Geometric broken line closure	+	++	+++	+++

for insertion of expanders is not always straightforward; several factors must be considered. Ordinarily, remote incision for insertion of the expander is preferable (see Fig. 34-11). The implant is then tunneled into a pocket adjacent to the defect. When planning the remote incision, one must consider the orientation of future flaps that will be required to rotate and/or advance the expanded tissue into the defect. Failure to do so may result in flap necrosis during flap insult. To avoid inadvertent puncturing of the expander during inflation, the inflation port is located away from the expander.

The level of implant placement in the face is in the subcutaneous plane. In the scalp, the subgaleal plane is used. The first injection should be delayed for 1 to 2 weeks after implantation, but not longer, because formation of a capsule around the implant can impede expansion. Once sufficient tissue expansion has occurred, the scar is excised and the expander is removed. The capsule that has formed around the expander may be removed to enable more advancement of the tissue. The tissue is then advanced into the defect. Rotation flaps and cutback techniques may also be necessary to optimally close the defect.

Complications of tissue expansion include hematoma, seroma, and neuropraxia. The overall infection rate is 2% when intraoperative IV antibiotics and antibiotic wound irrigations are used. Implant failure rate and induced skin necrosis are less than 1%. Implant extrusion is more of a concern, with a rate of 5% in the head and neck area.[56]

Nonlinear Surgical Revision

The most commonly used irregularization techniques are Z-plasty, W-plasty, and geometric broken line closure. They all produce irregularization and reorientation of the scar, but differ in their effects on lengthening, tissue sparing, camouflage, and complexity (Table 34-7).

Z-PLASTY

The Z-plasty is a time-honored technique. It is simply a triangular shaped double transposition flap across a scar. The scar itself is often excised with no margin. The excised scar (ellipse) becomes the central limb of the Z-plasty with two peripheral limbs of equal length placed parallel to each other at varying angles (dependent on degree of lengthening or angle of reorientation required). Wide undermining is necessary to transpose the two flaps. A two-layer, tension-free closure is executed. Once the two flaps are transposed, the scar will lengthen and the central limb will be reoriented (aiming for the RSTLs). Instead of the single preexisting scar, the resultant scar has three limbs, shaped as a Z.

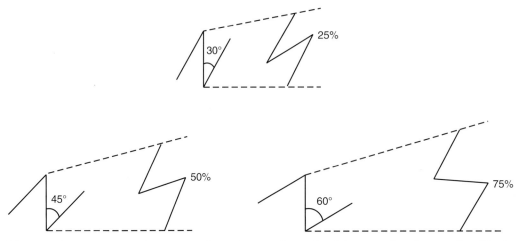

Fig. 34-12   The length of increase is dependent on the angle of the central to the peripheral limb.

Indications

The Z-plasty has three effects. It lengthens a scar (Fig. 34-12) and releases a contracture, camouflages a linear scar, and realigns a scar toward the RSTLs. Indications for Z-plasty include webbed scars, trapdoor deformities, and small linear scars not amenable to fusiform excision, and scars greater than 30 degrees to the RSTLs. This is the procedure of choice for scars greater than 30 degrees to the RSTLs on eyelids, lips, and nasolabial folds.

Z-plasty is particularly useful in realigning scars in the eyelid and lips, because unlike a W-plasty and a geometric broken line closure, the tissue is entirely preserved. Even small amounts of tissue deficiency near these mobile structures can cause secondary distortion of landmarks, such as ectropion.

When a Z-plasty is chosen, there are several variables to be considered, including single or multiple Zs, the length of limbs, the angles of limbs, and the desired orientation of the final scar.

On the face, one limits the limbs of the Z-plasty to 10 mm or less, even with longer scars. Multiple Z-plasties are employed when necessary to keep the limbs below this 10 mm, but not smaller than 5 mm. One large Z-plasty is often too conspicuous.

The use of wider angles at the junction between the two lateral limbs and the central limb of the Z-plasty results in increased length and a wider distribution of tension across the scar, but increases standing cutaneous deformity. There are general guidelines for degree of lengthening depending on the size of angle used (see Fig. 34-12).

Z-plasty to Reorient Scar Toward the Relaxed Skin Tension Lines

When a Z-plasty is used to reorient a scar parallel to the RSTLs, the angle of the lateral limbs in relation to the central limb determines the amount the central limb will be rotated after transposition of the flaps. Most commonly, a 60-degree angle is used; the resulting change in central limb orientation is predictable (90 degrees). This 60-degree angle ensures vascularity of the triangles, while permitting easy mobilization and transposition of the flaps. However, different angles may be chosen according to specific needs. If the scar direction is off the RSTLs from 90 degrees to 60 degrees, the angle between the central and peripheral limb should be reduced from 60 degrees to 45 degrees. This reorients the final central limb after transposi-

Table 34-8   Relationship Between Scar Angle to RSTL and Revision Design

Angle of Scar to RSTL (degrees)	Orientation of Peripheral to Central Limb
90	60-degree angle of central to peripheral limb
90-60	60- to 45-degree angle of central to peripheral limb
60-30	Peripheral limbs follow the RSTLs as closely as possible
<30	Fusiform excision

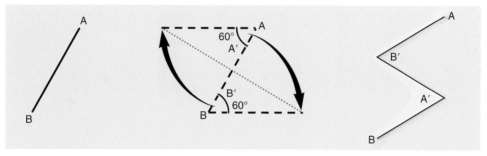

Fig. 34-13   Using the rule of thumb, one can predict the resulting orientation of the central limb after flap transposition.

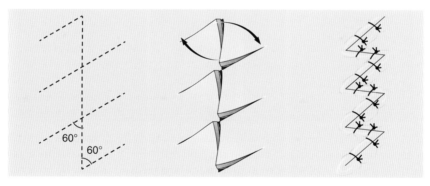

Fig. 34-14   Multiple Z-plasty.

tion of the Z-plasty parallel to the RSTLs. If the scar is less than 30 degrees off the RSTLs, fusiform excision should be employed instead of Z-plasty (Table 34-8). To predict final scar orientation, the surgeon must bear in mind that a line drawn between the ends of the two Z-plasty limbs will predict the resultant final position of the central limb of the scar after flap transposition (Fig. 34-13).

Multiple Z-plasty and Double Opposing Z-plasty

If there is a long scar, a multiple Z-plasty can be used to avoid limbs greater than 10 mm on the face. It is relatively easy to plan and execute, because the geometry is repetitive and all sequential angles and limb lengths are equal (Fig. 34-14). Double opposing Z-plasty is a more complex design (Fig. 34-15). It uses mirror image Z-plasties to recruit more tissue and to allow greater lengthening. This can be advantageous in areas in which there is little space and significant amounts of tissue lengthening is required, such as in webbing of the medial canthus (Fig. 34-16).

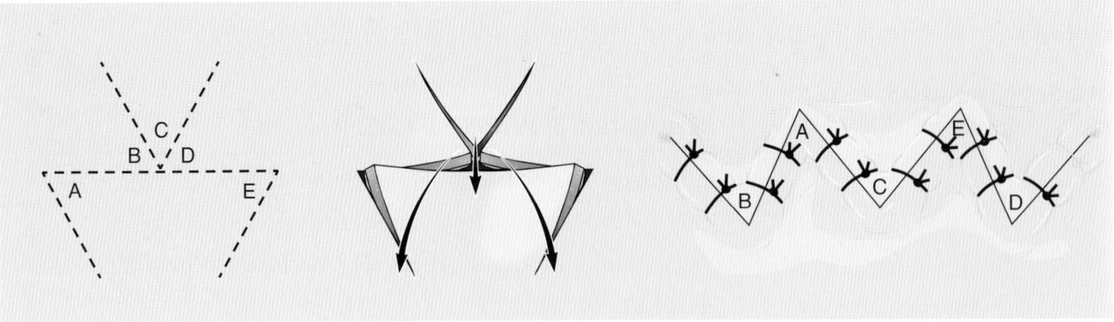

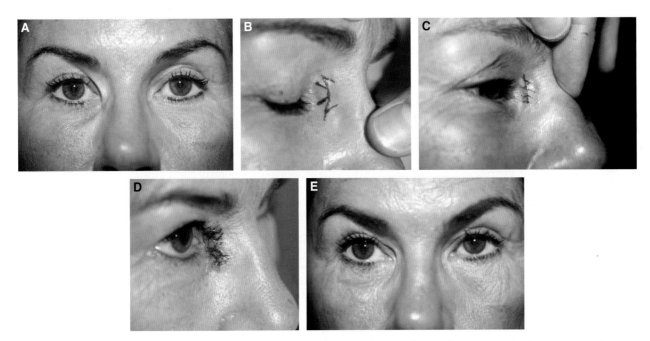

Fig. 34-15   Double opposing Z-plasty oriented around the medial canthus.

Fig. 34-16   Webbing in the right medial canthus is a classic indication for Z-plasty repair. **A,** Preoperative view. **B,** One option is a double opposing Z-plasty. Note how the limbs nicely conform around the medial canthus. **C,** An alternative approach is a multiple Z-plasty with limbs closer to the medial canthus. **D,** After transposition of the double opposing Z-plasty. **E,** Postoperative result. Z-plasty involves preservation and recruiting of tissue from the surrounding tissues. Apart from excision of the scar, no tissue was discarded.

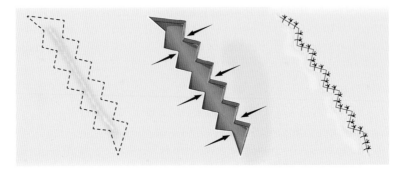

Fig. 34-17   W-plasty arc. Orientation of the W-plasty depends on the angle between the scar and the RSTLs.

W-PLASTY

A W-plasty involves creating two interdigitating advancement flaps (Fig. 34-17). The purpose of a W-plasty is to reorient the greater part of the incision toward the RSTLs. This helps create a longer, but less obvious, scar. The W-plasty involves not only excising the scar, but also discarding normal tissue. Therefore sufficient tissue laxity is required.

A W-plasty is generally indicated in long scars oriented more than 30 degrees from the RSTLs in areas of skin laxity, such as the forehead, temples, nose, cheeks, and chin.[3,57] W-plasty is also useful in mildly depressed scars.

Although a W-plasty and a Z-plasty both produce zigzag scars, there are appreciable differences. First, in a W-plasty there is only advancement but no flap transposition. Second, because there is no flap transposition in a W-plasty, it avoids the development of standing cutaneous deformities that can be observed with a Z-plasty. Finally, there is minimal scar lengthening in a W-plasty, and no tissue is discarded with a Z-plasty.

TIPS IN PLANNING A W-PLASTY

The length of the limbs should be 5 to 6 mm or longer. The angle of the apex of each triangle should be determined by the relationship of the angle of the scar to the RSTLs. For scars at an orientation of 90 to 60 degrees to the RSTLs, the angle of the multiple triangles should be 60 degrees (with neither limb following the RSTL), whereas for scars at an orientation of 60 to 45 degrees to the RSTLs, the angles of the W-plasty should increase from 60 to 90 degrees. One limb will be parallel to the RSTL. For scars at an orientation of 45 to 30 degrees to the RSTLs, the W-plasty angle will be 90 degrees. One limb will be parallel to the RSTLs, producing a stair-step W-plasty. For scars at an orientation of 30 degrees or less to the RSTLs, a Z-plasty is indicated. If the scar more closely follows the RSTL, a fusiform excision is the procedure of choice.[3] Reducing the size of the triangles at either end of the scar will permit a 30-degree angle excision to avoid dog-ear formation. The addition of an M-plasty at the end of the incision prevents scar lengthening (Fig. 34-18).

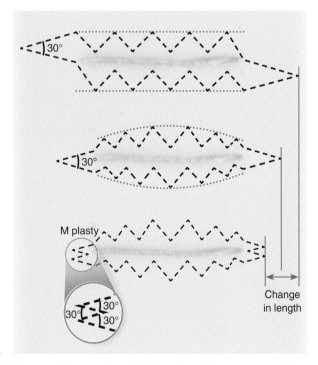

Fig. 34-18   Reducing the length of the W-plasty limbs and performing an M-plasty reduces overall scar length.

GEOMETRIC BROKEN LINE CLOSURE

Geometric broken line closure is a variation of the W-plasty that involves a more complex irregularization technique using not only triangles but also squares and semicircles. The indications for geometric broken line closure and W-plasty are similar. The key to geometric broken line closure design is that it has an irregular pattern, as opposed to the W-plasty, which has a regular pattern with repeating *V*s. With the geometric broken line closure scar the observer has difficulty following the less predictable, irregular pattern, which is better camouflaged than the alternative W-plasty.[58] The irregular pattern is produced by the random combination of triangles, rectangles, squares, and curved geometric shapes of different sizes along the scar.[59] The curved geometric shapes that irregularize the scar in geometric broken line closure can lead to pin-cushioning and should be minimized if possible (Fig. 34-19). When planning the geometric broken line closure, an attempt should be made to place as much of the new scar within the RSTLs as possible. As in a W-plasty, the lock and key effect of the mirror-image geometric shaped flaps helps to prevent scar depression (Fig. 34-20).[52]

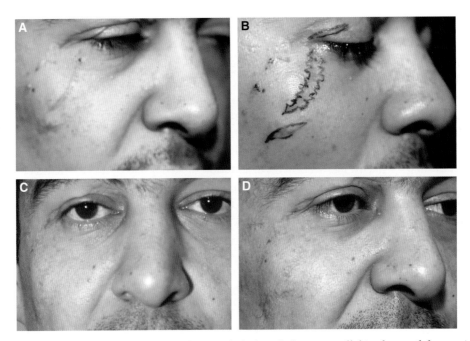

Fig. 34-19 Scar oriented 90 degrees to the RSTLs cephalad, and almost parallel in the caudal part. A small additional cheek scar is to be excised and closed in linear fashion. **A,** Preoperative view. **B,** A geometric broken line closure is planned, with the lower portion of the scar excised as an ellipse at less than 30 degrees off the RSTL. **C,** Result 6 months after surgery. **D,** The scar is well camouflaged.

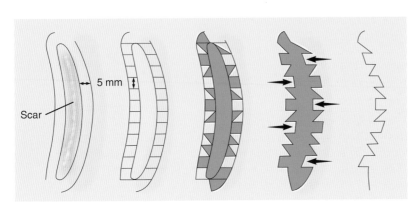

Fig. 34-20 Stepwise planning of a geometric broken line closure.

In curvilinear scars, there is an inevitable size disparity between the design on the inner curve (smaller) and outer curve (larger). The squares, circles, and rectangles will be different sizes, and this presents a risk of bunching of tissue and standing cutaneous deformities. A running W-plasty is preferred to a geometric broken line closure for scar revision in curvilinear scars.[58]

IRREGULARIZED W-PLASTY

A hybrid of the W-plasty and geometric broken line closure, the irregularized W-plasty (Fig. 34-21) offers the advantages of both techniques. The approach uses only triangles, as in a W-plasty, but it borrows from geometric broken line closure in that each sequential shape (triangle) is of a different geometry to irregularize the pattern. This modification combines the advantages of geometric broken line closure (unpredictable pattern) and still maintains the advantages of the W-plasty (ease of planning and execution).

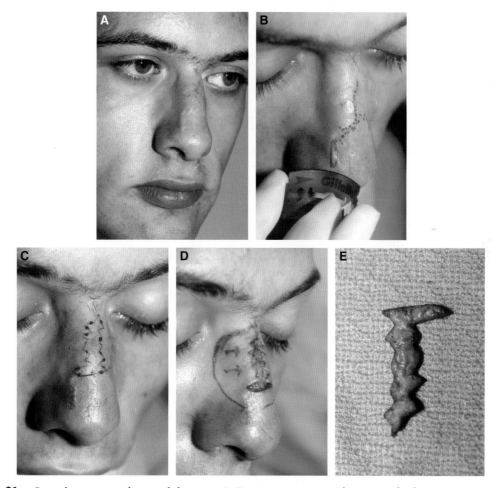

Fig. 34-21   Complex scar on the nasal dorsum. **A,** Preoperative view. The patient had an overprojection of the bony-cartilaginous dorsum. **B,** The scar outlined. Note that the scar had raised and depressed areas. The most caudal part was reduced by shave excision and dermabrasion. **C,** Irregularized W-plasty marked with one limb approximately 60 degrees to the RSTL. Limbs were 4 to 5 mm. The excision blended into a fusiform excision in the RSTL of an oblique part of the scar. **D,** As tissue was excised, wide undermining was necessary to close the wound primarily without excessive tension. A rhinoplasty was performed through the excisional defect to assist in closure. The cartilaginous dorsum was lowered at the time of scar correction. **E,** Scar and skin excision.

Continued

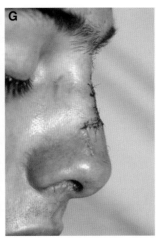
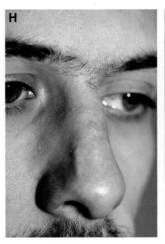
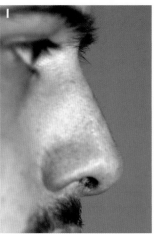

Fig. 34-21, cont'd   **F,** Overprojection of the bony-cartilaginous dorsum. **G,** View after bony-cartilaginous profile reduction through the skin incision to aid tension-free closure and cosmesis. **H,** Results 3 months after surgery with a well-camouflaged scar. There was some minor recurrence of the elevated scar, but the patient declined further minor revision. **I,** Improvement in bony-cartilaginous profile.

PLANNING A GEOMETRIC BROKEN LINE CLOSURE, W-PLASTY, OR IRREGULARIZED W-PLASTY

Planning both a geometric broken line closure and a W-plasty can be time consuming, and errors are easily made. A template (to scale) should be completed on paper before surgery to reduce intraoperative time and reduce unforseen errors. The surgeon can simplify planning by drawing out the W-plasty/geometric broken line closure stepwise as follows:

1. The scar outline is marked.
2. Circumferential margins of 5 mm are outlined.
3. Horizontal lines are marked (usually parallel to the RSTL).
4. A 5 mm distance is marked between to produce 5 mm squares.
5. The squares are filled in with a random selection of triangles, rectangles, or semicircles.
6. Areas to be excised are shaded.
7. The shaded areas are excised.
8. The area then undergoes wide 360-degree undermining and appropriate closure.

FREE GRAFTS

Skin and cartilage grafts play an important role in scar revision. Both cartilage grafts and composite skin-cartilage grafts offer support in critical areas. For example, distortion of the lower eyelid in ectropion or alar collapse/stenosis may be improved by the introduction of structural elements. Composite grafts can be taken from various parts of the ear, although the helical root and concha cymba are preferred.

In a Z-plasty two small flaps, one intranasal and one below the scar, are mobilized to recruit tissue into the base of the external nasal valve to widen the aperture. This can be technically difficult to perform if the scar is thick, because only very small flaps are produced with little tissue laxity. Alternatively, perinasal flaps from around the alar base may bring in fresh additional tissue, but often fail to reliably lateralize the ala. A free composite skin-cartilage graft will provide skin cover and structure after scar excision and therefore lateralize the ala and resist restenosis (Fig. 34-22).

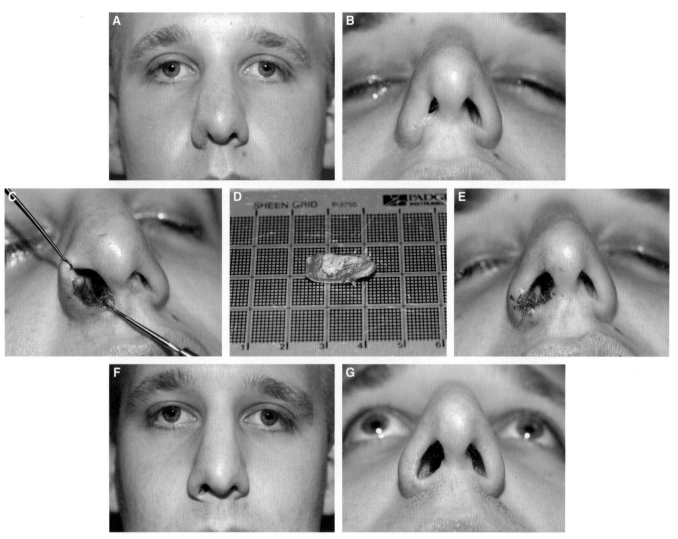

Fig. 34-22   External nasal valve stenosis from prior traumatic injury with tissue loss. This scar produced distortion of the ala, with resulting functional impairment of ipsilateral nasal breathing. The aim of scar revision was to correct the distorted landmark and prevent restenosis. A true cutaneous tissue deficiency existed; this tissue had to be restored. Because of the concave nature of this area, scars in this location tend to contract and web, and this must be accounted for in the revision. Options included a Z-plasty or free composite skin-cartilage graft. **A,** Scar band in the right vestibule. **B,** Right external valve stenosis causing ipsilateral nasal obstruction. **C,** The scar band was vertically incised to release the scar contraction, and the true tissue deficiency became apparent. **D,** A free skin-cartilage composite graft was harvested, with the skin on the concave aspect from the cymba concha. Note that the cartilage extends over a larger aspect than the skin to fit securely into subcutaneous pockets developed in the ala and nostril sill toward the nasal septal/spine area. This cartilage helped lateralization of the ala, increasing the vestibule entrance. **E,** Graft in situ. Note overcorrection to account for a possible occurrence of a degree of restenosis. **F,** View 3 months after surgery. **G,** Postoperative basal view. Note that further contraction is still to be expected over the next year.

RECONSTRUCTION OF A FACIAL SUBUNIT WITH A FOREHEAD FLAP

The nasal subunits are the areas in which flap reconstruction of facial unit/subunit in scar revision is most frequently employed (see Chapter 20). If excess scarring is present in one or more of the nasal subunits, it may be preferable to excise the whole subunit than to attempt scar revision (Fig. 34-23). Another common site for flap reconstruction is the medial cheek, where a laterally based cheek advancement/rotation flap is used to replace defects on the medial half of the cheek.

The incisions are hidden in the melolabial crease, nasal cheek facial unit border, and the cheek lower eyelid border. The cheek advancement flap is expandable to the cervicofacial facial flap for recruitment of more tissue, which can recruit enough tissue to replace the entire cheek subunit.[60,61] Upper lateral lip subunit can also be similarly replaced with a transposition flap from the medial cheek or alternatively an island advancement flap from the melolabial fold[62] (see Chapter 35).

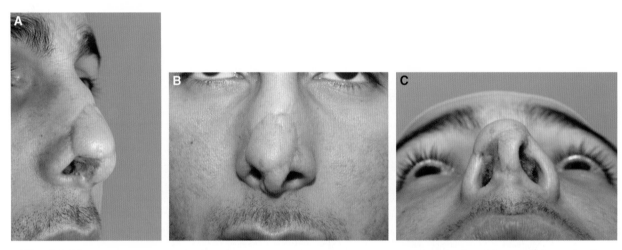

Fig. 34-23   War victim who had undergone immediate reconstruction with a forehead flap, which resulted in unacceptable scars and scar contractures. The normal contour and position of the ala and nasal tip were completely absent. The entire lower two thirds of the nose required cartilage restructuring. The retracted alar sidewalls presented through-and-through defects in need of lining reconstitution. Simple scar revision techniques would not be effective in this complex case. Subunit excision of the ala, soft triangle, dorsum, and tip was planned. The aim was to place the incisions in the borders of the aesthetic subunits to help camouflage them. The lining was replaced by local turn-in flaps. Note that cartilage was used to recreate the whole alar-tip framework and additional grafts were placed in extraanatomic sites such as alar rim. Skin coverage was reconstituted with a second flap harvested from the forehead. **A,** Complex scarring with pin-cushioning of the previous forehead flap. There is alar retraction because of insufficient buttressing of the alar margin from the primary repair and complete loss of tip structure. **B,** Cartilage support in the lower third (tip) is deficient, except for some part of columella. The appearance is unaesthetic, with significant asymmetry of alar margins and alar retraction. **C,** Basal view, showing distorted columella from scar contracture.

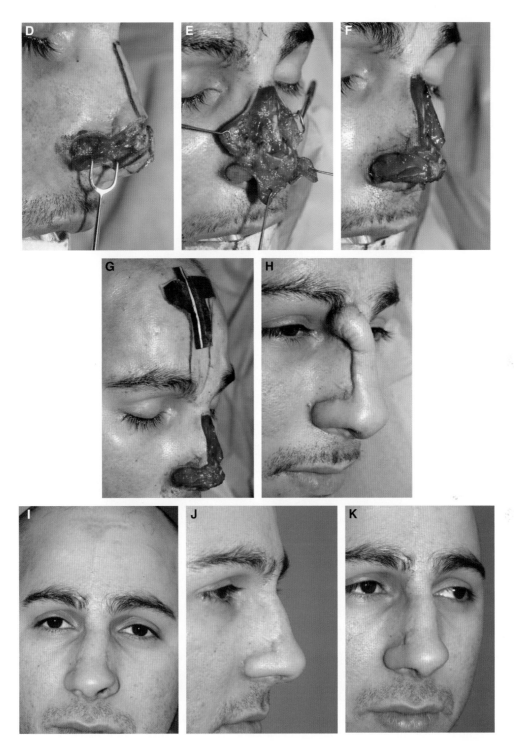

Fig. 34-23, cont'd **D,** Subunit excision of ala, soft triangle, dorsum, and tip was planned. Incisions were planned in the borders of the aesthetic subunits to help camouflage them. **E,** Scarred skin from the previous forehead flap was folded over to re-create the inner lining. **F,** Free cartilage grafts were placed to give support to the framework. **G,** A second forehead flap was planned, a paramedian design based on the right supratrochlear artery after Doppler location. **H,** The beginning of stage three demonstrates the importance of thinning the flap at the second stage. **I,** View 17 months after surgery, showing good alar symmetry without alar retraction or notching. Donor site morbidity was minimal. **J,** Aesthetic profile view with re-creation of the supratip break point, tip defining, and columella break point. **K,** Right oblique view showing good outcome of the reconstructed alar and soft triangle using the subunit principle.

MINIMALLY INVASIVE SURGICAL ADJUNCTIVE TECHNIQUES

SHAVE EXCISION

Shave excision is a straightforward and useful technique that is ideally suited to treat uneven scars (step-off) to reduce the contour deformity under local anesthetic in the office setting. A scalpel or razor blade is used to shave off the raised portion of an uneven scar (Fig. 34-24). This technique is not indicated in pin-cushion deformity, in which case Z-plasty with or without reduction of subcutaneous tissues is indicated. Additional skin resurfacing therapies include dermabrasion (mechanical or manual with scratch pad) and carbon dioxide laser therapy (see Chapter 41).

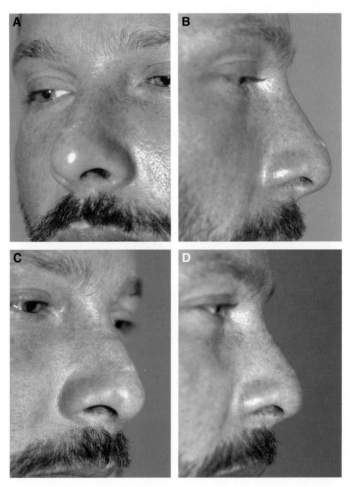

Fig. 34-24   Raised scar on the dorsum and tip. **A,** Preoperative view. **B,** Lateral view. **C,** Scar shaved flush with the surrounding skin. **D,** Final outcome, with the scar in the same plane as the surrounding tissue.

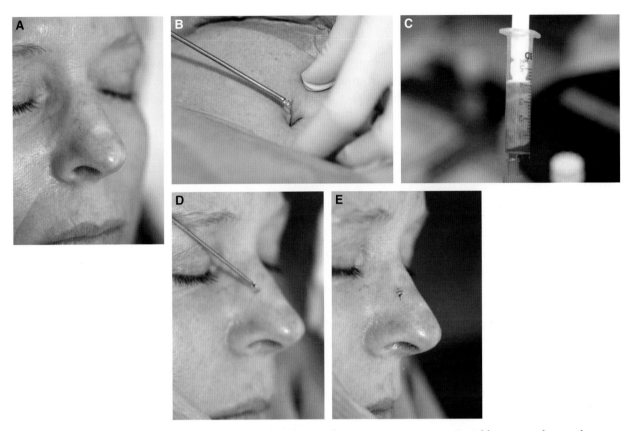

Fig. 34-25   Unaesthetic contour deformity after skin graft. **A,** Preoperative view. **B,** A blunt-tipped cannula was placed through a stab incision adjacent to the umbilicus. **C,** Fat was separated into its layers after placement in a centrifuge for 3 minutes at 300 rpm. **D,** A cannula was placed over the dorsum following stab incision. **E,** Immediate postoperative result.

LIPOFILLING AND FAT GRAFTING

Lipofilling for scar revision was first described more than 100 years ago to fill scars of the forearm.[63] Fat transplantation has a survival rate of 50%, occurring mainly through diffusion and neovascularization.[64] Generally, fat grafting can be applied in cases of depressed scars, or if replacement of missing volume is required (with deep tissue deficiency)[65] (Fig. 34-25).

NONSURGICAL

LASERS

Lasers used for scar revision can be classified broadly into ablative, nonablative (pulsed dye laser), and fractional laser therapy (see Chapter 41 for comprehensive discussion). Briefly, CO_2 laser therapy is an ablative therapy that causes tissue vaporization and may be used on uneven or depressed scars or to help skin grafts blend into surroundings. Prospective nonrandomized studies between CO_2 laser and dermabrasion demonstrate similar effectiveness for scar revision. However, CO_2 laser therapy for scar revision did offer a more bloodless field and a more precise method of tissue ablation.[66] The use of CO_2 laser in hypertrophic and keloid scarring has led to unacceptable rates of recurrence.[67] Atrophic scarring may be improved from 25% to 90%.[68]

PULSED DYE LASER THERAPY

Pulsed dye laser (PDL) therapy is a nonablative laser therapy. Its main indications are in the treatment of hypertrophic or erythematous scars. A systematic review has shown a moderate level of efficacy for the treatment of hypertrophic scarring.[69] It results in selective photothermolysis, in which the thermal injury to the scar is isolated to the microcirculation, with resulting destruction of the vasculature of the scar, preserving the skin components. These lasers have a low side effect profile, the most troublesome issue being occasional posttreatment purpura, which spontaneously settles within 7 to 10 days.[70] Single modality PDL therapy for keloids yields questionable results. Although some series suggest a high response rate in 57% to 83% of cases,[71] other investigators have noted rapid recurrence.[72]

FRACTIONAL LASER THERAPY

Fractional laser therapy avoids the confluent area of epidermal damage with thousands of pin-point lasers that produce localized thermal areas of injury to create microscopic thermal zones. In a comparison of fractional CO_2 laser therapy versus dermabrasion for scar revision, each was equivalent, but fractional therapy had reduced side effects.[73] In a recent comparison study, fractional nonablative laser therapy also outperformed PDL when used to improve cosmesis from surgical scars.[74] It is possible that further developments in fractional laser therapy will play an expanded role in scar revision.

ALGORITHM APPROACH TO SCAR REVISION

A working algorithm assists in decision-making in the management of scars (Fig. 34-26).

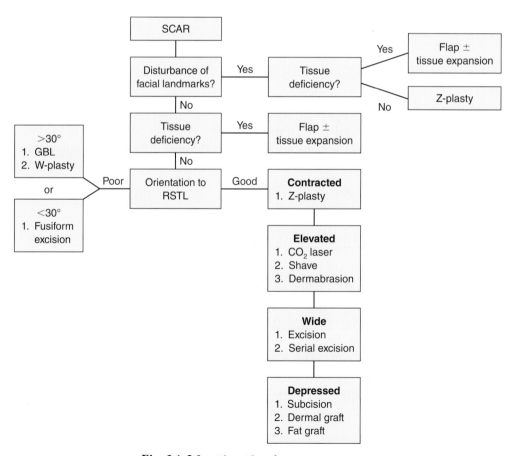

Fig. 34-26   Algorithm for scar assessment.

Complex cases (Figs. 34-27 and 34-28) benefit from such an algorithmic approach, although each plan is customized based on individual patient factors. Scar revision is a challenging endeavor. Scar revision merges seamlessly into areas that are considered facial reconstructive procedures. As with most areas of medicine, prevention is better than treatment. In many instances successful reduction of abnormal scarring by preoperative, intraoperative, and postoperative measures can prevent the requirements for scar revision.

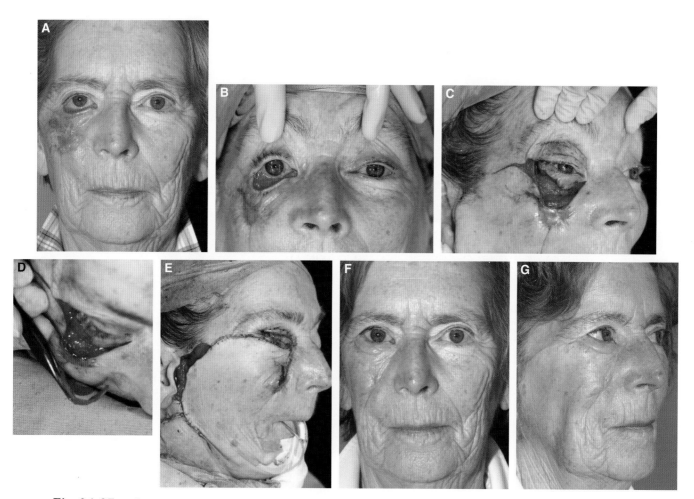

Fig. 34-27   This patient presented after a failed full-thickness skin graft of the cheek after basal cell carcinoma tumor excision. **A,** She had scarring of the anterior and middle lamella (orbital septum) with ectropion. **B,** Surgical release of cicatricial ectropion of the right lower eyelid. **C,** The true deficiency of the anterior lamella and cheek became apparent after release of the cheek and preseptal periocular skin and division of adhesions. Most of the skin deficiency was in the preorbital skin. **D,** A curved piece of conchal cartilage was used as a spacer to support the middle lamella. **E,** A large cheek rotation flap was developed to reconstruct the lower eyelid and medial cheek. Note the laterally based skin-muscle transposition flap from the upper eyelid to the lower eyelid. Its purpose is to produce an excess of skin in the lower eyelid to prevent recurrent ectropion in the postoperative healing phase, when further fibrosis and shortening of the anterior lamella can be predicted. **F,** Result 6 months after surgery, with no further revision. Ectropion was fully corrected and there is no lower eyelid malposition. Removal of excess skin from the lower eyelid (with a simple skin pinch blepharoplasty technique) will be delayed 1 year until the result is stable. **G,** The well-placed scars in the borders of the aesthetic subunits will continue to fade over the next 6 months and become increasingly well camouflaged with time. Persistent erythema could be treated with PDL laser therapy.

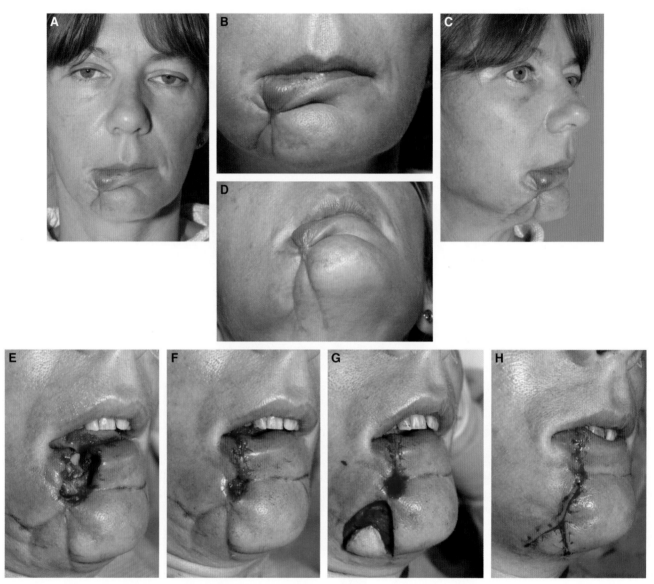

Fig. 34-28 A significant portion of this woman's cheek facial unit was affected by a complex scar. Tissue had to be recruited from adjacent areas, by a regional flap. The cheek subunit was fortuitous in that it had a great deal of adjacent tissue that could be recruited from the neck and chest (adjacent facial units), if required. **A,** Distortion of anatomic landmark (lower lip) leading to a disfiguring, unacceptable result and a minor degree of oral incompetence. **B,** Long linear scar: wide, depressed (greater than 2 mm), and hyperpigmented scar with areas of hypertrophic scarring in upper third. **C,** Scar within 30 degrees of the RSTL. **D,** Pin-cushion deformity and tethering with obvious contour deformity. **E,** After scar excision and release of any remaining fibrous bands, the true (superficial and deep) tissue deficiency could be appreciated. **F,** The tissue deficiency was less than one third of the lower lip and can be closed directly without concerns for microstomia. The vector of closure was purely horizontal to avoid any inferior pull on the lower lip. The vermilion margin was carefully realigned. **G,** The triangular flap was released and produced a second area of tissue deficiency. **H,** The lower portion was closed in a V-Y fashion with two-layer closure with vertical mattress sutures. Again, the tension had to be reoriented in a horizontal fashion to avoid vertical vector of pull on the lower lip. The result was correction of the depressed scar and contour deformity of the lateral mental area.

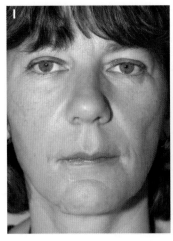
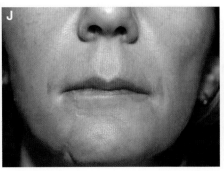
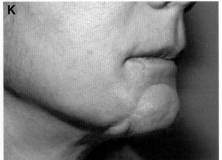

Fig. 34-28, cont'd **I,** Result 1 year after surgery. **J,** Lip in correct position with good alignment of the vermilion, and the upper third of the scar in RSTL. **K,** The lower third of the triangular portion of the scar demonstrates some persistent pin-cushion deformity. The patient declined further revision, but multiple Z-plasties with peripheral limbs oriented in RSTL may be helpful in this situation.

KEY POINTS

- Healing is a dynamic process that is not complete for up to one year.
- Collagen formation and remodeling aberrations can lead to poor scar tensile strength and hypertrophic or keloid scarring.
- To optimize healing, the surgeon must control for medical factors (diabetes, steroid use, nutrition), surgical factors (tension, surgical technique, correct orientation), and wound factors (dressing, moisture, silicone sheeting).

REFERENCES

1. Kocher T. Textbook of Operative Surgery. London: Adam & Charles Black, 1911.
2. Kurtin A. Corrective surgical planing of skin; new technique for treatment of acne scars and other skin defects. AMA Arch Derm Syphilol 68:389-397, 1953.
3. Borges A. Elective Incisions and Scar Revision. Baltimore: Lippincott Williams & Wilkins, 1985.
    Landmark book describing in-depth the planning and execution of Z-plasty and W-plasty for scar revision.
4. McCurdy SL. Manual of Orthopedic Surgery. Pittsburgh: Nicholson Press, 1898.
5. Berger P. Autoplastie par dédoublement de la palmure et échange de lambeaux. In Berger P, Banzet S, ed. Chirurgie Orthopédique. Paris: G. Steinheil, 1904.
6. Borges AF. Improvement of antitension-lines scar by the "W-plastic" operation. Br J Plast Surg 12:29-33, 1959.
7. Webster RC. Cosmetic concepts in scar camouflaging—serial excisional and broken line techniques. Trans Am Acad Ophthalmol Otolaryngol 73:256-265, 1969.
8. Neumann CG. The expansion of an area of skin by progressive distention of a subcutaneous balloon; use of the method for securing skin for subtotal reconstruction of the ear. Plast Reconstr Surg 19:124-130, 1957.
9. Manstein D, Herron GS, Sink RK, et al. Fractional photothermolysis: a new concept for cutaneous remodeling using microscopic patterns of thermal injury. Lasers Surg Med 34:426-438, 2004.
10. Singer AJ, Clark RA. Cutaneous wound healing. N Engl J Med 341:738-746, 1999.
11. Frodel E. Wound Healing, ed 2. New York: Thieme, 2002.
12. Terris D. Dynamics of Wound Healing, ed 2. Philadelphia: Lippincott-Raven, 1998.

13. Singer AJ, Quinn JV, Thode HC Jr, et al. Determinants of poor outcome after laceration and surgical incision repair. Plast Reconstr Surg 110:429-435; discussion 436-427, 2002.

14. Ogawa R, Akaishi S, Izumi M. Histologic analysis of keloids and hypertrophic scars. Ann Plast Surg 62:104-105, 2009.

15. Tredget EE. The molecular biology of fibroproliferative disorders of the skin: potential cytokine therapeutics. Ann Plast Surg 33:152-154, 1994.

16. Kose O, Waseem A. Keloids and hypertrophic scars: are they two different sides of the same coin? Dermatol Surg 34:336-346, 2008.

17. Marneros AG, Norris JE, Olsen BR, et al. Clinical genetics of familial keloids. Arch Dermatol 137:1429-1434, 2001.

18. Omo-Dare P. Genetic studies on keloid. J Natl Med Assoc 67:428-432, 1975.

19. Niessen FB, Spauwen PH, Schalkwijk J, et al. On the nature of hypertrophic scars and keloids: a review. Plast Reconstr Surg 104:1435-1458, 1999.

20. Bahar Dasgeb TP. Scar Revision. Philadelphia: Elsevier, 2006.

21. Thomas J. Facial Scars: Incisions, Revisions and Camouflage. St Louis: Mosby, 1989.

22. Al-Abdullah T, Plint AC, Fergusson D. Absorbable versus nonabsorbable sutures in the management of traumatic lacerations and surgical wounds: a meta-analysis. Pediatr Emerg Care 23:339-344, 2007.

23. van der Eerden PA, Lohuis PJ, Hart AA, et al. Secondary intention healing after excision of nonmelanoma skin cancer of the head and neck: statistical evaluation of prognostic values of wound characteristics and final cosmetic results. Plast Reconstr Surg 122:1747-1755, 2008.

24. Hom DB, Sun GH, Elluru RG. A contemporary review of wound healing in otolaryngology: current state and future promise. Laryngoscope 119:2099-2110, 2009.

25. Winter GD. Formation of the scab and the rate of epithelization of superficial wounds in the skin of the young domestic pig. Nature 193:293-294, 1962.

26. Alvarez OM, Mertz PM, Eaglstein WH. The effect of occlusive dressings on collagen synthesis and re-epithelialization in superficial wounds. J Surg Res 35:142-148, 1983.

27. Franz MG, Robson MC, Steed DL, et al. Guidelines to aid healing of acute wounds by decreasing impediments of healing. Wound Repair Regen 16:723-748, 2008.

28. Panuncialman J, Falanga V. The science of wound bed preparation. Clin Plast Surg 34:621-632, 2007.

29. O'Brien L, Pandit A. Silicon gel sheeting for preventing and treating hypertrophic and keloid scars. Cochrane Database Syst Rev 1:CD003826, 2006.

30. Tandara AA, Mustoe TA. The role of the epidermis in the control of scarring: evidence for mechanism of action for silicone gel. J Plast Reconstr Aesthet Surg 61:1219-2125, 2008.

31. Chang CC, Kuo YF, Chiu HC, et al. Hydration, not silicone, modulates the effects of keratinocytes on fibroblasts. J Surg Res 59:705-711, 1995.

32. Mustoe TA, Cooter RD, Gold MH, et al. International clinical recommendations on scar management. Plast Reconstr Surg 110:560-571, 2002.

33. Gassner HG, Brissett AE, Otley CC, et al. Botulinum toxin to improve facial wound healing: a prospective, blinded, placebo-controlled study. Mayo Clin Proc 81:1023-1028, 2006.

34. Gassner HG, Sherris DA, Otley CC. Treatment of facial wounds with botulinum toxin A improves cosmetic outcome in primates. Plast Reconstr Surg 105:1948-1953; discussion 1954-1955, 2000.

35. Ogawa R. The most current algorithms for the treatment and prevention of hypertrophic scars and keloids. Plast Reconstr Surg 125:557-568, 2010.

36. Brissett AE, Sherris DA. Scar contractures, hypertrophic scars, and keloids. Facial Plast Surg 17:263-272, 2001.

37. Leventhal D, Furr M, Reiter D. Treatment of keloids and hypertrophic scars: a meta-analysis and review of the literature. Arch Facial Plast Surg 8:362-368, 2006.

38. Engrav LH, Gottlieb JR, Millard SP, et al. A comparison of intramarginal and extramarginal excision of hypertrophic burn scars. Plast Reconstr Surg 81:40-45, 1988.

39. Tan KT, Shah N, Pritchard SA, et al. The influence of surgical excision margins on keloid prognosis. Ann Plast Surg 64:55-58, 2010.

40. Ardehali B, Nouraei SA, Van Dam H, et al. Objective assessment of keloid scars with three-dimensional imaging: quantifying response to intralesional steroid therapy. Plast Reconstr Surg 119:556-561, 2007.

41. Manuskiatti W, Fitzpatrick RE. Treatment response of keloidal and hypertrophic sternotomy scars: comparison among intralesional corticosteroid, 5-fluorouracil, and 585-nm flashlamp-pumped pulsed-dye laser treatments. Arch Dermatol 138:1149-1155, 2002.

42. Maguire HC Jr. Treatment of keloids with triamcinolone acetonide injected intralesionally. JAMA 192:325-326, 1965.

43. Berman B, Bieley HC. Adjunct therapies to surgical management of keloids. Dermatol Surg 22:126-130, 1996.

44. Lawrence WT. In search of the optimal treatment of keloids: report of a series and a review of the literature. Ann Plast Surg 27:164-178, 1991.

45. Asilian A, Darougheh A, Shariati F. New combination of triamcinolone, 5-fluorouracil, and pulsed-dye laser for treatment of keloid and hypertrophic scars. Dermatol Surg 32:907-915, 2006.

46. Darougheh A, Asilian A, Shariati F. Intralesional triamcinolone alone or in combination with 5-fluorouracil for the treatment of keloid and hypertrophic scars. Clin Exp Dermatol 34:219-223, 2009.

47. Hatamipour E, Mehrabi S, Hatamipour M, et al. Effects of combined intralesional 5-fluorouracil and topical silicone in prevention of keloids: a double blind randomized clinical trial study. Acta Med Iran 49:127-130, 2011.

48. Draaijers LJ, Tempelman FR, Botman YA, et al. The patient and observer scar assessment scale: a reliable and feasible tool for scar evaluation. Plast Reconstr Surg 113:1960-1965; discussion 1966-1967, 2004.

49. Sullivan T, Smith J, Kermode J, et al. Rating the burn scar. J Burn Care Rehabil 11:256-260, 1990.

50. Vercelli S, Ferriero G, Santorio F, et al. How to assess postsurgical scars: a review of outcome measures. Disabil Rehabil 31:2055-2063, 2009.

51. Mostafapour SP, Murakami CS. Tissue expansion and serial excision in scar revision. Facial Plast Surg 17:245-252, 2001.

52. Cupp CL, Johnson MB, Larrabee WF Jr, et al. Scar revision: a simplified method to design geometric broken line closures. Facial Plast Surg Clin North Am 6:195-201, 1998.
    Excellent paper simplifying the planning and execution of geometric broken line closure.

53. Burget GC, Menick FJ. The subunit principle in nasal reconstruction. Plast Reconstr Surg 76:239-247, 1985.

54. Borges AF. Principles of scar camouflage. Facial Plast Surg 1:181-190, 1984.

55. Ronert MA, Hofheinz H, Manassa E, et al. The beginning of a new era in tissue expansion: self-filling osmotic tissue expander—four-year clinical experience. Plast Reconstr Surg 114:1025-1031, 2004.

56. Sasaki G. Tissue Expansion in Reconstructive and Aesthetic Surgery. St Louis: Mosby, 1998.

57. Borges AF. The W-plastic versus the Z-plastic scar revision. Plast Reconstr Surg 44:58-62, 1969.

58. Wolfe D, Davidson TM. Scar revision. Arch Otolaryngol Head Neck Surg 117:200-204, 1991.
    Different scar revision techniques are compared on similar scars, all on the same patient. Comparison of the final results is unique and interesting, and provides insight into choosing the optimal technique for these procedures.

59. Webster CC, Davidson TM, Smith RC. Broken line scar revision. Clin Plast Surg 4:263-274, 1977.

60. Moore BA, Wine T, Netterville JL. Cervicofacial and cervicothoracic rotation flaps in head and neck reconstruction. Head Neck 27:1092-1101, 2005.

61. Juri J, Juri C. Advancement and rotation of a large cervicofacial flap for cheek repairs. Plast Reconstr Surg 64:692-696, 1979.

62. Griffin GR, Weber S, Baker SR. Outcomes following V-Y advancement flap reconstruction of large upper lip defects. Arch Facial Plast Surg 14:193-197, 2012.

63. Neuber F. Fettransplantation. Chir Kongr Verhandl Deutsche Gesellschaft für Chirurgie 22:66-68, 1893.

64. Peer LA. The neglected free fat graft, its behavior and clinical use. Am J Surg 92:40-47, 1956.

65. Clauser LC, Tieghi R, Galie M, et al. Structural fat grafting: facial volumetric restoration in complex reconstructive surgery. J Craniofac Surg 22:1695-1701, 2011.

66. Nehal KS, Levine VJ, Ross B, et al. Comparison of high-energy pulsed carbon dioxide laser resurfacing and dermabrasion in the revision of surgical scars. Dermatol Surg 24:647-650, 1998.

67. Apfelberg DB, Maser MR, White DN, et al. Failure of carbon dioxide laser excision of keloids. Lasers Surg Med 9:382-388, 1989.

68. Jordan R, Cummins C, Burls A. Laser resurfacing of the skin for the improvement of facial acne scarring: a systematic review of the evidence. Br J Dermatol 142:413-423, 2000.

69. Vrijman C, van Drooge AM, Limpens J, et al. Laser and intense pulsed light therapy for the treatment of hypertrophic scars: a systematic review. Br J Dermatol 165:934-942, 2011.

70. Lupton JR, Alster TS. Laser scar revision. Dermatol Clin 20:55-65, 2002.

71. Alster TS. Improvement of erythematous and hypertrophic scars by the 585-nm flashlamp-pumped pulsed dye laser. Ann Plast Surg 32:186-190, 1994.

72. Shih PY, Chen HH, Chen CH, et al. Rapid recurrence of keloid after pulse dye laser treatment. Dermatol Surg 34:1124-1127, 2008.

73. Jared Christophel J, Elm C, Endrizzi BT, et al. A randomized controlled trial of fractional laser therapy and dermabrasion for scar resurfacing. Dermatol Surg 38:595-602, 2012.

74. Tierney E, Mahmoud BH, Srivastava D, et al. Treatment of surgical scars with nonablative fractional laser versus pulsed dye laser: a randomized controlled trial. Dermatol Surg 35:1172-1180, 2009.

35

Local Flaps for Facial Reconstruction, Including Cheek and Lip Defects

Jon-Paul Pepper ▪ *Jennifer Kim*

Descriptions of cheek and lip reconstruction extend into antiquity.[1] Although *Sushruta Samhita* (600 BC) is often credited with providing the first written descriptions of lip reconstruction, this text was in fact a seminal description of nasal reconstruction and became a foundation for modern rhinoplasty; however, it included few formal descriptions of lip reconstruction.[2] Celsus (25-50 AD) documented the use of local flaps for the reconstruction of lip defects.[3] The principle of flap undermining to improve tissue movement and reapproximation was recommended by Paulus Aegineta[4] in the seventh century AD. Tagliacozzi introduced the concept of staged nasal reconstructions using skin from the upper extremities in the seventeenth century, and many of the nasal defects he described also included lip deformities.[5]

The next two centuries were a period of many significant surgical advances. One of the first known wedge excisions with linear reapproximation was described by Louis in 1768. Dieffenbach (Fig. 35-1) described the first cheek advancement flap techniques in 1834.[1]

Bernard[6] and von Burow introduced skin triangle excisions for advancement and closure in the 1850s. The first axial flap used for lip reconstruction was published by Pietro Sabattini[7] in 1838. This technique was also published in English and popularized by Robert Abbé[8] in 1898. Because of the circumstances of Sabattini's practice and limited circulation of his published work, Abbé had no exposure to Sabattini's published works and therefore appears to have developed the concept independently some 60 years later. In a similar period, Finnish surgeon Jakob Estlander[9] described his use of a vascularized lower lip flap used to repair upper lip defects that involved the oral commissure.

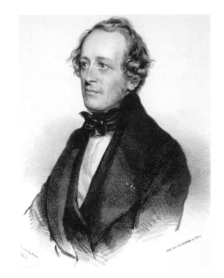

Fig. 35-1 Johann Friedrich Dieffenbach (1792-1847). German surgeon who specialized in cutaneous surgery.

Although Sabattini's work likely represented the first documented myocutaneous flap,[5] it was Gillies[10] who provided a detailed description of the use of myocutaneous flaps for large lip defects in 1920. This seminal work was modified by Karapandzic[11] in 1974, in an effort to preserve the neurovascular supply of the lip and improve functional outcome. Subsequent study of this concept has brought into question the degree to which neuromuscular function is preserved when performing the Karapandzic technique.[12] Bernard, Webster,[13] and McGregor[14] separately published technical refinements that described various methods of pivoting or rotating cheek tissue into lip defects.

Facial defects have a significant impact on the way an observer perceives an individual, with central defects having a larger perceptual impact than those located more laterally.[15-17] Even small central lesions may be perceived as significantly disfiguring.[16] Facial defects can affect the perception of a patient's honesty, employability, trustworthiness, and overall capability.[17] The cheek is the largest subunit of the face, and the lip is a key region for emotive expression and oral articulation. Cutaneous defects in these locations can therefore significantly affect the patient's quality of life.

Given the rise in incidence of cutaneous malignancies of the head and neck,[18] repair of facial defects through local tissue flaps has become an increasingly important skill in facial reconstruction. A discussion of this topic links the principles of wound healing with the principles of head and neck neurovascular anatomy and requires knowledge of the physiology of speech and swallowing and a solid understanding of soft tissue relationships in the youthful and aging face.

Surgeons who treat lip and cheek defects must possess a comprehensive knowledge of the local flaps commonly employed in the reconstruction of cheek and lip defects. Terminology employed in local flap reconstruction is standard (Table 35-1). A methodical approach to the selection, design, and execution of local flap reconstruction of cheek and lip defects will improve the ultimate outcome.

Table 35-1 Terminology Used in Local Flap Reconstruction

Local cutaneous flap	Area of skin and subcutaneous tissue with a direct vascular supply that is transferred from its in situ position to a site located immediately adjacent to or near the flap.
Regional flap	Tissue is harvested from a site not located on the face, scalp, or neck; however, the pedicle is sufficiently long to enable the flap to reach the primary defect.
Primary defect	Wound to be closed by a local cutaneous flap.
Secondary defect	Wound created when a skin flap is transferred to repair the primary defect.
Primary tissue movement	Motion of the flap into the primary defect.
Secondary tissue movement	Displacement of skin surrounding the defect toward the center of the primary defect.
Wound closure tension	Amount of stress (per unit area) along the suture line of a repaired wound; tension depends on the vector forces of the tissue involved with primary and secondary movement.

Pivotal flap	Rotates about a point at its base, and in the purest form is not stretched; thus are not subjected to wound closure tension greater than the natural tension of the remaining facial skin, although the repair of the donor site of the flap is subjected to increased skin tension.
	There are four types of pivotal flaps: *rotation, transposition, interpolated,* and *island.*
Advancement flap	Has a linear configuration and is moved by sliding toward the defect; in the majority of situations, depends on stretching the flap skin in the direction of flap movement. Such flaps are subjected to an increase in wound closure tension.
Hinge flap	Sometimes referred to as a *trapdoor, turn-in,* or *turn-down* flap; may be designed in a linear or curvilinear shape with the pedicle based on one border of the primary defect. The flap is dissected in the subcutaneous plane and turned over onto the defect like a page in a book.

ANATOMY

The cheek is typically divided into zygomatic, lateral (parotidomasseteric), medial (infraorbital), and buccal subunits (Fig. 35-2).

The borders between these subunits are not well defined. The anterior border of the lateral (parotidomasseteric) subunit roughly describes the location of the underlying anterior edge of the masseter muscle. The posterior border of the medial (infraorbital) subunit corresponds to the zygomaticus major muscle. The border between the zygomatic and buccal subunits is demarcated by a horizontal line at the level of the masseteric retaining ligament. The peripheral boundaries of the cheek span from the lateral canthus to root of helix, preauricular sulcus, inferior border of mandible, labiomental crease, melolabial fold, nasofacial sulcus, and lid-cheek junction.

The lateral retaining ligaments of the cheek include the zygomatic, orbital, masseteric, and mandibular ligaments. The zygomatic ligament is the strongest of the lateral retaining ligaments.[19] The ligaments are arranged in a roughly linear vertical orientation. Therefore the skin is more fixed to the deep tissues laterally, and there is greater mobility and more generous subcutaneous fat medially. In addition, Moss, Mendelson, and Taylor[20] described a portion of the superficial musculoaponeurotic system (SMAS) in the preauricular region as the platysma-auricular fascia, which refers to a layer of immobile, relatively fixed fascia that is often used to anchor SMAS flaps in rhytidectomy.

In addition to its two-dimensional compartments, the cheek is a region of complex three-dimensional topography. The static contour of the cheek is largely determined by compartmentalized subcutaneous and deep fatty layers. The subcutaneous fat of the cheek, or *malar* fat, was subdivided by Rohrich and Pessa[21] into medial, middle, and lateral temporal-cheek segments. Buccal fat composes a deeper fatty layer.[22] The medialmost fat of the cheek is actually a melolabial extension of buccal fat and is a prominent feature of normal cheek anatomy. This fat is responsible for the melolabial bulge that descends with age and increasing tissue laxity.

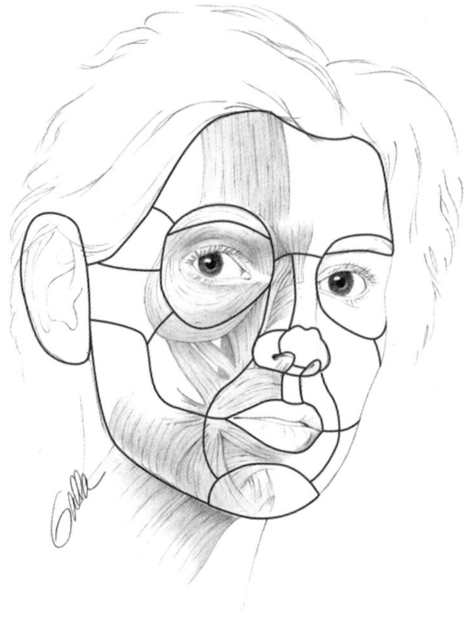

Fig. 35-2   Anatomic subunits of the face.

The SMAS was first described by Mitz and Peyronie,[23] and correction of its laxity with aging provides the basis for many modern face-lift techniques. It is found in a tissue layer corresponding to the temporoparietal fascia and zygomaticus major muscles, and is confluent with the platysma muscle. Although earlier reports maintained that the SMAS envelops the zygomaticus and midface muscles,[23] more recent anatomic study found that the SMAS simply terminates lateral to the zygomaticus major muscle.[22] The same study found no direct insertion of the SMAS into the dermis of the melolabial fold; instead, the SMAS forms a newly described *zone of fusion* with the buccinator muscle in the region of the modiolus.

Accurate reconstruction of the cheek relies on the re-creation of near-normal cheek volumes[24]; Understanding the complicated soft tissue relationships is critical to accomplishing this aim. The convexity of the cheek prevents ideal scar camouflage in relaxed skin tension lines. The lid-cheek junction is one of the thinnest dermal layers in the body[25] and requires specialized reconstructive approaches to avoid ectropion of the lower lid caused by secondary tissue movement after a local flap is moved into the defect. Additionally, there is an accessory fat layer that lies deep to the orbicularis oculi muscle (the suborbicularis oculi fat pad [SOOF]) and is distinct from the subcutaneous malar fat.[20]

The lip spans the lower third of the face from subnasale to the mental crease in vertical dimension and between the melolabial and labiomental creases in horizontal dimension. The upper lip is subdivided into two paired lateral compartments, with the *philtrum* inserted between them. The upper lip mimics an elongated lazy M, with apices that are the base of philtral columns, separated by the concave base of the philtral groove. Together the apices and philtral base make up the *cupid's bow*. The *tubercle* refers to the prominence at the center of upper lip. Philtral columns extend into the columella, separated by the philtral groove. The *vermilion* is composed of stratified epithelium adapted for external exposure and is highly vascular. There are no glandular tissues or hair follicles in this location. The anterior and posterior vermilion lines separate the vermilion from the cutaneous lip and the labial mucosa, respectively (Fig. 35-3).

The orbicularis oris muscle is commonly conceptualized as a circular sphincter, although its true action is significantly more complex because of the demands of articulation and emotive expression that define individualized lip movement. The superficial aspect of the muscle receives contribution from 21 facial muscles that help to fine-tune movement. The orbicularis oris muscle consists of four quadrants of muscle subdi-

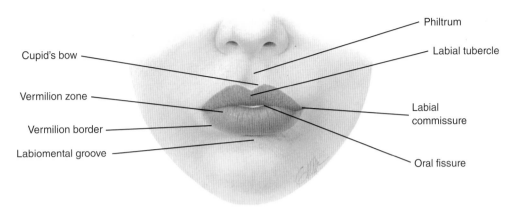

Fig. 35-3   Anatomy of the lips.

vided into a pars marginalis and pars peripheralis. The marginal component lies anterior and inferior to the peripheral component, and the junction between these distinct portions is responsible for the distinct white roll noted near the vermilion-cutaneous junction.[26,27] Although classically the marginal component was thought to underlie only the red portion of the lip, more recent analysis has shown that it does extend several millimeters beyond the vermilion.[27] The modiolus has three-dimensional subtleties, such as the insertion of the buccinator muscle posterior to the pars marginalis. Finally, the orbicularis fibers decussate 4 to 5 mm from the midline philtral columns.[28] These decussating fibers attach to the dermis and form the philtral columns. Centrally these decussations are absent, which creates the concave philtral groove.

The majority of the cheek is perfused by the transverse facial artery; the facial artery and infraorbital arteries are lesser contributors.[29,30] Significant anastomoses are found between the lip region and terminal branches of the internal maxillary artery in the nasal cavity.[30] The superficial temporal artery pierces the parotidomasseteric fascia approximately 1.0 cm anterior and 1.75 cm superior to the external auditory canal.[29] The transverse facial artery arises from the superficial temporal artery deep to the parotid gland, coursing along the superficial surface of the masseteric fascia.[29,31] Most of the lateral vascular supply arises from septocutaneous perforators of the transverse facial artery.

The anterior face, particularly the perioral and perinasal regions, are supplied by hundreds of musculocutaneous perforators that arborize directly from the facial artery and its terminal branches.[29] The facial artery typically emerges from the external carotid artery as a distinct branch, although a common lingual-facial trunk occurs in approximately 10% to 15% of cases.[30] After emerging from the parenchyma of the submandibular gland, the facial artery gives off its largest cervical branch, the submental artery.[32] The facial artery has anastomoses with the lingual, inferior alveolar, inferior labial, and mental arteries at its most distal extent. The facial artery has on average five dominant musculocutaneous perforators.[33] Perforators are found in highest density in a 1 cm diameter circle centered on a point 1.5 cm lateral to the oral commissure. The lip is perfused predominantly by the superior and inferior labial arteries. There is a distinct cascade of vessels that perfuses the philtrum separately as a terminal branch of the superior labial artery.[34]

Sensory innervation of the cheek and lip is supplied by terminal branches of the second and third divisions of the trigeminal nerve (see Chapter 1). Motor innervation is provided by the facial nerve. In most cases, the branches of the facial nerve penetrate their target muscles on the deep aspect of the muscles, which allows safe dissection superficial to the muscle layer. However, three paired muscles of the face receive neural input on their superficial aspect: the buccinator, levator anguli oris, and mentalis muscles.

EPIDEMIOLOGY AND CLASSIFICATION

The incidence of cutaneous malignancies is rapidly rising.[18] Commensurate with the rise in skin cancers, Mohs surgery has become the mainstay of cutaneous malignancy management.[35] The incidence of cutaneous malignancy is distinct from the referral pattern for reconstruction; cutaneous lip defects may be disproportionately referred to facial reconstructive surgeons based on the functional consequences of inadequate reconstruction.

Cheek and lip defects may be classified according to their aesthetic subunit location. Although algorithms for reconstruction based on defect size and location are conceptually useful, in reality the reconstructive technique chosen depends on numerous factors. Reconstructive algorithms must be considered in the context of the large number of variables that influence the choice of local flap to use for a given clinical situation. Thus both reconstructive techniques and their application in each aesthetic subunit will be discussed in the next section.

PATIENT PREPARATION AND PREOPERATIVE PLANNING

Candidates for Mohs microsurgery include those with large anticipated defects and those with lesions in anatomically and aesthetically sensitive areas. Additionally, patients with preinvasive melanoma (melanoma in situ) lesions are often referred to the facial reconstructive surgeon before margin control, after excision of the tumor periphery only (the so-called square-blade technique). Based on the anticipated defect size, depth, and location, the patient is shown representative photographs of each reconstructive option. This patient education is particularly important for any staged reconstruction, because the temporary disfigurement can be disturbing.[36]

Tumor histology is an important factor to consider in reconstructive planning. For example, although it is amenable to Mohs microsurgery, aggressive squamous cell carcinoma (SCC) may have a higher risk of occult regional metastases; in some cases these patients are referred for sentinel lymph node biopsy, which would affect incision placement for wound closure. For lower lip tumors, SCC is the most common pathology, and evaluation of the regional lymph node basin is critical. For instance, in midfacial cutaneous SCC and melanoma, the perifacial nodes are considered to be an important potential site of regional metastasis.[37] The need for concomitant neck dissection often requires ligation of the facial artery for thorough removal of the submandibular lymphatics. Details such as these can drastically alter the reconstructive plan for unexpectedly large defects or aggressive tumor types.

Evaluation of the patient's adjacent skin is a critical component of preoperative planning. Assessment of overall skin elasticity and skin integrity should be performed. Active immunosuppression with glucocorticoids or other pharmacologic agents, prior radiotherapy, and extensive photodamage caused by excessive sun exposure can significantly alter the ability of the skin to advance or pivot into a defect. Likewise, anticoagulation status is clarified, as is the safety of temporarily withholding anticoagulants in the perioperative period. Larger lesions are often addressed with flaps that require extensive undermining. This may require a temporary suction or passive drain, or in some instances a topical hemostatic agent may be used. For large surface area lip reconstruction, assessing the dentition is helpful, since patients may be unable to reinsert dentures because of postoperative microstomia.

Finally, an accurate assessment of the patient's goals for reconstruction is important. His or her vocation and lifestyle should be considered, and in men, distortion of the hair-bearing cutaneous lip will create disfigurement.

TECHNIQUE

As in all local flap reconstructions, the primary goal is to place incisions on natural skin creases or borders between facial subunits while avoiding distortion of the lower lid, upper lip vermilion-cutaneous junction, and nostril margin. If it is not possible to camouflage incisions along a unit border, incisions should be oriented parallel to relaxed skin tension lines. For nearly all flaps in these locations, wide subcutaneous undermining and aggressive excision of any standing cutaneous deformity are critical. On the cheek and lip, standing cutaneous deformities are unlikely to flatten over time and should be aggressively removed during initial reconstruction.

Unlike nasal reconstruction, cheek and lip reconstruction does not involve cartilaginous grafts, which might serve as a stabilizing semirigid scaffold for tissue placement. Thus significant soft tissue distortion through wound contracture is possible as the reconstruction heals. The lip in particular has unique tissue qualities—color, texture, and elasticity—that are difficult to match with flaps from other aesthetic units or distant sites.

The dynamic motility of the oral region makes restoration of sphincter function challenging. Also, subtle changes in lip orientation during emotive expression can easily be altered because of scar contracture.

CHEEK RECONSTRUCTION: SELECTED FLAPS
Bilateral Advancement Flap

The key landmark for repair of medial cheek defects is the melolabial crease (Fig. 35-4). The soft tissue lateral to the crease is mobile, and excising extensive standing cutaneous deformities superior and inferior to the lesion facilitates cosmetically acceptable primary repair within the crease. Although this approach often distorts the melolabial bulge and makes it asymmetrical to the contralateral side, this distortion is difficult to perceive on anterior view. For medial cheek defects, the preferred method of repair is by asymmetrical advancement flap. Advancement flaps are designed to asymmetrically recruit tissue from the lateral soft tissue, with the final closure placed in the melolabial and/or labiomandibular crease.

Transposition Flap: Note Flap

Fig. 35-5 shows a central and infraorbital cheek defect repaired with a modified *note flap*. The note flap was originally described by Walikee and Larrabee[38] for the repair of circular defects. This is a transposition flap designed to resemble a musical eighth note. The tangential limb has a length 1.5 times the diameter

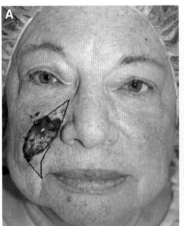
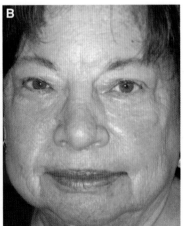

Fig. 35-4   Advancement flap closure. **A,** Preoperative defect in the medial cheek adjacent to the right melolabial crease. The defect is amenable to bilateral advancement flap closure. **B,** Final postoperative result.

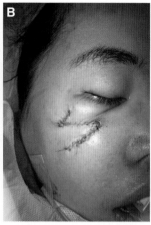

Fig. 35-5   Infraorbital and central cheek defect repaired with a modified note flap. **A,** Preoperative view, with flap design. **B,** Postoperative view after closure. The primary and secondary tissue movements are mostly in the transverse vector, which reduces inferior pulling on the lower lid and lessens the risk of ectropion.

of the circular defect. At an angle of 60 degrees, a second limb is drawn that enables a triangular pivoting flap to transpose into the defect. A standing cone is removed from the base of the flap. This design may be modified by shortening the tangent limb and making a larger standing cutaneous deformity at the base of the transposition flap. Given the frequent occurrence of circular defects after Mohs microsurgery, the note flap is a very useful reconstructive technique.

Cervicofacial Advancement Rotation Flap

Large defects that span multiple cheek subunits require commensurately large local flaps for reconstruction. Fig. 35-6 illustrates a management strategy for a patient with a large medial cheek lesion that has had prior margin control and presents for central lesion excision and reconstruction.

For large medial cheek defects adjacent to the melolabial crease and nasofacial sulcus, the cervicofacial advancement rotation flap is the reconstructive technique of choice. Key points include careful placement of the standing cutaneous deformity, the use of periosteal or bone-anchoring sutures to prevent lid retraction, and incorporation of a superior curvilinear arc above the lateral canthus to lateralize the vector of secondary tissue movement and resultant wound tension on closure. An inferior vector of secondary tissue movement is never acceptable, because lid retraction will result. The superior limb of the flap should be placed at the bony orbital rim. Subciliary incisions are reserved for occasions where the lower lid skin is clearly involved in the defect. Even then, skin grafting of the lower lid skin as a separate subunit may be preferable.

Although some authors report good results with deep plane cervicofacial flaps, standard cervicofacial flaps elevated in the subcutaneous plane are usually generously vascularized, and the deeper dissection with its attendant risks may not provide enough benefit to offset these risks. An anteriorly based flap (see Fig. 35-6) receives its vascular supply from the facial artery and its submental perforators. This approach permits a backcut in the neck or submandibular region and provides the flap a larger arc of rotation while preserving the vascular supply of the flap. A final consideration for cervicofacial flaps is postoperative hemostasis and prevention of fluid accumulation deep to a widely undermined flap. Placing a drain or applying a topical thrombin-based hemostatic to decrease the risk of postoperative hematoma may decrease the likelihood of this accumulation. Bipolar cautery is helpful for obtaining meticulous hemostasis, and a postoperative pressure wrap is routinely used.

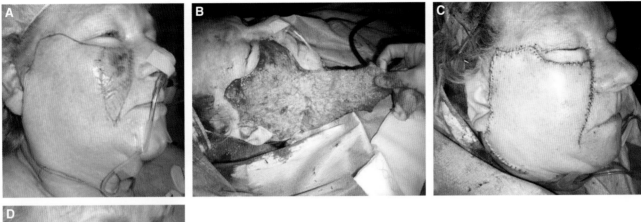

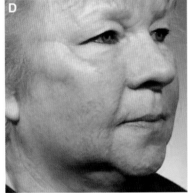

Fig. 35-6   Cervicofacial advancement for a melanoma in situ lesion with clear margins. **A,** Flap design; note the curvilinear arc of the superior limb of the flap and the inferior backcut in a natural skin crease of the neck. **B,** Flap elevated. **C,** Appearance at closure. **D,** Eight-week postoperative result with normal postoperative scar hyperemia. No revision surgery was required.

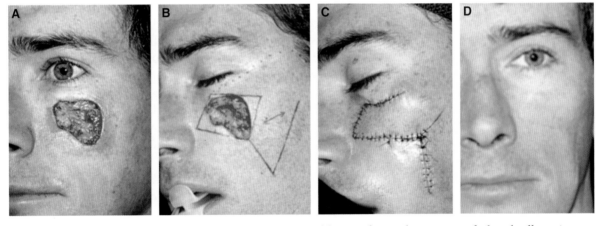

Fig. 35-7   Rhomboid flap. **A,** Cheek defect in a 35-year-old man after Mohs excision of a basal cell carcinoma. **B,** Rhomboid flap designed with the axis of tension indicated. **C,** Transfer of rhomboid flap for reconstruction of the cheek defect. **D,** Result after 6 months. Note the good position of the lower eyelid.

Rhomboid Flap

Laterally based rhomboid flaps represent an excellent option for cheek defects, particularly for rectangular defects such as the one shown in Fig. 35-7.

The buccal aesthetic subunit consists of the skin of the central cheek just lateral to the skin of the melolabial fold. Defects of this region may be reconstructed with cutaneous flaps harvested from cheek skin lateral or inferior to the buccal region. Medially based flaps will distort the oral commissure, melolabial crease, or

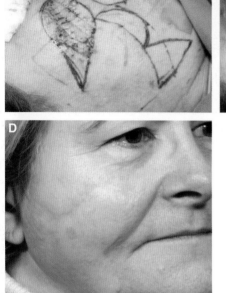
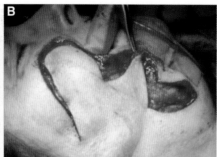
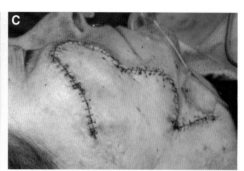

Fig. 35-8   Bilobed flap to repair a cheek defect involving infraorbital and zygomatic subunits of the cheek. **A,** Flap design. **B,** Flap before undermining. **C,** Flap after inset and closure. **D,** Final postoperative result.

labiomental sulcus and therefore are not used. Small defects (approximately 1 to 2 cm, depending on tissue laxity) can be closed primarily in the form of an ellipse that parallels relaxed skin tension lines. Medium sized defects (2 to 4 cm) that have a linear axis parallel to relaxed skin tension lines can often be repaired primarily. For defects of the buccal and lateral cheek subunits, a cervicofacial flap would create long and linear scars that traverse the center of an aesthetic unit, thus large transposition flaps for buccal subunit defects are more useful. The disadvantage of such flaps is that the resulting scars often lie in the center of the aesthetic unit and are oriented in several different directions; portions of the scar are not aligned with the relaxed skin tension lines.

Bilobed Flaps

Bilobed flaps are useful when more straightforward rotation or transposition flaps will not provide sufficient tissue for repair (Fig. 35-8). This occurs when the defect is large and located in the midcheek, lateral to the central part of the face. In this situation, the amount of remaining adjacent cheek skin may be insufficient to reconstruct the defect and still permit closure of the donor site.

A superolaterally based bilobed flap designed to recruit upper cervical skin can overcome this problem. The major downside to this reconstructive technique is that the incision lines do not fall along the relaxed skin tension lines, though the aesthetic penalty for this is usually minor. It is important to verify that the donor site of the second lobe can be closed.

V-Y Subcutaneous Tissue Pedicle Island Advancement Flap

The V-Y subcutaneous tissue pedicle island advancement flap is frequently used for repairing larger medial cheek defects at or below the level of the nasal ala. The primary movement of the flap is designed to be parallel to the vertical axis of the melolabial crease. The trailing half of the skin island tapers to a point to facilitate donor site closure in a V-Y fashion, ideally within the melolabial and labiomental creases. The technique for V-Y subcutaneous tissue pedicle island advancement flaps for lateral lip reconstruction is discussed later, but it is equally useful for medial cheek reconstruction.

Lip Reconstruction: Selected Flaps

Lip tissue is a composite of skin, muscle, and mucosa. The major feature of the upper and lower lips is the vermilion, which is composed of modified mucosa. The vermilion represents the mucocutaneous junction between the inner labial mucosa and outer skin and is a critical aesthetic landmark. The boundaries of the lip include the nasal base superiorly, melolabial folds laterally, and the mental crease inferiorly. The upper lip is divided into three aesthetic subunits: the central philtrum and the paired lateral units. The lower lip is composed of a single subunit. The body of the lips is made up principally of the orbicularis oris muscle, which decussates at the oral commissures. The melolabial and labiomandibular creases represent the sites where the muscles of facial expression attach to the orbicularis muscle and are ideal sites for incision placement. The relaxed skin tension lines of the lip are present in a radial pattern around the oral aperture. Centrally, the lines are vertically oriented; they become increasingly oblique on the lateral portion of the lip.

Conversion to Full Thickness With Direct Closure

Depending on the lip laxity, cutaneous defects approaching half of the width of the lip may be converted to full-thickness excisions of the lip, followed by primary wound closure (Fig. 35-9).

Optimal reconstruction involves carefully approximating four tissue layers: mucosa, muscle, dermis, and epithelium. The anterior vermilion is marked preoperatively with ink, or intraoperatively with methylene blue dye (Fig. 35-10). In either case, it is critical to mark the vermilion-cutaneous junction before injection of a local anesthetic. The vertical height of the vermilion is matched by careful approximation of the orbicularis muscle to prevent notching or retraction of the vermilion. Scars are placed along the relaxed skin tension lines, and W-plasty incisions can be employed to avoid extending the incision beyond aesthetic subunit borders such as the mental crease and melolabial fold (Fig. 35-11). Most skin defects of the central upper and lower lips that cannot be closed primarily can be repaired using bilateral advancement flaps. Releasing incisions for the advancement flaps are placed in the mental crease for the lower lip and the melolabial crease for the upper lip. Because of the highly mobile nature of the lip's soft tissue, there is an increased tendency for scar hypertrophy. Aggressive use of postoperative steroid injections is recommended and should be begun 1 month after repair. Perioperative chemodenervation with botulinum toxin may also improve scar outcomes for lip reconstructions.

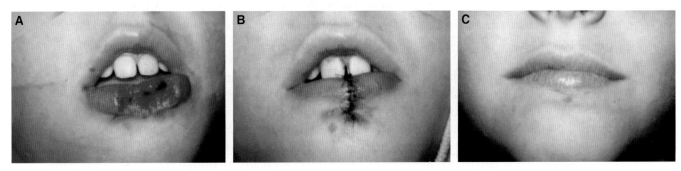

Fig. 35-9   Primary lip closure. **A,** Dog bite to the lower lip, with full-thickness tissue loss. **B,** Primary closure using mucosal advancement. **C,** Final result.

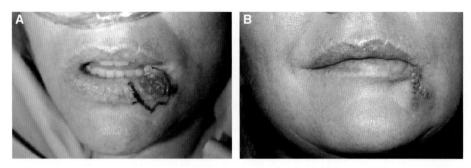

Fig. 35-10 **A,** Anticipated defect of a squamous cell carcinoma of the lower lip vermilion. **B,** W-plasty used to shorten the inferior aspect of the standing cutaneous deformity.

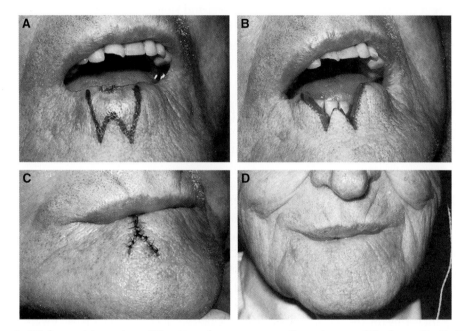

Fig. 35-11 **A,** Wedge excision using a W-pattern for squamous cell carcinoma of the lower lip. **B,** Defect. **C,** Primary closure. **D,** Final result.

Labial Mucosal Advancement Flaps

Labial mucosal advancement flaps are indicated usually for shallow vermilion defects and vermilionectomy-type defects. Elevation is performed in a plane deep to minor salivary glands and superficial to the orbicularis oris muscle (Fig. 35-12).

Care is taken to safeguard small neurovascular structures during elevation to preserve a sensate flap. For large defects, the vermilion advancement can be interpolated to the primary defect and delayed. The bridge of mucosa and submucosa is then divided and inset in 2 to 3 weeks. Advantages include an acceptable tissue match and a reliable vascular supply. Disadvantages include the deeper red pigmentation, which some male patients may perceive as feminizing. Moreover, the vermilion is often flattened by this flap, and the tissue volume advanced into the defect can be insufficient, particularly on profile view. Scar contraction can cause posterior displacement of the anterior vermilion line and upward displacement of hair follicles.

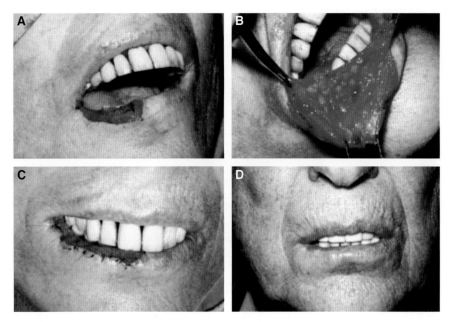

Fig. 35-12   Mucosal advancement flap. **A,** Mucosal defect after excision of a squamous cell carcinoma of the lower lip. **B,** The mucosal advancement flap is mobilized from the intraoral mucosa. **C,** The inset flap has reestablished the vermilion border. **D,** Final result.

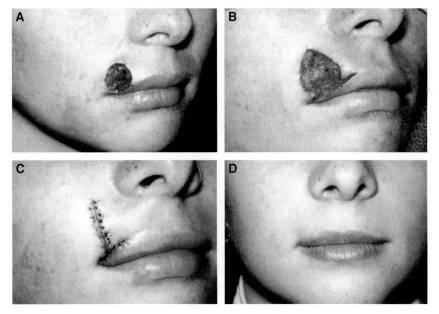

Fig. 35-13   Inverted O to T flap for closure of a combined vermilion and cutaneous defect of the upper lip. **A,** Defect after Mohs surgery. **B,** Advancement flaps along the vermilion border. **C,** Flap elevation and inset. **D,** Final result.

Advancement Flaps

Partial-thickness cutaneous defects can be closed using a multitude of local advancement or transposition flaps (Fig. 35-13). These flaps are elevated as subcutaneous flaps with the underlying facial musculature left intact. Lip skin, although highly elastic, is tightly adherent to the orbicularis oris muscle. The skin must be dissected sharply from the muscle to provide adequate release for tissue mobilization. For small defects, primary closure is usually possible with incision placement along the relaxed skin tension lines.

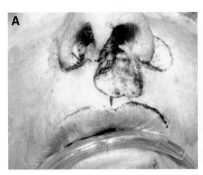
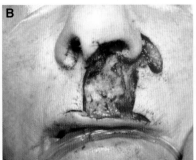
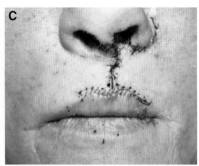

Fig. 35-14   Bilateral advancement flaps with a perialar crescent. **A,** Asymmetrical bilateral advancement flaps for closure of an upper lip defect approximately 2 cm in diameter. Note the incorporation of the right perialar crescent and the left nostril sill to promote a symmetrical closure along aesthetic subunit boundaries. Care must be taken to excise sill tissue conservatively to minimize the risk of vestibular stenosis. **B,** Flap after undermining. **C,** Final closure.

O to T horizontal advancement flaps can be used when the defect is adjacent to the vermilion or nasal sill. For partial-thickness central lip defects 1 to 2 cm in diameter, bilateral advancement flaps offer the best method of repair (Fig. 35-14).

Larger advancement flaps achieve a better overall result when accompanied by a crescent-shaped excision of perialar skin to reduce a standing cutaneous deformity and alar distortion (see Fig. 35-14). For the upper lip, incisions for opposing advancement flaps are made along the vermilion-cutaneous border and immediately below the nasal sill. For the lower lip, incisions are placed in the vermilion-cutaneous border and the mental crease.

V-Y Subcutaneous Tissue Pedicle Island Advancement Flap

V-Y subcutaneous tissue pedicle island advancement flaps are ideally suited for repair of large lateral upper lip defects (Fig. 35-15).

Here, the surgeon can take advantage of the loose melolabial cheek skin, with excellent movement based on a subcutaneous pedicle to reconstruct fairly sizable upper lip defects without causing lip distortion, but preserving the nasolabial border. These flaps are not as effective for defects of the lower lip. The flap is freed from its attachments to the orbicularis muscle near the oral commissure and is based on the abundant subcutaneous fat in this region. The flap can be partially undermined safely, preserving approximately 50% of the deep central attachments to the richly vascularized fat. The V-Y flap is typically designed to have a length that is twice its width. The width is determined by the width of the primary defect. The adjacent tissue of the cheek is undermined for 1 to 2 cm to provide a tension-free closure.

For larger defects, it is helpful to excise a perialar crescent of skin and replace it with a portion of the flap. The result is a more subtle scar that follows the natural line of the melolabial crease to a position lateral to the nasal ala. In general, minor revisions are common with the V-Y subcutaneous tissue pedicle island advancement flap. The circumferential scar line makes it somewhat prone to trapdoor deformity. Patients with large defects in this area should be counseled that revision surgery may be helpful to optimize the outcome of the scar.[39]

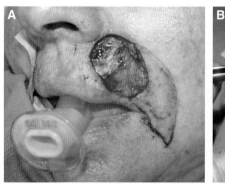

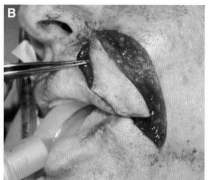

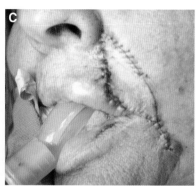

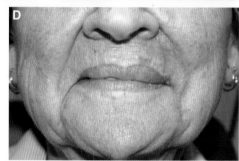

Fig. 35-15   V-Y subcutaneous tissue pedicle island advancement flap. **A,** Primary defect with planned flap. **B,** Flap being advanced on its subcutaneous pedicle. **C,** Flap after advancement. **D,** Patient photo at 6-week postoperative visit.

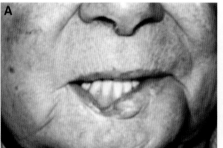

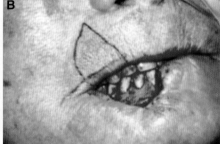

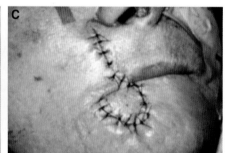

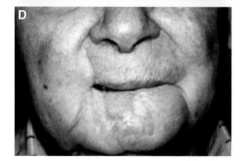

Fig. 35-16   Abbé flap. **A,** Distortion of lower lip after excision of a basal cell carcinoma with primary closure. **B,** Abbé flap based on the labial artery. **C,** Flap rotated and transferred into the defect. **D,** Final result after pedicle division.

Abbé Flap (Sabattini-Abbé Flap)

The Abbé flap is an extremely useful technique for large lip defects (Fig. 35-16). This flap is an interpolated axial flap based on the superior (or inferior) labial artery (Fig. 35-17).

The Abbé flap is indicated for 30% to 60% of full-thickness defects of the upper or lower lip in which the oral commissure is spared, but indications for this flap can be extended to larger defects, depending on the elasticity of adjacent tissue. Disadvantages to this flap include an upper lip donor site scar. It is impor-

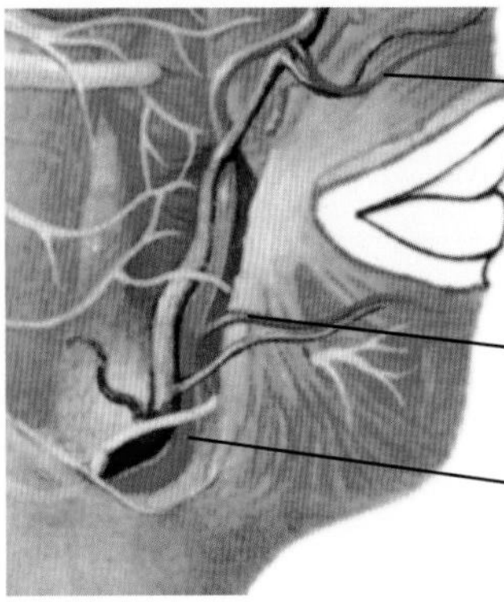

Superior labial artery

Inferior labial artery

Facial artery

Fig. 35-17   Anatomic course of the superior and inferior labial arteries.

tant to avoid distortion of the philtral columns when harvesting the flap from the upper lip; therefore the flap is best designed lateral to the philtral ridge. The flap is drawn with a donor site base width that is half the width of the defect. The height of the donor and defect site should be equal. The pedicle is routinely divided after 3 weeks. The labial artery runs deep to orbicularis oris muscle, so it is safe to extend the incision slightly into the vermilion on the side of the pedicle.

As the superior and inferior labial arteries course medially, their course becomes more predictable within the substance of the vermilion. Laterally, the course of the vessel is less unpredictable with respect to the vermilion, thus laterally based Abbé flaps run the risk of injuring the arterial pedicle. Additionally, medially based flaps possess a more favorable arc of rotation for inset. For central upper lip defects repaired with an Abbé flap, it is best to convert the defect to include the entirety of the philtral column, and conceal the superior incision in the nasal sill. Soft tissue of the submental region is well perfused by the inferior labial artery.[40] Therefore mental and submental soft tissue may be incorporated into Abbé flap design for defects of the upper lip that also effect perialar skin, the cheek, or the columella.

In general, functional outcomes after an Abbé flap procedure are favorable. Motor function will either be spared or, if the tissue is temporarily denervated, will return to baseline within 1 year. Sphincter restoration is routinely complete and oral incompetence is rare. Sensory function returns after inset, with pain (2 months), then tactile (3 months), then temperature (cold at 6 months, warm at 9 months), to baseline in 2 years. Abbé flaps may temporarily appear thickened, because the full-thickness scar impedes lymphatic drainage.

Estlander Flap

The Estlander flap is an axial interpolated rotation flap based on the labial artery and is used to repair defects that involve the oral commissure (Fig. 35-18).

Unlike Abbé flaps, the Estlander flap is single staged; the pivoted tissue includes the commissure and therefore no tissue interpolation is required. However, the Estlander flap may distort any remaining commissure, and some of these flaps will require revision commissuroplasty to normalize the appearance and function of the commissure. Patients are most likely to note the blunting of the commissure with the mouth open.

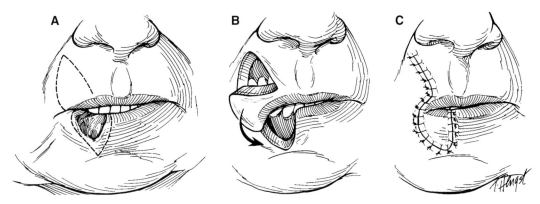

Fig. 35-18   Design of the Estlander flap. **A,** Flap design. **B,** Rotation of the flap into the defect. **C,** Final inset. Note the 180-degree rotation required.

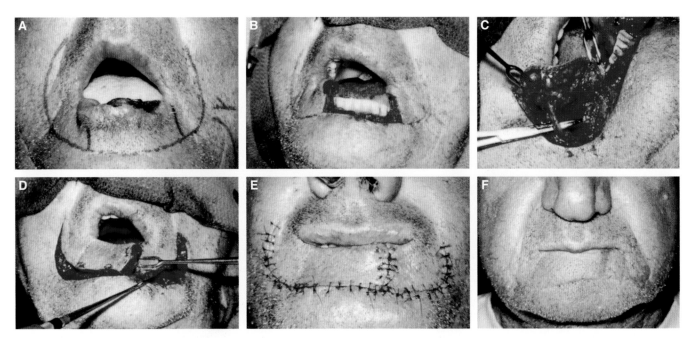

Fig. 35-19   Karapandzic technique. **A,** Squamous cell carcinoma of the lower lip. **B,** Excision of the lesion. **C,** The Karapandzic flap designed with preservation of the neurovascular pedicle. **D,** Advancement and midline closure of flap. **E,** Immediate result, showing microstomia. **F,** Final result.

Karapandzic Flap

The Karapandzic technique is a variation of a Gillies flap, in which a circumoral composite rotation-advancement flap is performed (Fig. 35-19).

Estlander flaps are indicated for full-thickness defects that encompass approximately 80% of the lip. Although ideal for large central lower lip defects, these flaps are slightly less effective for large central upper lip defects. The Karapandzic flap has largely replaced the Gillies technique because of the theoretical benefit that careful dissection of the neurovascular supply of the lip provides for a superior functional and reconstructive outcome. The major disadvantages are circumoral scars that violate boundaries of aesthetic subunits, microstomia, and blunting of the oral commissure.

For lower lip reconstruction, first the defect is carefully measured. The height of the defect dictates the distance of the flap incisions from the oral commissure. Circumoral incisions are made in the melolabial creases bilaterally. For large defects, an extension of the incision along the alar-facial sulcus and below the nasal sill can provide further tissue movement. After the incisions are made into the subcutaneous tissue, the dissection begins to identify perforating vessels and nerve fibers. The overall goal is to free the orbicularis attachment to the subcutaneous fat. Blunt spreading in the subcutaneous plane will accomplish this, and the attachments of the zygomatic muscles from the orbicularis oris muscle require release to provide additional soft tissue mobilization.

All patients will have profound microstomia postoperatively, but this will partially resolve with time and physical therapy. Patients are counseled to expect microstomia to be pronounced for 6 months. If this is persistent, bilateral commissuroplasties are performed to create a neocommissure in the appropriate location. A Karapandzic technique may be performed unilaterally, and combined with a contralateral Abbé flap (Fig. 35-20). The rationale for this combination of techniques is that their combined use will result in minimal distortion of the commissures, in contrast to bilateral Karapandzic techniques for repair.

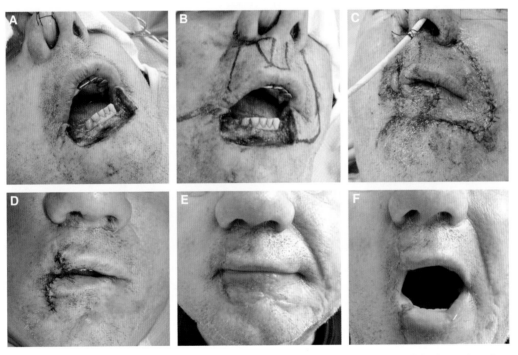

Fig. 35-20   Combined Karapandzic technique with an Abbé flap. **A,** A large defect of the lower lip after excision of a T2N0M0 squamous cell carcinoma of the lower lip. **B,** Flap design. Note that a right-sided Abbé flap that preserves the philtral ridges (marked) is designed in combination with a left-sided Karapandzic flap. **C,** Closure of the primary defect and donor sites. **D,** Closure after division of the pedicle and inset at 3 weeks after the primary surgery. **E,** One week after pedicle division with mouth closed. **F,** Mouth open, demonstrating mild microstomia. Patient did not seek additional adjunctive treatments.

POSTOPERATIVE CARE

A pressure dressing is applied with Telfa and Hypafix tape, which provides excellent pressure without the need for a cumbersome circumferential wrap. This dressing is routinely removed 24 hours after the procedure. Patients resume a normal diet as tolerated. For interpolated flaps that cause temporary microstomia or functional impairment, a temporary feeding tube is necessary very occasionally. This supplemental feeding should be considered, however, in a severely malnourished patient who presents after excision of a large cutaneous malignancy of the lip.

COMPLICATIONS

Possible complications from local flap reconstruction of the cheek and lip include hematoma, flap necrosis, unanticipated revision, loss of oral competence, sensory or motor nerve injury, and eyelid or lip asymmetry. Fortunately, these are rare with careful flap planning and meticulous execution. Adjunctive procedures are frequently necessary and should be planned for from the outset, particularly with larger local flaps.

ADJUNCTIVE PROCEDURES

Postoperative triamcinolone acetonide (Kenalog) injections have a beneficial effect on hypertrophic scars in the lip (see Chapter 34) and administration is encouraged at the first sign of hypertrophic scarring. The constant movement and prominent location of these scars merits an aggressive approach. Aside from persistent scar hyperemia and scar hypertrophy, a mismatch of the vermilion-cutaneous junction may occur after reconstruction. A Z-plasty is the single most effective technique for scar revision in this instance. Dermabrasion may be employed to resurface the perioral region. This approach is reserved for persistent scar hypertrophy more than 3 months after initial surgery.

KEY POINTS

- Cheek reconstruction is dictated by the subunit principle.
- Effective planning of local flaps for cheek reconstruction involves careful and sometimes creative placement of the standing cutaneous deformity.
- Secondary tissue movement should be preferentially distributed laterally, avoiding vectors of force that displace the lower lid and upper lip.
- Lip reconstruction should be planned by considering involvement of vermilion, depth of the lesion, and the degree of tissue elasticity.
- Adjunctive Kenalog injections, dermabrasion, and secondary surgical revision optimize outcome after cheek and lip reconstruction.

REFERENCES

1. Santoni-Rugiu P, Sykes PJ. Who was the first? Misconceptions and precedents in lip reconstruction. Ann Plast Surg 63:236-239, 2009.
2. Bhishagratna KK. The Sushruta Samhita. English Translation of the Original Sanskrit Text XI. Varanasi, India: The Chowkhamba Sanskrit Series, 1963.
3. Celsus. De Medicina. English translation by WG Spencer. Cambridge, MA: Harvard University Press, 1989.

4. Aegineta P. The Seven Books of Paulus Aegineta. English translation by F. Adams. London: Sydenham Society, 1847.

5. Santoni-Rugiu P, Sykes PJ. Nasal reconstruction. In A History of Plastic Surgery. Heidelberg: Springer-Verlag, 2007.

6. Bernard C. Cancer de la lèvre inférieure; restauration a l'aide de lambeaux quadrataires-latéreaux. Scalpel 5:162-165, 1852.

7. Sabattini P. Cenno Storico dell'Origine e Progressi della Rinoplastica e Cheiloplastica. Bologna: Belle Arti, 1838.

8. Abbé R. A new plastic operation for the relief of deformity due to double harelip. Med Rec 53:477, 1898.

9. Estlander JA. Eine Methode aus der einen lippe Substanzverluste der Anderen zu Ersetzen. Arch Klin Kir 14:622, 1872.

10. Gillies HD. Plastic Surgery of the Face. London: Gower Medical Publishers, 1983.

11. Karapandzic M. Reconstruction of lip defects by local arterial flaps. Br J Plast Surg 27:93-97, 1974.

12. Civelek B, Celebioglu S, Unlu E, et al. Denervated or innervated flaps for the lower lip reconstruction? Are they really different to get a good result? Otolaryngol Head Neck Surg 134:613-617, 2006.

13. Webster RC, Coffey RJ, Kelleher R. Total and partial reconstruction of the lower lip with innervated muscle bearing flaps. Plast Reconstruct Surg 25:360-371, 1960.

14. McGregor IA. Reconstruction of the lower lip. Br J Plast Surg 36:40-47, 1983.

15. Furr LA, Wiggins O, Cunningham M, et al. Psychosocial implications of disfigurement and the future of human face transplantation. Plast Reconstr Surg 120:559-565, 2007.

16. Godoy A, Ishii M, Byrne PJ, et al. How facial lesions impact attractiveness and perception: differential effects of size and location. Laryngoscope 121:2542-2547, 2011.

17. Rankin M, Borah GL. Perceived functional impact of abnormal facial appearance. Plast Reconstr Surg 111:2140-2146; discussion 2147-2148, 2003.

18. Rogers HW, Weinstock MA, Harris AR, et al. Incidence estimate of nonmelanoma skin cancer in the United States, 2006. Arch Dermatol 146:283-287, 2010.

19. Brandt MG, Hassa A, Roth K, et al. Biomechanical properties of the facial retaining ligaments. Arch Facial Plast Surg 14:289-294, 2012.

20. Moss CJ, Mendelson BC, Taylor GI. Surgical anatomy of the ligamentous attachments in the temple and periorbital regions. Plast Reconstr Surg 105:1475-1490; discussion 1491-1498, 2000.
    Detailed description of the osteocutaneous and musculocutaneous ligaments of the periorbital region and lateral midface. Essential for understanding both rhytidectomy and local flap anatomy.

21. Rohrich RJ, Pessa JE. The fat compartments of the face: anatomy and clinical implications for cosmetic surgery. Plast Reconstr Surg 119:2219-2227; discussion 2228-2231, 2007.
    Excellent analysis of the frequently misunderstood midface fat compartments. Important for understanding normal soft tissue distribution and sources of tissue laxity.

22. Gassner HG, Rafii A, Young A, et al. Surgical anatomy of the face: implications for modern face-lift techniques. Arch Facial Plast Surg 10:9-19, 2008.
    Essential update to classic work of Mitz and Peyronie, demonstrates that the SMAS terminates anterior to the masseter and does not envelop the zygomaticus muscles as previously described. Also provides beautiful description of the modiolus.

23. Mitz V, Peyronie M. The superficial musculo-aponeurotic system (SMAS) in the parotid and cheek area. Plast Reconstr Surg 58:80-88, 1976.

24. Dobratz EJ, Hilger PA. Cheek defects. Facial Plast Surg Clin North Am 17:455-467, 2009.

25. Kakizaki H, Malhotra R, Madge SN, et al. Lower eyelid anatomy: an update. Ann Plast Surg 63:344-351, 2009.

26. Mulliken JB, Pensler JM, Kozakewich HP. The anatomy of Cupid's bow in normal and cleft lip. Plast Reconstr Surg 92:395-403, 1993.

27. Hwang K, Huan F, Kim DJ. Muscle fiber types of human orbicularis oculi muscle. J Craniofac Surg 22:1827-1830, 2011.

28. Briedis J, Jackson IT. The anatomy of the philtrum: observations made on dissections in the normal lip. Br J Plast Surg 34:128-132, 1981.

29. Whetzel TP, Mathes SJ. Arterial anatomy of the face: an analysis of vascular territories and perforating cutaneous vessels. Plast Reconstr Surg 89:591-603, 1992.

30. Soikkonen K, Wolf J, Hietanen J, et al. Three main arteries of the face and their tortuosity. Br J Oral Maxillofac Surg 29:395-398, 1991.

31. Schaverien MV, Pessa JE, Saint-Cyr M, et al. The arterial and venous anatomies of the lateral face lift flap and the SMAS. Plast Reconstr Surg 123:1581-1587, 2009.

32. Mağden O, Edizer M, Atabey A, et al. Cadaveric study of the arterial anatomy of the upper lip. Plast Reconstr Surg 114:355-359, 2004.

33. Qassemyar Q, Havet E, Sinna R. Vascular basis of the facial artery perforator flap: analysis of 101 perforator territories. Plast Reconstr Surg 129:421-429, 2012.

34. Garcia de Mitchell CA, Pessa JE, Schaverien MV, Rohrich RJ. The philtrum: anatomical observations from a new perspective. Plast Reconstr Surg 122:1756-1760, 2008.

35. Viola KV, Jhaveri MB, Soulos PR, et al. Mohs micrographic surgery and surgical excision for nonmelanoma skin cancer treatment in the Medicare population. Arch Dermatol 148:473-477, 2012.

36. Pepper JP, Asaria J, Moyer JS, et al. Quality of life in patients undergoing nasal reconstruction. Plast Reconstr Surg 129:430-437, 2012.

37. Netterville JL, Sinard RJ, Bryant GL Jr, et al. Delayed regional metastasis from midfacial squamous carcinomas. Head Neck 20:328-333, 1998.

38. Walike JW, Larrabee WF Jr. The 'note flap'. Arch Otolaryngol 111:430-433, 1985.

39. Griffin GR, Weber S, Baker SR. Outcomes following V-Y advancement flap reconstruction of large upper lip defects. Arch Facial Plast Surg 14:193-197, 2012.

    One of the few notable pieces of outcomes research after local flap reconstruction that includes a large series of patients. This is a well-written analysis of predictors of subsequent revision surgery.

40. Kriet JD, Cupp CL, Sherris DA, et al. The extended Abbé flap. Laryngoscope 105(9 Pt 1):988-992, 1995.

36

Pedicled Flaps
for Facial Reconstruction

Marc W. Herr ▪ *Kevin S. Emerick*

The reconstruction of major head and neck defects continues to be a challenge, both because of the anatomic complexity of the region and the critical role it plays in function, communication, and appearance. Therefore reconstructive surgeons must be versatile and innovative when addressing facial defects. The introduction, integration, and eventual dominance of microvascular free tissue transfer as the primary reconstructive tool for major defects of the head and neck is a response to the need for versatility and innovation in managing these defects. However, free flaps are often inferior aesthetically, with poor color and texture match to the surrounding skin and soft tissues. Additionally, many patients are not appropriate candidates for free tissue transfer because of severe medical comorbidities or lack of donor vessels for anastomosis. Chronically immunosuppressed patients and transplant recipients represent groups that manifest these issues. These medically complex patients are at high risk of developing locally and regionally advanced head and neck malignancies, especially those of cutaneous origin. Surgical extirpation of these lesions often requires parotidectomy and comprehensive neck dissection and results in large skin defects. Multiple medical comorbidities and incompetent wound healing produce significant reconstructive challenges, and more straightforward surgical options should be considered before using microvascular free tissue transfer. In these cases, pedicled flaps provide an important reconstructive tool.

CLINICAL EVOLUTION OF PEDICLED FLAPS IN FACIAL RECONSTRUCTION

DELTOPECTORAL FLAP

For more than 50 years pedicled flaps have been reliable tools for the reconstruction of large ablative defects of the face and neck. Initially, fasciocutaneous flaps such as the deltopectoral flap were used. Popularized by Bakamjian[1] in the early 1960s for pharyngoesophageal reconstruction, the deltopectoral flap is based on the second and third perforators of the internal mammary artery.[2] Thus the primary blood supply originates from the medial aspect of the flap, which has an axial architecture; the distal portion of the flap is more random and less reliable. The surface area of the flap extends laterally from the parasternal area over the upper chest to the level of the clavicle and onto the deltoid muscle (Fig. 36-1).

The deltopectoral flap is thin and pliable, with good color match to the head and neck, making it equally well suited for reconstruction and contouring of external soft tissue and skin defects. It has been used successfully in the neck, cheek, auricular region, and mentum.[3] The distal portions of the flap may be unreliable if they are extended past the deltoid muscle, and several large series report flap failure rates that range from 9% to 16%.[4-6] To avoid this complication, definitive reconstruction often requires two stages, including interpolation followed by delayed takedown of the pedicle. The second stage using pedicle division is typically performed 21 days later (Fig. 36-2). The donor site is addressed using a split-thickness skin graft.

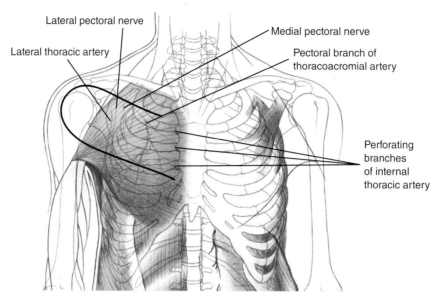

Fig. 36-1 Vascular anatomy and outline of the deltopectoral flap. Note that the primary blood supply is from the medial aspect of the flap via perforators of the internal mammary artery.

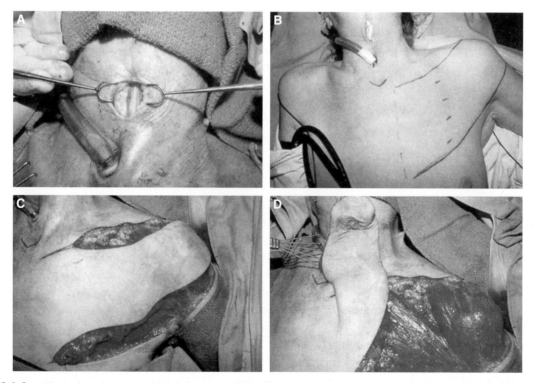

Fig. 36-2 Clinical application of the deltopectoral flap for repair of a pharyngocutaneous fistula. **A,** Pharyngocutaneous fistula. **B,** Outline of deltopectoral flap. **C,** Flap elevation from lateral to medial in a subfascial plane. **D,** Flap rotation into the defect.

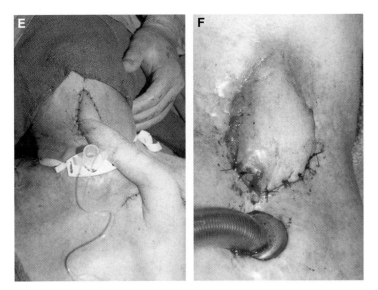

Fig. 36-2, cont'd   **E,** Stage one: the flap is tubulated and inset. **F,** Stage two: the pedicle is divided and inset is completed at day 21 postoperatively.

TRAPEZIUS MYOCUTANEOUS FLAPS

Stimulated by the work of Owens,[7] surgeons began using the pedicled myocutaneous flap more frequently. Conley[8] was the first to introduce the concept of the trapezius muscle as a carrier for skin in a single-stage flap. The trapezius is a large, triangular muscle that overlies the central portion of the upper back and posterior neck. It can be divided into three separate functional units. The superior portion of the trapezius muscle originates from the superior nuchal line, the external occipital protuberance, and the ligamentum nuchae, and inserts into the lateral third of the clavicle. The midportion of the trapezius muscle originates from the seventh cervical and upper six thoracic vertebrae. These fibers insert on the medial edge of the acromion and the upper border of the scapula. The lower portion of the muscle originates from the lower six thoracic vertebrae and inserts on the medial edges of the acromion and upper border of the scapula.

In addition to describing a myocutaneous trapezius flap, Conley[8] also developed a composite flap that included a segment of vascularized clavicle. Additional work with the trapezius system produced three distinct myocutaneous flaps based on combinations of the paraspinous perforators, transverse cervical vessels, and the dorsal scapular artery[9-11] (Fig. 36-3).

The superior trapezius myocutaneous flap is based on paraspinous perforators and the transverse cervical artery, which most commonly originates as a branch of the thyrocervical trunk. The length and width of the flap are determined by the size and distance of the defect from the flap base. The minimum width of the flap should be 10 cm to capture an adequate blood supply. The anterior border of the trapezius muscle establishes the anterior incision and a parallel incision is made posteriorly. The lateral aspect of the flap may extend as far as 10 cm beyond the trapezius muscle onto the deltoid fascia. Elevation of the flap proceeds from lateral to medial and incorporates a full-thickness section of trapezius muscle, which is separated

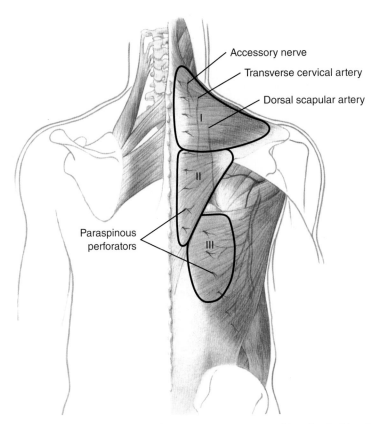

Fig. 36-3 The angiosomes of the trapezius muscle. The primary angiosome *(I)* is divided by the paraspinous perforators, which supply the medial aspect, and the transverse cervical artery, which supplies the lateral portion. The secondary angiosome *(II)* is supplied by the paraspinous perforators and the dorsal scapular artery, which courses deep to the levator scapulae and rhomboid minor muscles before sending branches to the undersurface of the trapezius muscle. Angiosome *III* is located at the junction of the inferior border of the trapezius muscle and the superomedial aspect of the latissimus dorsi muscle. Skin paddles incorporating this region inferior to the trapezius muscle rely primarily on the paraspinous perforators and dorsal scapular artery.

from the supraspinous and scapular muscles. The flap is transposed into the recipient defect, and the donor site is closed primarily or with a split-thickness skin graft (Fig. 36-4). Although generally reliable, the superior trapezius flap has a short arc of rotation, and its utility is limited to reconstruction of defects in the posterolateral neck and lower face. It is particularly useful in patients with an exposed carotid artery in a previously operated or irradiated field.

The lateral island trapezius myocutaneous flap is based exclusively on the transverse cervical artery. The flap is outlined overlying the superior aspect of the trapezius muscle, with dimensions ranging from 25 to 250 cm². After the position and patency of the vascular pedicle is confirmed with Doppler ultrasonography, the flap is incised to the trapezius fascia and elevated from laterally to medially. During elevation, branches of the dorsal scapular artery may be ligated after there is confirmation that the transverse cervical artery has been incorporated into the flap. The donor site is generally closed primarily.

The lower trapezius island myocutaneous flap extends from the medial border of the scapula to the midline. The flap may be designed as far distally as 15 cm below the tip of the scapula, although the blood supply becomes increasingly more random in this location. The skin paddle is incised and the surrounding skin is elevated off the latissimus dorsi and trapezius muscles. After the trapezius muscle is fully exposed, flap elevation is begun inferiorly and deep to the trapezius. As the harvest proceeds superiorly and approaches

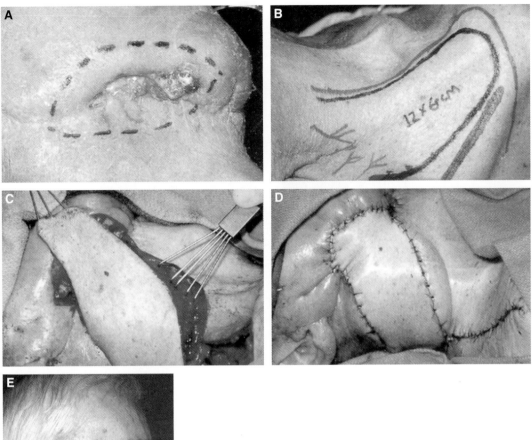

Fig. 36-4   Clinical application of the superior trapezius myo-cutaneous flap for closure of an orocutaneous fistula. **A,** The oro-cutaneous fistula is marked for repair. **B,** Outline of the superior myocutaneous trapezius flap, including the paraspinous perfora-tors. **C,** Flap elevated. **D,** Flap inset into the ablative defect. **E,** Re-sult 6 months postoperatively.

the rhomboid major muscle, the distal branches of the dorsal scapular vessels are identified. These vessels usually pass from deep to the rhomboid minor muscle, and ramify on the undersurface of the trapezius muscle. If additional pedicle length is needed, branches deep to the rhomboid major muscle are ligated. In cases where further pedicle length is required, the rhomboid minor muscle may be divided on either side of the vascular pedicle. The donor site is closed primarily in most cases.

The lateral and inferior trapezius flaps have significantly greater rotational excursion than the superiorly based flap, and may be used for defects of the anteriolateral neck, lateral skull base, midface, and oral cav-ity.[12] However, the harvest of these flaps requires careful dissection and preservation of the transverse cer-vical vessels. This may be technically difficult given the anatomic variability of these vessels, which com-monly arise from the thyrocervical trunk, but may also originate from the suprascapular, subclavian, or dorsal scapular arteries.[12] The transverse cervical vessels are also susceptible to injury in the setting of a previous neck dissection on the ipsilateral side.[11]

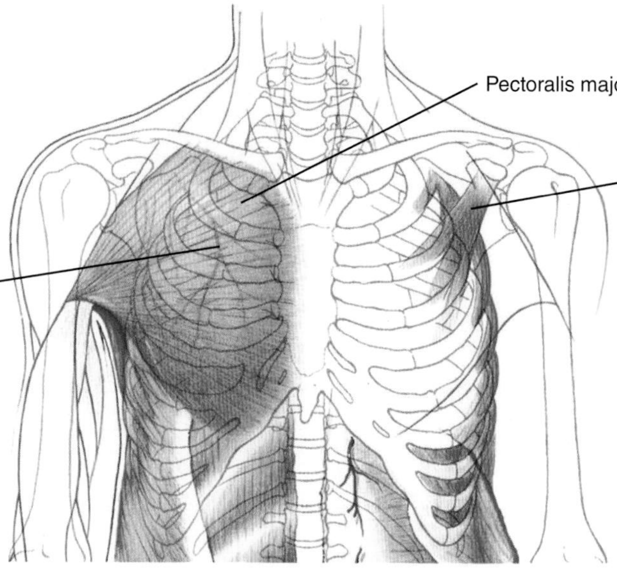

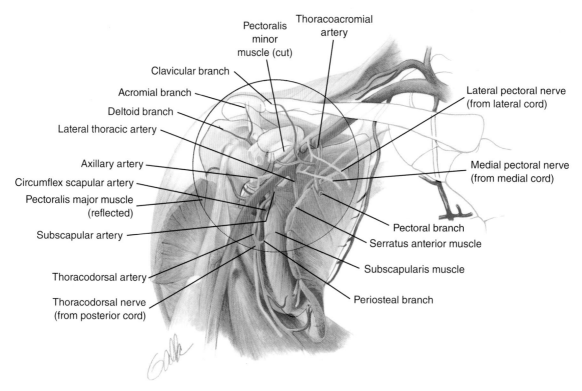

Fig. 36-5   The anatomy of the pectoralis major muscle.

Fig. 36-6   Detailed vascular anatomy of the pectoralis muscle and shoulder. The thoracoacromial artery is a branch off the second portion of the axillary artery. It gives rise to four branches in the shoulder, of which the pectoral branch is the largest. The subscapular artery is a branch from the third portion of the axillary artery. It divides into the circumflex scapular artery, which courses over the scapular bone, and the thoracodorsal artery, which continues inferiorly into the axilla along the undersurface of the latissimus dorsi muscle.

Pectoralis Major Myocutaneous Flap

In 1979, Ariyan[13] and Baek et al[14] simultaneously described using the pectoralis major myocutaneous flap for single-stage reconstruction of head and neck defects. Since that time, its ease of harvest and reliability have made this flap a workhorse for reconstructive surgeons. It has successfully been employed for the repair of a wide variety of oropharyngeal, oral cavity, lateral skull base, periauricular, cervical esophageal, and hypopharyngeal defects.[15-21]

The pectoralis major flap is supplied by the pectoral branch of the thoracoacromial artery (Figs. 36-5 and 36-6). It is a large fan-shaped muscle that originates from the medial half of the clavicle, sternum, and upper six ribs. Its muscular fibers condense to insert on the intertubercular sulcus of the humerus. The muscle receives motor innervation from the medial and lateral pectoral nerves and functions to adduct and medially rotate the humerus. The primary vascular pedicle is the pectoral branch of the thoracoacromial artery and vein.

The vascular pedicle is located by drawing a line from the acromion to the xyphoid. A vertical line is then drawn from the midpoint of the clavicle and should intersect the xiphisternal angle. The pectoral branch of the thoracoacromial artery follows this line and continues medially. The skin paddle is designed on the anterior chest wall medial to the nipple. The dimensions of the paddle permit transfer of 100 to 200 cm^2 of skin. An incision is carried from the superolateral aspect of the skin paddle obliquely into the axilla. This facilitates elevation of the pectoralis flap and spares the medially based vascular perforators of the ipsilateral deltopectoral flap. Inferiorly, up to a third of the skin paddle can be extended over the rectus sheath and will remain viable with a random blood supply.

Harvest begins by incising the skin paddle down to the level of the muscular fascia. Temporary sutures are used to stabilize the dermis to the muscular fascia and prevent shearing of the cutaneous paddle from the underlying muscle. The skin overlying the pectoralis major muscle, excluding the cutaneous paddle, is elevated. The lateral and inferior borders of the pectoralis muscle are identified and elevated superiorly to expose the underlying pectoralis minor muscle. A plane is bluntly developed between the pectoralis major and minor muscles. The pedicle is visualized on the undersurface of the pectoralis major muscle. The muscular attachments to the sternum and humerus are divided, and elevation of the pectoralis muscle continues superiorly until the clavicle is reached. The medial and lateral pectoral nerves are identified and transected to increase the arc of rotation and prevent strangulation of the blood vessels. The flap is then transposed into the defect and the donor site is closed primarily.

Despite its versatility and reliability, there are disadvantages to using the pectoralis flap. Substantial soft tissue movement produces significant bulkiness, making its use less ideal for the primary reconstruction of external soft tissue defects of the face or neck. Moreover, the color and texture match of the chest wall skin to that of the head and neck is suboptimal. In addition, closure of the donor site results in a large visible scar and medial displacement of the areolar complex. Furthermore, the pectoralis major muscle is the major adductor and medial rotator of the upper extremity; thus the potential for ipsilateral shoulder girdle weakness exists after flap harvest. Given these limitations, the pectoralis major myocutaneous flap has been relegated to a salvage role in most modern reconstructive algorithms. Recent series recommend its use for (1) the protection of great vessels or free flap pedicles in patients with compromised wound healing or wound breakdown caused by fistula or infection, (2) secondary reconstruction of defects after free flap complication, and (3) obliteration of dead space and closure of recalcitrant pharyngeal defects.[22,23]

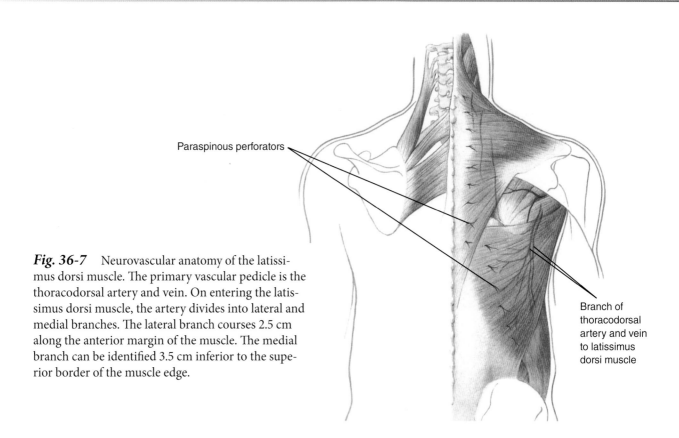

Paraspinous perforators

Branch of thoracodorsal artery and vein to latissimus dorsi muscle

Fig. 36-7 Neurovascular anatomy of the latissimus dorsi muscle. The primary vascular pedicle is the thoracodorsal artery and vein. On entering the latissimus dorsi muscle, the artery divides into lateral and medial branches. The lateral branch courses 2.5 cm along the anterior margin of the muscle. The medial branch can be identified 3.5 cm inferior to the superior border of the muscle edge.

Latissimus Dorsi Flap

Although not as popular as the pectoralis major flap for the reconstruction of lateral skull base defects, the latissimus dorsi muscular or myocutaneous flap has been used successfully for resurfacing the neck when carotid coverage is necessary, such as for pharyngeal reconstruction, and tongue reconstruction after total glossectomy. It may also be used as a free flap for scalp resurfacing. The latissimus dorsi is a broad, flat muscle that originates from the spinous processes of the lower six thoracic vertebrae and posterior iliac crest and inserts into the intertubercular groove of the humerus. It is supplied by the thoracodorsal vessels, which originate from the subscapular system. Contributions from the dorsal branches of the intercostal arteries establish a secondary pedicle (Fig. 36-7). The muscular innervation is from the thoracodorsal nerve.

The flap may be harvested with a skin paddle or as a muscle-only flap; it has an advantage in the versatility in the amount of tissue that can be harvested, ranging from a small amount of muscle under the skin paddle to the entire muscle. Other advantages include a long pedicle, large-caliber vessels, and the ability to design a bilobed flap based on the medial and lateral branches of the thoracodorsal artery.

A primary disadvantage of this flap is that it must be harvested with the patient in the lateral decubitus position, which precludes the more efficient strategy of a two-team approach. If the serratus anterior is included with the flap, there is potential for winging of the scapula and chronic shoulder pain. Furthermore, the donor site is prone to seroma formation, and if a large skin island is harvested, skin grafting of the donor site is susceptible to breakdown. Although the pedicled flap continues to have a role, its use is more limited in the modern reconstruction of soft tissue defects of the face and neck. Two emerging reliable and versatile pedicled flaps, the supraclavicular artery flap and submental flap, offer distinct advantages over the pedicled flaps mentioned and over most free flaps.

SUPRACLAVICULAR ARTERY FLAP

HISTORICAL BACKGROUND

Kazanjian and Converse[24] described the precursor of the modern supraclavicular artery flap in 1949. They named it the *acromial* or *in charretera* flap, which in Spanish refers to the strip of cloth on the shoulder to which military honors are attached. Thirty years later, Mathes and Vasconez[25] modified the acromial flap and described both the vascular territory and clinical applications of the cervicohumeral flap. However, the flap had a high incidence of distal necrosis, and its reliability remained controversial throughout the 1980s.[26] Lamberty and Cormack[27-29] jointly published several reports describing the anatomy of the supraclavicular artery and demonstrating its anatomic reliability. Renewed interest in the flap emerged in the late 1990s, when Pallua et al[30] performed detailed anatomic studies and defined the vascular patterns of the supraclavicular island flap. These detailed vascular studies gave reconstructive surgeons the confidence needed to reconsider this flap as a realistic option. This, in turn, has produced a dramatic increase in the use of the supraclavicular artery flap during the past 10 years.

The supraclavicular artery flap found initial success in the release of postburn mentosternal contractures.[30-33] In these cases, the flap was transferred in continuity with the defect. Pallua et al[34] subsequently described the supraclavicular artery island flap for reconstruction of oncologic defects in the head and neck using a tunneled approach to the wound. Soon thereafter, Di Benedetto et al[35] demonstrated the flap's reliability for lining the oral cavity. More recently, Chiu et al[36-42] have employed the flap in the reconstruction of partial and total pharyngectomy defects, posterolateral skull base defects, postparotidectomy contouring irregularities, and oropharyngeal defects. These series, as well as our own experience, have demonstrated that this flap is an excellent (and frequently the primary) option for reconstructing large skin and soft tissue defects of the face and neck. It offers excellent color and thickness match for most of these defects. Additionally, it can be harvested efficiently, with limited morbidity.

ANATOMY

The supraclavicular artery flap is a fasciocutaneous flap based on the SCA. It arises from the transverse cervical artery in 93% of patients and the suprascapular artery in the remaining cases.[33,36,43-45] The vascular pedicle of the supraclavicular artery flap is reliably found in a triangle formed by the dorsal edge of the sternocleidomastoid muscle anteriorly, the external jugular vein posteriorly, and the medial clavicle, which forms the base of this triangle (Fig. 36-8). The artery typically arises 3 to 4 cm from the origin of the transverse cervical artery and has a pedicle length varying from 1 to 7 cm.[34,36] The vessel diameter ranges from 1.1 to 1.5 mm. Two veins drain the flap, one into the transverse cervical vein and the other into the external jugular or subclavian vein.[34]

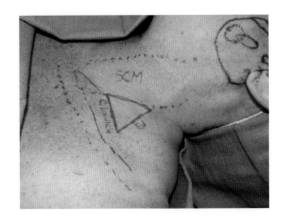

Fig. 36-8   The vascular pedicle of the supraclavicular artery flap is found in a triangle formed by the dorsal edge of the sternocleidomastoid muscle anteriorly, the external jugular vein posteriorly, and the medial part of the clavicle, which forms the base of this triangle.

The vascular territory of the supraclavicular artery extends from the supraclavicular region to the shoulder cap and distally to the ventral surface of the deltoid muscle.[34] CT angiography studies corroborate these findings and demonstrate that the distal portion of the flap is dependent on interperforator flow from direct linking vessels and recurrent flow through the subdermal plexus.[46,47] The area of this angiosome ranges from 8 to 16 cm in width by 22 to 35 cm in length.[34,35,43,46] Therefore the skin paddle of the supraclavicular artery flap should be centered over the ventrolateral aspect of the deltoid muscle and may include the region overlying the deltopectoral groove and superior border of the pectoralis major muscle. The distal aspect of the flap should extend no farther than the inferolateral border of the deltoid muscle. On occasion, the reconstructive requirements of the defect will exceed safe dimensions of the cutaneous portion of the flap, pushing the limits of the angiosome. In these cases it may be beneficial to incorporate additional skin into the proximal aspect of the flap. The extra skin will capture additional proximal perforators, and increase the viability of distal skin segments that rely on random vascular inflow.[21] Extra skin can be deepithelialized when inset.

Indications and Limitations

The supraclavicular artery flap provides a versatile reconstructive option for facial defects that cannot be definitively addressed with local flaps, including cutaneous defects whose location or surface area limit local tissue options, and those that require additional bulk to manage concomitant underlying soft tissue loss (Fig. 36-9). Well-vascularized regional pedicled flaps are ideal for reconstruction in this postradiation setting, compared to extensive cervicofacial advancement flaps. Although microvascular free flaps also provide well-vascularized tissue for these defects, they require surgical expertise in microsurgical techniques, recipient vessels for anastomosis, additional operative time, donor site morbidity, and special postoperative

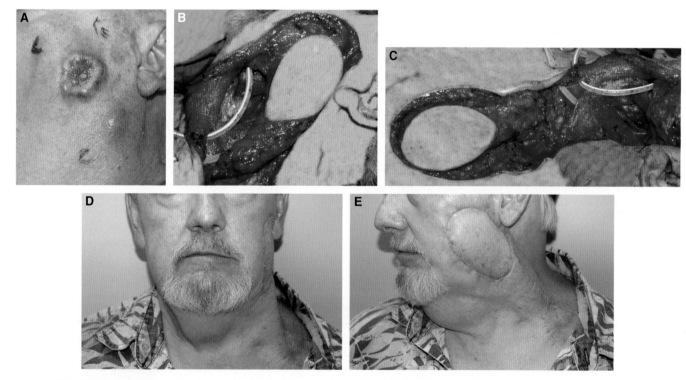

Fig. 36-9   **A,** Large cutaneous squamous cell carcinoma of the left midface and obvious dermal metastases. **B,** Intraoperative image demonstrating the ablative defect and the harvested supraclavicular artery flap. **C,** The supraclavicular artery flap has been rotated into the midface defect. **D** and **E,** Frontal and lateral images of the patient 6 weeks after surgery.

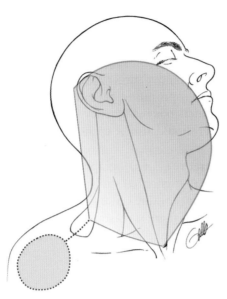

Fig. 36-10   Schematic depicting both the cutaneous distribution of the supraclavicular flap *(blue)* and the extensive potential arc of rotation *(orange)*. Note the extensive potential reach of the skin paddle.

monitoring. High-risk individuals with significant medical comorbidities are not good candidates for such procedures and the supraclavicular artery flap offers an appropriate surgical alternative for these patients.

Good color and texture match make the supraclavicular artery flap an excellent option for covering cutaneous defects of the face and neck. Its arc of rotation permits reach as far superiorly as the lateral canthus, medial cheek, temporal, and occipital regions, and anteriorly into the submentum and contralateral neck (Fig. 36-10). In cosmetically important facial zones like these, the color and texture match is significantly superior to free tissue transfer options such as the forearm or anterolateral thigh. The supraclavicular artery flap is also thin and pliable, lending itself to the correction of ablative contour irregularities, including those produced by parotidectomy, posterolateral skull base, and temporal bone defects. There is some variability to the thickness of the supraclavicular artery flap, thus preoperative assessment of the area is necessary to determine if the flap will provide a reasonable reconstructive option.

The supraclavicular artery island flap requires a donor site that has not sustained previous injury from surgery or trauma.[46] Particular caution is warranted if the patient has had a previous ipsilateral neck dissection. Lymphadenectomy, including levels IV and V, places the transverse cervical vessels, and consequently the flap pedicle, at risk. Additionally, although the supraclavicular artery flap has diverse applications, its arc of rotation limits its use for defects of the midface, forehead, or scalp. Anecdotally, the flap has been used to reconstruct a large defect of the medial cheek, nose, and forehead; however, this required interpolation and should only be considered as a last resort. Furthermore, the size of the supraclavicular artery flap is constrained by the angiosome of the supraclavicular artery[48] (see Fig. 36-10).

In rare cases in which a thin or cachectic patient has a very deep lateral skull base or extensive soft tissue defect, the supraclavicular artery flap may not provide enough bulk to address the contour defect. This bulk deficiency may be addressed by harvesting a skin paddle larger than the dimensions of the defect, and deepithelializing a segment and folding it into the wound, thereby providing additional bulk. The surgeon should consider primary closure of the donor site. Although the precise limitations to primary closure in this location have yet to be clearly defined, primary closure of donor sites up to 16 cm wide has been reported.[34]

Patient Evaluation and Preoperative Planning

A critical aspect of preoperative evaluation is assessing the status of the shoulder and supraclavicular fossa, with particular attention to previous shoulder surgery, trauma to the area, previous neck dissections, or radiation to the region. In immunocompromised patients, all suspicious cutaneous lesions should be scrutinized to avoid transferring a cutaneous malignancy into the head and neck defect. The presence of a pacemaker or Port-A-Cath catheter should also be evaluated.

Several series describe using preoperative CT angiography to assess the presence and integrity of the supraclavicular artery.[36,43,44] However, experience has shown the vascular anatomy to be consistent and reliable, which likely precludes the need for routine CT angiography. In specific cases, such as patients with previous head and neck operations or if there is reason to suspect the vessels may no longer be present, imaging may be a useful adjunct for surgical planning. Doppler ultrasonography, a less invasive alternative, could also be used in the preoperative setting to confirm the presence of the supraclavicular vessels.

Surgical Technique

With the patient in the supine position, the neck and arm down to the elbow are sterilized appropriately. A Doppler probe is used to mark the location of the supraclavicular artery and vein, both within the triangular fossa (bordered by the sternocleidomastoid muscle, external jugular vein, and clavicle) and as they course over the clavicle. A fusiform skin paddle is designed over the ventral aspect of the deltoid with its axis aligned on the proximally auscultated Doppler signal (Fig. 36-11). Incisions are made circumferentially around the skin paddle and from the medial apex of the skin paddle to the clavicle. Bilateral subdermal skin flaps are subsequently raised adjacent to the proximal incision and extended to the approximate width of the skin paddle. The flap is raised in a subfascial plane over the deltoid muscle using monopolar electrocautery and/or jeweler tipped bipolar forceps. Dissection proceeds in a distal to proximal direction to prevent inadvertent injury to the vascular pedicle[36] (Fig. 36-12).

Dissection remains inferior to the clavicle and extends posteriorly to the external jugular vein. A fascial pedicle approximating the width of the skin paddle is maintained. This maneuver protects the flap vasculature by preventing kinking, partial compression, and excessive tension.[35] The fascial pedicle should extend from the lateral attachment of the sternocleidomastoid muscle to a point approximately 3 cm lateral to the identified vascular pedicle at the clavicle, providing adequate tissue to protect the vasculature without additional dissection or exposure. Once dissection reaches the clavicle, the subcutaneous tunnel is created. A subdermal flap is raised proximal to the lateral border of the sternocleidomastoid muscle. At this point, the dissection continues medial and superficial to the pedicle, which remains safely tethered deep in the neck. Approximately 2 cm above the clavicle, the platysma muscle is transected to connect the tunnel into the anterior neck (Fig. 36-13). Frequently, this dissection has already been performed during the ablative surgery; if not, a subplatysmal tunnel from the defect to this area is created.

Flap elevation into the supraclavicular fossa is performed next. The periosteum of the inferior border of the clavicle is incised and subperiosteal dissection continues superiorly into the supraclavicular fossa. The elevated periosteum is then incised, allowing access into the soft tissue component of the supraclavicular fossa (Fig. 36-14).

This maneuver releases the flap, increasing its maximal excursion. If additional length is required, the middle plane of the deep cervical fascia is released, with meticulous attention to protecting the underlying transverse cervical vessels and their branches. The distal aspect of the EJ system is identified and preserved. If this maneuver does not provide sufficient additional length, a back cut may be created at the medial soft tissue pedicle at the clavicular head, over the sternocleidomastoid muscle, which is in a safe location medial to the takeoff of the pedicle. Finally, if even further length or rotation is required, the medial pedicle

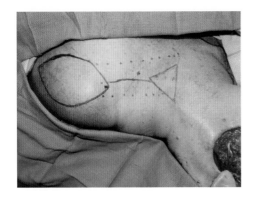

Fig. 36-11   The location of the supraclavicular artery and vein is marked within the triangular fossa and as they course over the clavicle. A fusiform skin paddle is designed over the ventral aspect of the deltoid with its axis aligned on the proximally auscultated Doppler signal.

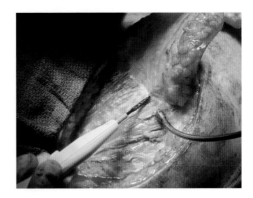

Fig. 36-12   Subfascial dissection proceeds over the deltoid in a distal to proximal direction.

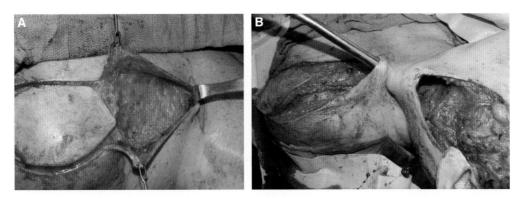

Fig. 36-13   **A,** A subdermal flap is raised proximal to the lateral border of the sternocleidomastoid muscle. **B,** Approximately 2 cm above the clavicle, the platysma muscle is transected to connect the tunnel into the anterior neck.

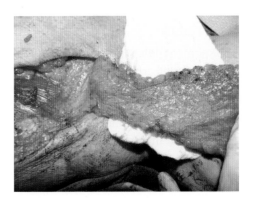

Fig. 36-14   The periosteum of the inferior border of the clavicle is incised, and subperiosteal dissection continues superiorly into the supraclavicular fossa. The elevated periosteum is then incised, allowing access into the soft tissue component of the supraclavicular fossa.

and transverse cervical vessels may be further isolated and mobilized; this maneuver is rarely necessary. The supraclavicular artery flap is then brought through the tunnel and rotated into the defect.

Closure of the donor site is accomplished with wide undermining, both posteriorly over the shoulder and trapezius and anteriorly onto the chest. Primary closure can routinely be accomplished with adjacent tissue advancement.[35,36] In rare instances where this is not possible, skin grafting may be used.

POSTOPERATIVE CARE

Flaps may be monitored clinically with no need for Doppler ultrasonography or other sophisticated testing. Two suctions drains are routinely placed in the donor site, one extending into the subcutaneous tunnel. Patients are evaluated by physical therapists on postoperative day 2, to begin range-of-motion therapy.

RESULTS AND COMPLICATIONS

In more than three decades of use, the supraclavicular artery flap has emerged as a reliable flap for a wide variety of facial defects. In a large series of 103 supraclavicular artery flaps used to reconstruct postburn mentosternal contractures, 94.2% survived completely.[33] Other series had similar rates of flap survival.[36,40,41,43]

Donor site complications such as incisional dehiscence and seroma formation have been reported in 0% to 15% of cases.[33,36,43,49] These are typically self-limiting and resolve with aspiration and local wound care. However, negative pressure wound therapy closure followed by skin grafting has occasionally been necessary.[43] Widening of the donor site scar has been reported, but most series note acceptable cosmetic results and good overall patient satisfaction.[33,36,43] Patients have reported a nonirritating, referred sensation to the shoulder with touching of the flap.[36,43] There have been no documented cases of prolonged or permanent functional morbidity at the donor site.

SUBMENTAL FLAP

HISTORICAL BACKGROUND

Martin et al[50] developed the submental flap in 1993 as a reconstructive alternative for cutaneous defects of the middle and lower third of the face.[51] Since that time, it has been successfully used to repair a variety of facial defects, including those of the cheek and preauricular skin, external auditory canal and mastoid, lip and chin, nasal ala, and forehead.[52-57] Over the years, the flap's versatility and reliability have led to additional applications, including to transfer hair-bearing skin for mustache and beard restoration in men.[58] Over the past decade, the submental flap has also seen increasing use in reconstruction of oral cavity defects.[52,57,59,60]

ANATOMY

The submental flap is a fasciocutaneous flap based on the submental artery, a branch of the facial artery. The submental artery consistently arises 5 to 6.5 cm from the origin of the facial artery as it exits from the superior aspect of the submandibular gland.[50] It then runs medially superficial to the mylohyoid muscle and inferior to the mandible. In 70% to 81% of patients the submental artery travels deep to the anterior belly of the digastric muscle, while in the remaining cases it courses superficial to the muscle.[61,62] It terminates behind the mandibular symphysis, and has a pedicle length of approximately 8 cm[50,53] (Fig. 36-15). The diameter of the submental artery ranges from 1 to 2 mm.[50,61] Venous drainage is from the submental vein, a tributary of the facial vein. Anatomic studies have also demonstrated at least one anastomosing

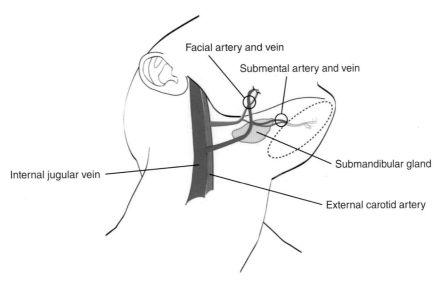

Fig. 36-15   Vascular anatomy of the submental flap. The flap is based on the submental artery, a branch of the facial artery. The submental artery consistently arises 5 to 6.5 cm from the origin of the facial artery as it exits from the superior aspect of the submandibular gland. It then runs medially, superficial to the mylohyoid muscle and deep to the anterior belly of the digastric muscle.

vein between the facial and external jugular systems. This may be used for flap drainage in some cases.[50] The diameter of the submental vein ranges from 1.0 to 2.9 mm.[52,63]

Several perforators from the submental artery supply the surrounding muscles and overlying skin. Four types of collateral vessels have been described: branches to the submandibular gland; branches to the platysma, digastric, and mylohyoid muscle; branches to the subplatysmal fatty layer; and one to four cutaneous perforators.[50] Two major cutaneous perforators are consistently described, one emerging proximal and one distal to the digastric muscle.[61] A detailed anatomic study identified only one reliable perforator per side in 87.5% of cases.[63] The location of this perforator is variable and may be medial or lateral to the anterior belly of the digastric muscle.

In their landmark study on the arterial anatomy of the face, Whetzel and Mathes[64] used ink injections to define 11 vascular territories of the face, scalp, and neck. They described the angiosome of the submental artery as measuring 5 by 5 cm and extending from just lateral to oral commissure to 2 cm anterior to the sternocleidomastoid muscle and 3 cm below the border of the mandible. Additional work by Martin et al,[50] and also Faltaous and Yetman,[61] demonstrates a larger angiosome that includes the submandibular region, extending medially over the chin past midline and superiorly to the lower lip. Dimensions of this skin territory range from 4 by 5 cm to a maximum of 7 by 15 cm. Clinical experience with the submental flap has confirmed the more robust findings of these latter studies. Skin paddles are frequently extended from the mandibular angle to the contralateral angle without compromising viability.

INDICATIONS AND LIMITATIONS

Indications for the submental flap are similar to those for the supraclavicular artery flap; the excellent color and texture match is ideal for reconstruction of cutaneous facial defects. The arc of rotation allows use of the flap in the lower and midface (Fig. 36-16). The submental flap is particularly well suited to the repair of hair-bearing defects, including those of the upper lip, the temporal hairline, and in the beard distribution.[52] Conversely, this characteristic may be undesirable for reconstruction of oral cavity defects or other glabrous regions of the face or neck.

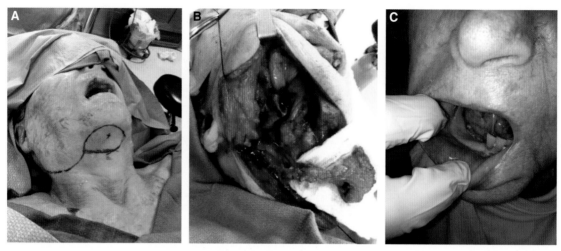

Fig. 36-16   **A,** The anterior border of the skin paddle is drawn at least 1 cm inferior to the margin of the mandible to hide the scar as much as possible. The lower border of the skin paddle is determined by a pinch test of the submental skin. The length of the flap is tailored to the size of the defect, but may extend from mandibular angle to angle. **B,** Harvest proceeds deep to the digastric muscle and the submental vessels are released from the underlying mylohyoid muscle. Dissection continues until sufficient length of vascular pedicle is obtained or until the junction of the submental and facial vessels is reached. **C,** Postoperative result 6 weeks after inset of a submental flap for an anterior oral cavity defect. (Courtesy of Daniel Deschler, MD.)

As a pedicled flap, the submental flap does not reach the upper third of the face. However, this limitation can potentially be overcome by mobilization of the pedicle using reverse flow from the distal facial artery or by converting it to a free flap. Older patients may possess excess submental fat that may result in excess flap bulk, which may be further compounded by including the anterior belly of the digastric and mylohyoid muscles in flap harvest. Finally, safe flap harvest may limit complete level I lymphadenectomy and caution must be exercised in oncologic cases where this region is at risk for metastatic involvement.

Patient Evaluation and Preoperative Planning

If a level I neck dissection has been performed previously, the vascular pedicle will not be intact and an alternate reconstructive option should be employed. If the patient's surgical history is uncertain, a CT scan of the neck should be obtained. If the ipsilateral submandibular gland is present, the submental vessels are likely intact. CT angiography may also confirm the integrity of the facial and submental vessels. The patient should be questioned regarding any previous radiation to the region. Finally, a clinical history of the patient's swallowing function should be obtained, since resection of the suprahyoid strap muscles may produce or worsen dysphagia and lead to aspiration.

Surgical Technique

The patient is placed in the supine position with the neck extended. The anterior border of the skin paddle is outlined at least 1 cm inferior to the margin of the mandible to hide the scar as much as possible.[59] The maximum flap width should allow primary closure, and thus the lower border of the skin paddle is determined by a pinch test of the submental skin. The length of the flap is tailored to the size of the defect, but may extend from mandibular angle to angle.

Descriptions of the harvesting technique vary among institutions, but most surgeons harvest the flap in a subplatysmal plane from distal to proximal.[50-54,59,65-66] Whether the vascular pedicle is identified and skeletonized in an anterograde fashion from the facial vessels or in a retrograde manner from the submental vessels, the overlying anterior belly of the digastric muscle is released from its attachments and incorporated into the flap.[52] This maneuver protects the submental vessels and preserves the cutaneous and musculocutaneous perforators as they pass deep to the muscle.

An initial incision is made along the inferior aspect of the skin paddle. The submandibular gland and intermediate tendon of the digastric muscle are identified and dissection proceeds superiorly and posteriorly. The facial vessels are identified and traced to the origin of the submental vessels. The submandibular gland is then removed, taking care to preserve the submental pedicle. The marginal mandibular branch of the facial nerve should also be identified and preserved during this portion of the procedure. After removal of the gland, the submental vessels are followed to the lateral border of the mylohyoid muscle.

The superior skin incision is then executed and the harvest proceeds from the contralateral side toward the midline in a subplatysmal plane. At the midline, careful dissection identifies the submental artery and vein at the medial border of the anterior belly of the digastric muscle on the pedicle side.[59] The anterior belly of the digastric muscle is released from its attachments to the mandible and hyoid bone and elevated with the flap. The traditional flap harvest continues deep to the digastric muscle, and the submental vessels are released from the underlying mylohyoid muscle. Care must be taken not to separate the skin paddle from the submental vessels as the harvest proceeds laterally. Dissection continues until sufficient length of the vascular pedicle is obtained, or until the junction of the submental and facial vessels is reached[59,66] (see Fig. 36-16).

A modification of the harvest technique has been described that provides additional protection for the submental vessels.[66] The pedicle is dissected in an anterograde fashion after removal of the submandibular gland, as described earlier. From the contralateral side, dissection proceeds to the midline and down to the mylohyoid muscle. The mylohyoid muscle is then detached from the mandible and hyoid bone and is bluntly separated from the ipsilateral geniohyoid muscle.[66] At this point the flap is completely mobilized and may be rotated into the defect. This technique protects the submental vessels between the anterior belly of the digastric and mylohyoid muscle and minimizes dissection of the terminal branches off the mylohyoid muscle, thus preventing inadvertent injury. The donor defect is closed primarily. Skin mobilization should only be performed on the cervical side to prevent eversion of the lower lip.[54] The cervicomental angle may be preserved by hitching the cervical platysma to the hyoid bone.[53]

If additional pedicle length or arc of rotation is required, elongation of the flap pedicle may be achieved by raising the flap with a reverse flow technique. Initially described by Sterne et al[67] in 1996, the modification involves ligation of the facial vessels distal to the origin of the submental artery, followed by division of the submental vein with anastomosis to the common facial vein or a nearby recipient vein. This overcomes any valves within the facial venous system and provides an additional 1 to 2 cm of pedicle length.[52,67] Maximal length is then achieved by dividing the facial vessels proximal to the origin of the facial artery. A clinical series using this technique found that the facial vein (running adjacent to the artery) has sufficient connection with the neighboring veins to adequately overcome the reversed venous flow against valves within the system, and concluded that ligation and anastomosis to the common facial vein is not necessary.[63]

POSTOPERATIVE CARE

Like the supraclavicular artery flap, the submental flap may be monitored clinically with no need for Doppler ultrasonography or other advanced testing. Typically, a suction drain is placed in the donor site to limit hematoma or seroma formation. Hair growth on the skin paddle may be addressed after complete healing, using laser hair removal or other dermatologic methods (see Chapter 41).

RESULTS AND COMPLICATIONS

In the two decades since its first description, the submental flap has established itself as a reliable reconstructive tool for facial defects. Total flap loss is extremely uncommon. Incidences of partial flap loss are reported in several large series and occur in 0% to 11% of cases.*

Although injury to the marginal mandibular branch of the facial nerve is an inherent risk during the harvest of the submental flap, documented cases are very rare. Hematomas can occur and should be promptly addressed to minimize the risk of flap compromise.[50,54] Donor site morbidity is otherwise uncommon and self-limited. The donor defect is universally closed primarily and the resulting scar remains well concealed if the incision is properly designed behind the lower border of the mandible. Blunting of the cervicomental angle can occur, but can be prevented by attaching the cervical platysma to the hyoid bone before closure.

TEMPOROPARIETAL FASCIA FLAP

HISTORICAL BACKGROUND

Since its introduction by Golovine in 1898, the temporoparietal fascia flap (TPFF) has been used extensively for the reconstruction of a variety of head and neck defects.[68,69] It is composed of thin, pliable, and well-vascularized tissue that readily accepts a skin graft and molds to complex facial defects, with minimal donor site morbidity.

ANATOMY

The temporoparietal fascia is a 2 to 4 mm thick layer of connective tissue that represents the superior continuation of the superficial musculoaponeurotic system and continues cranially to become the galea. The temporoparietal fascia is deep and firmly adherent to the subcutaneous tissue underneath the skin of the scalp and is separated from the underlying temporalis muscle and fascia by a layer of loose areolar tissue.[69] This loose connective tissue layer is a mobile, avascular plane that allows the overlying skin, subcutaneous tissue, and temporoparietal fascia to be moveable relative to the firmly adherent pericranium.

The temporoparietal fascia flap derives its blood supply from the superficial temporal artery—a terminal branch of the external carotid artery that follows a tortuous course in the preauricular region after arising from within the parotid tissue immediately anterior to the tragus. The vessels traverse distally within the temporoparietal fascia and divide into anterior and posterior branches approximately 2 to 3 cm superior to the zygomatic arch. In addition, the superficial temporal artery is the source of the middle temporal artery at the level of the zygomatic arch. The middle temporal artery courses deep to supply the temporalis muscular fascia and then anastomoses with branches of the deep temporal vessels. The superficial temporal vein runs anterior and superior to the artery (Fig. 36-17).

---

*References 50, 53, 54, 59, 63, 66, 67.

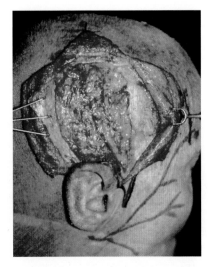

Fig. 36-17   The vascular anatomy of the temporoparietal fascia flap. (Courtesy of Mack Cheney, MD.)

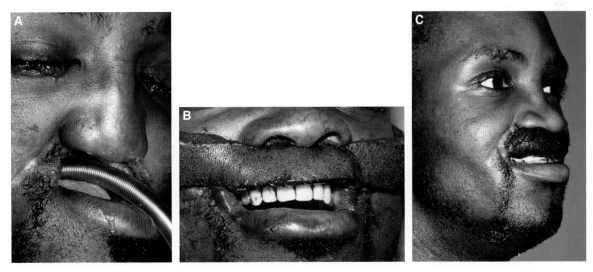

Fig. 36-18   **A,** Preoperative complete upper lip defect. **B,** Reconstruction of upper lip with a bilateral temporoparietal fascia flap elevated in bucket-handle fashion. **C,** Final result.

INDICATIONS AND LIMITATIONS

The temporoparietal fascia flap is useful for the repair of the external ear, defects of the scalp, defects of the nose and orbit, and obliteration of the mastoid after surgery for chronic otitis media or lateral temporal bone resection.[51,70-75] The flap may be transferred with fascia only or in combination with skin and calvarial bone.[68,74,75] The temporoparietal fascia flap may also be harvested with an island of overlying hair-bearing scalp, which can be used for reconstruction of the eyebrow, mustache, or other hirsute facial areas (Fig. 36-18, see also Fig. 7-17).

The flap can be used as either a pedicled or free tissue flap. As a pedicled flap, the temporoparietal fascia flap is limited by its arc of rotation, which allows for excursion to the ipsilateral orbitomaxillary region,

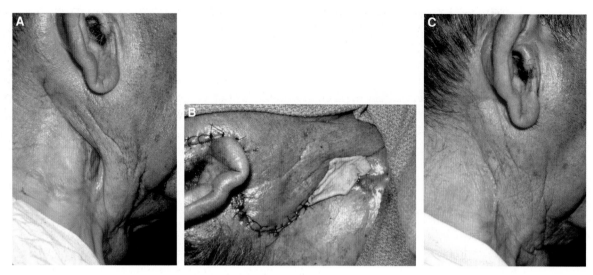

Fig. 36-19   **A,** Preoperative orocutaneous fistula. **B,** Closure of the defect with a temporoparietal fascia flap. **C,** Final result.

posterior oral cavity, lateral skull base, and lateral mandible (Fig. 36-19). If necessary, identification of the facial nerve and mobilization of the parotid gland can be performed to increase pedicle length.[68,69] A flap of 14 by 17 cm may be elevated safely.

PATIENT EVALUATION AND PREOPERATIVE PLANNING

The primary preoperative evaluation for a temporoparietal fascia flap focuses on the adequacy of the vascular pedicle. Previous radiation to the head and neck, prior neck dissection or parotid surgery, or external carotid embolization may compromise the superficial temporal system and are considered relative contraindications to the use of the temporoparietal fascia flap.[76] This flap should be considered with caution in patients who have a history of trauma to the temporal or zygomatic region or a history of temporal arteritis.[69] On physical examination, the patient should be evaluated for evidence of a face lift, and coronal and neck incisions. The most important preoperative test is Doppler auscultation of the superficial temporal artery to confirm its patency and sufficient inflow. This can be performed in the office with a handheld device, or through formal assessment with ultrasonographic color flow studies.

SURGICAL TECHNIQUE

The temporoparietal fascia flap is typically harvested without shaving the overlying hair. The superficial temporal artery is outlined preoperatively using handheld Doppler ultrasonography. The standard approach is an extension of a face-lift incision. This may be terminated superiorly in a Y-shaped incision to allow greater exposure of the superiormost aspect of the TPF above the superior temporal line.

The initial skin incision is made to the level of the subcutaneous tissue. The flap is elevated anteriorly, superiorly, and posteriorly in a plane below the hair follicles. This aspect of the dissection is the most tedious and is critical to successful flap elevation. Dissection deeper than this level risks injury to the superficial temporal vessels, and dissection in too superficial a plane will result in alopecia. As dissection continues anteriorly, care must be taken not to injure the frontal branch of the facial nerve. This nerve travels within the TPF layer and lies approximately 1.5 cm lateral to the orbital rim.

Both the anterior and posterior branches of the superficial temporal artery are identified and included in the flap. Elevation of the temporoparietal fascia flap begins superiorly, at the level of the superior temporal line and continues as far inferiorly as necessary to transpose the flap into the recipient site. The width of the flap base is typically 2.0 to 2.5 cm. The deep plane of dissection is the avascular plane of loose alveolar tissue, which separates the TPF from the underlying layer of muscular fascia. Once the elevation is complete, a suction drain is placed in the scalp and the incision is closed primarily.

POSTOPERATIVE CARE

There are no special requirements for postoperative monitoring of the temporoparietal fascia flap. Careful hemostasis should be obtained with bipolar cautery. A suction drain is generally used, and should be positioned superiorly to avoid inadvertent contact with the vascular pedicle of the transposed flap.[76] A bulky compressive dressing is typically applied to the donor site for 24 hours.

RESULTS AND COMPLICATIONS

The temporoparietal fascia is well established as a versatile and reliable flap for the reconstruction of a wide variety of facial defects. Total flap loss is extremely uncommon with flap survival rates ranging from 95% to 100%.[68,74,77,78] The incidence of partial flap loss is reported to occur in 0% to 14% of cases and often heals without additional surgical intervention.[68,74,77,78]

The most commonly described complication associated with temporoparietal fascia flap harvest is alopecia, which results from thermal damage to the hair follicles and/or elevation of the flap in too superficial of a plane.[69]

Injury of the frontal branch of the facial nerve is another potential complication of temporoparietal fascia flap harvest, although the incidence is very low, with several large series reporting no cases of permanent frontal nerve injury.[68,74,77,78] Contour deformity in the temporoparietal area has also been reported.[77]

CONCLUSION

Pedicled flaps play an important role in reconstruction of major face and neck defects. Because of the complexity of these defects, reconstructive surgeons should tailor flap selection to provide the most functional repair, optimize aesthetic outcomes, and balance the potential morbidities of flap harvest and operative time. Historic fasciocutaneous and myocutaneous flaps produce acceptable outcomes, particularly for a salvage reconstruction. Recent innovations permitted the addition of several other flaps to the reconstructive armamentarium.

The supraclavicular, submental, and temporoparietal fascia flaps provide thin, pliable tissue with a reliable blood supply. They have been employed to address a multitude of facial defects with high rates of success and minimal morbidity. These flaps also have relatively rapid and straightforward harvest procedures and minimal postoperative requirements. Consequently, they offer an important reconstructive alternative to free tissue transfer for medically complex patients with multiple comorbidities. They also provide excellent color and texture match that is often superior to free tissue options.

KEY POINTS

- Historic fasciocutaneous and myocutaneous pedicled flaps, such as the deltopectoral, trapezius, pectoralis major, and latissimus dorsi flaps, have an important (although limited) role in head and neck reconstruction. They are primarily used in the salvage setting.
- The supraclavicular artery flap is a fasciocutaneous flap well suited to reconstruction of cheek and auricular defects, defects of the lower lip, and cutaneous defects of the neck and submentum.
- The supraclavicular artery is located in a triangle formed by the dorsal edge of the sternocleidomastoid muscle anteriorly, the external jugular vein posteriorly, and the medial part of the clavicle.
- The fasciocutaneous submental artery flap may be employed for defects in the lower and midface, including the cheek and preauricular skin, external auditory canal and auricle, lip and chin, and nasal ala.
- The submental artery flap is based on the submental artery and its perforators, which have a variable anatomy with respect to the anterior belly of the digastric muscle.
- Harvest of a submental artery flap requires incorporation of the ipsilateral anterior belly of the digastric muscle into the flap. The mylohyoid muscle may also be included to provide additional protection of the vascular pedicle.
- The temporoparietal fascia flap is based on the superficial temporal artery and is composed of thin, pliable, well-vascularized tissue that readily accepts a skin graft and molds to a variety of complex facial defects.

REFERENCES

1. Bakamjian VY. A two-staged method for pharyngoesophageal reconstruction with a primary pectoral skin flap. Plast Reconstr Surg 36:173-184, 1965.
2. Urken ML. Deltopectoral. In Urken ML, Cheney ML, Blackwell KE, et al, eds. Atlas of Regional and Free Flaps for Head and Neck Reconstruction: Flap Harvest and Insetting. Philadelphia: Lippincott Williams & Wilkins, 2012.
3. McGregor I, Jackson I. The extended role of the deltopectoral flap. Br J Plast Surg 23:173-185, 1970.
4. Bakamjian VY, Long M, Rigg B. Experience with the medially based deltopectoral flap in reconstructive surgery of the head and neck. Br J Plast Surg 24:174-183, 1971.
5. Mendelson B, Woods J, Masson J. Experience with the deltopectoral flap. Plast Reconstr Surg 59:360-365, 1977.
6. Park JS, Sako K, Marchetta FC. Reconstructive experience with the medially based deltopectoral flap. Am J Surg 128:548-552, 1974.
7. Owens N. Compound neck pedicle designed for repair of massive facial defects. Plast Reconstr Surg 15:369-389, 1955.
8. Conley J. Use of composite flaps containing bone for major repairs in the head and neck. Plast Reconstr Surg 49:522-526, 1972.
9. McCraw JB, Dibbell DG. Experimental definition of independent myocutaneous vascular territories. Plast Reconstr Surg 60:212-220, 1977.
10. Baek SM, Biller HF, Krespi YP, et al. The lower trapezius island myocutaneous flap. Ann Plast Surg 5:108-114, 1980.
11. Urken ML. Trapezius system. In Urken ML, Cheney ML, Blackwell KE, et al, eds. Atlas of Regional and Free Flaps for Head and Neck Reconstruction: Flap Harvest and Insetting. Philadelphia: Lippincott Williams & Wilkins, 2012.
12. Netterville JL, Panje WR, Maves MD. The trapezius myocutaneous flap. Arch Otolaryngol Head Neck Surg 113:271-281, 1987.
13. Ariyan S. The pectoralis major myocutaneous flap: a versatile flap for reconstruction in the head and neck. Plast Reconstr Surg 63:73-81, 1979.

14. Baek SM, Biller HF, Krespi Y, et al. The pectoralis major myocutaneous island flap for reconstruction of the head and neck. Head Neck Surg 1:293-300, 1979.

15. Withers EH, Franklin JD, Madden JJ, et al. Immediate reconstruction of the pharynx and cervical esophagus with pectoralis major myocutaneous flap following laryngopharyngectomy. Plast Reconstr Surg 68:898-904, 1981.

16. Ariyan S. The pectoralis major for single-stage reconstruction of difficult wounds of the orbit and pharyngo-esophagus. Plast Reconstr Surg 72:468-477, 1983.

17. Cusumano RJ, Silver CE, Brauer RJ, et al. Pectoralis myocutaneous flap for replacement of cervical esophagus. Head Neck Surg 11:450-456, 1989.

18. Spriano G, Pellini R, Roselli R. Pectoralis major myocutaneous flap for hypopharyngeal reconstruction. Plast Reconstr Surg 110:1408-1413, 2002.

19. Liu R, Gullane P, Brown D, et al. Pectoralis major myocutaneous pedicled flap in head and neck reconstruction: retrospective review of indications and results in 244 consecutive cases at the Toronto General Hospital. J Otolaryngol 30:34-40, 2001.

20. McLean JN, Carlson GW, Losken A. The pectoralis major myocutaneous flap revisited: a reliable technique for head and neck reconstruction. Ann Plast Surg 64:570-573, 2010.

21. Resto VA, McKenna MJ, Deschler DG. Pectoralis major flap in composite lateral skull base defect reconstruction. Arch Otolaryngol Head Neck Surg 133:490-494, 2007.

22. Zbar RI, Funk GF, McCulloch TM, et al. Pectoralis major myofascial flap: a valuable tool in contemporary head and neck reconstruction. Head Neck 19:412-418, 1997.

23. Schneider DS, Wu V, Wax MK. Indications for pedicled pectoralis major flap in a free tissue transfer practice. Head Neck 34:1106-1110, 2012.

24. Kazanjian VH, Converse J. The Surgical Treatment of Facial Injuries. Baltimore: Williams & Wilkins, 1949.

25. Mathes SJ, Vasconez LO. The cervicohumeral flap. Plast Reconstr Surg 67:7-12, 1978.

26. Blevins PK, Luce EA. Limitations of the cervicohumeral flap in head and neck reconstruction. Plast Reconstr Surg 66:220-224, 1980.

27. Cormack GC, Lamberty BG. The anatomical vascular basis of the axillary fascio-cutaneous pedicled flap. Br J Plast Surg 36:425-427, 1983.

28. Lamberty BG, Cormack GC. Misconceptions regarding the cervico-humeral flap. Br J Plast Surg 36:60-63, 1983.

29. Cormack GC, Lamberty BG. A classification of fascio-cutaneous flaps according to their patterns of vascularisation. Br J Plast Surg 37:80-87, 1984.

30. Pallua N, Machens HG, Rennekampff O, et al. The fasciocutaneous supraclavicular artery island flap for releasing postburn mentosternal contractures. Plast Reconstr Surg 99:1878-1884, 1997.

31. Pallua N, Demir E. Postburn head and neck reconstruction in children with the fasciocutaneous supraclavicular artery island flap. Ann Plast Surg 60:276-282, 2008.

32. Vinh BQ, Ogawa R, Van Anh T, et al. Reconstruction of neck scar contractures using supraclavicular flaps: retrospective study of 30 cases. Plast Reconstr Surg 119:130-135, 2007.

33. Vinh BQ, Ogawa R, Van Anh T, et al. Anatomical and clinical studies of the supraclavicular flap: analysis of 103 flaps used to reconstruct neck scar contractures. Plast Reconstr Surg 123:1471-1480, 2009.

34. Pallua N, Magnus NE. The tunneled supraclavicular island flap: an optimized technique for head and neck reconstruction. Plast Reconstr Surg 105:842-851, 2000.

    In this landmark paper, the authors describe detailed anatomic studies of the supraclavicular artery and its angiosome. They introduce the concept of a tunneled island flap and successfully use this technique to reconstruct defects in the head and neck.

35. Di Benedetto G, Auinati A, Pierangeli M, et al. From the "charretera" to the supraclavicular fascial island flap: revisitation and further evolution of a controversial flap. Plast Reconstr Surg 115:70-76, 2005.

36. Chiu ES, Liu PH, Friedlander PL. Supraclavicular artery island flap for head and neck oncologic reconstruction: indications, complications, and outcomes. Plast Reconstr Surg 124:115-123, 2009.

37. Liu PH, Chiu ES. Supraclavicular artery flap: a new option for pharyngeal reconstruction. Ann Plast Surg 62:497-501, 2009.

38. Henderson MM, Chiu ES, Jaffer AS. A simple approach of tubularizing the supraclavicular flap for circumferential pharyngoesophageal defects. Plast Reconstr Surg 126:28-29, 2010.

39. Chiu ES, Liu PH, Baratelli R, et al. Circumferential pharyngoesophageal reconstruction with a supraclavicular artery island flap. Plast Reconstr Surg 125:161-166, 2010.

40. Levy JM, Eko FN, Hilaire HS, et al. Posterolateral skull base reconstruction using the supraclavicular artery island flap. J Craniofac Surg 22:1751-1754, 2011.

41. Epps MT, Cannon CL, Wright MJ, et al. Aesthetic restoration of parotidectomy contour deformity using the supraclavicular artery island flap. Plast Reconstr Surg 127:1925-1931, 2011.

42. Anand AG, Tran EJ, Hasney CP, et al. Oropharyngeal reconstruction using the supraclavicular artery island flap: a new flap alternative. Plast Reconstr Surg 129:438-441, 2012.

43. Sandu K, Monnier P, Pasche P. Supraclavicular flap in head and neck reconstruction: experience in 50 consecutive patients. Eur Arch Otolaryngol 269:1261-1267, 2012.

44. Chen WL, Zhang D, Yang Z, et al. Extended supraclavicular fasciocutaneous island flap based on the transverse cervical artery for head and neck reconstruction after cancer ablation. J Oral Maxillofac Surg 68:2422-2430, 2010.

45. Nthumba PM. The supraclavicular artery flap: a versatile flap for neck and orofacial reconstruction. J Oral Maxillofac Surg 70:1997-2004, 2012.

46. Kim RJ, Izzard ME, Patel RS. Supraclavicular artery island flap for reconstructing defects in the head and neck region. Curr Opin Otolaryngol Head Neck Surg 19:248-250, 2011.

47. Chan JW, Wong C, Ward K, et al. Three- and four-dimensional computed tomographic angiography studies of the supraclavicular artery island flap. Plast Reconst Surg 125:525-531, 2009.

48. Cormack GC, Lamberty, BG. The Arterial Anatomy of Skin Flaps, ed 1. London: Churchill Livingstone, 1989.

49. Alves HR, Ishida LC, Ishida LH, et al. A clinical experience of the supraclavicular flap used to reconstruct head and neck defects in late-stage cancer patients. J Plast Reconstr Aesthet Surg 65:1350-1356, 2012.

50. Martin D, Pascal JF, Baudet J, et al. The submental island flap: a donor site. Anatomy and clinical applications as a free or pedicled flap. Plast Reconstr Surg 92:867-873, 1993.

   The authors describe the original anatomic studies and clinical application of the submental flap. Their harvest technique and flap use remain the standard on which all additional work has been founded.

51. Urken ML. The submental island. In Urken ML, Cheney ML, Blackwell KE, et al, eds. Atlas of Regional and Free Flaps for Head and Neck Reconstruction: Flap Harvest and Insetting. Philadelphia: Lippincott Williams & Wilkins, 2012.

52. Parmar PS, Goldstein DP. The submental island flap in head and neck reconstruction. Curr Opin Otolaryngol Head Neck Surg 17:263-266, 2009.

53. Merten S, Jiang R, Caminer D. The submental artery island flap for head and neck reconstruction. Aust N Z J Surg 72:121-124, 2002.

54. Pistre V, Pelissier P, Martin D, et al. Ten years of experience with the submental flap. Plast Reconstr Surg 108:1576-1581, 2001.

55. Akan I, Ozdemir R, Uysal A, et al. The submental artery flap. Eur J Plast Surg 24:134-139, 2001.

56. Abouchadi A, Capon-Degardin N, Patenotre P, et al. The submental flap in facial reconstruction: advantages and limitations. J Oral Maxillofac Surg 65:863-869, 2007.

57. Sebastian P, Thomas S, Varghese B, et al. The submental island flap for reconstruction of intraoral defects in oral cancer patients. Oral Oncol 44:1014-1018, 2008.

58. Demir Z, Kurtay A, Sahin U, et al. Hair-bearing submental artery island flap for reconstruction of mustache and beard. Plast Reconstr Surg 112:423-429, 2003.

59. Vural E, Suen J. The submental island flap in head and neck reconstruction. Head Neck 22:572-578, 2000.

60. Chow TL, Chan TT, Chow TK, et al. Reconstruction with submental flap for aggressive orofacial cancer. Plast Reconstr Surg 120:431-436, 2007.

61. Faltaous AA, Yetman RJ. The submental artery flap: an anatomic study. Plast Reconstr Surg 97:56-60, 1996.

62. Madgen O, Edizer M, Tayfur V, et al. Anatomic study of the vasculature of the submental artery flap. Plast Reconstr Surg 114:1719-1723, 2004.

63. Kim JT, Kim ST, Koshima I. An anatomic study and clinical applications of the reversed submental artery island flap. Plast Reconstr Surg 109:2204-2210, 2002.

64. Whetzel TP, Mathes SJ. Arterial anatomy of the face: an analysis of vascular territories and perforating cutaneous vessels. Plast Reconstr Surg 89:591-603, 1992.

65. Yilmaz M, Menderes A, Barutcu A. Submental artery island flap for reconstruction of the lower and mid face. Ann Plast Surg 39:30-35, 1997.

66. Patel UA, Bayles SW, Hayden RE. The submental flap: a modified technique for resident training. Laryngoscope 117:186-189, 2007.

   The authors provide an excellent anatomic review of the submental vasculature and introduce a useful technical modification that improves the safety and efficiency of flap harvest.

67. Sterne G, Januszkiewicz J, Hall P, et al. The submental island flap. Br J Plast Surg 49:85-89, 1996.

68. Cheney ML, Varvares MA, Nadol JB. The temporoparietal fascial flap in head and neck reconstruction. Arch Otolaryngol Head Neck Surg 119:618-623, 1993.

   This paper provides the foundation for using the TPFF for the reconstruction of multiple head and neck defects. It offers an excellent description of indications for the use of the flap as well as detailed descriptions of the salient anatomy and harvest technique.

69. Jaquet Y, Higgins KM, Enepekidis DJ. The temporoparietal fascia flap: a versatile tool in head and neck reconstruction. Curr Opin Otolaryngol Head Neck Surg 19:235-241, 2011.

70. Chiarelli A, Baldelli A, DiVincenzo A, et al. Utilization of the superficial temporoparietal fascia in reconstructive plastic surgery: a clinical case. Ophthal Plast Reconstr Surg 5:274-276, 1989.

71. Brent B, Byrd HS. Secondary ear reconstruction with cartilage grafts covered by axial, random, and free flaps of temporoparietal fascia. Plast Reconstr Surg 72:141-151, 1983.

72. East CA, Brough MD, Grant HR. Mastoid obliteration with the temporoparietal fascia flap. J Laryngol Otol 105:417-420, 1991.

73. Cheney ML, Megerian CA, Brown MT, et al. Mastoid obliteration and lining using the temporoparietal fascial flap. Laryngoscope 105:1010-1013, 1995.

74. Lai A, Cheney ML. Temporoparietal fascia flap in orbital reconstruction. Arch Facial Plast Surg 2:196-201, 2000.

75. McCarthy JG, Zido BM. The spectrum of calvarial bone grafting: introduction of the vascularized calvarial bone graft. Plast Reconstr Surg 74:10-18, 1984.

76. Cheney ML, Lindsay RW, Hadlock TA. Temporoparietal fascia. In Urken ML, Cheney ML, Blackwell KE, et al, eds. Atlas of Regional and Free Flaps for Head and Neck Reconstruction: Flap Harvest and Insetting. Philadelphia: Lippincott Williams & Wilkins, 2012.

77. Kim JY, Buck DW, Johnson SA, et al. The temporoparietal fascial flap as an alternative to free flaps for orbito-maxillary reconstruction. Plast Reconstr Surg 126:880-888, 2010.

78. Davison SP, Mesbahi AN, Clemens MW, et al. Vascularized calvarial bone flaps and midface reconstruction. Plast Reconstr Surg 122:10e-18e, 2008.

37

Free Flaps for Facial Skin and Soft Tissue Reconstruction

Marc W. Herr ▪ *Daniel Deschler*

Soft tissue defects of the head and neck present a multitude of challenges related to the geometric complexity of the region, the critical nature of the underlying structures, the intricate functional interplay, and the potential for long-term, visible disfigurement. In recent decades microvascular free tissue transfers have become the preferred method of reconstruction for these difficult defects. These techniques allow reliable, single-stage, and immediate reconstruction in this challenging patient population.[1] During the past half-century more than 20 free flap donor sites have been described for use in the head and neck, and improved techniques have resulted in success rates as high as 95% to 99%.[1-5]

The first surgery performed using a microscope to aid in the repair of blood vessels was described by Jacobson and Suarez in 1960.[6,7] Their concepts were extrapolated into contemporary reconstructive microsurgery several years later by Buncke and Schulz[8] and Hoffman et al.[9] In the 1970s McGregor and Jackson[10] and Taylor and colleagues[11,12] published their work on free flaps of the groin and iliac region based off the iliac arterial system. Yang et al[13] introduced the radial forearm flap to reconstructive surgery in the early 1980s. Soutar and McGregor[14] and others[9,15] popularized the technique in their subsequent studies and promoted its use in oral soft tissue reconstruction. Continued innovation and progress have seen a number of subsequent landmark reports published on free flap reconstruction of the head and neck.[16-20] Reconstructive surgeons have adopted these techniques, continue to modify them, and introduce new flaps for the reconstruction of complex and diverse defects.

ANATOMY AND EPIDEMIOLOGY

Most defects in the head and neck (93% to 95%) are produced by surgical ablation of malignancies. The remainder (5% to 7%) result from traumatic or congenital causes or from the excision of benign neoplasms.[1,2] Facial skin and soft tissue defects are approximately 6% of the total.[2]

The regions of the head and neck are divided into aesthetic subunits for the purposes of simplifying analysis and surgical planning. The major units traditionally include the forehead, eyes, nose, lips, chin, ears, and neck (Fig. 37-1).

These subunits are based on skin thickness, color, texture, and underlying structural contour.[21] Thus the specific free flap used depends on the characteristics of the defect, including surface area of skin loss, volume of soft tissue loss, status of underlying remnant bony framework, and the facial subunit involved. In addition to aesthetic outcomes, surgeons must consider the functional requirements of each subunit. These functions include patency of the nasal and oral airway, oral competence, oral-nasal separation, velopharyngeal competence, bolus transfer and deglutition, articulation, facial mimetic function and symmetry, and ocular hygiene related to eyelid function.

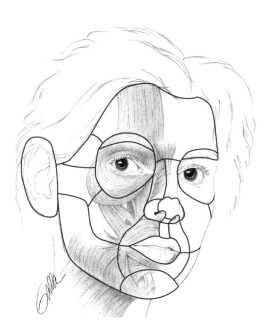

Fig. 37-1   Subunits of the head and neck.

The most commonly employed flaps are the radial forearm (40% to 67%), the anterolateral thigh (2% to 8%), the rectus abdominis (1% to 8%), and the latissimus dorsi (1% to 8%).[1,2,5] The temporoparietal fascia flap, which may be used as pedicled or free flap, also continues to play an important role in the reconstruction of soft tissue defects of the head and neck.[22,23]

PATIENT EVALUATION AND PREOPERATIVE PLANNING

As microvascular experience and technical expertise have increased, free tissue transfer is being used for more diverse defects and in an expanding population of patients. Patients requiring this type of reconstruction are typically older and demonstrate significant comorbidities. Although overall surgical success rates remain excellent, the procedures are lengthy and physiologically demanding. Documented medical complications after microvascular surgery include pulmonary embolism, supraventricular tachycardia, myocardial ischemia/infarction, mental status changes, cerebrovascular accident, pulmonary edema, pneumonia, renal insufficiency, and deep venous thrombosis.[1,2,24-26]

Several large series have reported patient comorbidity to be a significant risk factor for medical complications after microvascular reconstruction. Typically this parameter is quantified with the American Society of Anesthesiologists (ASA) system, an index used by anesthesiologists to evaluate patients preoperatively with regard to their general state of health and the severity of underlying diseases. Specific criteria are used to define each class. Class I denotes a healthy patient, class II describes a patient with mild systemic disease, class III describes a patient with severe systemic disease with definite functional limitations, class IV describes a patient with severe systemic disease that is a constant threat to life, and class V describes a moribund patient who is not expected to survive without operative intervention.[1,26] Shestak et al[27] and others[1,25,26] reported an increased incidence of medical complications in patients with ASA classifications of III and higher, and these findings were corroborated in several subsequent reviews. Farwell et al[24] analyzed more specific individual comorbidities and found the presence of hepatitis to be a significant risk factor for medical complications on multivariate analysis.

The effect of age on perioperative complications has also been examined with varying results. Singh et al[28] noted that age older than 70 years was associated with increasing severity of complications. Researchers in subsequent reviews identified a significant relationship between the incidence of major medical complications and patients age older than 55 years[2] or 65 years.[26] In contrast, several other investigators concluded that age does not affect the likelihood of perioperative complications and thus should not influence decisions regarding a patient's candidacy for free flap reconstruction.[24,25,27] Other notable factors that may increase the likelihood of complications include aggressive intraoperative administration of intravenous crystalloid[2,26] and operative times of more than 8 hours.[24]

Although some discrepancies exist, most medical literature suggests that comorbidity is the most important factor in determining the risk of perioperative complications. In their retrospective comparison of free flap outcomes in 1999 versus 2009, Kakarala et al[29] noted similar complication rates despite significantly higher comorbidities in the more recent patient cohort. They concluded that this likely resulted from their consistent and systematic use of medical consultation conducted both preoperatively and as an integral part of the postoperative pathway in their 2009 patients. Therefore such consultations should be considered a routine part of preoperative planning for patients requiring microvascular reconstructive procedures.

MICROVASCULAR FLAP ANATOMY AND HARVEST TECHNIQUE

CLASSIFICATION OF FLAPS

Blood supply to the skin island is critical to flap survival, and classification schemes emphasize the anatomy of these tissues. The cutaneous portion of each free tissue flap is supplied by the main vascular pedicle through perforating vessels. These small-caliber perforators branch off the pedicle in relatively predictable locations and ramify in the subcutaneous plexus, which in turn provides the vascular supply to the skin. The perforating vessels may take a direct route to the skin paddle. Alternatively they may travel through the fascial septum between muscles (septocutaneous perforators) or through the muscles themselves (musculocutaneous perforators). Each perforator supplies a limited area of the skin (or angiosome), therefore the number of these vessels included in each flap design is determined by the required size and shape of the cutaneous paddle.[30]

Multiple classification systems have been proposed for cutaneous free tissue flaps. Cormack and Lamberty[31] used the term *fasciocutaneous* to describe all soft tissue flaps with a blood supply depending on a fascial plexus of perforating vessels; they described three types of flaps based on the arborization of this perforator as it enters the fascia.[32] Mathes and Nahai[33] described a similar tripartite classification scheme based on the type of deep fascial perforator: direct cutaneous, septocutaneous, and musculocutaneous.[32] In 1986 Nakajima et al[34] developed a classification system for skin flaps that included five types of flaps: (1) cutaneous, (2) fasciocutaneous, (3) adipofascial, (4) septocutaneous, and (5) musculocutaneous flaps. They further characterized six types of fasciocutaneous flaps, each based on distinct perforators of the deep fascia. Thus, with subtle differences, these systems characterize soft tissue flaps based on circulation; however, for these categories to be complete, other flap characteristics should be considered.[32] Tolhurst accounted for these secondary characteristics and described flaps based on their tissue composition.[35]

For ease of description throughout this chapter, we will simplify this system further and identify flaps by the tissues they contain: skin *(cutaneo-)*, fascia *(fascio-)*, and/or muscle *(myo-)*. For example, a flap that is primarily composed of skin and fascia would be characterized as a *fasciocutaneous flap.*

Studies over the past three decades have shown that neither a passive muscle carrier nor the underlying fascial plexus of vessels is absolutely necessary for flap survival if careful dissection of the myocutaneous or fasciocutaneous perforators is accomplished.[36,37] In the past decade, further refinements in our understanding of microvascular anatomy and surgical technique have given rise to the design and implementation of true perforator flaps. As these flaps are harvested, the muscle through which the perforator travels is separated and not included in the flap elevation. This technique allows greater customization of the soft tissue elements. The surgeon can tailor skin and subcutaneous tissue segments to the specific defect rather than including unwanted tissue bulk to maintain a viable pedicle. Furthermore, limiting the harvest of excess tissue may also minimize donor site morbidity. Although perforator flaps are more technically demanding to harvest, they are extremely versatile, and their use has become increasingly widespread.[36] Nevertheless, care must be taken not to overcustomize the transferred tissue, because contracture, atrophy, and settling caused by the effects of gravity and adjoining tissues can significantly alter the appearance and function of a free tissue reconstruction. The ultimate goals of reconstruction are often best served by transferring slightly more soft tissue than is required; the tissue can be debulked and revised secondarily once wound stability is achieved.

FASCIAL AND FASCIOCUTANEOUS FLAPS
Radial Forearm Free Flap

The radial forearm free flap (RFFF) is a fasciocutaneous flap composed of a thin, pliable skin island, varying amounts adipofascial tissue, and a long, consistent vascular pedicle (Table 37-1).

The RFFF was first introduced by Yang et al[13] in 1981 based on their work at the Shenyang Military Hospital. They reported a series of 60 flaps with only one documented failure. Soutar and colleagues[14,15] described its use for reconstruction of the oral cavity. Since that time, the RFFF has become the workhorse flap for reconstruction of defects throughout the head, neck, and upper aerodigestive tract. In addition to external defects, tongue, floor of the mouth, buccal, pharyngeal, and laryngopharyngeal defects have

Table 37-1   Anatomy and Clinical Applications for Fascial and Fasciocutaneous Flaps

Type of Flap	Neurovascular Anatomy	Advantages	Disadvantages	Clinical Applications
Radial forearm	Radial artery and venae comitantes Cephalic and basilic veins Lateral and medial antebrachial nerves	Thin and pliable Long pedicle	Limited surface area Delayed healing of donor site Unsightly donor site	Forehead reconstruction Lateral skull base reconstruction fold over Orbitomaxillary and orbital exenteration, including eyelids Full-thickness lip and chin Neck
Temporoparietal fascia	Superficial temporal artery and vein Auriculotemporal nerve	Thin and pliable Robust vascularization	No bulk Requires skin grafting if used for external coverage	Orbitomaxillary and auricular reconstruction Orbital exenteration, with eyelids preserved
Anterolateral thigh	Lateral circumflex femoral artery Venae comitantes Lateral femoral cutaneous nerve	Substantial volume of skin and soft tissue Separate skin paddles possible Minimal donor site morbidity	Anatomic variability of the perforators Short vascular pedicle Small vessel diameter	Forehead reconstruction Lateral skull base reconstruction Orbitomaxillary and orbital exenteration, including eyelids Full-thickness lip and chin Neck

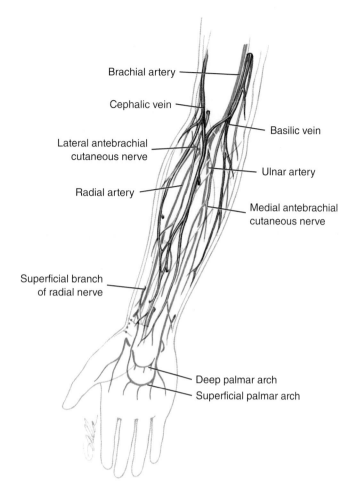

Fig. 37-2   The neurovascular anatomy of the radial forearm free flap. The radial artery supplies inflow. Outflow is through the cutaneous veins of the forearm (usually the cephalic vein) and/or the vena comitantes of the radial artery. The lateral antebrachial cutaneous nerve provides the primary sensory innervation to the region.

all been successfully reconstructed with the RFFF. The RFFF is based on the radial artery and its associated venae comitantes. Venous drainage is also facilitated by a superficial system of large cutaneous veins, including the cephalic and basilic veins. Along the length of the forearm there are multiple connections between the venae comitantes and the superficial veins, which allow either system to serve as the primary drainage system of the flap. Therefore only one venous anastomosis is required in the majority of cases. In general, however, the veins of the superficial system tend to have thicker walls and be of larger caliber, thus facilitating microvascular anastomosis.[38] The lateral antebrachial cutaneous nerve runs in close proximity to the cephalic vein and provides sensory innervation to the region of the forearm that is typically harvested. Sensory neural coaptation is possible in cases in which an applicable donor nerve exists in the head and neck (Fig. 37-2).

The main advantages of the RFFF are its thin and pliable tissue and its long vascular pedicle. The greatest shortcoming of the RFFF is the somewhat limited surface area, which makes it unsuitable for resurfacing larger defects. Tendon exposure at the harvest site with delayed wound healing is a common postoperative complication. Although this is almost always self-limited and resolves with basic wound care, reports indicate that the use of a suprafascial harvest technique can significantly decrease the incidence of tendon exposure.[39,40] Other postoperative issues include numbness along the distribution of the superficial radial nerve in the region of the anatomic snuffbox, and temporary limitations in hand strength and mobility. These problems typically resolve without further intervention.

The most devastating complication after transfer of an RFFF is the potential for hand ischemia after sacrifice of the radial artery. The hand receives a dual blood supply. The radial artery terminates in the deep palmar arch, which supplies the thumb and index finger, whereas the ulnar artery supplies the third, fourth, and fifth digits through the superficial palmar arch (see Fig. 37-2). The ulnar artery may supply the entire hand through either a complete superficial palmar arch, which sends arterial branches to all five digits, or through communication with the deep palmar arch.[38] In a study of 265 cadaveric specimens, Coleman and Anson[41] found a complete superficial arch in only 77.3% of cases. In 12% of specimens, vascular anomalies were present that would have placed the lateral hand at risk for ischemia after radial artery occlusion or sacrifice. Therefore preoperative evaluation with an Allen's test is critically important in preventing ischemic complications.

Temporoparietal Fascial Flap

The temporoparietal fascia flap (TPFF) has been a versatile and adaptable tool for the reconstructive surgeon since Golovine introduced it in 1898.[22,42] It is composed of thin, pliable, well-vascularized tissue, allowing it to mold to complex facial defects. The flap comprises the temporoparietal fascia (TPF), which is a 2 to 4 mm thick layer of connective tissue that represents the superior continuation of the superficial musculoaponeurotic system (SMAS) and continues cranially to become the galea. The TPF is deep and firmly adherent to the subcutaneous tissue underneath the skin of the scalp and is separated from the underlying temporalis muscle and fascia by a layer of loose areolar tissue[42] (Fig. 37-3).

The TPFF derives its blood supply from the superficial temporal artery and vein, which course within the fascia and divide into anterior and posterior branches approximately 2 to 3 cm superior to the zygomatic arch (see Fig. 37-3). The flap can be used as either a pedicled or free flap and may be transferred independently or in combination with skin and calvarial bone.[22,23,43] As a fascial flap the TPFF is particularly well

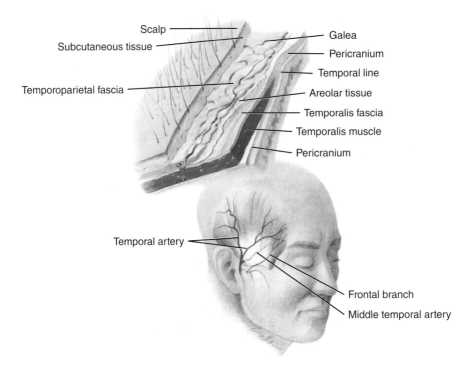

Fig. 37-3   The anatomy of the scalp and the superficial temporal artery system in the temporal fossa as it relates to the temporoparietal fascial flap.

suited to orbitomaxillary and auricular reconstructions.[22,23] The TPFF may also be harvested with an island of overlying hair-bearing scalp, which can be used for reconstruction of the eyebrow, mustache, or other hirsute facial areas.

Anterolateral Thigh Flap

The anterolateral thigh (ALT) flap has been in widespread use in Asia for almost 30 years and has gained popularity in Europe and North America over the past decade.[19,20,44-46] The flap is based on septocutaneous or septomyocutaneous perforators from the descending branch of the lateral circumflex femoral artery and its associated vena comitantes. The vascular pedicle travels between the rectus femoris and vastus lateralis muscles until giving off perforating branches to the overlying skin. The perforators consistently lie along a line drawn from the anterior superior iliac spine to the superolateral border of the patella. If a cutaneous paddle is planned the vessels are mapped by handheld Doppler centered over the midpoint of this line, with most of the skin perforators located within a 3 cm radius of this midpoint[45] (Fig. 37-4).

A significant advantage of the ALT flap is the availability of a substantial amount of skin and soft tissue. This makes the flap particularly well suited for the reconstruction of large orbitomaxillary and lateral skull base defects.[47-50] The flap also produces minimal donor site morbidity because primary closure of the donor site is usually achievable. The donor site for the ALT is also easily accessible for a two-team surgical approach, and its location on the anterior aspect of the leg permits a much simpler harvest than the previously described lateral thigh flap. The primary disadvantage of the ALT flap is the anatomic variability of the perforating vessels. However, as experience with the flap harvest increases, perforator anatomy becomes less problematic. The surgeon can also simplify the harvest by taking a cuff of vastus lateralis muscle to safely incorporate the myocutaneous perforators.[50] Other disadvantages of the flap include a relatively short vascular pedicle and a somewhat small vessel diameter.

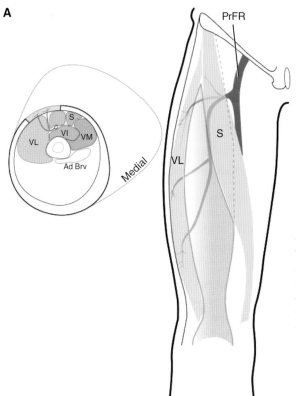

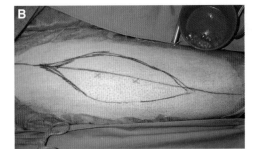

Fig. 37-4   The anterolateral thigh flap. **A,** The neurovascular anatomy of the anterolateral thigh flap. (*Ad Brv,* Adductor brevis; *PrFR,* profunda femoris artery; *S,* sartorius; *VI,* vastus intermedius; *VL,* vastus lateralis; *VM,* vastus medialis.) **B,** Intraoperative view of the marked location of the arterial perforators from the descending branch of the lateral circumflex femoral artery.

MYOGENOUS AND MYOCUTANEOUS FLAPS

Rectus Abdominis Myocutaneous Flap

With its large size and long, consistent vascular pedicle the rectus abdominis myocutaneous (RAM) flap is the historic workhorse for the reconstruction of the head, neck, and skull base[51-58] (Table 37-2).

The blood supply is provided by the inferior epigastric artery and vein, which enter the lateral border of the rectus muscle posteriorly just below the arcuate line and halfway between the pubis and umbilicus (Fig. 37-5). The rectus abdominis muscle may be transferred alone, with overlying fascia and subcutaneous tissue, or as a composite flap consisting of muscle, fascia, skin, and subcutaneous tissue.[59]

If a skin paddle is incorporated, the primary disadvantage of the RAM flap is potential bulkiness caused by the width of the subcutaneous tissues of the abdominal wall. This is particularly true in women and obese patients. There is also a long-term postoperative risk of abdominal wall weakness and ventral hernia development. This risk is minimized with meticulous closure of the anterior rectus sheath below the arcuate line, although it may also require the use of surgical mesh. In addition, postoperative rehabilitation can be prolonged as a result of abdominal wall disruption.

Myogenous and Myocutaneous Latissimus Dorsi Flap

The latissimus dorsi muscle is a broad, flat muscle that originates from the thoracic spinous processes and posterior iliac crest and inserts into the posterior portion of the humerus. It is supplied by the thoracodorsal vessels, which originate from the subscapular system. The muscular innervation is from the thoracodorsal nerve (Fig. 37-6).

Free latissimus dorsi flaps have been used for head and neck reconstruction since Watson et al[60] initially described them in 1979. The flap can be harvested with a skin paddle or as a muscle only flap. An advantage of the flap is the versatility in the amount of tissue that can be harvested, ranging from a small amount of muscle under the skin paddle to the entire muscle. Other advantages include a long pedicle, large caliber vessels, and the ability to design a bilobed flap based on the medial and lateral branches of the thoracodorsal artery.

Table 37-2 Anatomy and Clinical Applications for Myogenous and Myocutaneous Flaps

Type of Flap	Neurovascular Anatomy	Advantages	Disadvantages	Clinical Applications
Rectus abdominis	Inferior epigastric artery and vein	Substantial volume of skin and soft tissue Long pedicle	Excessive bulkiness in obese patients Risk of abdominal hernia	Scalp reconstruction Skull base reconstruction Orbitomaxillary and orbital exenteration including eyelids
Latissimus dorsi	Thoracodorsal artery and vein Thoracodorsal nerve	Large volume of tissue available Long pedicle Large caliber vessels	Patient repositioning for harvest Volume loss as a result of tissue atrophy	Scalp reconstruction

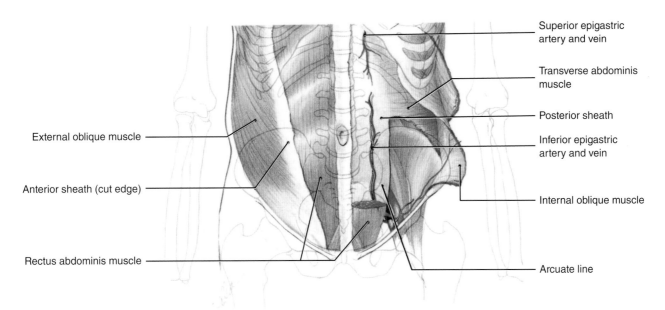

Fig. 37-5   The vascular anatomy of the rectus abdominis myocutaneous flap. The rectus abdominis muscle has been removed from the rectus sheath. Note that the epigastric vessels are deep to the muscle. The arcuate line is midway between the umbilicus and the pubis.

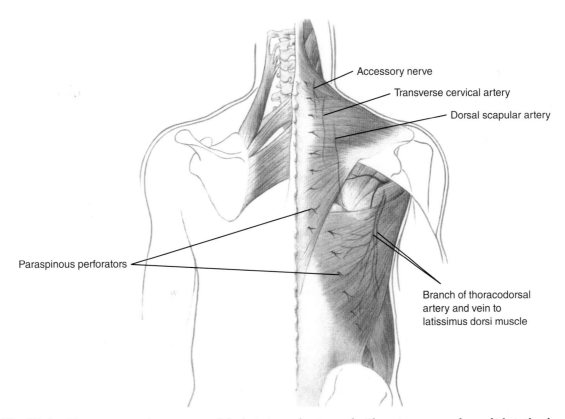

Fig. 37-6   The neurovascular anatomy of the latissimus dorsi muscle. The primary vascular pedicle is the thoraco-dorsal artery and vein.

The primary disadvantage of this flap is the need to harvest it with the patient in the lateral decubitus position, making a two-team approach impossible. If the serratus anterior is included with the flap, there is the potential for winging of the scapula and chronic shoulder pain. Furthermore, the donor site can be prone to seroma formation with the large degree of undermining that is required. If a large skin island is harvested, skin grafting of the donor site is subject to breakdown. Additionally, the latissimus dorsi is one of the thinnest muscles in the body, which makes it ideal for resurfacing, but the muscle atrophy that occurs after denervation may compromise the flap's ability to fill dead space and provide stable, long-term contouring.[61]

Subunit Approach to Facial Reconstruction
Scalp, Forehead, and Orbit

The correction of soft tissue defects of the scalp and forehead is challenging because of the convexity of the skull and inelastic nature of the underlying tissues. In regions of the hair-bearing scalp, tissue expanders can be used to incorporate a maximal amount of hirsute tissue into local flaps. However, free tissue transfer is required in cases in which local or regional options are inadequate, such as in cases of reoperation, previously irradiated or scarred wound beds, infected wounds, and defects with large surface areas (greater than 50 to 100 cm^2).[62-64] In general, defects are addressed with either fasciocutaneous flaps or my-

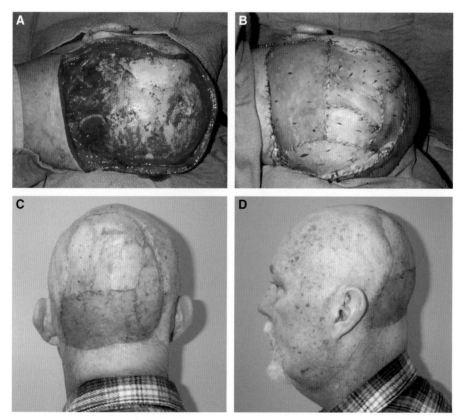

Fig. 37-7 **A,** A large defect of the occipital scalp after excision of a carcinoma. **B,** A muscle-only latissimus dorsi free flap has been inset and covered with a split-thickness skin graft. **C** and **D,** Results 3 months after surgery.

ogenous flaps in conjunction with a split-thickness skin graft. The most commonly employed flap in this region is the myogenous or myocutaneous latissimus dorsi flap.[62-65] Although the RAM flap is also used,[66,67] it has largely been replaced by alternate flaps in several recent series.[62-64,67]

No clear differences appear to exist in terms of flap reliability or complications when a comparison is made between myogenous free flaps covered with split-thickness skin grafts and free flaps with a skin paddle.[62] Thus flap selection is based on the characteristics and requirements of the wound. Myogenous flaps with an overlying split-thickness skin graft are more commonly employed for defects of the scalp, especially the occipital and parietal regions (Fig. 37-7). In more aesthetically sensitive locations such as the forehead, defects are reconstructed with fasciocutaneous flaps (such as the RFFF).[62,67] Larger defects (greater than 200 cm^2) are more readily addressed with latissimus dorsi or RAM flaps, whereas defects less than 100 cm^2 are amenable to coverage with an RFFF.[67]

Involvement of the orbit may necessitate orbital exenteration in conjunction with the creation of a scalp, forehead, or temple defect. In such instances, it is critical to obliterate the orbital defect and simultaneously provide soft tissue coverage. The radial forearm can be effective if the defect is not too extensive and bulk is not essential. The long vascular pedicle also facilitates microvascular anastomosis in the neck. Defects with extensive resurfacing requirements are better served by the latissimus dorsi myogenous flap with a split-thickness skin graft (Fig. 37-8).

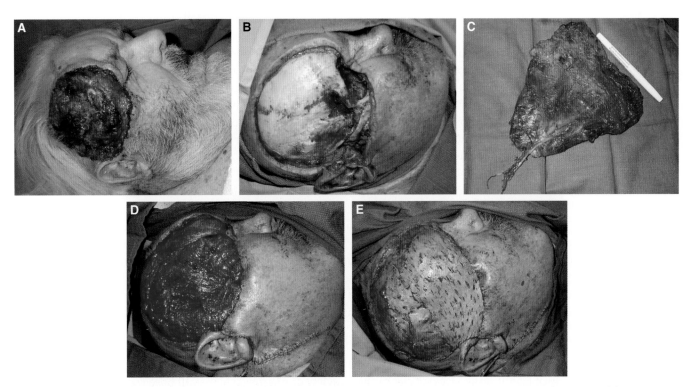

Fig. 37-8   **A,** This patient had a cutaneous basal cell carcinoma involving the parietal scalp, infratemporal fossa, and right orbit. **B,** Postablative defect after a composite resection and orbital exenteration. **C,** A muscle-only latissimus dorsi flap was harvested. **D,** The latissimus dorsi flap was inset to provide coverage of the scalp defect and obliteration of the right orbit. **E,** A split-thickness skin graft was placed over the myogenous flap.

Continued

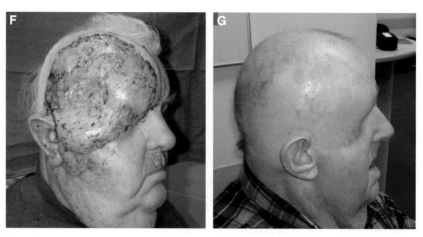

Fig. 37-8, cont'd   **F,** Results 4 weeks after surgery. **G,** The appearance of the reconstruction after complete healing.

Lateral Skull Base and Temporal Bone

Defects of the lateral skull base involve soft tissue and/or bone loss in the region of the temporal bone. They are often associated with large cutaneous defects that involve the preauricular and postauricular skin and potentially the entire auricle. Frequently they also result in exposed cranial bone and dura.[51]

Outcomes of skull base reconstruction have been compared using local, pedicled, and free flaps[52]; in the free flap group there was a lower overall complication rate (33.5% versus 75%), less risk of compromised healing (10% versus 36.3%), and less incidence of flap failure (0 patients versus 3 patients).[52] This finding is likely because the size and location of lateral skull base defects often approximate or exceed the excursional limits of pedicled flaps. Thus the distal tip of the flap, where the blood supply is most tenuous, is responsible for coverage of the defect,[51] which places the most critical area of the reconstruction at greatest risk for breakdown and wound exposure. Nevertheless, when necessary, a pedicled pectoralis major flap and pedicled latissimus dorsi myocutaneous flap can be used dependably for large lateral skull base defects if additional intraoperative maneuvers are employed.[68]

Free flaps are relatively unrestricted by the anatomic constraints of pedicled flaps and can provide well-vascularized soft tissue to cover cutaneous and bony defects and obliterate underlying dead space.[51] Thus vascularized free tissue has largely replaced regional flaps as the preferred modality for reconstructing defects of the lateral skull base and temporal bone.[51,53,69,70] Most patients require external skin[51]; therefore reconstruction is generally performed with myocutaneous or fasciocutaneous flaps that include large skin paddles and significant underlying fascial and adipose tissue. In several large series the RAM flap has been successfully employed as the primary reconstructive option.[51-55,71] The flap's long vascular pedicle and sizable soft tissue component make it ideal for defects in this region (Fig. 37-9). The ALT flap offers similar advantages.[48,49]

With a long, consistent vascular pedicle and adequate skin paddle the RFFF provides an excellent alternative for repair of lateral skull base defects. In their review of microvascular skull base reconstructions, Nouraei et al[72] employed the RFFF in 30 patients, with favorable results. Additionally, dead space from underlying bony defects may be obliterated by folding the RFFF over onto itself. In this orientation, the pedicle creates extra bulk while the skin paddle provides coverage of the external defect (Fig. 37-10). In these cases the overall bulk of the flap, and specifically the pedicled portion, requires careful consideration at the time of harvest. Subdermal skin flaps are elevated to allow inclusion of the fat in the more proximal region of the forearm, and care is taken to preserve perforators from the main pedicle to this proximal component of the flap.

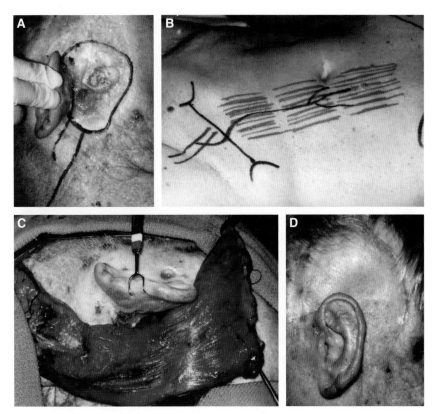

Fig. 37-9 **A,** This patient presented with chronic osteoradionecrosis of the temporal bone after multiple excisions of cutaneous carcinomas and radiotherapy. **B,** The planned rectus abdominis muscle free flap for coverage of the area. **C,** After debridement the rectus abdominis free flap was revascularized and used to obliterate the defect. A split-thickness skin graft was placed overlying the muscle to allow rapid reepithelialization of this area. **D,** Appearance of the reconstruction after complete healing.

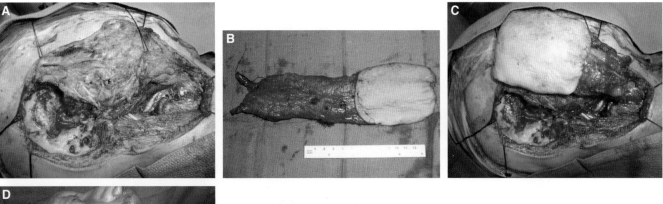

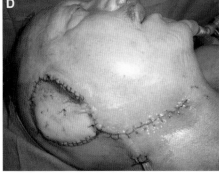

Fig. 37-10 **A,** An ablative defect of the lateral skull base after total auriculectomy, total parotidectomy, and lateral temporal bone resection for recurrent squamous cell carcinoma of the external auditory canal. **B,** A radial forearm flap was harvested. **C,** The radial forearm flap was folded over onto itself, providing bulk to obliterate the underlying dead space while the skin paddle was used to address the cutaneous defect. **D,** Intraoperative appearance of the flap after inset.

Finally, in cases in which there is no external or cutaneous defect, a myogenous, myoadipose, or myofascial rectus abdominis flap or ALT flap may be employed to provide protection for underlying structures and obliterate dead space. Similarly, a deepithelialized radial forearm fascial flap with optimized proximal bulk can be used.

Orbitomaxillary and Cheek Defects

Defects of the cheek, including the orbitomaxillary complex, can vary widely in terms of size and involved tissues. Defects must be evaluated and addressed based on the amount of cutaneous loss, the volume of soft tissue removed, and the potential need to separate or support structures of the orbit and upper aerodigestive tract. If an orbital exenteration is performed additional consideration must be given to the presence or absence of the eyelids. Furthermore the potential deleterious effects of wound closure and scar contraction must be anticipated and avoided, including traction on the oral commissure or nasal ala and lower lid ectropion.[73] Whereas smaller defects may be addressed with local tissue flaps, microvascular free flap reconstruction is the preferred option for surgical defects that require a large amount of soft tissue replacement and/or tissue lining in multiple areas.[74]

Although the RAM flap has been used in a more historical context (Fig. 37-11), the RFFF and ALT flaps are considered the workhorse free flaps for soft tissue defects of the midface. The RFFF is thin and pliable, making it ideal for preserving facial contouring while providing soft tissue coverage (Fig. 37-12). The RFFF may also be used for full-thickness defects of the cheek, including defects that involve the oral commissure. In these cases, the flap is folded over onto itself, permitting inset into both sides of the defect and creation of a new commissure.[73] The distal component is usually rolled intraorally with care taken to provide adequate redundancy, which limits intraoral contracture and trismus (Fig. 37-13).

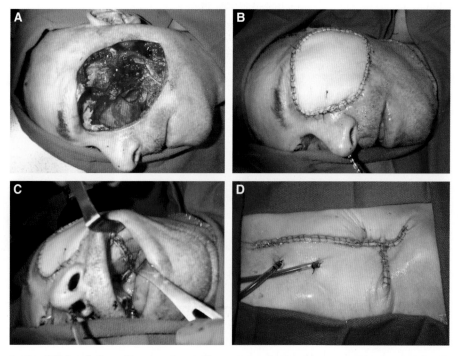

Fig. 37-11   **A,** An ablative defect after a total maxillectomy and orbital exenteration for sinonasal squamous cell carcinoma. **B,** A rectus abdominis myocutaneous flap was harvested. The distal portion of the skin paddle was used to reconstruct the external cutaneous defect while the underlying soft tissue obliterated the dead space of the orbit. **C,** The distal portion of the skin paddle was inset to repair the palatal defect. **D,** The rectus abdominis flap donor site was closed primarily.

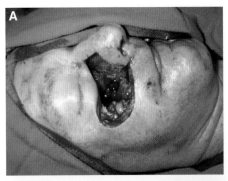

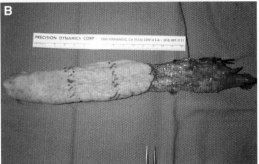

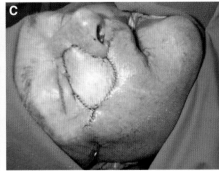

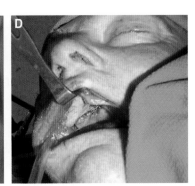

Fig. 37-12   **A,** An ablative defect after a total maxillectomy including overlying skin with preservation of the orbit. **B,** A radial forearm flap was harvested; the skin paddle has been marked to show the plan for inset, with the more distal segment to be used for external coverage. The middle segment was deepithelialized and folded to allow inset of the proximal segment in the palatal defect. **C,** Inset of the external skin paddle. **D,** Inset of the proximal portion of the skin paddle to reconstruct the hard palate defect.

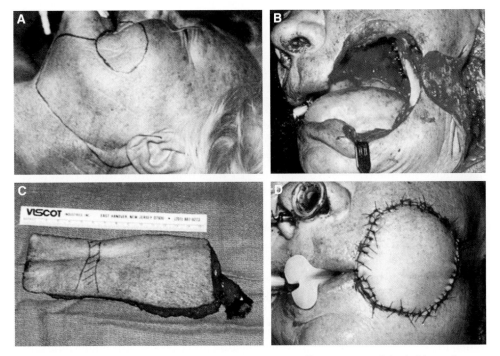

Fig. 37-13   **A,** This patient presented with recurrent squamous cell carcinoma of the left buccal mucosa with extensive involvement of the subcutaneous tissues of the left cheek adjacent to the oral commissure. **B,** Ablation included a through-and-through defect of the skin of the cheek and buccal mucosa, superficial parotidectomy, and supraomohyoid neck dissection. **C and D,** A radial forearm free flap was selected for reconstruction of the defect and was designed with an inner and outer skin paddle. A segment of the flap was deepithelialized to fold onto itself for reconstruction of the buccal mucosal and the facial skin defect.

Continued

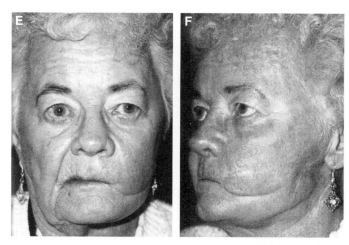

Fig. 37-13, cont'd   **E** and **F,** Appearance of the patient postoperatively after flap debulking.

In addition to a potentially larger skin paddle the ALT flap also possesses substantial soft tissue volume. Thus the ALT flap can simultaneously restore deficient facial bulk and provide coverage for cutaneous defects in the lateral face.[47,73] Additionally, unlike muscular and myocutaneous flaps the ALT is primarily a fascioadipocutaneous flap and does not tend to lose bulk because of atrophy. Kuo et al[75] reported a series of 15 patients with extensive defects involving the cheek and oral commissure who were successfully reconstructed with ALT flaps. Vascularized fascia lata was used to suspend the flap and remaining orbicularis oris muscle, thereby restoring adequate oral competence. Other series have described the application of ALT flaps in cheek reconstruction after burns and trauma.[47,73,76,77]

The arterial perforators of the ALT flap increase its flexibility, allowing for numerous variations in skin paddle design and orientation. Rodriguez-Vegas et al[78] took advantage of this versatility to provide oronasal separation for patients with maxillary defects. They describe an ALT flap that consists of two skin islands, a proximal one for palatal reconstruction and a distal one for nasal lining. The authors created two separate skin islands if two adequate perforators were present; otherwise a small strip of skin was deepithelialized to serve as a hinge between the skin paddles. Chou et al[79] further refined this technique when they repaired bilateral buccal defects by harvesting two separate ALT flaps from a single thigh. Each fasciocutaneous flap was based on a distinct perforator from the descending branch of the lateral femoral circumflex artery.

Maxillectomy defects become more complex in cases in which critical structures such as the orbit, globe, and cranial base are resected.[74] In these cases, reconstructive options are based on the volume and type of tissue lost and the structures preserved. When the eyelids are involved and must be included in the resection, the external defect may be addressed with the cutaneous portion of a free flap. If the use of an ocular prosthesis is planned the orbit needs enough bulk to maintain the prosthesis in proper position.[80] Flaps composed primarily of muscle eventually atrophy. The resulting loss of tissue volume may make prosthetic use difficult or impossible.[80] Thus a thin, pliable fasciocutaneous flap such as the RFFF is ideal for reconstruction. When the eyelids are preserved they may be used for coverage. Although some reports endorse suturing the lids together and allowing them to retract into the orbital socket,[74] this technique is not advocated; there is often insufficient tissue for coverage of the apex. In such cases, the orbital defect can be lined with a TPFF or temporalis muscle flap to provide bulk at the apex and facilitate healing[23] (Fig. 37-14).

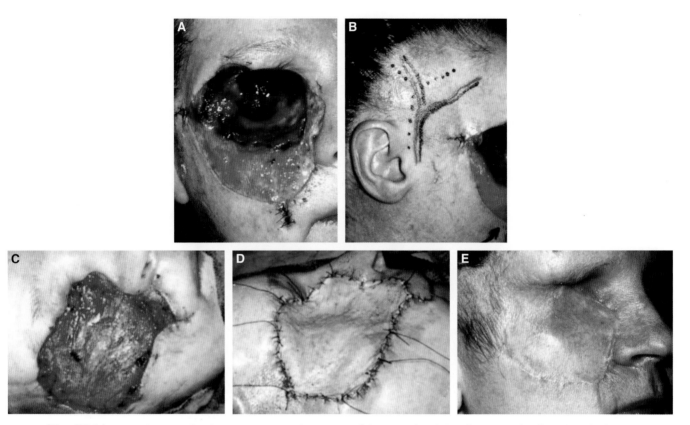

Fig. 37-14   **A,** After an orbital exenteration and excision of the periorbital skin for a morpheaform basal cell carcinoma. **B,** The proposed temporoparietal flap incision site and the superficial temporal vascular pedicle. **C,** The temporoparietal fascial flap rotated into the orbital and periorbital defect. **D,** The overlying split-thickness skin graft that allows reepithelialization of the defect. **E,** Final result.

Lip and Chin Defects

The lips are composed of skin, intrinsic and extrinsic muscles, and mucosa. The intrinsic muscle of the lips is the sphincteric orbicularis oris, which provides oral competence. The extrinsic facial muscles insert into the lips and contribute to speech modulation and facial expression. The lips are divided into several aesthetic subunits. The upper lip is divided into three subunits: two lateral subunits and one medial subunit, the *philtrum*. The lower lip is a single subunit.[81]

The goals of lip and chin reconstruction involve restoration of function, taking into consideration the aesthetic units, vermilion borderlines, and hair-bearing skin. The result should achieve a competent oral sphincter with complete skin coverage, oral lining, and the semblance of a vermilion. The nature of the defect ultimately determines the feasibility of achieving these goals. Lip defects less than one third in size can be closed primarily. Defects greater than one third require the importation of new tissue. This new tissue can be borrowed from the remaining lip, the opposite lip, the adjacent cheek, or local flaps may be used[81] (see Chapter 35). Distant flaps are considered if the defect involves the whole lower lip, the entire upper lip, or half of each with the oral commissure.[80] Such defects may also extensively involve the chin, the cheek, and the base of the nose. These large, full-thickness defects are best repaired with free vascularized fasciocutaneous flaps.

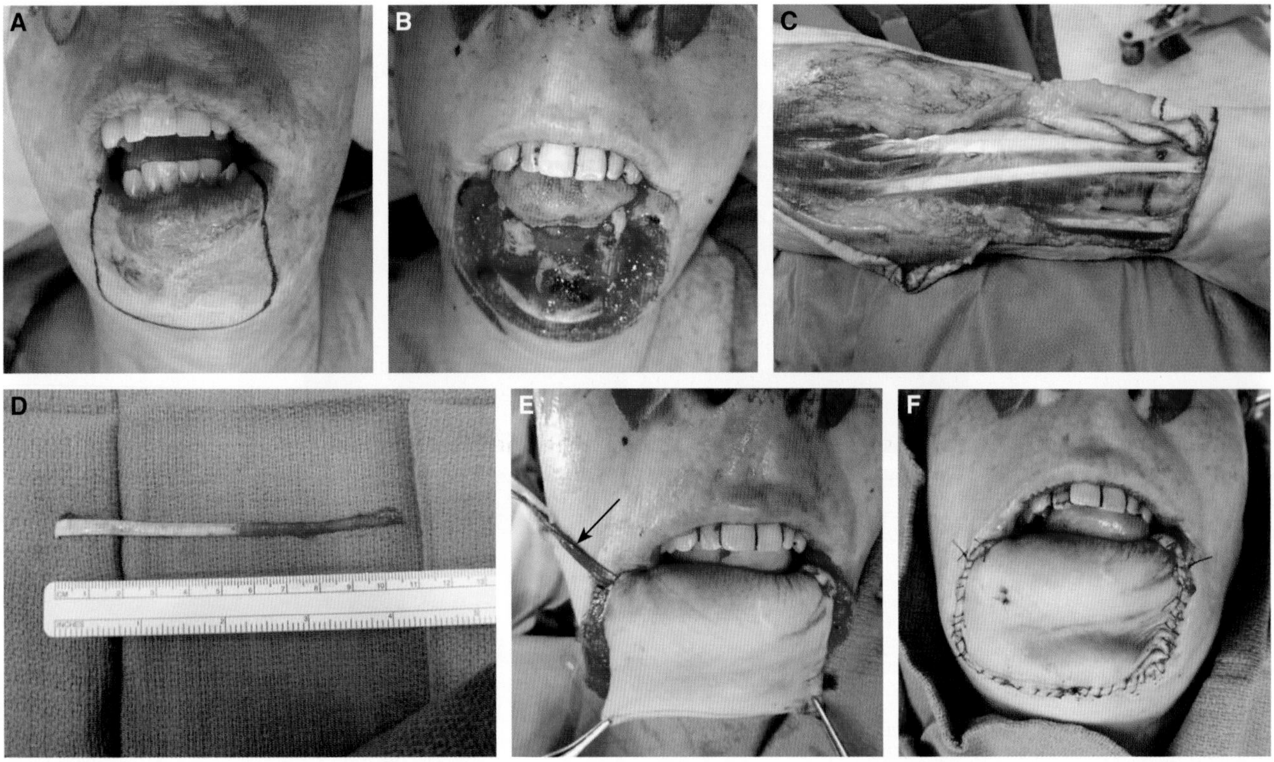

Fig. 37-15   **A,** A planned surgical resection for a patient who presented with squamous cell carcinoma involving nearly all of the mucosa of the lower lip with an extension into the gingivolabial sulcus and onto the alveolar ridge. **B,** An ablative defect after a total lower lip resection and marginal mandibulectomy. **C,** The palmaris longus tendon during harvest of the radial forearm free flap. **D,** The palmaris tendon after harvest. **E,** Insetting of the intraoral component of the radial forearm free flap. The flap is folded over and suspended over the palmaris longus tendon *(arrow).* **F,** Completion of inset and suspension of the flap.

In 1989 Sakai et al[83] described the use of the RFFF in the reconstruction of large lip defects. Since that time several reports have described the successful application of the RFFF for the restoration of total lip defects.[81,83-86] As with the cheek, the thin and pliable tissue of the RFFF readily contours to the defect and in cases of full-thickness defects can even be folded over onto itself to simultaneously provide external coverage and mucosal lining. An alternative to the RFFF is the ALT, which is used for defects that require thicker, bulkier tissue.[82] Composite defects that include portions of the mandible can be addressed with osteocutaneous free tissue flaps.

In general, the RFFF provides well-vascularized, pliable tissue that can easily be molded to accommodate three-layer lip defects. Another important consideration is the restoration of oral competence. The palmaris longus tendon provides a reliable static sling and can easily be harvested in conjunction with an RFFF (Fig. 37-15).

Harvest of a composite radial forearm-palmaris longus tendon free flap was first described by Sakai et al[83] in 1989, and several other series report the merits of this flap technique.[81,87,88] During harvest the palmaris longus tendon is transected 2 to 5 cm from the edges of the flap. The skin of the flap is then draped over the tendon and inset to properly recreate the sulcus and lip.[88] The ends of the tendon are then passed intramuscularly at the angles of the mouth and anchored to the remaining orbicularis oris and facial muscles with nonabsorbable suture.[81,88] The tendon is stretched tight enough to achieve proper support of the lower lip and restore oral competence. The palmaris longus tendon is absent in 7% to 10% of the population. In these cases, the flexor carpi radialis tendon may be harvested with the RFFF. Fascia lata may also be used, although its harvest requires an additional procedure in the thigh. The surgeon can accomplish static support of the lower lip by fixing the palmaris tendon or fascial sling to the zygoma if inadequate facial musculature is present to secure the tendon.

Neck

Soft tissue defects of the neck have many causes, including oncologic ablation, radiotherapy, and trauma, specifically burn injuries. If local or rotational flaps cannot provide adequate coverage, free tissue transfer may be required, and the flap selected must be tailored to the size and location of the defect. Because most tissue defects in this region are best reconstructed with thinner tissue, the RFFF is an ideal choice. This flap provides reliable coverage of critical neurovascular and aerodigestive structures while contouring to the neck. Another application for the RFFF is in the release of neck scar contractures in burn victims. Similar to the scalp, the free flap tissue in these cases can be used in conjunction with native tissue expansion. The ALT can be used for very large defects. Although the initial bulk may be significant, delayed debulking procedures can yield quite favorable results.

POSTOPERATIVE CARE

In addition to the general health of the patient, the most critical aspects of postoperative care focus on the viability of the free flap. Although the exact protocol for postoperative flap monitoring varies among institutions, a consistent and rational monitoring program should be strictly adhered to in the immediate postoperative setting. Monitoring may be conducted with clinical observation, conventional or implantable Doppler ultrasonography, pinprick testing, or a combination of these.[3,4] The goal of monitoring is to expeditiously identify features that are suggestive of arterial or venous compromise, so that intervention, such as reexploration and microvascular revision, can be undertaken in a timely fashion.

Monitoring examination is typically performed on an hourly basis for the first 48 to 72 hours and extended to 4- to 8-hour intervals thereafter. Kroll et al[89] studied the timing of pedicle thrombosis in their series of 990 consecutive free flaps. They observed that 80% of thrombi occurred within the first 48 hours postoperatively, and 90% of arterial thromboses occurred within the first 24 hours. They concluded that 3 to 4 days was optimal for the postoperative monitoring period after microvascular free tissue transfer.[4,89] Another large series identified that 76% of the head and neck free flaps requiring reexploration demonstrated vascular compromise within 5 days postoperatively.[4]

Similar to monitoring protocols, postoperative pharmacologic therapy is empiric and institutionally based. There have been no consistent data demonstrating a significant improvement in outcomes with the use of therapeutic anticoagulation using low-molecular-weight heparin or low-dose unfractionated heparin. The use of intravenous dextran infused in the immediate postoperative period has not proven to increase microvascular patency rates and may actually increase the risk for anaphylactoid reactions, adult respiratory distress syndrome, postoperative hemorrhage, and renal failure.[90] Although clopidogrel (Plavix) decreased the rate of thrombosis in a rat tuck model, no definitive regimen has been developed for postoperative microvascular free flap patients.[91] Studies have shown that low-dose aspirin inhibits anastomotic venous thrombosis and improves microcirculatory perfusion.[92,93] Therefore most patients are given a daily aspirin (81 or 325 mg) for 5 to 14 days postoperatively.

Despite the paucity of conclusive data, a surgeon may give special consideration to the use of adjuvant thrombopreventive agents (such as heparin, low-molecular-weight heparin, and platelet inhibitors) if the microvascular anastomosis is believed to be at increased risk for thrombosis at the time of surgery. Such situations would include recent "take-back" cases requiring microvascular revision, poor vessel condition (both donor and recipient) with intimal fragility, and numerous attempts to achieve flow during the initial anastomosis.

COMPLICATIONS

Over the past several decades, microvascular free tissue transfer has become an extremely reliable and widely used technique for head and neck reconstruction. Technological advancements in magnification, suture material, and surgical instruments and increasing surgical experience have produced success rates ranging from 96% to 99%.* Nevertheless there is a small risk of flap compromise, and reexploration rates ranged from 2% to 14% in several large series.[1,2,4,5,94] Most complications in free tissue transfer are related to circulatory compromise of the vascular pedicle, which may occur for a variety of reasons.

Thrombus formation within the pedicle is a common cause of arterial or venous occlusion, but it is more frequent within the venous system because of its low pressure, low flow characteristics.[92] Venous thrombi typically form within the first 48 to 72 hours postoperatively and tend to evolve over several hours. A flap that has venous congestion will become tense and appear dusky or bluish. Capillary refill will be brisk with a rapid return of dark blood on pinprick testing. Arterial occlusion presents more rapidly and produces a cool, mottled, cyanotic flap with poor capillary refill and scant blood return on pinprick testing. Both situations require urgent reexploration in the operating room. Furthermore the likelihood of successful flap salvage increases if the vascular compromise is corrected within 4 to 6 hours.[4] However even with timely identification and rapid correction, overall flap salvage rates after thrombotic occlusion typically range from 40% to 87%.[1,4,5,94] Survival rates after venous occlusion and thrombectomy tend to be more favorable (60% to 71%) in contrast to arterial thrombosis and thrombectomy (15% to 40%).[4,91,95] Even when the threatened flap is salvaged, as many as 50% manifest partial flap loss, which requires wound care and debridement.

External influences may also produce vascular compromise. Unfavorable geometry of the pedicle may result in kinking of the vessels or produce excessive tension on the anastomoses. Postoperative hematomas can cause compression of the vascular pedicle, resulting in venous congestion. This situation should be corrected with open exploration and evacuation. Meticulous hemostasis should be employed to prevent hematomas; drain placement within the wound bed can alert the surgeon to ongoing bleeding and potentially prevent large collections of blood and clot.

Other flap complications include wound dehiscence, fistula formation, and infection. The frequency of these reconstructive complications ranges from 13% to 29%.[1,2,5]

CONCLUSION

Microvascular free tissue transfer is a reliable and versatile tool for the reconstructive surgeon. The variability and complexity of defects in the head and neck require tailoring the selection of a specific flap to the characteristics of the wound. Defects should be evaluated based on the facial subunits and anatomic structures involved. Reconstructive goals should focus on providing adequate tissue coverage while restoring function and optimizing aesthetic results. The five flaps are most commonly used for the reconstruction of facial skin and soft tissues are the radial forearm flap, the temporoparietal fascia flap, the anterolateral thigh flap, the rectus abdominis flap, and the latissimus dorsi flap. These have been employed with high success rates, and reconstructive techniques continue to be refined.

---

*References 1, 2, 4, 5, 9, 25, 94.

Key Points

- Free flaps are reliable and versatile options for the reconstruction of facial skin and soft tissue. The most commonly used flaps are the radial forearm flap, the anterolateral thigh flap, the rectus abdominis flap, the latissimus dorsi flap, and the temporoparietal fascia flap.
- The specific free flap used depends on the aesthetic and functional characteristics of the defect, including the surface area of skin loss, the volume of soft tissue loss, the status of underlying remnant bony framework, and the functional requirements of each subunit involved.
- Defects of the scalp, forehead, and orbit are frequently addressed with a myogenous or myocutaneous latissimus dorsi flap. Rectus abdominis flaps are also used, but their role is more historic in nature.
- Currently, the anterolateral thigh flap and radial forearm free flap offer excellent options for reconstruction of lateral temporal bone and skull base defects and orbitomaxillary and cheek defects.
- Lip and chin defects are amenable to reconstruction with a radial forearm free flap. The palmaris longus tendon or fascia lata may be incorporated in total lip reconstruction to improve oral competence and aesthetic results.
- Postoperative monitoring is essential to the early identification of flap compromise and the prevention of flap loss. The most critical period is within the first 48 to 72 hours.
- With appropriate patient selection, meticulous surgical technique, and aggressive postoperative monitoring, success rates for free flap reconstruction of facial defects range from 96% to 99%.

REFERENCES

1. Suh JD, Secarz JA, Abemayor E, et al. Analysis of outcomes and complications in 400 cases of microvascular head and neck reconstruction. Arch Otolaryngol Head Neck Surg 130:962-966, 2004.
2. Haughey BH, Wilson E, Kluwe L, et al. Free flap reconstruction of the head and neck: analysis of 241 cases. Otolaryngol Head Neck Surg 125:10-17, 2001.
3. Spiegel JH, Polat JK. Microvascular flap reconstruction by otolaryngologists: prevalence, postoperative care, and monitoring techniques. Laryngoscope 117:485-490, 2007.
4. Bui DT, Cordeiro PG, Hu QY, et al. Free flap reexploration: indications, treatment, and outcomes in 1193 free flaps. Plast Reconstr Surg 119:2092-2100, 2007.
    This is an excellent discussion of the management and outcome of microvascular complications based on the authors' experience with a robust patient cohort.
5. Rosenthal E, Carroll W, Dobbs M, et al. Simplifying head and neck microvascular reconstruction. Head Neck 26:930-936, 2004.
6. Jacobson JH II, Suarez EL. Microsurgery in anastomosis of small vessels. Surg Forum 11:243-245, 1960.
7. Jacobson JH II, Suarez EL. Microvascular surgery. Dis Chest 41:220-224, 1962.
8. Buncke HJ Jr, Schulz WP. Total ear reimplantation in the rabbit utilising microminiature vascular anastomoses. Br J Plast Surg 19:15-22, 1966.
9. Hoffman GR, Islam S, Eisenberg RL. Microvascular reconstruction of the mouth, jaws, and face: experience of an Australian oral and maxillofacial surgery unit. J Oral Maxillofac Surg 70:e371-e377, 2012.
10. McGregor IA, Jackson IT. The groin flap. Br J Plast Surg 25:3-16, 1972.
11. Taylor GI, Watson N. One-stage repair of compound leg defects with free, revascularized flaps of groin skin and iliac bone. Plast Reconstr Surg 61:494-506, 1978.
12. Taylor GI, Townsend P, Corlett R. Superiority of the deep circumflex iliac vessels as the supply for free groin flaps: clinical work. Plast Reconstr Surg 64:745-759, 1979.
13. Yang G, Chen B, Gao Y, et al. Forearm free skin flap transplantation. Natl Med J China 61:139-141, 1981.
14. Soutar DS, McGregor IA. The radial forearm flap in intraoral reconstruction: the experience of 60 consecutive cases. Plast Reconstr Surg 78:1-8, 1986.
15. Soutar DS, Scheker LR, Tanner NS, et al. The radial forearm flap: a versatile method for intraoral reconstruction. Br J Plast Surg 36:1-8, 1983.

16. Hidalgo DA, Disa JJ, Cordeiro PG, et al. A review of 716 consecutive free flaps for oncologic surgical defects: refinement on donor-site selection and technique. Plast Reconstr Surg 102:722-732, 1998.

17. Urken ML, Turk JB, Weinberg H, et al. The rectus abdominis free flap in head and neck reconstruction. Arch Otolaryngol Head Neck Surg 117:857-866, 1991.

18. Deschler DG, Hayden RE. Lateral thigh free flap. Facial Plast Surg 12:75-79, 1996.

19. Wei FC, Jain V, Celik N, et al. Have we found an ideal soft-tissue flap? An experience with 672 anterolateral thigh flaps. Plast Reconstr Surg 109:2219-2227, 2002.

20. Gedebou TM, Wei FC, Lin CH. Clinical experience of 1284 free anterolateral thigh flaps. Handchir Mikrochir Plast Chir 34:239-244, 2002.

21. Zimbler MS. Aesthetic facial analysis. In Flint PW, Haughey BH, Lund VJ, et al, eds. Cummings Otolaryngology—Head & Neck Surgery, ed 5. Philadelphia: Elsevier, 2010.

22. Cheney ML, Varvares MA, Nadol JB. The temporoparietal fascia flap in head and neck reconstruction. Arch Otolaryngol Head Neck Surg 119:618-623, 1993.

23. Lai A, Cheney ML. Temporoparietal fascia flap in orbital reconstruction. Arch Facial Plast Surg 2:196-201, 2000.

24. Farwell DG, Reilly DF, Weymuller EA, et al. Predictors of perioperative complications in head and neck patients. Arch Otolaryngol Head Neck Surg 128:505-511, 2002.

    This is an excellent and insightful prospective analysis of medical and surgical factors affecting postoperative complications in patients undergoing microvascular procedures.

25. Serletti JM, Higgins JP, Moran S, et al. Factors affecting outcome in free-tissue transfer in the elderly. Plast Reconstr Surg 106:66-70, 2000.

26. Clark JR, McCluskey SA, Hall F, et al. Predictors of morbidity following free flap reconstruction for cancer of the head and neck. Head Neck 29:1090-1101, 2007.

27. Shestak KC, Jones NF, Wu W, et al. Effect of advanced age and medical disease on the outcome of microvascular reconstruction for head and neck defects. Head Neck 14:14-18, 1992.

28. Singh B, Cordeiro PG, Santamarie E, et al. Factors associated with complications in microvascular reconstruction of head and neck defects. Plast Reconstr Surg 103:403-411, 1999.

29. Kakarala K, Emerick KS, Lin DT, et al. Free flap reconstruction in 1999 and 2009: changing case characteristics and outcomes. Laryngoscope 122:2160-2163, 2012.

30. Taylor GI, Palmer JH. The vascular territories (angiosomes) of the body: experimental study and clinical applications. Br Plast Surg 40:113-141, 1987.

31. Cormack GC, Lamberty BGH. A classification of fascio-cutaneous flaps according to their patterns of vascularisation. Br J Plast Surg 37:80-87, 1984.

32. Hallock GG. Classification of flaps. In Wei FC, Mardini S, eds. Flaps and Reconstructive Surgery. Philadelphia: Saunders Elsevier, 2009.

33. Mathes SJ, Nahai F. Flap selection: analysis of features, modifications, and application. In Mathes SJ, Nahai F, eds. Reconstructive Surgery: Principles, Anatomy, & Technique. St Louis: Quality Medical Publishing, 1998.

34. Nakajima H, Fujino T, Adachi S. A new concept of vascular supply to the skin and classification of skin flaps according to their vascularization. Ann Plast Surg 16:1-17, 1986.

35. Tolhurst, DE. A comprehensive classification of flaps: the atomic system. Plast Reconstr Surg 80:608-609, 1987.

36. Geddes CR, Morris SF, Neligan PC. Perforator flaps: evolution, classification, and applications. Ann Plast Surg 50:90-99, 2003.

37. Koshima I, Soeda S. Inferior epigastric artery skin flaps without rectus abdominis muscle. Br J Plast Surg 42:645-648, 1989.

38. Urken ML, Harris JR. Radial forearm. In Urken ML, Cheney ML, et al, eds. Regional and Free Flaps for Head and Neck Reconstruction. Philadelphia: Lippincott Williams & Wilkins, 2012.

39. Lutz BS, Wei FC, Chang SC, et al. Donor site morbidity after suprafascial elevation of the radial forearm flap: a prospective study in 95 consecutive cases. Plast Reconstr Surg 103:132-137, 1999.

40. Emerick KS, Deschler DG. Incidence of donor site skin graft loss requiring surgical intervention with the radial forearm free flap. Head Neck 29:573-576, 2007.

41. Coleman SS, Anson BJ. Arterial patterns in the hand based upon a study of 650 specimens. Surg Gynecol Obstet 113:409-424, 1961.

42. Jaquet Y, Higgins KM, Enepekidis DJ. The temporoparietal fascia flap: a versatile tool in head and neck reconstruction. Curr Opin Otolaryngol Head Neck Surg 19:235-241, 2011.

43. McCarthy JG, Zido BM. The spectrum of calvarial bone grafting: introduction of the vascularized calvarial bone graft. Plast Reconstr Surg 74:10-18, 1984.

44. Makitie AA, Beasley NJ, Neligan PC, et al. Head and neck reconstruction with anterolateral thigh flap. Otolaryngol Head Neck Surg 129:547-555, 2003.

45. Yu P. Characteristics of the anterolateral thigh flap in a western population and its application in head and neck reconstruction. Head Neck 26:759-769, 2004.

46. Lin DT, Coppit GL, Burkey BB. Use of the anterolateral thigh flap for reconstruction of the head and neck. Curr Opin Otolaryngol Head Neck Surg 12:300-304, 2004.

47. Ali RS, Bluebond-Langner R, Rodriguez ED, et al. The versatility of the anterolateral thigh flap. Plast Reconstr Surg 124:395e-407e, 2009.

48. Hanasono MM, Sacks JM, Goel N, et al. The anterolateral thigh free flap for skull base reconstruction. Otolaryngol Head Neck Surg 140:155-160, 2009.

49. Malata CM, Tehrani H, Kumiponjera D, et al. Use of anterolateral thigh and lateral arm fasciocutaneous free flaps in lateral skull base reconstruction. Ann Plast Surg 57:169-175, 2006.

50. Lueg EA. The anterolateral thigh flap: radial forearm's "big brother" for extensive soft tissue head and neck defects. Arch Otolaryngol Head Neck Surg 130:813-818, 2004.

51. Disa JJ, Rodriguez VM, Cordeiro PG. Reconstruction of lateral skull base oncological defects: the role of free tissue transfer. Ann Plast Surg 41:633-639, 1998.

52. Neligan PC, Mulholland S, Irish J, et al. Flap selection in cranial base reconstruction. Plast Reconstr Surg 98:1159-1168, 1996.

53. Califano J, Cordeiro PG, Disa JJ, et al. Anterior cranial base reconstruction using free tissue transfer: changing trends. Head Neck 25:89-96, 2003.

54. Chang DW, Langstein HN, Gupta A, et al. Reconstructive management of cranial base defects after tumor ablation. Plast Reconstr Surg 107:1346-1355, 2001.

55. Izquierdo R, Leonetti JP, Origitano TC, et al. Refinements in using free-tissue transfer from complex cranial base reconstruction. Plast Reconstr Surg 92:567-574, 1993.

56. Meland N, Fisher J, Irons G, et al. Experience with 80 rectus abdominis free-tissue transfers. Plast Reconstr Surg 83:481-487, 1989.

57. Pennington DG, Pelly AD. The rectus abdominis myocutaneous free flap. Br J Plast Surg 33:277-282, 1980.

58. Urken ML, Catalano PJ, Sen C, et al. Free tissue transfer for skull base reconstruction: analysis of complications and a classification scheme for defining skull base defects. Arch Otolaryngol Head Neck Surg 119:1318-1325, 1993.

59. Urken ML, Blackwell KE. Rectus abdominis. In Urken ML, Cheney ML, et al, eds. Regional and Free Flaps for Head and Neck Reconstruction. Philadelphia: Lippincott Williams & Wilkins, 2012.

60. Watson JS, Craig RD, Orton CI. The free latissimus dorsi myocutaneous flap. Plast Reconstr Surg 64:299-305, 1979.

61. Schmalbach CE, Webb DE, Weitzel EK. Anterior skull base reconstruction: a review of current techniques. Curr Opin Otolaryngol Head Neck Surg 18:238-243, 2010.

62. Chao AH, Yu P, Skoracki RJ, et al. Microsurgical reconstruction of composite scalp and calvarial defects in patients with cancer: a 10-year experience. Head Neck 34:1759-1764, 2012.

63. Van Driel AA, Mureau MAM, Goldstein DP, et al. Aesthetic and oncologic outcome after microsurgical reconstruction of complex scalp and forehead defects after malignant tumor resection: an algorithm for treatment. Plast Reconstr Surg 126:460-470, 2010.

64. Shonka DC, Potash AH, Jameson MJ, et al. Successful reconstruction of scalp and skull defects: lessons learned from a large series. Laryngoscope 121:2305-2312, 2011.

65. O'Connell DA, Teng MS, Mendez E, et al. Microvascular free tissue transfer in the reconstruction of scalp and lateral temporal bone defects. J Craniofac Surg 22:801-804, 2011.

66. Newman MI, Hanasono MM, Disa JJ, et al. Scalp reconstruction: a 15-year experience. Ann Plast Surg 52:501-506, 2004.

67. Sweeny L, Eby B, Magnuson JS, et al. Reconstruction of scalp defects with the radial forearm free flap. Head Neck Oncol 4:21, 2012.

68. Resto VA, McKenna MJ, Deschler DG. Pectoralis major flap in composite lateral skull base defect reconstruction. Arch Otolaryngol Head Neck Surg 133:490-494, 2007.

69. Pusic AL, Chen CM, Patel S, et al. Microvascular reconstruction of the skull base: a clinical approach to surgical defect classification and flap selection. Skull Base 17:5-15, 1997.

70. Newman J, O'Malley BW, Chalian A, et al. Microvascular reconstruction of cranial base defects: an evaluation of complication and survival rates to justify the use of this repair. Arch Otolaryngol Head Neck Surg 132:381-384, 2006.

71. Chiu ES, Kraus D, Bui DT, et al. Anterior and middle cranial fossa skull base reconstruction using microvascular free tissue techniques: surgical complications and functional outcomes. Ann Plast Surg 60:514-520, 2008.

72. Nouraei SA, Ismail Y, Gerber CJ, et al. Long-term outcome of skull base surgery with microvascular reconstruction for malignant disease. Plast Reconstr Surg 118:1151-1158, 2006.

73. Jowett N, Mlynarek AM. Reconstruction of cheek defects: a review of current techniques. Curr Opin Otolaryngol Head Neck Surg 18:244-254, 2010.

74. Suarez C, Ferlito A, Lund VJ, et al. Management of the orbit in malignant sinonasal tumors. Head Neck 30:242-250, 2008.

75. Kuo YR, Jeng SF, Wei FC, et al. Functional reconstruction of complex lip and cheek defect with free composite anterolateral thigh flap and vascularized fascia. Head Neck 30:1001-1006, 2008.

76. Lee JC, St-Hilaire H, Christy MR, et al. Anterolateral thigh flap for trauma reconstruction. Ann Plast Surg 64:164-168, 2010.

77. Lee JT, Hsiao HT, Tung KY, et al. Successful one-stage resurfacing and contouring of an extensively burned cheek by using a scar template free anterolateral thigh flap: a case report and literature review. J Trauma 65:E1-E3, 2008.

78. Rodriguez-Vegas JM, Angel PA, Manuela PR. Refining the anterolateral thigh free flap in complex orbitomaxillary reconstructions. Plast Reconstr Surg 121:481-486, 2008.

79. Chou EK, Ulusal BG, Ulusal A, et al. Using the descending branch of the lateral femoral circumflex vessel as a source of two independent flaps. Plast Reconstr Surg 117:2059-2063, 2006.

80. Funk GF, Laurenzo JF, Valentino J, et al. Free-tissue transfer reconstruction of midfacial and cranio-orbito-facial defects. Arch Otolaryngol Head Neck Surg 121:293-303, 1995.

81. Carroll CM, Pathak I, Irish J, et al. Reconstruction of total lower lip and chin defects using the composite radial forearm-palmaris longus tendon free flap. Arch Facial Plast Surg 2:53-56, 2000.

82. Godefroy WP, Klop WM, Smeele LE, et al. Free-flap reconstruction of large full-thickness lip and chin defects. Ann Oto Rhino Laryngol 121:594-603, 2012.
    This is a modern and thorough review of free flap reconstruction for large lip and chin defects. A classification scheme for these defects is provided, as are numerous case examples.

83. Sakai S, Soeda S, Endo T, et al. A compound radial artery forearm flap for the reconstruction of lip and chin defect. Br J Plast Surg 42:337-338, 1989.

84. Wei FC, Tan BK, Chen IH, et al. Mimicking lip features in free-flap reconstruction of lip defects. Br J Plast Surg 54:8-11, 2001.

85. Lee JW, Jang YC, Oh SJ. Esthetic and functional reconstruction for burn deformities of the lower lip and chin with free radial forearm flap. Ann Plast Surg 56:384-386, 2006.

86. Ozdemir R, Ortak T, Koçer U, et al. Total lower lip reconstruction using sensate composite radial forearm flap. J Craniofac Surg 14:393-405, 2003.

87. Sadove RC, Luce EA, McGrath PC. Reconstruction of the lower lip and chin with the composite radial forearm-palmaris longus free flap. Plast Reconstr Surg 88:209-214, 1991.

88. Jeng SF, Kuo YR, Wei FC, et al. Total lower lip reconstruction with a composite radial forearm-palmaris longus tendon flap: a clinical series. Plast Reconstr Surg 113:19-23, 2004.

89. Kroll SS, Schusterman MA, Reece G, et al. Timing of pedicle thrombosis and flap loss after free-tissue transfer. Plast Reconstr Surg 98:1230-1233, 1996.

90. Sun TB, Chien SH, Lee JT, et al. Is dextran infusion as an antithrombotic agent necessary in microvascular reconstruction of the upper aerodigestive tract? J Reconstr Microsurg 19:463-466, 2003.

91. Moore MG, Deschler DG. Clopidogrel (Plavix) reduces the rate of thrombosis in the rat tuck model for microvenous anastomosis. Otolaryngol Head Neck Surg 136:573-576, 2007.

92. Budd ME, Evans GR. Postoperative care. In Wei FC, Mardini S, eds. Flaps and Reconstructive Surgery. Philadephia: Saunders Elsevier, 2009.

93. Peter FW, Franken RJ, Wang WZ. Effect of low dose aspirin on thrombus formation at arterial and venous microanastomoses and on the tissue microcirculation. Plast Reconstr Surg 99:1112-1121, 1997.

94. Disa JJ, Pusic AL, Hidalgo DH, et al. Simplifying microvascular head and neck reconstruction: a rational approach for donor site selection. Ann Plast Surg 47:385-389, 2001.

95. Nakatuska T, Harii K, Asato H, et al. Analytic review of 2372 free flap transfers for head and neck reconstruction following cancer resection. J Reconstr Microsurg 19:363-368, 2003.

38

Benign and Malignant Cutaneous Neoplasms

Jessica L. Fewkes

While Frederic Mohs was a medical student in 1932, he tried to induce a leukocytic reaction in normal and cancerous skin using zinc chloride paste. He noticed that when excised, the tumors were already fixed and could be examined under the microscope without further preparation. As serendipity, astute observation, and original thinking have led to many discoveries, Dr. Mohs[1] reasoned that these properties could be used to examine tumor margins immediately after excision with application of this fixative paste. This would give quick feedback to the surgeon, thus allowing continued extirpation of clinically negative—but histologically positive—tissue and removal of the entire tumor. In the 1960s Drs. Stegman and Tromovitch[2] spent several weeks with Dr. Mohs to learn his technique. In 1974 they published their landmark article showing that the technique could be equally effective without the use of zinc chloride paste, using frozen sections, and thus began the evolution of the Mohs technique as it is used today worldwide (Fig. 38-1).

For anyone who examines the skin, knowledge of the spectrum of cutaneous neoplasms is essential. This chapter will address both benign and malignant lesions, with the exception of melanoma (see Chapter 39) and vascular lesions (see Chapter 47). A benign cutaneous neoplasm is defined as a dysregulated proliferation of cells and supportive stroma derived from components found in normal skin, without potential to metastasize or cause death. Because the skin is readily accessible for both inspection and tissue sampling, myriad benign cutaneous growths have been cataloged. Although most benign cutaneous neoplasms are of minor clinical significance, many tumors are indicators of important systemic syndromes or precursors to malignancies.

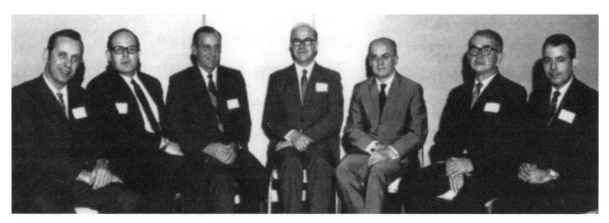

Fig. 38-1 Pioneers in dermatologic surgery. *Left to right:* Theodore Tromovitch, Perry Robins, R. Raymond Allington, Frederic Mohs, George Vavruska, William R. Buckley, Richard Moraites. (From Robins P. 44 years in dermatologic surgery: a retrospective. J Drugs Dermatol 8:519-525, 2009.)

BENIGN CUTANEOUS NEOPLASMS

Benign cutaneous neoplasms may be classified by the tissue elements from which they arise: keratinocytes, melanocytes, nerves, blood vessels, connective tissue, sebaceous glands, eccrine sweat glands, apocrine glands, hair follicles, smooth muscle, and fat. Another classification schema divides cutaneous neoplasms by the location within the skin of the proliferative component, be it epidermal, dermal, or subcutaneous, as outlined in Box 38-1, or by color (Box 38-2).

Classification alone will not distinguish benign from malignant cutaneous neoplasms. Histopathologic examination is required for making this distinction. Factors favoring a benign process include very slow, regular growth or stability over time, well-circumscribed borders, and preservation of cutaneous appendages. A history of rapid growth, disruption of appendages, poorly defined borders, ulceration, and tissue firmness suggest malignancy.

EPIDERMAL NEOPLASMS

Biopsy may definitively establish the diagnosis of a cutaneous lesion. In general, tangential or shave biopsy is appropriate for epidermal lesions or papular lesions that rise above the skin surface. A deep tangential or saucerization biopsy may be necessary for an actinic keratosis or cutaneous horn because possible malignant transformation in a deeper part of the growth could be missed by a cut made too superficially. In cases where examination of the overall architecture or the base of the lesion is essential, or in which the lesion is too deep for tangential biopsy, a punch or incisional biopsy is preferred. Examples of lesions in which punch biopsy is preferable include macular (flat) lesions, nevi, squamous cell carcinoma (SCC), and most dermal neoplasms. If melanoma or keratoacanthoma is a consideration, the optimal approach is an excisional biopsy, because the entire lesion is required for adequate diagnosis.

Box 38-1   Classification of Benign Cutaneous Neoplasms by Location in the Skin

Epidermal Neoplasms
Actinic keratosis
Cutaneous horn
Epidermal nevus
Keratoacanthoma
Seborrheic keratosis
Solar lentigo
Warts

Epidermal/Dermal Neoplasms
Blue nevus
Compound nevus
Congenital nevus
Dermal nevus
Dysplastic nevus
Junctional nevus

Dermal Neoplasms
Acrochordon
Adenoma sebaceum
Angiokeratoma
Capillary hemangioma
Cavernous hemangioma
Cherry hemangioma
Cylindroma
Dermatofibroma
Epidermoid cyst
Fibrous papule
Keloid
Lipoma

Milium
Neurofibroma
Nevus sebaceous
Pilar cyst
Port-wine stain
Pyogenic granuloma
Sebaceous adenoma
Sebaceous hyperplasia
Syringoma
Trichilemmoma
Trichoepithelioma
Venous lake

Most benign cutaneous neoplasms need no treatment; they require only reassurance of the patient. However, some lesions cause discomfort because of their location, size, and/or growth. In those situations a variety of treatment modalities are available such as topical chemotherapy, cryosurgery, electrodessication with or without curettage, and laser (Box 38-3).

Seborrheic Keratosis

Rarely seen in patients younger than age 30, seborrheic keratoses are extremely common benign, epidermal, keratinocytic neoplasms that may be transmitted in an autosomally dominant pattern. More than 80% of adults have at least one seborrheic keratosis, whereas some patients develop hundreds. Although they are rarely symptomatic, pruritus, bleeding or discomfort may develop. The sudden appearance of numerous, pruritic seborrheic keratoses, called the *sign of Leser-Trelat*, may be an indicator of underlying malignancy.

Box 38-2   Differentiation of Benign Cutaneous Neoplasms by Color

Skin-Colored Neoplasms
Acrochordon
Angiolipoma
Epidermal inclusion cyst
Keloids
Lipoma
Milium
Neurofibroma
Pilar cyst
Syringoma
Trichilemmoma
Trichoepithelioma

Red Neoplasms
Angiokeratoma
Capillary hemangioma
Cavernous hemangioma
Cherry hemangioma
Pyogenic granuloma

White/Scaly Neoplasms
Actinic keratosis
Cutaneous horn
Keratoacanthoma

Brown-Black Neoplasms
Compound nevus
Congenital nevus
Dermal nevus
Dermatofibroma
Dysplastic nevus
Epidermal nevus
Junctional nevus
Seborrheic keratosis
Solar lentigo

Blue Neoplasms
Blue nevus
Hemangiomas
Venous lake

Yellow Neoplasms
Nevus sebaceous
Sebaceous adenoma
Sebaceous hyperplasia

Box 38-3   Treatment of Cutaneous Lesions

- Topical
  - Imiquimod (Aldara, Zyclara)
  - 5-Fluorouracil (Efudex, Carac)
- Cryosurgery
- Electrodessication and curettage
- Excision
- Mohs surgery
- Photodynamic therapy
- Laser
- Injection (intralesional chemotherapy)

Seborrheic keratoses present with a wide range of clinical appearances, with colors ranging from brown, black, red, yellow, tan, and gray, to skin colored. Typical lesions are slightly to significantly elevated papules, plaques, or nodules that appear stuck on with a distinctive warty or papillomatous surface (Fig. 38-2). Smooth variants are common. A waxy or greasy character is apparent with small round horn cysts visible with magnification. Round or oval lesions with a predilection for the face, trunk, and upper extremities ranging from 0.2 to 3 cm may be isolated or multiple. One variant of seborrheic keratoses, commonly seen on the temples and cheeks, appears as 1 to 3 mm, pedunculated, brown papules that mimic acrochorda.

The differential diagnosis of seborrheic keratoses includes verruca, nevus, lentigo, actinic keratosis, SCC, pigmented basal cell carcinoma (BCC), and malignant melanoma. Although treatment is usually unnecessary unless symptomatic, cryosurgery or light curettage and electrodesiccation are effective means of removal.

Actinic Keratosis

Seen primarily on sun-exposed skin in patients with Fitzpatrick skin phototypes I through III, actinic or solar keratoses are common in middle-aged and elderly patients who have a history of prolonged and repeated sun exposure. These discrete, adherent papules are 1 to 10 mm, scaly, rough, pink, red, yellow, or white, and often grow with summer solar exposure, recede during winter, and recur for months or years (Fig. 38-3). They may also be pigmented. Often, actinic keratoses are appreciated more effectively by palpation than by visual inspection. Although usually asymptomatic, lesions may become inflamed and tender, and may bleed, especially in men who shave over this compromised tissue. The most common sites of involvement correlate with sun exposure, including the nose, forehead, cheeks, ears, lower lip, upper chest, forearms, and dorsal hands.

Actinic keratoses are atypical keratinocytic neoplasms that are considered precursor lesions for the development of SCC. The annual risk of an actinic keratosis transforming into an SCC is uncertain, but estimates vary from 0.025% to 20%.[3] Ultraviolet radiation B (UVB) in the 290 to 320 nm range is considered the primary pathogenic factor. There may be a delay of 10 to 40 years between the sun exposure and the appearance of actinic keratoses on the skin. Epidemiologic risk factors for actinic keratoses include older age, blue eyes, childhood freckling, southern latitude, extensive solar exposure through occupation or recreation, immunosuppression, and the use of tanning booths. The differential diagnosis of an actinic keratosis includes seborrheic keratosis, verruca, discoid lupus erythematosus, eczema, BCC, and SCC.

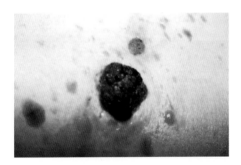

Fig. 38-2   Typically waxy, stuck-on, papillomatous appearance of a seborrheic keratosis, surrounded by smaller, less developed variants of the same lesion.

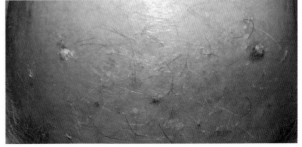

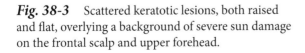

Fig. 38-3   Scattered keratotic lesions, both raised and flat, overlying a background of severe sun damage on the frontal scalp and upper forehead.

Actinic damage can be prevented by using sunscreens and protective clothing and avoiding sun exposure. However, once present, isolated lesions may be treated with cryotherapy. Diffuse, widespread involvement may be managed with topical application of 5-fluorouracil, imiquimod, chemexfoliation, or photodynamic therapy.[4] If actinic keratoses persist despite adequate treatment, biopsy should be considered to rule out SCC. Extensive involvement of the lower lip, referred to as *actinic cheilitis,* may be treated with these same modalities and with laser and surgical excision.[5]

Solar Lentigo

Solar lentigo lesions consist of a proliferation of normal melanocytes in the basal epithelial layer of skin, occurring in sun-exposed areas, usually in fair-skinned individuals (Fig. 38-4). They differ from lentigo simplex, which share the same clinical appearance but are not limited to sun-exposed areas and may be present at birth. The presence of those lesions may suggest an underlying multiple lentigines syndrome, such as Peutz-Jeghers or LEOPARD (*l*entigines, *E*CG abnormalities, *o*cular hypertelorism/obstructive cardiomyopathy, *p*ulmonary valve stenosis, *a*bnormalities of genitalia in males, *r*etardation of growth, and *d*eafness) or neurofibromatosis. The differential diagnosis includes seborrheic keratosis, nevus, lentigo maligna, and pigmented actinic keratosis. Lesions may be treated with cryosurgery, topical hydroquinone, and lasers.[6]

Epidermal Nevus

The verrucous or linear epidermal nevus is a congenital or early onset hamartomatous proliferation of epidermal structures presenting as a sharply marginated collection of discrete or coalescent verrucoid or papillomatous skin-colored, brown, or gray papules and plaques, commonly in a linear arrangement (Fig. 38-5). They often follow relaxed skin tension lines and may be limited, segmental, or generalized. When prominent epidermal nevi are localized to the midforehead, the possibility of the epidermal nevus syndrome with underlying CNS or skeletal abnormalities should be entertained. There are rare reports of BCC and SCC manifesting as localized nodular or ulcerative changes within verrucous epidermal nevi. The differential diagnosis of verrucous epidermal nevi includes verruca (warts), seborrheic keratosis, nevus sebaceous, lichen striatus, the verrucous phase of incontinentia pigmenti, linear psoriasis or lichen planus, and linear porokeratosis.[7] For extensive lesions, removal is often impractical. However, if removal is desired, excision is the most definitive mode of therapy. Alternative modalities include laser, electrodesicca-

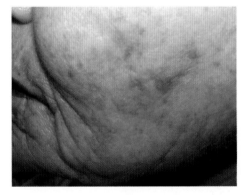

Fig. 38-4   Light brown macular pigmentation, widespread over the cheek occurring amid other signs of dermatoheliosis, such as telangiectasias and rhytids.

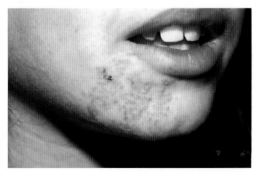

Fig. 38-5   Multifocal, tan-pink, irregular plaques with peripheral inflammation characteristic of an inflamed epidermal nevus.

tion, dermabrasion, cryosurgery, or chemical exfoliation. In general, these techniques achieve only partial responses. Recurrences after treatment are common. Any changing area within an epidermal nevus should be biopsied to rule out malignant transformation.

Keratoacanthoma

Keratoacanthomas are dome-shaped, erythematous papules or nodules with a central keratinous plug, when mature. These keratinocytic tumors are rapidly growing, benign, and are found in areas of sun exposure, most often in elderly patients (Fig. 38-6). The history is typically of rapid growth over 2 to 6 weeks, followed by gradual spontaneous regression over 2 to 12 months. There are also reports of giant, recurring keratoacanthomas. Clinically and histologically, differentiation from SCC is difficult. By definition, keratoacanthomas are benign and regress spontaneously. However, if a rapidly growing, epidermal tumor is found in a critical location—such as periorally—local destruction to vital structures can be avoided by early surgical removal.[8]

The differential diagnosis of keratoacanthomas includes SCC, hypertrophic actinic keratosis, molluscum contagiosum, and irritated seborrheic keratosis. Because clinical differentiation of keratoacanthoma from SCC is difficult, and because of the need for adequate cross-sectional biopsy for histologic diagnosis, it is appropriate to perform either narrow excisional biopsy or full-thickness wedge biopsy whenever possible. If histological findings reveal keratoacanthoma, then the variety of treatment options available are the same for other benign lesions. If histologic findings indicate SCC or if the findings are equivocal, then the treatment chosen is that for SCC. Some clinicians think that given the clinical and histologic similarities between this pseudocarcinoma and true SCC, conservative excision is the optimal approach at initial presentation. Mohs micrographic surgery may be appropriate for large, recurrent, or aggressive lesions. The final cosmetic result from excision is also often superior to the depressed scar left after spontaneous involution.[9]

Cutaneous Horn

Cutaneous horns are compact, white-yellow, filiform, hornlike projections that measure 1 to 15 mm and appear on sun-exposed skin of older patients (Fig. 38-7). The term *cutaneous horn* refers to clinical ap-

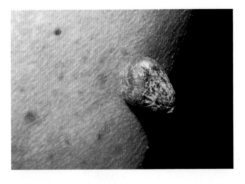

Fig. 38-6 Dome-shaped, keratin-filled nodule consistent with keratoacanthoma.

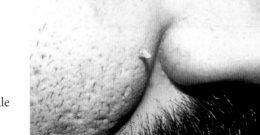

Fig. 38-7 Compact, hornlike, exophytic scale of a cutaneous horn, formed by a verruca.

pearance; the underlying histologic findings can reveal verruca, actinic keratosis, seborrheic keratosis, SCC or BCC, and rarely, Kaposi's sarcoma, sebaceous carcinoma, renal cell carcinoma, or granular cell tumor. Because of the latter possibilities, it is advisable to do a deep tangential biopsy, including the base, to determine the nature of the lesion. Therapy is guided by the underlying histologic findings.[10]

Epidermal/Dermal Neoplasms
Nevus

Nevi are benign, nested proliferations of nevomelanocytes and are categorized by the site within the skin from which the nests arise. Junctional nevi are composed of nests of nevomelanocytes in the lower epidermis, whereas the nevomelanocytes in the dermal nevi are located entirely within the dermis. Compound nevi comprise nests of nevomelanocytes within both the epidermis and dermis. Numerous nevi may be a marker for increased susceptibility to malignant melanoma. Patients with numerous or large nevi, a personal or family history of melanoma, history of significant sun exposure, skin phototype I or II with sun-induced freckling, immunosuppression, or atypical features to their nevi should generate a higher degree of suspicion for new or changing nevi (Fig. 38-8).

The differential diagnosis of nevi includes lentigo simplex, solar lentigo, dermatofibroma, pigmented BCC, molluscum contagiosum, juvenile xanthogranuloma, and malignant melanoma. Normal-appearing nevi require no treatment. Criteria for the removal of acquired nevomelanocytic nevi include a history of change; asymmetry; an irregularly irregular border; color variegation; atypical appearance or behavior; unusual sensation, including itching, pain, and bleeding; and location in a site that cannot be monitored, such as the scalp, and posterior ear and mucous membranes. A history of change in a nevus must be taken seriously, but it should also be considered that because people generally are not born with nevi, all nevi are in fact changing, but in a very slow, regular way. Another important aspect to consider when evaluating nevi is the uniformity of a patient's nevus pattern. If a patient has dozens of nevi with similar atypical features, then excision of multiple nevi may not be necessary and close clinical observation, perhaps with the aid of serial photographs, should be considered. Alternatively, if one particular nevus stands out as distinctly different from the others, then consideration should be given to removal. A noninvasive tool for evaluating nevi is the dermatoscope or *epiluminescence microscopy,* which has demonstrated its usefulness

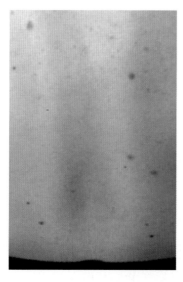

Fig. 38-8   Multiple nevi on the back of various shapes, sizes, and colors.

Box 38-4   Variable Configurations Seen With Epiluminescence Microscopy (Dermatoscope)

- Atypical pigment network
- Gray-blue areas
- Atypical vascular pattern
- Radial streaming (streaking)

- Blotches
- Irregular dots and globules
- Regression

Box 38-5   Criteria for Suspicion in Nevi

A	Asymmetry
B	Border
C	Color
D	Diameter/different
E	Elevation/evolving

---

in diagnosing benign nevi versus melanoma.[11] With or without the use of immersion oil and at 10 times magnification, it increases both the sensitivity and specificity of the clinical diagnosis of melanoma.[12] There are various ways to analyze what is seen using the easy handheld device, including pattern analysis (Box 38-4), ABCDE rules (Box 38-5), and the seven-point checklist.[13] A dermatologist can be helpful in assessing the degree of clinical atypia and in formulating a therapeutic strategy in patients with numerous nevomelanocytic nevi. In all patients, especially those with multiple or atypical nevi, education should be provided concerning the regular use of sunscreens with a sun protection factor of 30 or greater; the use of protective clothing, including long-sleeved shirts, pants, broad-brimmed hats, and sunglasses; and the limitation of outdoor activities during peak hours of the day (10 AM to 4 PM).

If removal of a nevomelanocytic nevus is indicated and there is any possibility of atypia or malignancy, excisional biopsy is appropriate. If a lesion is very large, then removal of the most clinically atypical area is recommended. Only if there is no suspicion of atypia is tangential biopsy acceptable as a cosmetic modality. Nevi occasionally recur with unusual pigmentation after tangential removal. Destructive therapies, such as electrodesiccation and curettage, dermabrasion, cryotherapy, or laser, are unacceptable modalities for the management of atypical nevomelanocytic nevi. Surgical specimens should routinely be submitted for histologic examination.

Junctional Nevus

Junctional nevi appear as smooth, well-defined, brown to tan macules, with more uniform and sharply marginated pigmentation (Fig. 38-9). Junctional nevi have only a slight papular component, if any, because they are primarily an epidermal lesion; instead, they show fine stippling of their surface.

Compound Nevus

Unlike junctional nevi, compound nevi are by definition elevated, have a smooth or papillomatous surface, are tan to brown in color, and have fairly regular borders (Fig. 38-10).

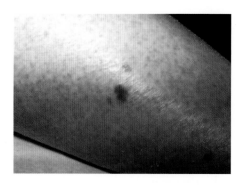

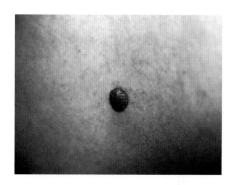

Fig. 38-9   Typical brown, well-circumscribed, macular junctional nevus.

Fig. 38-10   Compound nevus with fleshy, pink-brown, papular appearance.

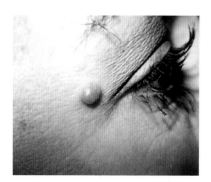

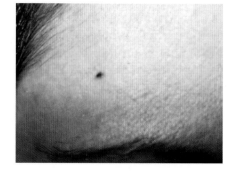

Fig. 38-11   Dome-shaped, flesh-colored papule with fine telangiectasia characteristic of dermal nevus.

Fig. 38-12   Characteristic blue-gray pigmentation of a blue nevus.

Dermal Nevus

Commonly arising in the second or third decade, dermal nevi often persist for life. They are characteristically raised, skin colored or opalescent, with telangiectasias (Fig. 38-11). Dermal nevi are commonly seen on the face and neck. Because of their pearly telangiectatic appearance, dermal nevi may be difficult to distinguish from BCC. One helpful differential point is that, in dermal nevi, normal skin lines are relatively preserved, as opposed to BCC, in which skin markings are effaced; this effacement is more readily identified by inspection using a magnifying lens. Furthermore, dermal nevi are often more dome shaped, whereas BCCs tend to be flat topped or centrally depressed. The evolution of the lesion, if it has bled or changed significantly, may help distinguish benign from malignant lesions, although biopsy is sometimes necessary for differentiation.

Blue Nevus

As a result of tissue-light interactions, the spindle-shaped, dermal nevomelanocytes of a blue nevus display a distinctive blue-gray color (Fig. 38-12). Blue nevi are acquired, benign, firm, papular lesions that usually arise in late adolescence. In addition to those entities discussed for nevi in general, the differential diagnosis of blue nevi includes traumatic lead or radiation tattoo, dermatofibroma, pigmented spindle cell nevus, and glomus tumor. In general, blue nevi have no greater propensity for malignant transformation than other nevomelanocytic processes, and the decision to excise should be based on atypical clinical appearance or a history of change.

Dysplastic Nevus

Junctional and compound nevi have the potential to become dysplastic nevi, which are simply nevomelanocytic nevi with clinical and histologic features of atypia. Dysplastic nevi may also arise de novo from normal skin. Dysplastic nevi may arise sporadically or, more often, be transmitted in an autosomal dominant pattern. They arise somewhat later than commonly acquired nevi, continue to develop even in elderly patients, and tend not to regress spontaneously.[14,15] Sunlight is considered an inducing agent for the development or transformation of some dysplastic nevi. The dermatoscope assists in diagnosis of nevi, so dermatologic referral is appropriate when this lesion is suspected.

The degree of clinical histologic atypia may be graded on a scale from mild to severe, with higher grades conferring increasing risk of transformation into malignant melanoma. Dysplastic nevi can be considered clinical markers of patients at increased risk for the development of melanoma. The differential diagnosis of dysplastic nevi includes normal nevus, lentigo and lentigo maligna, seborrheic keratosis, dermatofibroma, blue nevus, and malignant melanoma (Fig. 38-13).

Congenital Nevus

Present at birth or arising soon thereafter, congenital nevi are benign proliferations of nevomelanocytes that have an increased risk of transformation into malignant melanoma. Congenital nevi are present in less than 1% of newborns, usually are less than 3 cm, and may rarely involve large portions of the body. As the size of the nevus increases, there is an increased risk of development of malignant melanoma. Large congenital nevi may be associated with leptomeningeal melanocytosis, a condition referred to as neurocutaneous melanosis, which carries significant risk of mortality from obstructive hydrocephalus and melanoma. Many congenital nevi may be distinguished from acquired nevi by a history of early onset as well as by large size, increased terminal hair, and a rough, flat-topped, opaque morphologic structure (Fig. 38-

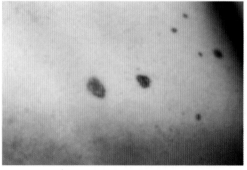

Fig. 38-14   Dark brown papillomatous, papular congenital nevus with increased terminal hair.

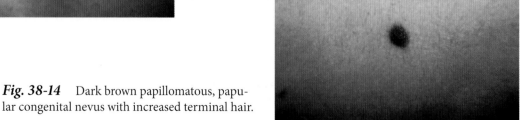

Fig. 38-13   Asymmetrical, color-variegated, light and dark brown, papular dysplastic nevi with mild border irregularity.

14). However, if an accurate history is unavailable, clinical differentiation between acquired and congenital nevi may be difficult. The differential diagnosis of congenital nevi includes acquired nevus, dysplastic nevus, mongolian spot, nevus of Ota, nevus spilus, café-au-lait, Becker's nevus, and epidermal nevus.[16,17]

Nevus of Ota is a pigmentation disorder that is more commonly seen in Asian women. It occurs around the eyes, cheeks, and/or temples; in the distribution of the trigeminal nerve; imparting a blue-gray, purple, brown, or black coloring to small, even stippled, or large smooth areas of skin. It may be bilateral and encroach on the eye, affecting multiple different esthetic subunits. Treatment is not mandatory, but the pigmentation may be successfully treated with lasers. Nevus of Ota should be watched for rare—but reported—changes suggestive of melanoma.[18]

Dermal Neoplasms
Cystic Hamartomas
Epidermoid and Epidermal Inclusion Cysts

Epidermoid cysts are cystic invaginations of the epidermis into the dermis that become filled with dead keratinocytes. An epidermal inclusion cyst is structurally similar, with a history of traumatic implantation of the epidermis within the dermis. Epidermoid cysts are the most common cutaneous cysts, usually occurring in young and middle-aged adults. Clinically they appear as firm, well-circumscribed, mobile, nontender, dermal or subcutaneous nodules, often with an overlying pore from which foul, cheeselike keratinous debris can be expressed (Fig. 38-15). They range from 0.5 to 5 cm and occur predominantly on the upper trunk, face, neck, and scrotum. Epidermoid cysts may remain stable, grow, or regress. Because the cyst lining is thin, rupture of the keratinous contents into the dermis often occurs with resultant intense inflammation that mimics cellulitis. Multiple epidermal inclusion cysts are a feature of Gardner's syndrome, which is an autosomal dominant syndrome comprising epidermal cysts, osteomas, fibromas, and small intestinal polyps with a propensity for malignant degeneration.

The differential diagnosis of epidermoid cysts includes pilar cyst, lipoma, pilomatrixoma, metastatic nodule, neurofibroma, or malignant dermal tumor. Treatment of epidermoid cysts is unnecessary if they are asymptomatic. If there is diagnostic uncertainty, expression of keratinous material through the overlying pore is diagnostic. If this is not possible and a diagnosis is unclear, then close clinical observation, incision, and drainage, or excisional biopsy may be indicated. Surgery should be avoided during episodes of rupture and acute inflammation, which are managed with warm compresses. The use of systemic antibiotics is reserved for the uncommon instances of superinfection because these cysts are usually sterile. If removal is elected, several methods are possible. Surgical excision with blunt dissection to remove the cyst with the wall intact is optimal, although cyst walls can sometimes be extracted through small incisions with the aid of a curette.

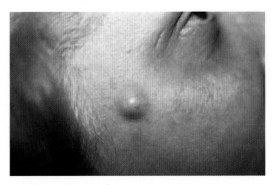

Fig. 38-15   Subcutaneous nodule with central pore characteristic of epidermal inclusion cyst.

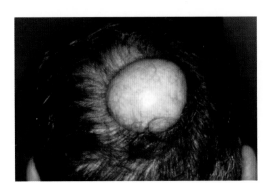

Fig. 38-16   Large, tense, protuberant, flesh-colored pilar cyst of the scalp.

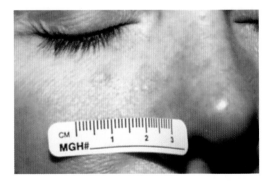

Fig. 38-17   Two 2 mm white superficial papular milia.

Pilar Cyst

Pilar, or *trichilemmal,* are the second most common cutaneous cysts and arise from the isthmus of hair follicles; they may be inherited in an autosomal dominant pattern. Pilar cysts usually appear on the scalp of middle-aged adults and can be distinguished from epidermoid cysts by the lack of a central pore. Clinically they appear as firm, smooth, skin-colored nodules ranging from 0.5 to 5 cm (Fig. 38-16). As with epidermoid cysts, rupture into the dermis results in acute inflammation. The differential diagnosis of pilar cysts includes epidermoid cyst, lipoma, pilomatrixoma, metastatic nodule, neurofibroma, or malignant dermal tumor. Management is identical to that of epidermoid cysts.

Milium

Milia are tiny variants of epidermoid cysts, ranging from 1 to 2 mm, seen both in newborns and adults, most often on the face (Fig. 38-17). They also may form in response to a variety of traumatic stimuli, including abrasions, burns, dermabrasion, corticosteroid atrophy, and radiotherapy, and during the healing of certain primary subepidermal blistering skin diseases, including bullous pemphigoid, porphyria cutanea tarda, and epidermolysis bullosa. The differential diagnosis of the milia includes sebaceous hyperplasia, syringoma, osteoma cutis, and molluscum contagiosum. As with other benign cysts, treatment is not required. Milia of infancy spontaneously resolve. Incision and drainage with a No. 11 blade and cotton swabs is usually effective for cosmetic treatment.

Follicular Hamartoma
Trichilemmoma

The importance of trichilemmomas is that these nondescript facial papules are the hallmark of significant underlying hereditary syndromes, such as Cowden's syndrome. Cowden's syndrome is an autosomal dominant disorder characterized by facial trichilemmomas, oral mucosal cobblestoning, acral (extremity) keratoses, high-arched palate, and other benign cutaneous neoplasms in association with increased risk of breast, thyroid, and gastrointestinal cancer. Trichilemmomas are benign intradermal proliferations of follicular epithelium and appear as skin-colored 1 to 4 mm papules that occur over the cheeks and nose. Biopsy is necessary for diagnosis. Solitary trichilemmomas unassociated with Cowden's syndrome occur as well. The differential diagnosis of trichilemmomas includes milia, molluscum contagiosum, verruca, trichoepithelioma, BCC, and adenoma sebaceum of tuberous sclerosis.[19] They are clinically indistinguishable from trichoepitheliomas.

Trichoepithelioma

Trichoepitheliomas are follicular-derived, hamartomatous proliferations that appear as nondescript, 1 to 4 mm, skin-colored, smooth, round papules distributed over the cheeks, nose, and nasolabial folds as an autosomal dominant inherited trait. They also occur as solitary, sporadic neoplasms in adults (Fig. 38-18). The differential diagnosis of trichoepitheliomas includes nevus, epidermal inclusion cyst, BCC, trichilemmoma, adenoma sebaceum, and neurofibroma. Treatment with excision, cryosurgery, or laser may produce acceptable results, although there is a high rate of recurrence.

Sebaceous Neoplasms
Sebaceous Hyperplasia

Sebaceous hyperplasia is simply the hypertrophy of normal sebaceous glands around a hair follicle and appears as a 1 to 5 mm, yellow, centrally depressed, cauliflower-like papule frequently with visible telangiectasias (Fig. 38-19). Most often these lesions are localized to the forehead and cheeks of adult patients. The primary differential diagnosis is BCC. Aside from a history of stability and the appearance of multiple, similar lesions, the distinctive yellow color and central dell or depression may help differentiate sebaceous hyperplasia from BCC. Biopsy is sometimes necessary, however. Treatment is usually unnecessary, although light cautery, laser, or cryosurgery may be used to improve cosmesis.

Sebaceous Adenoma

The importance of sebaceous adenomas is magnified by their association with Muir-Torre syndrome, a primarily autosomal dominant syndrome of multiple sebaceous neoplasms, including sebaceous adenomas, sebaceous hyperplasia, sebaceous epitheliomas, and sebaceous carcinomas, in addition to keratoacanthomas and visceral tumors such as colon, laryngeal, urinary tract, and endometrial cancer. Sebaceous adenomas are benign proliferations of sebaceous glands that appear as smooth, round, firm, sometimes

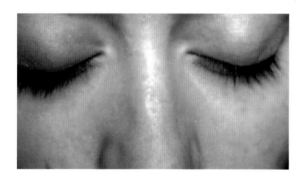

Fig. 38-18   Solitary trichoepithelioma with depressed biopsy site as a nondescript, 4 mm, skin-colored, smooth papule. (Courtesy of Suzanne Olbricht, MD.)

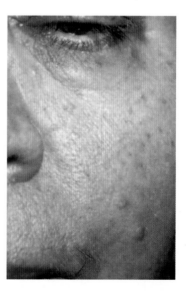

Fig. 38-19   Sebaceous hyperplasia presents as multiple 3 mm, pearly yellow, centrally depressed papules. (Courtesy of Richard A. Johnson, MD.)

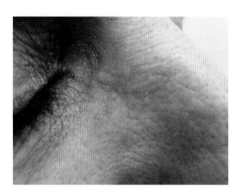

Fig. 38-20   Sebaceous adenomas appearing as several small red papules on the nose.

Fig. 38-21   Waxy, orange-yellow-tan, papillomatous plaque on the scalp characteristic of nevus sebaceous.

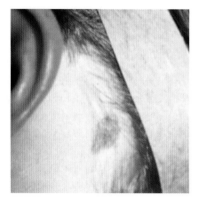

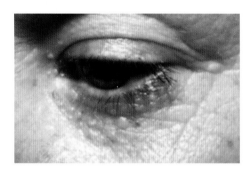

Fig. 38-22   Syringomas presenting as 1 to 3 mm, skin-colored papules on the eyelid.

pedunculated papules, usually on the face or scalp of adults. The differential diagnosis of sebaceous adenomas includes sebaceous hyperplasia, trichilemmoma, trichoepithelioma, syringoma, neurofibroma, and acrochorda. The presence of sebaceous neoplasms other than typical sebaceous hyperplasia should prompt investigation for visceral malignancy[19] (Fig. 38-20).

Nevus Sebaceous

Nevus sebaceous, hamartomatous proliferation of sebaceous glands and other appendageal elements, is a congenital hairless, orange-yellow, slightly verrucoid plaque occurring on the scalp or face of infants (Fig. 38-21). As the child reaches puberty, the sebaceous component of nevus sebaceous hypertrophies under the influence of androgenic hormones and manifests as increased thickness with a more corrugated surface. Extensive midline nevus sebaceous may be associated with underlying skeletal and neurologic abnormalities and, when coupled, are known as *epidermal nevus* or *nevus sebaceous syndrome*. The differential diagnosis of nevus sebaceous includes epidermal nevus and xanthoma. Approximately 10% to 25% of these nevi develop into BCC or other malignant neoplasms during a patient's lifetime; prophylactic excision around puberty is often recommended.[20]

Eccrine Neoplasms
Syringoma

Syringomas are benign intradermal proliferations of eccrine sweat glands that occur singly, as a familial condition, or in a widespread, eruptive form usually manifesting at puberty. They are more common in women than in men, and are seen primarily on the eyelids, face, upper chest, neck, axillae, and lower abdomen. The clinical appearance is not specific, with discrete 1 to 3 mm, skin-colored, round, moderately firm papules (Fig. 38-22). The differential diagnosis of syringomas includes eruptive vellus hair cyst, steatocystoma multiplex, acne scar, eruptive xanthoma, and milium. Treatment options include light electrodesiccation, cryosurgery, or punch excision.

Fibrous Neoplasms
Fibrous Papule

These small, usually white, firm papules are most characteristically found on the nose (Fig. 38-23). They are benign but may be confused with milium, cysts, and BCCs. Biopsy is diagnostic.

Dermatofibroma

The differential diagnosis of dermatofibroma includes blue nevus, epidermoid cyst, scar, dermatofibrosarcoma protuberans, metastatic carcinoma, dermal fibrous tumors, melanoma, and Kaposi's sarcoma. These are small, 5 to 10 mm, usually brownish papules that may occur anywhere on the body with a propensity for the lower extremities. A diagnostic "dimple" sign occurs when lateral pressure on the papule causes it to invaginate. Treatment is usually unnecessary. Pruritus may be relieved with intralesional injections of corticosteroids. Cryosurgery has been used for treatment of dermatofibromas. Excision may result in scarring less cosmetically acceptable than the original lesion. If biopsy or excision is undertaken, elliptical excision to include the entire lesion is preferable as the overall, histologic pattern is important for differentiating dermatofibroma from dermatofibrosarcoma protuberans, which is a malignant tumor.

Keloids and Hypertrophic Scars

Commonly seen in black and Asian patients, keloids are overgrowths of excessive scar tissue beyond the confines of the original site of injury. Hypertrophic scars, in contrast, remain localized, albeit in an exuberant way, to the site of injury and usually resolve or soften with time. In genetically predisposed individuals, keloids and hypertrophic scars occur as a result of lacerations, puncture wounds, abrasions, acne lesions, vaccination sites, surgical incisions, cryosurgery, or electrodesiccation. Although usually asymptomatic, a significant percentage will be pruritic or tender. Commonly involved areas include earlobes, chest, shoulders, and upper back (Fig. 38-24). Keloids may continue to grow for years, whereas hypertrophic scars tend

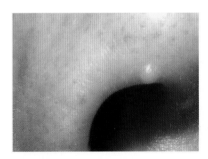

Fig. 38-23   A fibrous papule is a small white lesion on the alar rim that may be confused with a basal cell carcinoma.

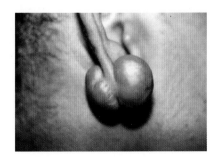

Fig. 38-24   Keloids are exuberant, indurated, shiny nodules that exceed the boundary of the original trauma, most commonly occurring on the torso or earlobes.

to improve with time. The differential diagnosis of keloids and hypertrophic scars includes dermatofibroma, foreign body granulomas, scar, sarcoidosis, and dermatofibrosarcoma protuberans.[21]

Patients who form keloids must be advised to avoid unnecessary or cosmetic surgical procedures, including ear piercing. Once formed, keloids and hypertrophic scars can often be flattened and made less erythematous with intralesional injection of corticosteroids, such as triamcinolone acetonide, in concentrations of 10 to 40 mg/ml. Pretreatment with cryotherapy permits easier injection; however, cryotherapy and the intralesional corticosteroid may cause obvious and permanent depigmentation in pigmented skin. The pruritus responds favorably to intralesional injections. Silastic sheeting may be helpful for treating both hypertrophic scars and keloids.[22] Keloids have a high propensity for recurrence after therapy, often with increased size. Recurrence may be delayed by years. If excision is performed, minimal intraoperative tissue trauma, regular postoperative intralesional corticosteroid injections, and postoperative pressure therapy should be employed. Adjuvant postoperative radiotherapy should be considered; it is associated with control rates of approximately 70%,[23] better than other reported therapies.

Adenoma Sebaceum

Adenoma sebaceum are nondescript, 2 to 5 mm, skin-colored or erythematous, dome-shaped round papules that occur on the face of 75% of patients with tuberous sclerosis, an autosomal dominant disorder characterized by seizures, mental retardation, and skin lesions (Fig. 38-25). They also occur sporadically in otherwise healthy adults. Histologically, they represent angiofibromas; thus the term "adenoma sebaceum" is misleading. The onset of adenoma sebaceum occurs by age 4. Other types of cutaneous lesions seen in tuberous sclerosis include hypomelanotic macules, shagreen patches that are collagenomas over the lumbosacral spine, and periungual fibromas. Internal manifestations include cardiac rhabdomyomas, retinal plaques, bone and lung cysts, and hamartomas of mixed cell types. Management of patients who have tuberous sclerosis includes genetic counseling, anticonvulsants, and careful follow-up. The differential diagnosis of adenoma sebaceum includes acne, trichoepithelioma, trichilemmoma of Cowden's syndrome, milium, molluscum contagiosum, and verruca.

The key to managing patients with angiofibroma is to consider the diagnosis of tuberous sclerosis and thus to connect these patients with appropriate specialists, including neurologists, pediatricians, and genetic counselors. The treatment of adenoma sebaceum can be performed with dermabrasion, tangential excision, electrodesiccation, and CO_2 laser. Adenoma sebaceum tend to recur.[24]

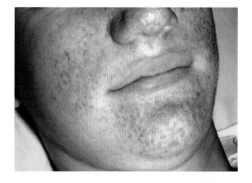

Fig. 38-25   Confluent and discrete, erythematous, shiny papules in a typical distribution for adenoma sebaceum of tuberous sclerosis. (Courtesy of Joannes Grevelink, MD.)

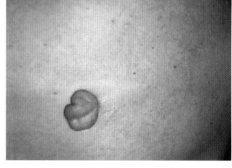

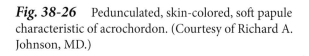

Fig. 38-26   Pedunculated, skin-colored, soft papule characteristic of acrochordon. (Courtesy of Richard A. Johnson, MD.)

Acrochordon

Acrochorda, or skin tags, are very common, asymptomatic, benign, pedunculated outpouchings of skin, often in a familial pattern, seen in the middle-aged and elderly. They range in size from 1 mm to greater than 1 cm, are soft and usually skin-colored, tan, or brown (Fig. 38-26). Acrochorda display a predilection for the eyelids, axillae, neck, groin, and inframammary regions. If traumatized, they may become crusted or even necrotic as a result of strangulation. Acrochorda often become more numerous and large with time. The differential diagnosis of acrochorda includes pedunculated seborrheic keratosis, neurofibroma, and dermal nevus. Generally, biopsy is unnecessary for diagnosis. Although for most patients assurance of the benign nature of acrochorda is sufficient, some request removal for cosmetic reasons or because of irritation. If treatment is desired, removal at the base with a scissor or light electrodesiccation with or without anesthesia is effective. Large, solitary, inflamed, or atypical lesions should be submitted for histologic examination.

Chondrodermatitis Nodularis Helicis

Chondrodermatitis nodularis helicis affects the cartilage in the ear and appears as one or more firm, painful, usually erythematous papules overlying cartilage (Fig. 38-27). The papules are thought to consist of degenerated collagen that has extruded through the epidermis. The degeneration may be a result of ischemia and/or pressure, or perhaps ultraviolet lights or cold temperatures. The differential diagnosis includes a skin cancer, keratoacanthoma, rheumatoid nodules, clavus, and tophus. Treatment includes removal of any sources of pressure such as headphones or firm pillows. If the problem continues, treatment options include injection with steroids, laser ablation, or excision. Recurrence after any of these techniques is common.[25]

Venous Lake

Venous lakes are common, asymptomatic, 2 to 8 mm, soft, compressible, blue to purple vascular dilations occurring on the lips, face, and ears of adult patients (Fig. 38-28). They undergo a period of growth followed by stability with rare involution. The differential diagnosis includes angiokeratoma, blue nevus, tattoo, hemangioma, pyogenic granuloma, and nodular melanoma. No treatment is required, although pulsed-dye laser is effective at eliminating them, as are electrocoagulation and excision.

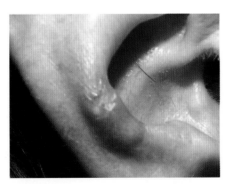

Fig. 38-27 A red, tender papule on the antihelical protuberant cartilage that is a classic example of active chondrodermatitis nodularis helicis.

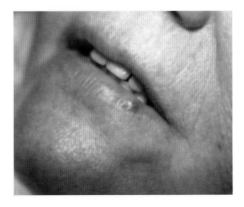

Fig. 38-28 A compressible, dome-shaped, purple-blue papule characteristic of venous lake.

Lipocyte Neoplasms
Lipoma

Lipomas are common, painless, soft, well-circumscribed subcutaneous tumors composed of lipocytes surrounded by a fibrous sheath. In contradistinction to epidermoid cysts, lipomas are not attached to the epidermis, and therefore are more mobile as well as softer and smoother (Fig. 38-29). They appear on the trunk, neck, scalp, and extremities. A variant of lipoma with a prominent vascular component, known as *angiolipoma*, is often tender or painful. Another variant often occurring on the forehead is labeled *infiltrating*, because it goes into muscle and is not encapsulated, thus complicating surgical removal.[26] Lipomas may be seen as part of syndromes, including Gardner's syndrome, which is an autosomal dominant syndrome composed of multiple cysts, lipomas, fibromas, osteomas, and intestinal polyps or Dercum's disease, in which obese middle-aged persons have numerous, painful lipomas. The differential diagnosis includes epidermoid cyst, angiolipoma, and metastatic dermal tumor. If there is any doubt about the possibility of a malignant neoplasm, biopsy should be performed. No treatment is required, although excision and liposuction are usually curative.

Neural Neoplasms
Neurofibromas

Neurofibromas are benign proliferations of neurons, Schwann cells, and fibroblasts. They appear as skin colored to violaceous, soft to firm, 3 to 30 mm papules, often pedunculated, which characteristically invaginate with fingertip pressure (the buttonhole sign) (Fig. 38-30). Affected individuals have between one and thousands of lesions that may be distributed randomly or segmentally. Neurofibromas may be attached to underlying nerves and may be pruritic. Neurofibromas may occur sporadically or in association with systemic von Recklinghausen's neurofibromatosis 1, an autosomal dominant syndrome characterized by café-au-lait macules, peripheral and CNS neurofibromas, skeletal abnormalities, and pheochromocytomas. Diagnosis is based on specifically defined clinical criteria. The differential diagnosis of neurofibromas includes nevus, dermatofibroma, and acrochordon.

The management of neurofibromas requires inquiry into family history of neurofibromatosis, examination for café-au-lait macules, axillary or inguinal freckling, consideration of evaluation for Lisch nodules of the iris, and auditory and skeletal abnormalities. If a diagnosis of neurofibromatosis is established, coordination of care with a neurologist, orthopedic surgeon, and facial plastic surgeon should be established. Ge-

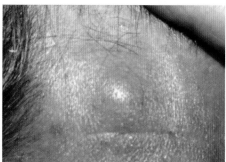

Fig. 38-29   Lipomas appear as soft, smooth, mobile subcutaneous nodules without central pores.

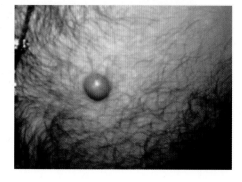

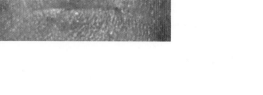

Fig. 38-30   Shiny, skin-colored papule suggestive of neurofibroma.

Box 38-6   Inflammatory and Infiltrative Pseudotumors

- Lymphoma
- Molluscum contagiosum
- Orf/Milker's nodule
- Lichenoid keratosis
- Morphea
- Lichen sclerosus et atrophicus
- Prurigo nodularis

- Nodular amyloidosis
- Panniculitis
- Lymphoma/leukemia cutis
- Juvenile xanthogranuloma
- Mastocytoma
- Cylindromas

- Tophus
- Bacillary angiomatosis
- Kaposi's sarcoma
- Xanthoma
- Osteoma cutis
- Warts

---

netic counseling is paramount, and the patient should be regularly monitored for signs of malignant transformation. Affected individuals may require special education and social services. Individual neurofibromas are managed effectively by standard surgical excision.

INFLAMMATORY AND INFILTRATIVE PSEUDOTUMORS

A variety of inflammatory and infiltrative cutaneous diseases can masquerade as benign cutaneous neoplasms. Box 38-6 lists some of the more common pseudotumors that may enter the differential diagnosis of benign cutaneous neoplasms.

MALIGNANT CUTANEOUS NEOPLASMS

Nonmelanoma skin cancers (NMSCs) are the most common neoplasms in Fitzpatrick type I through III individuals. BCCs constitute slightly greater than three quarters of skin cancers, with the remainder being primarily SCCs.[27] There are several unusual NMSCs that arise from overproliferation of various adnexal structures and other cellular constituents of the skin. Microcytic adnexal carcinoma, dermatofibrosarcoma protuberans, various lymphomas, sebaceous carcinoma, and Merkel cell carcinoma are examples of unusual cutaneous neoplasms with unique histologic and clinical features that represent a small percentage of the total number of NMSCs.[28,29]

BCCs and SCCs share several features. They both have an overall predilection for sun-exposed sites, and are characteristically seen in light-skinned individuals, reflecting the importance of UV light in the ontogeny of the majority of them.[30] Furthermore, both appear to be more common in individuals with chronic sun exposure and photodamage, suggesting sustained UV damage as an important etiologic factor. Both tumors have an increased incidence in syndromes such as xeroderma pigmentosum, characterized by an inability to repair UV-induced damage adequately. It is sometimes difficult to distinguish BCC from SCC clinically, and occasionally, even with histologic evaluation, the distinction can be challenging.

There are also several essential differences between and among BCCs and SCCs, including their biologic and histologic origin, their clinical and morphologic presentations, and differences in anatomic distribution. These differences are crucial in selecting appropriate treatment modalities. Neither tumor type is monomorphic. For example, with respect to biologic behavior and treatment approaches, the superficial subtype of BCC has more in common with SCC in situ than it does with the morpheic-sclerosing subtype of BCC. An understanding of the epidemiologic factors, clinical characteristics, histologic findings, and treatment approaches to the various types of BCC and SCC is essential in approaching the diagnosis and treatment of these common tumors in a systematic and informed manner.

BASAL CELL CARCINOMA

Epidemiologic Factors

Basal cell carcinoma is the most common cancer in the United States, and its incidence is increasing. There are an estimated 3.5 million new cases of BCC and SCC in the United States each year, occurring in 2.2 million Americans (many patients have more than one); and numbers are increasing at an alarming rate. However, deaths caused by NMSC are decreasing, and estimated to be approximately 2000 per year.[31] The reasons for the increase in incidence have been postulated to involve factors such as damage to the protective ozone layer, increased surveillance, use of tanning parlors, and changing sociocultural patterns of leisure activities.[32] There are several factors that correlate with risk for developing BCC. Although all races develop the tumor, the overwhelming majority are in white individuals. Even among Europeans, those of northern European ancestry are at considerably higher risk than those originating from southern Europe. Skin type is independently associated with risk for developing BCC; individuals with a propensity to burn and a history of sunburns, and those with an inability to tan or who freckle easily (Fitzpatrick skin types I-II) are at higher risk (Box 38-7). It is estimated that 50% of people over the age of 60 with these skin types will develop a skin cancer.[32] People with greater exposure to the sun are at higher risk. Both living in a sunnier climate or an area closer to the equator and spending more time in the sun (for example, with an outdoor occupation or greater leisure time in the sun) are correlated with an increased risk for BCC. Persons who have markers of chronic photodamaged skin, such as telangiectasia, solar lentigines, rhytides, and atrophy, have an increased risk for BCC compared with those without such photodamage. Risk generally increases with age. Although earlier data showed a significantly higher incidence of BCC in men than in women, recent data suggest that the incidence is equalizing, perhaps reflecting changes in lifestyles.[33]

Box 38-7   Fitzpatrick Skin Phototypes

I	Always burns, never tans
II	Sometimes burns, rarely tans
III	Sometimes burns, tans
IV	Rarely burns, always tans
V	Almost never burns, always tans
VI	Never burns, always tans

Box 38-8   Risk Factors for Skin Cancers

- Light skin (types I-III)
- Radiation exposure
  - Recreation
  - Residence
  - Tanning booths
  - Therapy
- Immunosuppression
- Arsenic
- Burn scars
- Chronic ulcers

Basal cell carcinoma may occur anywhere on the body, but the majority (85%) are on the head and neck. Although BCC is often thought of as related directly to the degree of photoexposure, there are some paradoxical findings. BCC on the lips tend to be on the upper lip, which is relatively photoprotected compared with the lower lip, whereas most lip SCCs occur on the lower lip. Also of interest is the apparent tendency for aggressive BCCs to develop in the relatively photoprotected postauricular sulci. Further, unlike SCC, BCC is rare on the dorsal hands and fingers, which receive considerable direct sunlight.

Risk factors for BCC other than sun exposure include radiation exposure, long-term therapy with psoralens and UV light for skin diseases, arsenic exposure, immunosuppression,[34] burn scars, and chronic ulcers (Box 38-8). Patients who have a nevus sebaceous of Jadassohn, a cutaneous hamartoma most commonly located on the face or the scalp, have a 10% to 30% chance of developing malignancy within the nevus, with BCC being the most common tumor. There are also three inherited syndromes that often include the development of multiple BCCs: the nevoid BCC (basal cell nevus syndrome or Gorlin's syndrome), Bazex syndrome, and xeroderma pigmentation. A final risk factor for development of a BCC is a prior BCC.

Clinical Characteristics

Basal cell carcinomas are often found in the context of photodamaged skin. Evidence of chronic photodamage includes actinic keratoses, elastosis, xerosis, rhytids, telangiectasias, lentigines, freckles, and dyspigmentation. There is no direct clinical precursor lesion of BCC, but actinic elastosis and other evidence of actinic damage can suggest a patient and a location at risk. Most BCCs occur on the face. The tumor does not usually affect glabrous areas, such as mucous membranes and (with the exception of basal cell nevus syndrome) the palms and soles. The most prevalent sites are the nose, forehead/temple, cheek, and ears.[35] Basal cell carcinoma possesses clinicopathologic subtypes, with important ramifications in the clinical approach to the tumor. In addition to gross and microscopic appearance, the growth patterns, subclinical extent, and treatment approaches vary with subtype.

Nodular or noduloulcerative BCC is the most common subtype, constituting 45% to 60% of BCCs. Classically, it presents as a pearly, translucent, pink-white, dome-shaped papule, with telangiectasias (Fig. 38-31, *A*). It is most common on the face and is often ulcerated. A frequent complaint of patients with this lesion is that of a bump that bleeds and scabs, but never fully heals. Neglected tumors can become large (Fig. 38-31, *B*). Pieces of these tumors can fall out, leading to ulcers (called *rodent ulcers*) as the most prominent clinical feature (Fig. 38-31, *C*). Any nonhealing ulcer must be evaluated carefully and biopsied. The differential diagnosis of nodular BCC includes SCC and other cutaneous neoplasms, intradermal nevi, rosacea/acne lesions, sebaceous hyperplasia, or various causes of ulceration.

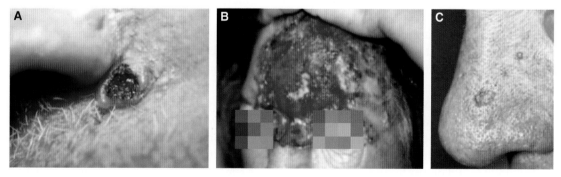

Fig. 38-31   **A,** Noduloulcerative basal cell carcinoma. **B,** Extensive basal cell carcinoma. **C,** A small "rodent ulcer" on the nose; a nodular basal cell carcinoma.

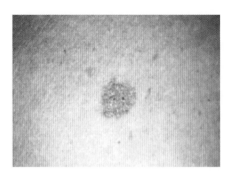

Fig. 38-32   Superficial basal cell carcinoma.

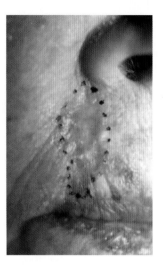

Fig. 38-33   Scarlike plaque; a morpheic basal cell carcinoma.

The other common subtype, superficial BCC, is 15% to 35% of this tumor group. They often present as slow-growing, scaly, erythematous patches on the trunk or extremities, although they are also frequently seen on the face (Fig. 38-32). Clinically, they can mimic dermatitis (nummular or contact), psoriasis, Bowen's disease, extramammary Paget's disease, or AKs. These tumors can also ulcerate and become crusted or scabbed.

Less common, but clinically important to recognize, are morpheic or sclerosing BCCs, which are 4% to 17% of all BCCs. Sometimes grouped with so-called infiltrative BCCs, these can be deceptively aggressive lesions. They often present as ill-defined, waxy, white-yellow indurated plaques with telangiectasias (Fig. 38-33). The pearly rolled edge of nodular BCCs is often absent. They may be slightly depressed or elevated and may mimic a scar. Although these are clinically the more subtle of BCCs, they are the most aggressive of the subtypes. One study showed an average subclinical extension of these tumors of greater than 7 mm.[36] Histologically, recurrent BCCs are infiltrative in a greater percentage of cases than primary BCCs. It is uncertain whether this is because of inadequate primary treatment of a more aggressive histologic subtype, or evolution of an infiltrative pattern in a recurrent BCC emerging through a scar.

Finally, 1% to 2% of BCCs are pigmented. This does not refer to a histologic subtype or a clinically unique or characteristic behavior, but is simply descriptive (often a nodular BCC with pigment) (Fig. 38-34). They are important to recognize clinically because they can resemble a seborrheic keratosis, nevus, and melanoma.

There are also rare variants of BCC recognized in diverse clinical contexts. Within scars or old irradiation sites, BCCs can be subtle, difficult to recognize, and aggressive. Cystic BCC can present as a small translucent papule and is usually diagnosed histologically rather than clinically. Fibroepithelioma of Pinkus has a characteristic histologic finding and clinically can be a pedunculated lesion, which can resemble a fibroma and is generally found on the lower back or buttocks. BCCs may develop in a nevus sebaceous, which in adults (when BCCs generally form) is usually a pebbly, yellow-orange, verrucous, hairless plaque, commonly found on the scalp.[20] The nevoid BCC syndrome is an autosomal dominant disorder characterized

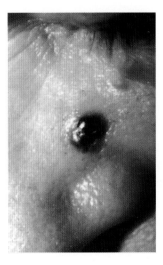

Fig. 38-34   Pigmented basal cell carcinoma.

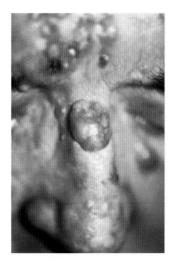

Fig. 38-35   Multiple basal cell carcinomas in a patient who has basal cell nevus syndrome.

by palmar pits, mandibular cysts, various skeletal and CNS abnormalities, and an increased incidence of ovarian fibromas and medulloblastomas. Patients with the syndrome develop multiple BCCs (sometimes hundreds or thousands) beginning at a young age (Fig. 38-35).

Clinically, these lesions often appear "nevoid" (small tan, fleshy papules). Other syndromes predisposing individuals to development of BCC include xeroderma pigmentosum and Bazex syndrome. In xeroderma pigmentosum, BCCs develop in the context of severe, early photodamage and other photo-induced cancers. Bazex syndrome is characterized by follicular atrophoderma, hypohidrosis, hypotrichosis, and multiple BCCs on the face. Finally, the rare linear unilateral basal cell nevus usually presents as a congenital unilateral linear or zosteriform array of nodules of BCC.

Giant BCCs are rare (1%). Defined as lesions that are 5 cm or more in diameter, they can be characterized by significant local invasion and often leave extensive disfiguring cutaneous defects. They may extend down to and through bone, invading the skull and penetrating the dura. The tumors have often been neglected for many years, and have a greater chance of having been previously treated. A history of radiation exposure/treatment and immunosuppression also increases risk (see Fig. 38-31, *B*).

Metastases from BCC are extremely rare; reported incidence ranges from 0.0028% to 0.55%. Patients at risk for metastasis include men, patients who have a history of radiation treatment, patients who have large locally invasive primary tumors, and patients who have primary location of BCCs on the ear or scalp. The most common site of metastasis is lymph nodes, followed by lung, bone, skin. A prolonged interval has been reported between tumor onset and metastasis. Hematogenous or lymphogenous modes of spread are equally common. BCC rarely results in death. Of NMSCs (most of which are BCC), it accounts for only 20% of deaths, the leading cause of which is direct extension into vital structures, not metastases. The most common sites are multiple sites on the head, periorbital area, and the ear. This is much more frequently a disfiguring tumor than a life-threatening tumor.

Histologic Evaluation of Basal Cell Carcinoma

The histologic subtype of a BCC is an important factor in influencing the therapeutic approach to a given tumor. BCC cells generally have large, basophilic, elongated nuclei and scant cytoplasm—in many ways reminiscent of cells of the basal layer of the epidermis. As opposed to many other neoplasms, neither variegation in nuclear size nor mitotic figures are common. Histologically, BCC consists of nest, cords, or masses of these epithelial basaloid cells within a characteristic connective tissue stroma. In superficial BCC, the typical palisading basaloid cells bud down from, or represent, a thickening of the lower epidermis with its upper dermal stroma. Nests of tumor in nodular BCC can be bland and monomorphic or can differentiate toward adnexal structures like hair or glands. Some show keratotic foci. Morpheic or sclerosing BCCs have a much greater proportion of dense, fibrotic connective tissue, enveloping elongated infiltrating strands of epithelial tumor cells, often only one cell layer thick. Micronodular tumors consist of multiple, small, infiltrating nodules of tumor, and may represent a degree of aggressiveness somewhere between a nodular and a sclerotic tumor.[37]

SQUAMOUS CELL CARCINOMA

Epidemiologic Factors

Cutaneous squamous cell carcinoma is the most deadly NMSC. Although it represents a minority of NMSCs, it is responsible for 59% of deaths from such cancers. The incidence of this tumor has been rising over the past decades.[38]

As with BCC, light-skinned white individuals with significant sun exposure are at highest risk for developing SCC. Host factors other than skin pigmentation that are important etiologic factors for SCC include age, immune status, chronic dermatoses (especially conditions leading to chronic ulcers), and genetic abnormalities (for example, xeroderma pigmentosum and albinism). Although patients who are immunosuppressed have increases in both BCC and SCC, the usual predominance of BCCs is reversed, and SCCs are three times more common than BCC. In renal transplant patients the incidence of SCC is up to 250 times that of the general population.[39] Although UV radiation is the major environmental factor in the development of SCC, other extrinsic factors can play a role. Chemical carcinogens (such as arsenic or organic hydrocarbons), chronic heat exposure to a single anatomic location, radiation exposure, and certain human papillomaviruses all correlate positively with the development of SCC.

Clinical Characteristics

SCC of the skin may arise de novo, from chronic skin diseases, or from common precursor lesions, AKs (or solar keratoses). They often develop in the context of photodamaged skin, and are most common on the head and neck. Unlike BCC, they are also common on the upper extremities, especially the chronically exposed dorsal hands. Further, unlike BCC, they develop on mucous membranes as well as nonglaborous skin.

SCCs often appear as hard, keratotic nodules on an indurated base (Fig. 38-36). They may appear in a scar, a chronic ulcer, a tattoo, or other chronic dermatoses. When arising from an AK, they are often scaly. The lesion can be the color of normal skin or slightly erythematous. AKs are rough, sometimes erythematous, flat papules, commonly seen in photodamaged skin of elderly white individuals (Fig. 38-37). They are markers for patients at risk for developing BCC, and are a precursor to SCC. One study demonstrated that 60% of cutaneous SCCs in a given population arose from preexisting actinic keratosis (the other 40% arose de novo). However, a given actinic keratosis probably has a low likelihood of malignant transformation, but serves as a marker for sun damage and an increased likelihood of developing SCCs.[40,41]

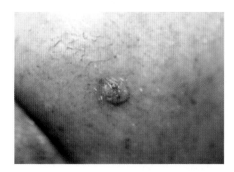

Fig. 38-36   Keratotic verrucous squamous cell carcinoma.

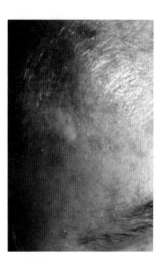

Fig. 38-37   Multiple rough erythematous actinic keratoses on the temple (the lesions can usually be better felt than seen).

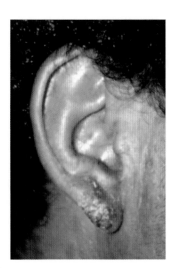

Fig. 38-38   A squamous cell carcinoma in situ on the ear lobe.

Fig. 38-39   Keratoacanthoma of the ear.

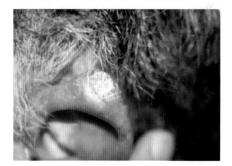

Another important precursor of SCC is squamous cell carcinoma in situ or *Bowen's disease*. This is a slow-growing, sharply demarcated, scaly, and crusted erythematous plaque and can be located anywhere on the integument (as well as mucous membranes) (Fig. 38-38). They are most common in sun-exposed areas. If untreated, they may evolve into invasive SCC.

Keratoacanthomas are a clinically and histopathologically distinct form of SCC. It is a tumor characterized by rapid growth (often with tenderness) of a dome-shaped keratotic nodule in photodamaged skin (Fig. 38-39). There is a tendency for many of these tumors to regress spontaneously, but some can persist and evolve into invasive SCC (see earlier discussion).

Box 38-9   Risk Factors for Metastases in Squamous Cell Carcinoma

- *Size:* Tumors larger than 2 cm are more likely to metastasize than those smaller than 2 cm.
- *Depth:* Risk increases with both anatomic and absolute depth.
- *Histologic differentiation:* Metastatic rate is triple in poorly differentiated tumors versus those well differentiated.
- *Site:* Tumors on the ear and lip have significantly increased risk for metastasis.
- *Scars:* Tumors arising within scars (such as from burns, chronic ulcers, and radiation dermatitis) have a significantly increased rate of metastasis when compared with sun-induced tumors.
- *Neurotropism:* Tumors with histologic evidence of perineural spread seem to be high risk.
- *Previously treated SCC:* Locally recurrent SCCs are at higher risk for metastasis.
- *Immunosuppression:* Transplant patients are at very high risk for developing multiple SCCs, generally in sun-exposed sites. Although individual tumors may not be high risk, the presence of multiple tumors puts the patient at higher risk for metastasis.

Although local invasion and destruction is usually the major concern with BCC, the potential for metastasis is the most serious consequence of SCC. Varying estimates of metastatic risk for cutaneous SCC range from 0.5% to 16%. Several factors have been identified as important in stratifying risk for patients who have developed metastatic SCC[42] (Box 38-9).

Histologic Evaluation of Squamous Cell Carcinoma

SCC is composed of epidermal keratinocytes proliferating beneath the dermal-epidermal junction into the dermis. Characteristic features include evidence for keratinization of the invasive cells. Broders' grading system defines four grades of severity based on the proportion of differentiated cells in the tumor. Other histologic factors important in grading tumors include the degree of atypicality of tumor cells and the depth and pattern of invasion. Some tumors show a spindle cell pattern without usual clearly identifying features of the keratinocyte. Immunoperoxidase staining for cytokeratins may help in the identification of these tumors.

MERKEL CELL CARCINOMA

Merkel cell carcinoma, originally called trabecular carcinoma,[43] is an aggressive lesion of neuroendocrine origins.[44] Although very rare, the incidence is increasing, especially in immunosuppressed patients. Recent elucidation of its association with a polyomavirus may shed light on its cause.[45] It presents as a nonulcerated; asymptomatic; flesh-colored, pink, or red papule often demonstrating rapid growth (Fig. 38-40).

However, its 5-year disease-free survival rate is approximately 60%. Its lethality is likely related to its rapid lymphatic dissemination and the inconspicuous nature of the cutaneous papules, allowing it to go unnoticed for years. Heath[46] coined a mnemonic for the features and presentation of a Merkel cell tumor (Box 38-10). Many patients who present with only a small facial papule will already have metastatic disease.

Once diagnosed, patients require care from a multidisciplinary team, including a dermatologist, surgeon, radiation oncologist, and medical oncologist.[47] Current recommendations are for wide local excision and sentinel lymph node biopsy, followed by radiotherapy.[48]

Box 38-10   Merkel Cell Carcinoma

A   *A*symptomatic/lack of tenderness
E   *E*xpanding rapidly
I   *I*mmune suppression
O   *O*lder than 50
U   *U*V-exposed skin

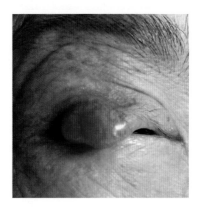

Fig. 38-40   A Merkel cell tumor, a rapidly growing pink nodule; nonulcerated and asymptomatic, except for location.

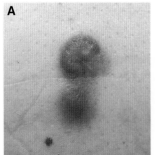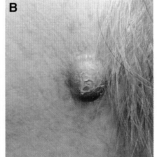

Fig. 38-41   **A,** Dermatofibroma sarcoma protuberans: a nodular dermal plaque with brownish red to purple coloring. **B,** Atypical fibrous xanthoma that had recently grown, although it was present for years as an asymptomatic, small reddish papule.

CUTANEOUS SARCOMAS

Dermatofibroma sarcoma protuberans and atypical fibrous xanthoma (AFX) are rare cutaneous sarcomas that may grow to significant size and bear the ability to metastasize, although they rarely do.[49,50] They present as smooth papules and plaques, often slightly pigmented, and may have been present for many years before they began to grow, prompting medical attention (Fig. 38-41, *A*). These tumors are being seen more frequently in immunosuppressed patients. AFX usually occurs on the head and neck in elderly patients[51] (Fig. 38-41, *B*). Recommended treatment is Mohs surgery, which offers the lowest recurrence rates. The number of recurrences is directly correlated with metastases. If wide local excision is employed, 3 cm margins are recommended. Since these tumors are radiosensitive, radiation may be considered as primary or adjuvant therapy in special circumstances.

Epidermotropic Metastases

Several cancers will metastasize to the skin and present as a reddish papule. The most common are ovary, colon, melanoma, lung, kidney, and breast. The last three have a predilection for the scalp. Melanoma me-

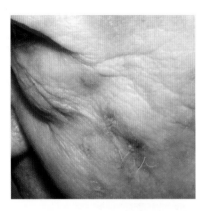

Fig. 38-42   A flat, yellowish-white, sclerotic plaque microcystic adnexal carcinoma on the left cheek, more palpable than visible and thought to be a scar.

tastases are usually blue or black, but can be amelanotic. As many as 7% of patients may have such a lesion as the first indicator of their disease.[52]

Microcystic Adnexal Carcinoma

Microcystic adnexal carcinoma, also called sclerosing sweat duct or syringoid carcinoma, is a rare tumor usually occurring midface, especially periorally, in adults—most often in women. It is a locally aggressive lesion with almost no potential to metastasize. However, because it has a subtle growth pattern, it is often quite large and invasive by the time it is diagnosed. Perineural involvement may cause paresthesia, prompting the patient to seek medical attention. A lesion appears as a firm, smooth, skin-colored or slightly yellowish plaque, more palpable than visible (Fig. 38-42). Histopathologic diagnosis may prove to be difficult. Immunohistochemical staining is very useful. Treatment is most effective using Mohs surgery because this tumor often possesses wide and deep subtle extensions.[53] This lesion's propensity for the midface often yields large defects with challenging reconstructions. Radiotherapy is not recommended. With the widespread use of immunosuppressive agents for many different disease entities, there is a significant rise in the occurrence of all NMSC, including these rare lesions.[54,55]

BIOPSY OF A NONMELANOMA SKIN CANCER

The appropriate approach to biopsy of a suspected skin cancer depends on the clinical scenario. Most commonly, a small, fairly superficial shave biopsy is sufficient for adequate histologic diagnosis. A piece of tumor nodule should be left behind or the location carefully photographed and/or measured and mapped, so that a positive biopsy can be followed by appropriate definitive treatment at the correct location. If a melanocytic neoplasm is in the differential diagnosis of a lesion, a full-thickness biopsy (punch or excisional) should be performed. In an apparent, ulcerated lesion with a necrotic center, the edge is ordinarily the best place to perform the biopsy.

TREATMENT OPTIONS FOR NONMELANOMA SKIN CANCER

The most appropriate mode of treatment for a skin cancer depends on several factors. Factors that are considered in tailoring treatment to an individual patient/tumor include: the histologic subtype, the size of the tumor, the location, whether the tumor is primary or recurrent, and individual patient considerations. For example, a small, primary, well-defined, histologically and clinically nodular BCC on the cheek would be approached differently from a recurrent, ill-defined, morpheic tumor on the upper lip. Those modalities include cryosurgery, topical creams, electrodessication and curettage, radiation, laser ablation, excisional surgery, Mohs surgery, photodynamic therapy, and intralesional injection (Table 38-1).

Table 38-1   Treatment Options for Nonmelanoma Lesions

Treatment Options	Advantages	Disadvantages
Topical creams	At home Repeatable No scarring	Long time Patient dependent Inflammation
Electrodessication and curettage	In office Local anesthesia	Scar No histologic evaluation
Cryosurgery	In office Local anesthesia	Scar No histologic evaluation
Surgery (excisional/Mohs)	Histologic evaluation	Standard for surgical procedures
Photodynamic therapy	In office No anesthesia	No histologic evaluation Postprocedure discomfort
Radiotherapy	No anesthesia No surgery	Multiple visits Radiation dermatitis
Intralesional	In office No surgery	Painful, multiple visits to histology

The two most frequently used topical creams to treat skin cancers are 5-fluorouracil (5FU) and imiquimod. 5FU is a structural analog of thymine that will block DNA synthesis when taken up by a cell. It is available in several different strengths that may be titrated to a patient's individual sensitivity; its use may cause significant inflammation and even erosion of the skin. It is FDA approved for the treatment of actinic keratosis, superficial basal cell carcinomas, and SCC in situ, anywhere and any size. Regimens vary widely; however, it is commonly prescribed once or twice per day for 3 to 6 weeks, with cure rates approaching 90% for superficial BCC and 27% to 85% for SCC in situ.[57]

Imiquimod is an immunomodulating drug that binds to cell surface receptors, causing apoptosis and activation of cell-mediated immunity. It is FDA approved for the treatment in immunocompetent adults of AKs and superficial BCCs less than 2 cm. Various regimens have been used, from 3 to 7 days per week, with clearance rates near 80%.[58] This pharmacologic approach may also be combined with other modalities to increase the cure rate.[59] The advantage of these topical treatment modalities is that they may be applied at home, treatment can be stopped and restarted to accommodate an individual, and requires infrequent office visits.

Electrodesiccation and curettage shares several features with cryosurgery. It is a tissue-destructive modality that allows wounds to heal by secondary intention, and does not histologically examine tissue margins. The curette can be an extremely valuable instrument in the treatment of BCC. The sharp edge scrapes away easily friable tissue. Tumor tissue (with the general exception of morpheaform tumors) is soft and easily removed, whereas the instrument does not affect uninvolved skin. This assists in debulking the tumor and helps to define its true borders. The base is then electrodesiccated, including a 1 to 2 mm rim of tissue around the erosion. The two-step procedure is repeated one to three times. For low-risk sites (from the neck down), one retrospective study showed a 5-year recurrence rate of 3.3% after electrodesiccation and curettage. Treatment of high-risk sites (nose, paranasal, nasolabial groove, ear, chin, mandible, perioral, and periocular) had a 5-year recurrence rate of 16.3% or more, and middle-risk sites (other areas above the neck) recurred in 10.7% to 13.4% of cases. If the data were limited to small tumors (5 mm) in high-risk sites, a 5-year recurrence rate of only 4% to 5% was noted.[60] This technique is best used only on head and neck sites where there is a firm base underlying the lesion, such as the forehead.

Cryosurgery destroys tissue by freezing it at tumoricidal temperatures ($-50°$ C), most commonly with liquid nitrogen. It has the advantage of being relatively safe, efficient, and easy to perform (in skilled hands). The mechanism of tumor destruction includes direct effects of freezing the cells (including permanent membrane damage) and microcirculation failure in the treated region, which leads to cell death. Generally, the region to be treated is anesthetized with lidocaine. Superficial BCC (approximately 60-second freeze) responds slightly better than nodular BCC (60- to 90-second freeze). Relative and absolute contraindications include poorly defined tumors, patients who have abnormal cold tolerance, very large tumors, morpheic tumors, and recurrent tumors. Special care should be taken in freezing tumors that overlie important nerves; are near the free margins of the eyes, vermilion border of the lip, and nasal ala; and tumors in the postauricular sulcus or on the scalp. Wounds essentially heal by secondary intention beneath an eschar of dead tissue, usually leaving hypopigmented scars. One disadvantage to this therapy is that treated tissue is not excised, and therefore cannot be evaluated histologically for margins. However, in experienced hands, results may be excellent. In some series, cure rates are as high as 95.5% to 97.5%. In certain clinical scenarios, and in experienced hands, cryosurgery represents an excellent therapeutic approach.[56]

Surgical excision of BCC is a well-accepted method of treatment. The tumor and an appropriate margin of clinically normal-appearing surrounding skin is excised into the subcutaneous fat, and the wound is closed (or left to heal by secondary intention). One difficulty with this method is defining and determining what margin of clinically normal skin to remove. Use of the curette to debulk the tumor before excision can help to find the extent of the tumor and improve the accuracy of excisional margins, and therefore the cure rate.[67] One study attempted to determine what constitutes appropriate margins using a review of the literature for tumors less than 2 cm and concluded that in clinically well-defined tumors, a 2 mm margin would eradicate 90% of tumors, a 3 mm margin 93.5%, and a 4 mm margin is necessary to extirpate 95.8% of tumors, although there is some variability among studies.[68] Using this guideline, a tumor may extend 4 mm in one direction (in which case the 4 mm margin was necessary for extirpation), but only 1 mm in the other direction (leading to removal of 3 mm of normal skin). However, it is clear that there is an incremental advantage of complete removal directly correlated with increasing size of the margin.[69]

A theoretical advantage of excisional surgery, as opposed to the field destructive modalities, is the opportunity for histopathologic evaluation of the excised tumor. This can be performed either with fresh frozen sections or permanent sections. Repair may be delayed until histopathologic evaluation confirms complete tumor removal, or an excision with an already closed positive margin may be reexcised. Recurrent tumors tend to be more aggressive and more difficult to extirpate.

Photodynamic therapy combines light technology with a chemical biologic reaction to treat superficial lesions on the skin. It is FDA approved for the treatment of AK and superficial BCCs. The area of concern is "painted" with 5-aminolevulinic acid (ALA) and remains undisturbed for approximately 1 hour. The ALA is converted intracellularly to protoporphyrin IX. When blue light is applied to the areas, a cytotoxic reaction occurs. With one or more treatments, this may clear the AKs for as long as a year. Clearance rates of approximately 80% have been achieved for superficial BCCs.[64] A newer regimen for use with immunocompromised patients describes frequent sessions to lessen the rate of appearance of multiple lesions in these patients.[65] The use of light technology (that is, lasers) as a single modality without ALA has not proven useful in NMSC other than for very superficial lesions.[66]

Radiotherapy is another field-destructive therapy applied to the area involved with tumor. Radiation is delivered to the area encompassed by the tumor and a small margin of clinically normal skin. Multiple treatments are usually required. Radiation dermatitis develops in the treated area, usually followed by an atrophic hypopigmented scar. Recurrences within a radiation scar may be more aggressive and difficult to eradicate. Further, radiation can induce tumors in the treated site. Overall, the 5-year recurrence rate at one center was 7.4% for treatment of primary tumors. BCCs with greater diameter did not respond as well. Patient satisfaction with the long-term cosmetic outcome (63%) was significantly lower than with electrodesiccation and curettage (91%) or surgical excision (84%). In selected well-defined tumors in elderly patients who wish to avoid surgical treatments, radiotherapy is a reasonable alternative. Brachytherapy is now being used in centers to avoid some of the negative aspects of radiation treatment.[61]

Several agents have been used over the years to treat NMSC in situations when other modalities are inappropriate or unavailable. However, there is little data to support therapeutic guidelines of even the most frequently used: methotrexate, 5FU, bleomycin, and interferon.[62] With the advent of new molecular targeted therapy, the development of new topical and systemic drugs may offer exciting new options for limited, widespread, or systemic disease in NMSC.[63]

Mohs Micrographic Surgery for Nonmelanoma Skin Cancers

The final major treatment modality is microscopically controlled surgery, or Mohs micrographic surgery. Mohs surgery addresses several problems that occur with standard tumor excision: the tumor may extend significantly beyond its clinically discernible margins, unidirectionally or through pseudopodial extensions that might be missed clinically or histopathologically.[70] In a Mohs procedure the surgeon does not have to unnecessarily remove even small amounts of normal skin around a tumor in critical locations such as the central face, eyelids, and orbit that might lead to significant cosmetic and/or functional compromise. There are two goals to Mohs micrographic surgery: to remove the tumor with all of its microscopic extensions completely, and to spare as much normal tissue as possible. These two goals are achieved with precise methods of tissue handling and evaluation (Fig. 38-43). The basic procedure involves the following steps:

1. The tumor is debulked with a curette to define its minimal margins (Fig. 38-43, *A*).
2. The tumor is excised with a narrow (approximately 1 mm) margin of normal skin, cut inward at an oblique angle (approximately 45 degrees) at the epidermis (cutting out a pie-shaped piece of tissue) (Fig. 38-43, *B*).
3. The peripheral intact skin edge on the patient is marked with small scores to orient the tissue anatomically (Fig. 38-43, *C*).
4. A map is drawn of the excised tissue and its orientation to the patient.
5. The tissue is cut into appropriately sized pieces for microscopic examination and inked so that when compared with the drawn map and the scores around the defect on the patient, precise correlation may be made between microscopic areas of the tissue and the corresponding area of the surgical defect that they reflect (Fig. 38-43, *D*).
6. While the tissue is being processed, bleeding is controlled and a temporary bandage is applied to the wound (Fig. 38-43, *E*).
7. The cut and inked pieces of tissue are mounted by the histotechnician in a manner that allows the entire bottom or undersurface of the piece and its peripheral epidermal edge to be examined. Thus the true surgical margin (the entire periphery of tissue removed) can be evaluated microscopically (Fig. 38-43, *F*).
8. The slides are stained and the surgeon, serving as pathologist, evaluates the deep and peripheral rim of tissue removed for residual tumor. Areas of tumor are marked on the drawn map (Fig. 38-43, *G*).
9. The Mohs surgeon returns to the patient, correlates the drawn map and marked tumor to the areas of the defect in the patient that they reflect, and removes another layer of skin only in those areas of the defect with remaining tumor, thus sparing areas free of tumor.
10. Steps 2 to 9 are repeated in stages until the entire tumor is removed.

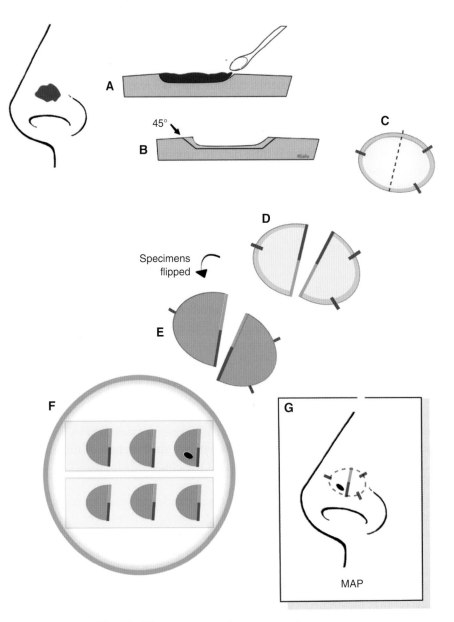

Fig. 38-43   Steps in Mohs micrographic surgery.

Removing a minimal margin around the tumor, followed by inking and orienting the tissue to define exactly where tumor persists (and removing only those areas), permits sparing as much normal tissue as possible. This sparing becomes especially important in cosmetically and functionally important areas. Sparing 3 or 4 mm of tissue near the nasal ala or lacrimal duct can significantly influence outcome. In addition, extirpating the tumor and evaluating it in a manner that permits full examination of the true surgical margin permits theoretically complete elimination of any contiguous tumor. Mohs techniques are generally performed on more aggressive and larger tumors in locations with higher rates of recurrence and the data suggest a better cure rate than with other modalities.

For purposes of analysis of cure rates of different treatment approaches to BCC, one useful distinction is the treatment of primary versus recurrent BCCs. An impressive meta-analysis of the literature, which has

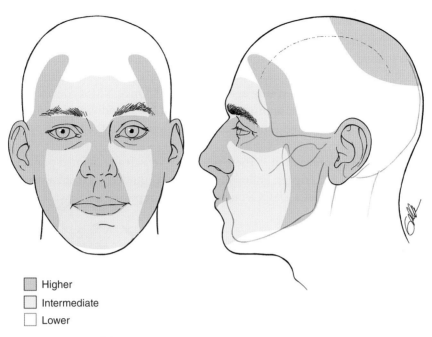

■ Higher
□ Intermediate
□ Lower

Fig. 38-44   The H distribution on the face.

stood the test of time on cure rates of different treatment approaches to primary BCC, demonstrates that tumors treated with non-Mohs modalities had a short-term (less than 5 years) recurrence rate approximately three times higher than tumors treated with Mohs micrographic surgery, which had a 1.4% rate. Long-term analysis showed an approximately nine times higher recurrence rate with non-Mohs treatment than with Mohs techniques.[71]

A further meta-analysis by the same group looked at outcomes of treatment of recurrent BCC. As expected, recurrence rates with all treatment modalities were significantly higher. Long-term recurrence rate for Mohs was 5.6%, compared with an aggregate of 19.9% with other modalities.[72]

Mohs surgery should be strongly considered as treatment for high-risk tumors. These include tumors in high-risk areas such as the H-zone of the face (Fig. 38-44), tumors with aggressive histologic findings (such as morpheic), large tumors, tumors with ill-defined clinical borders, and recurrent or incompletely excised tumors.[73]

Multidisciplinary Approach to Basal Cell Carcinoma Treatment

The aim of Mohs micrographic surgery is tumor extirpation. The Mohs surgeon aims to remove the tumor completely, separately from considerations of reconstruction. When BCC invades structures not easily amenable to its horizontal frozen section technique (such as bone, sinuses, or orbit), the Mohs surgeon works closely with the appropriate surgical specialist to establish cutaneous tumor-free margins and orient the surgical specialist to the location of deeper invasion. Further, for high-risk BCCs, the Mohs surgeon may collaborate closely with a reconstructive surgeon by reliably eliminating the tumor before complex reconstruction. The reconstructive surgeon may be reasonably confident that (1) cosmetically or functionally important structures not involved by tumor are left intact, (2) those same structures are removed when tumor extends into them, and (3) that the repair is not covering persistent tumor with a complex flap or graft.

CONCLUSION

NMSC is the most common cutaneous neoplasm. There is a strong relationship between exposure by genetically susceptible individuals to UV light and development of the tumor. Given this important and well-documented environmental risk, the optimal approach to it is prevention. Use of sunscreens and avoidance of intense sun exposure beginning at a young age are essential. Once NMSC develops, there are several reasonable approaches to treatment. The appropriate treatment for an individual tumor should be tailored to the patient as well as specific histologic and clinical characteristics of the tumor.

The best treatment for NMSC is prevention.[74] These tumors have a clearly defined population at risk, and a clear and avoidable environmental trigger. Following "sunsense" guidelines from a young age could theoretically influence the epidemic of BCCs/SCCs currently being reported worldwide (Box 38-11).

Box 38-11   Sunsense Guidelines

1. Use sunscreens daily, all year round.
   a. Apply 30 minutes before going outside.
   b. Reapply every 2 hours while outside.
   c. Use an SPF of 30 or above.
   d. Choose a broad spectrum that covers both UVA and UVB.
2. Wear broad-brimmed hats.
3. Wear sunglasses.
4. Wear sun-protective clothing.
5. Avoid the sun between the hours of 10:00 AM and 4:00 PM.
6. *Do not sunburn.*

KEY POINTS

- Neoplasms may be benign or malignant and are often difficult to distinguish clinically. Do not hesitate to biopsy a lesion that gives you or a patient any concern.
- Nonmelanoma skin cancers are the most common neoplasm in white individuals. Approximately 85% will occur on the head and neck.
- Treatment of a basal cell or squamous cell carcinoma should be individualized depending on several characteristics, including histologic subtype, location, and size.
- Mohs surgery has appropriate use criteria formulated by the American Academy of Dermatology, American College of Mohs Surgery, American Society for Dermatologic Surgery Association, and the American Society for Mohs Surgery.
- There is an exponential increase in many cutaneous benign and malignant lesions in our ever-increasing immunosuppressed population.

REFERENCES

1. Mohs FE. Chemosurgery: a microscopically controlled method of cancer excision. Arch Surg 42:279-295, 1941.

2. Tromovitch TB, Stegman SJ. Microscopically controlled excision of skin tumors. Arch Dermatol 110:231-232, 1974.

3. Del Rosso JQ. Current regimens and guideline implications for the treatment of actinic keratosis: proceedings of a clinical round table at the 2011 Winter Clinical Dermatology Conference. Cutis 88(Suppl):S1-S8, 2011.

4. Brodsky J. Management of benign skin lesions commonly affecting the face: actinic keratosis, seborrheic keratosis, and rosacea. Curr Opin Otolaryngol Head Neck Surg 17:315-320, 2009.

5. Jadot YT, Schwartz RA. Solar cheilosis: an ominous precursor: Part II. Therapeutic perspectives. J Am Acad Dermatol 66:187-198, 2012.

6. Polder KD, Landau J, Vergilis-Kalner I, et al. Laser eradication of pigmented lesions: a review. Dermatol Surg 37:572-595, 2001.

7. Brandling-Bennett HA, Morel KD. Epidermal nevi. Pediatr Clin North Am 57:1177-1198, 2010.

8. Pattee S, Silvis N. Keratoacanthoma developing in sites of previous trauma: a report of two cases and review of the literature. J Am Acad Dermatol 48(2 Suppl):S35-S38, 2003.

9. Karaa A, Khachemune A. Keratoacanthomas: a tumor in search of a classification. Int J Dermatol 46:671-678, 2007.

10. DiMaio D, Cohen P. Trichilemmal horn: case presentation and literature review. J Am Acad Dermatol 39:368-371, 1998.

11. Argenziano G, Fabbrocini G, Carli P, et al. Epiluminescence microscopy for the diagnosis of doubtful melanocytic skin lesions: comparison of the ABCD rule of dermatoscopy and a new 7-point checklist based on pattern analysis. Arch Dermatol 134:1563-1570, 1998.

12. Hirokawa D, Lee JB. Dermatoscopy: an overview of subsurface morphology. Clin Dermatol 29:557-565, 2001.

13. Annessi G, Bono R, Sampogna F, et al. Sensitivity, specificity, and diagnostic accuracy of three dermoscope algorithmic methods in the diagnosis of doubtful melanocytic lesions. J Am Acad Dermatol 56:759-767, 2007.

14. Duffy K, Grossman D. The dysplastic nevus: from historical perspective to management in the modern era: part I. Historical, histologic, and clinical aspects. J Am Acad Dermatol 67:e1-e16, 2012.

15. Duffy K, Grossman D. The dysplastic nevus: from historical perspective to management in the modern era: part II. Molecular aspects and clinical management. J Am Acad Dermatol 67:e1-e12, 2012.

16. Alikihan A, Ibrahimi OA, Eisen D. Congenital melanocytic nevi: where are we now? Part I. Clinical presentation, epidemiology, pathogenesis, histology, malignant transformation, and neurocutaneous melanosis. J Am Acad Dermatol 67:495-511, 2012.

17. Alikihan A, Ibrahimi OA, Eisen D. Congenital melanocytic nevi: where are we now? Part II. Treatment options and approach to treatment. J Am Acad Dermatol 67:515-627, 2012.

18. Park JM, Tsao H, Tsao S. Acquired bilateral nevus of Ota-like macules (Hori nevus): etiologic therapeutic considerations. J Am Acad Dermatol 61:88-93, 2009.

19. Kanitakis J. Adnexal tumors of the skin as markers of cancer-prone syndromes. J Euro Acad Dermatol Venereol 24:379-387, 2010.

20. Aguayo R. Squamous cell carcinoma developing in Jadassohn's sebaceous nevus: case report and review of the literature. Dermatol Surg 36:1763-1768, 2010.

21. Sidle DM, Kim H. Keloids: prevention and management. Facial Plast Surg Clin North Am 19:505-515, 2011.

22. Shatter JJ, Taylor SC, Cook-Bolden F. Keloidal scars: a review with a critical look at therapeutic options. J Am Acad Derm 46(2 Suppl Understanding):S63-S97, 2002.

23. DiKhimpar JC, Murray MA. Keloids treated with excision followed by radiation therapy. J Am Acad Dermatol 31:225-231, 1994.

24. Borkowska J, Schwartz RA, Kotulskak, et al. Tuberous sclerosis complex: tumors and tumorigenesis. Int J Dermatol 50:13-20, 2011.

25. Moncrieff M, Sassoon EM. Effective treatment of chondrodermatitis nodularis helicis using a conservative approach. Br J Dermatol 150:892-894, 2004.

26. Salasche SJ, McCullough ML, Angeloni V, et al. Frontalis-associated lipomas of the forehead. J Am Acad Dermatol 20:462-468, 1989.

27. Lear W, Dahkle E, Murray CA. Basal cell carcinoma: review of epidemiology, pathogenesis, and associated risk factors. J Cutan Med Surg 11:19-30, 2007.

28. Hollmig ST, Sachdev R, Cockerell CJ, et al. Spindle cell neoplasms encountered in dermatologic surgery: a review. Dermatol Surg 38:825-850, 2012.

29. Lee DA, Stanley JM. Nonmelanoma skin cancer. Facial Plast Surg Clin N Am 17:309-324, 2009.

30. Armstrong BK, Kricher A. The epidemiology of UV induced skin cancer. J Photochem Photobiol B 63:8-18, 2001.

31. American Cancer Society. Cancer Facts and Figures 2012. Available at: *www.cancer.org/Research/CancerFacts-Figures/CancerFactsFigures/2012-cancer-facts-and-figures.pdf.*

32. Bulliard JL, Panizzon RG, Levi F. [Epidemiology of epithelial skin cancer] Rev Med Suisse 5:882, 884-888, 2009.

33. Bentham G, Aase A. Incidence of malignant melanoma of the skin in Norway, 1955-1989: associations with solar ultraviolet radiation, income and holidays abroad. Internatl J Epidemiol 25:1132-1138, 1996.

34. Berg D, Otley CC. Skin cancer in organ transplant recipients: epidemiology, pathogenesis, and management. J Am Acad Dermatol 47:1-17, 2002.

35. Richmond-Sinclair NM, Pandeya N, Ware RS, et al. Incidence of basal cell carcinoma and detailed anatomic distribution: longitudinal study of an Australian population. J Invest Dermatol 129:323-328, 2009.

36. Salasche SJ, Amonette RA. Morpheaform basal-cell epitheliomas. A study of subclinical extensions in a series of 51 cases. J Dermatol Surg Oncol 7:387-394, 1981.

37. Sexton M, Jones DB, Maloney ME. Histologic pattern analysis of basal cell carcinoma: study of a series of 1039 consecutive neoplasms. J Am Acad Dermatol 23:1118-1126, 1990.

   This article separated the various forms of basal cell carcinoma seen histologically and heralded the era in which the behavior of the various types were studied and found to be different. This has significant impact on the choice of treatment modality. All pathology reports should subtype a basal cell carcinoma to provide the physician and the patient with necessary information to choose the best therapy.

38. Bumpous J. Metastatic cutaneous squamous cell carcinoma to the parotid and cervical lymph nodes: treatment and outcomes. Curr Opin Otolaryngol Head Neck Surg 17:122-125, 2009.

39. Alam M, Ratner D. Cutaneous squamous-cell carcinoma. N Engl J Med 344:975-983, 2001.

40. Martin G. The impact of the current United States guidelines on the management of actinic keratosis: is it time for an update? J Clin Aesthet Dermatol 3:20-25, 2010.

41. Criscione VD, Weinstock MA, Naylor MF, et al. Actinic keratosis: natural history and risk of malignant transformation in the Veterans Affairs Topical Tretinoin Chemoprevention Trial. Cancer 115:2523-2530, 2009.

42. Geist DE, Garcia-Moliner M, Fitzek MM, et al. Perineural invasion of cutaneous squamous cell carcinoma: raising awareness and optimizing management. Dermatol Surg 34:1642-1651, 2008.

43. Toker C. Trabecular carcinoma of the skin. Arch Dermatol 105:107-110, 1972.

44. Nghiem P, Jaimes N. Merkel cell carcinoma. In Wolff K, Goldsmith LA, Katz SI, et al, eds. Fitzpatrick's Dermatology in General Medicine, ed 7. New York: McGraw-Hill Professional, 2008.

45. Donepudi S, DeConti RC, Samlowski WE. Recent advances in the understanding of the genetics, etiology, and treatment of Merkel cell carcinoma. Semin Oncol 39:163-172, 2012.

46. Heath M, Jaimes N, Lemos B, et al. Clinical characteristics of Merkel cell carcinoma at diagnosis in 195 patients: the AEIOU features. J Am Dermatol 58:375-381, 2008.

47. Howle JR, Hughes M, Gebski B, et al. Merkel cell carcinoma: an Australian perspective and the importance of addressing the regional lymph nodes in clinically node-negative patients. J Am Acad Dermatol 67:33-40, 2012.

48. Nicolaidou E, Mikrova A, Antoniou C, et al. Advances in Merkel cell carcinoma pathogenesis and management: a recently discovered virus, a new international consensus staging system and new diagnostic codes. Br J Dermatol 166:16-21, 2012.

49. Angouridakis N, Panagiotis K, Waseem J, et al. Dermatofibrosarcoma protuberans with fibrosarcomatous transformation of the head and neck. Head Neck Oncol 3:1-7, 2011.

50. Iorizzo LJ, Brown MD. Atypical fibroxanthoma: a review of the literature. Dermatol Surg 37:146-157, 2011.

51. Withers AH, Brougham ND, Barber RM, et al. Atypical fibroxanthoma and malignant fibrous histiocytoma. J Plastic Reconstr Aesthet Surg 64:e273-e278, 2011.

52. Saeed S, Keehn CA, Morgan MB. Cutaneous metastasis: a clinical, pathological, and immunohistochemical appraisal. J Cutan Pathol 31:419-430, 2004.

53. Diamantis SA, Marks VJ. Mohs micrographic surgery in the treatment of microcystic adnexal carcinoma. Dermatol Clin 29:185-190, 2011.

54. Zwald FO, Brown M. Skin cancer in solid organ transplant recipients: advances in therapy and management: part 1. Epidemiology of skin cancer in solid organ transplant recipients. J Am Acad Derm 65:253-261, 2011.

>   *Today's immunocompromised patients, who are either transplant recipients or receiving new biologics, are challenging current detection and treatment methods with both local and metastatic occurrence of once extremely rare cutaneous neoplasms. This article summarizes some of the current approaches to this rapidly expanding patient population.*

55. McCoppin HH, Christiansen D, Stasko T, et al. Clinical spectrum of atypical fibroxanthomas and undifferentiated pleomorphic sarcoma in solid organ transplant recipients: a collective experience. Dermatol Surg 38:230-239, 2012.

56. Kokoszka A, Scheinfeld N. Evidence-based reviews of the use of cryosurgery in treatment of basal cell carcinoma. Dermatol Surg 29:566-571, 2003.

57. Love WE, Bernhard JD, Bordeaux JS. Topical imiquimod or fluorouracil therapy for basal and squamous cell carcinoma: a systematic review. Arch Dermatol 145:1431-1438, 2009.

58. Lien MH, Sondak VK. Nonsurgical treatment options for basal cell carcinoma. J Skin Cancer 2011:1-6, 2011.

59. MacFarlane DF, El Tal AK. Cryoimmunotherapy: superficial basal cell cancer and squamous cell carcinoma in situ treated with liquid nitrogen followed by imiquimod. Arch Dermatol 147:1326-1327, 2011.

60. Silverman MK, Kopf AW, Grin CM, et al. Recurrence rates of treated basal cell carcinomas. Part 2: Curettage-electrodesiccation. J Dermatol Surg Oncol 17:720-726, 1991.

61. Alam M, Nanda S, Mittal BB, et al. The use of brachytherapy in the treatment of nonmelanoma skin cancer: a review. J Am Acad Dermatol 65:377-388, 2011.

62. Kirby JS, Miller CJ. Intralesional chemotherapy for nonmelanoma skin cancer: a practical review. J Am Acad Dermatol 63:689-702, 2010.

63. Kudchadkar R, Lewis K, Gonzalez R. Advances in the treatment of basal cell carcinoma: hedgehog inhibitors. Semin Oncol 39:139-144, 2012.

64. Braathen LR, Szeimies RM, Basset-Seguin N, et al. Guidelines on the use of photodynamic therapy for nonmelanoma skin cancer: an international consensus. J Am Acad Dermatol 56:125-143, 2007.

65. Willey A, Metha S, Lee PK. Reduction in the incidence of squamous cell carcinoma in solid organ transplant recipients treated with cyclic photodynamic therapy. Dermatol Surg 36:652-658, 2010.

66. Choudhary S, Tang J, Elsaie ML, et al. Lasers in the treatment of nonmelanoma skin cancers. Dermatol Surg 37:409-425, 2011.

67. Chiller K, Passaro D, McCalmont T, et al. Efficacy of curettage before excision in clearing surgical margins of nonmelanoma skin cancer. Arch Dermatol 136:1327-1332, 2000.

68. Gulleth Y, Goldberg N, Silverman RP, et al. What is the best surgical margin for a basal cell carcinoma: a meta-analysis of the literature. Plast Reconstr Surg 126:1222-1231, 2010.

69. Bailey JS, Goldwasser MS. Surgical management of facial skin cancer. Oral Maxillofac Surg Clin North Am 17:205-233, 2005.

70. Tromovitch TA, Stegman SJ. Microscopic-controlled excision of cutaneous tumors: chemosurgery, fresh tissue technique. Cancer 41:653-658, 1978.

71. Rowe DE, Carroll RJ, Day CL. Long-term recurrence rates in previously untreated (primary) basal cell carcinomas: implications for patient follow up. J Dermatol Surg Oncol 15:315-328, 1989.

72. Rowe DE, Carroll RJ, Day CL. Mohs surgery is the treatment of choice for recurrent (previously treated) basal cell carcinoma. J Dermatol Surg Oncol 15:424-431, 1989.

73. Ad Hoc Task Force. AAD/ACMS/ASMS 2012 appropriate use criteria for Mohs micrographic surgery: a report of the American Academy of Dermatology, American College of Mohs Surgery, American Society for Dermatologic Surgery Association, and the American Society for Mohs Surgery. JAAD 67:531-550, 2012.

>   *A complete guide to Mohs surgery and its current approved use.*

74. van der Pols JC, Goldberg N, Silverman RP, et al. Prolonged prevention of squamous cell carcinoma of skin by regular sunscreen use. Cancer Epidemiol Bimarkers Prev 15:2546-2548, 2006.

39

Melanoma of the Head and Neck

Audrey Baker Erman ▪ *Kevin S. Emerick*

Melanoma is the most lethal of the skin cancers. Despite decades of dedicated research, community education platforms, and outreach, melanoma remains one of the few solid organ tumors without demonstrable advances in treatment and survival over the past four decades. The only current cure for melanoma is surgical extirpation; small gains in overall survival have been made because of increased identification and diagnosis of early stage, surgically resectable tumors.

Significant changes have occurred over the years regarding management of the lymph nodes, elective lymph node dissection, and sentinel node biopsy. Historically, head and neck melanoma has been managed by surgical oncologists who trained through general surgery pathways. Today there are a growing number of dedicated head and neck surgical oncologists whose familiarity with head and neck anatomy and experience with the lymphadenectomy procedures that are needed to best manage head and neck melanoma have contributed to improved care. There is now wide acceptance of sentinel lymph node biopsy in head and neck melanoma, although early reports suggested it was not as reliable in the head and neck as in other parts of the body.

From an anatomic, epidemiologic, and prognostic perspective, head and neck melanoma differs substantially from melanoma at other sites, leading some to consider head and neck melanoma as a distinct disease process (Fig. 39-1). For example, compared with melanoma at other sites, there are significant differences in risk factor assessment, age of patient at diagnosis, ultraviolet radiation exposure history, and prognosis.

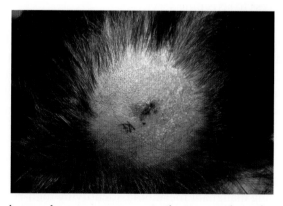

Fig. 39-1 Head and neck melanoma has an appearance similar to any other subsite on the body. However, it may have a unique behavior; scalp melanoma in particular may have a higher risk of metastasis and death.

EPIDEMIOLOGIC FACTORS

INCIDENCE

The incidence of cutaneous melanoma has been rising consistently in countries with white populations, at an annual increase of 3% to 7%,[1,2] and represents the most rapidly increasing cancer in white populations.[3] Australia and New Zealand have the highest incidence rates of melanoma in the world: up to 60 per 100,000 population.[4] In the United States, cutaneous melanoma is currently the fifth most commonly diagnosed cancer in men and the seventh in women.[5]

The lifetime risk of developing invasive melanoma has been steadily increasing.[6] One in 1500 individuals born in 1935 will develop malignant melanoma, whereas individuals born in 2010 have a lifetime probability of developing melanoma of 1 in 39 for men and 1 in 58 for women.[7] Trends in overall cancer rates have declined in the United States, yet melanoma remains one of the few with an increasing incidence.[7] In other countries this trend has been stabilizing in recent years,[8-10] perhaps as a result of primary prevention efforts.[11]

Melanoma incidence is dependent on race, age, and sex. White individuals have the highest rates globally, and in the United States whites have a lifetime risk of developing melanoma that is nearly 23 times higher than that of black individuals.[5] Incidence rises with age, and at a faster rate in men. Women have a slightly higher risk before the age of 40, after which men have a higher incidence. For men, the risk rises dramatically during life, eclipsing women at age 40 and doubling that of women by age 85.[12] Although pediatric melanoma is rare, its incidence has also increased by an average of 2% per year over the past 30 years.[13]

It is unclear why the incidence of melanoma is increasing. In the late 1920s, Coco Chanel popularized sunbathing with her famous words, "A girl simply has to be tanned." This social trend plus changes in the environment may cause increased ultraviolet (UV) exposure. Indoor tanning likely increases the risk of melanoma, in a dose-response relationship.[14] Climate change and ozone depletion have also been implicated in rising rates.[15-18] With heightened community outreach and education about skin cancers there has been a significant rise in the number of cases diagnosed, leading some to propose that the observed elevation in incidence is not a biological change, but instead represents increased identification patterns.[19,20] Expanded screening for melanoma may lead to the detection of thinner, less aggressive lesions.[20] A recent study identified the greatest incidence increase in individuals with the lowest socioeconomic status, who theoretically have the least access to screening services.[21]

Histologic interpretations may also lead to falsely elevated incidence rates.[22] Lesions previously described as benign melanocytic nevi may now be reclassified as early stage I melanoma by some pathologists, a phenomenon labeled *diagnostic drift*.[23] Although these findings clarify the increased incidence in melanoma, they do not explain increasing mortality rates. Although melanoma is only 4% of all cutaneous malignancies, it is responsible for more than 70% of skin cancer–related deaths,[5,7,24] and mortality is rising.[1]

RISK FACTORS

The interplay between a patient's inherent susceptibility to UV radiation and the amount of sun exposure determine the risk of developing malignant melanoma. Identifying high-risk individuals is important in tailoring public health efforts. These risk factors are summarized in Box 39-1.

Box 39-1   Risk Factors for Cutaneous Melanoma

Genetic Factors
Susceptibility genes: *CDKN2A, CDK4, MC1R*
Family history: first-degree relative with melanoma, atypical mole syndrome
Personal history of melanoma

Phenotypic Characteristics
Fair skin with inability to tan
Light or blue eyes
Red or blond hair

Nevi
Giant congenital nevus: greater than 5% of total body surface area
Common nevi: more than 100 (any size)
More than three dysplastic nevi

Environmental Factors
Solar UV radiation
Artificial UV radiation (tanning beds)

Genetic Factors

There is a strong genetic tendency for some individuals to develop melanoma, with approximately 5% of all cutaneous melanomas arising in patients with a family history of melanoma. Nomenclature has evolved over the years to accurately describe families with a higher than normal incidence of melanoma. First described by Clark as the "B-K mole syndrome,"[25] it is now referred to as *familial atypical mole-melanoma syndrome* (FAM-M),[26] or simply *dysplastic nevus* or *atypical mole* syndrome. The syndrome is inherited in an autosomal dominant fashion, and family members have multiple large moles that may vary in size and color. Patients have a lifetime cumulative incidence of melanoma of nearly 100%.[27] The most common mutation associated with familial melanoma is *CDKN2A,* or p16, an important regulator of cell cycle entry.[28] Multiple other chromosomal mutations have been identified in families prone to melanoma, although most families with cutaneous melanoma remain without a specific genetic diagnosis.[29]

Xeroderma pigmentosa is an autosomal recessive disease in which fibroblasts have a limited ability to repair DNA damaged by ultraviolet radiation.[30] Patients develop multiple cutaneous malignancies, including melanoma, basal cell carcinoma, and squamous cell carcinoma. Many patients are diagnosed with their first cancer before adolescence and die from the disease at a young age.[31]

Pigment Characteristics and Nevi

A patient's inherent susceptibility to the sun is a more significant risk factor than the amount of sun exposure. Melanin acts as a natural sunscreen and is a highly conjugated molecule produced by melanosomes in the basal layer of the dermis. High degrees of conjugation in both melanin and in commercially based chemical sunscreens allow UV energy to dissipate as kinetic energy. The risk of developing melanoma is strongly tied to skin pigmentation. Variation in skin color is based on the distribution of melanin within keratinocytes rather than the absolute number of melanosomes.[32] Melanin is located in supranuclear "caps" over surrounding keratinocytes, acting as an endogenous sunscreen by protecting the nucleus and enclosed DNA from environmental UV exposure.[33]

Pigmentary characteristics of the skin have long been associated with melanoma risk, with light skin color and high freckle density as significant risk factors.[34] In studies of multiethnic populations in a single environment, melanoma rates are 5 to 10 times higher in non-Hispanic whites than in Hispanic whites, and Hispanic white individuals have twice the risk of black individuals.[35] Hair and eye color are also noted as independent risk factors and are considered markers for skin phenotypes.[36,37]

Any single benign-appearing nevus may progress to malignant melanoma, but the overall risk is low. The lifetime risk of transformation of any selected mole into melanoma is 0.03% for men and 0.009% for women.[38] Patients with increased numbers of benign nevi are at increased risk of melanoma, but not because of each individual nevi's risk of transformation. Rather, the number of benign nevi acts as a surrogate marker for overall UV-induced skin damage, causing both the development of benign nevi and malignant melanoma as two distinct events.

Although the risk of transformation of benign-appearing nevi is low, the absolute number of benign-appearing nevi is an important predictive factor in determining melanoma risk. Patients with 50 to 100 nevi are at increased risk of developing melanoma, with a relative risk of 5/17.[39] This may not apply to the development of head and neck melanoma. A pooled analysis of case-control studies showed increasing numbers of nevi associated with trunk and extremity melanoma, but not melanoma of the head and neck.[40]

Patients with head and neck melanoma often have a different clinical history from those who have melanoma at other body sites. Melanomas developing on the trunk or extremities are often in a background of minimally sun-damaged skin in a patient with large numbers of benign nevi. Head and neck melanoma has more similarity to melanoma developing on the back of the hands: patients are older and the lesion develops in the setting of previous nonmelanoma skin cancers and sun-damaged skin. Whiteman[37] hypothesized two divergent pathways to melanoma. Individuals with large numbers of nevi may require less UV radiation to induce carcinogenesis in melanocytes and will develop melanomas on less sun-exposed sites, such as the trunk or legs. Individuals without large numbers of nevi are hypothesized to require more UV-induced injury before developing melanoma and will do so only on sun-exposed sites such as the head and neck. Pigmentary characteristics such as skin, hair, and eye color do not differ among body sites, which further supports this hypothesis.[41,42]

UV Exposure

After decades of research, the specific mechanisms by which UV radiation causes cutaneous melanoma remains unclear. A substantial body of epidemiologic evidence concludes that UV radiation causes melanoma,[35] and this is strongly supported by animal models.[43] The precise means by which UV radiation causes cutaneous malignant melanoma in humans and its dose-response curve remains elusive.

The sun is the main source of UV exposure for humans, although the ubiquity and heterogeneity of exposure makes this variable difficult to study. Studying patients with nonenvironmental, succinct UV radiation exposure, such as tanning bed use or in patients with psoriasis with UVA treatments, has helped delineate a dose-response curve between UV exposure and the development of melanoma in these two distinct patient populations. The cumulative dose of UV radiation from the sun is best studied by comparing populations at different latitudes. As predicted, the incidence of melanoma is highest in equatorial areas, decreasing proportionately with distance from the equator.[44] Timing of exposure, especially exposure early in life, is particularly important, as demonstrated by migration studies and the incidence of melanoma in Australia. In people who migrated to Australia before the age of 10, skin cancer rates equaled those of native Australians. Immigration after the age of 10 reduced the incidence by threefold.[35]

The pattern of exposure is also an important factor in developing melanoma. The literature divides exposure into occupational (chronic) and recreational (intense or intermittent), although there is much overlap between the two groups. Elwood et al[41] systematically reviewed the major case-controlled studies evaluating the incidence of melanoma and sun exposure. A history of multiple severe sunburns was a strong predictor of melanoma risk, especially on parts of the body with only sporadic sun exposure such as the legs or trunk.[45] They also found a small but significant reduction in the risk of melanoma associated with high amounts of occupational exposure, although this may be confounded by high intermittent sun exposure in the low occupational group. Chang et al[43] found occupational exposure to be positively associated with the development of head and neck melanoma, especially at low latitudes, but had no effect on melanoma at other sites.[46]

PREVENTION

It is unclear whether sunscreen prevents melanoma, although it has been shown to prevent nonmelanoma skin cancers. In fact sunscreen use may be positively associated with melanoma development as an independent risk factor,[47,48] although there are no convincing data to support this.

In the only randomized controlled trial of sunscreen use, even over a relatively short period of months regular sunscreen use was able to demonstrate a significant decrease in developing benign nevi, which are a known proxy for melanoma.[49]

CLINICAL CHARACTERISTICS

STAGING AND PROGNOSIS

The most recent version of the American Joint Commission on Cancer (AJCC) staging system was published in October 2009[50,51] (Table 39-1). The mitotic rate of the primary tumor proved to be a powerful indicator of survival and replaces level of invasion for defining T1b melanoma. The increasing acceptance and use of sentinel lymph node biopsy warranted verification of previous criteria for stage III disease. A fivefold increase in patients with stage IV disease provided information about the prognostic value of serum lactate dehydrogenase (LDH) level as an independent marker.

Table 39-1   AJCC 2009 TNM and Staging Categories for Cutaneous Melanoma

Tumor Classification		
T	**Tumor Thickness (mm)**	**Ulceration or Mitoses**
Tis	Melanoma in situ	NA
T1	$\leq$1.00	a: without ulceration and mitoses $<1/mm^2$ b: with ulceration or mitoses $\geq 1/mm^2$
T2	1.01-2.00	a: without ulceration b: with ulceration
T3	2.01-4.00	a: without ulceration b: with ulceration
T4	>4.00	a: without ulceration b: with ulceration

Continued

Table 39-1   AJCC 2009 TNM and Staging Categories for Cutaneous Melanoma—cont'd

Node Classification

N	Number of Metastatic Nodes	Nodal Metastatic Burden
N0	0	NA
N1	1	a: micrometastasis b: macrometastasis
N2	2-3	a: micrometastasis b: macrometastasis c: In transit metastases/satellites without metastatic nodes
N3	4+, or matted nodes, or in transit metastases/satellites with metastatic nodes	

Metastatic Classification

M	Site	Serum LDH
M0	No distant metastases	NA
$M1_a$	Distant skin, subcutaneous, or nodal metastases	Normal
$M1_b$	Lung metastases	Normal
$M1_c$	All other visceral metastases Any distant metastasis	Normal Elevated

Staging for Cutaneous Melanoma

Clinical Staging				Pathologic Staging			
Stage	T	N	M	Stage	T	N	M
0	Tis	N0	M0	0	Tis	N0	M0
IA	T1a	N0	M0	IA	T1a	N0	M0
IB	T1b, T2a	N0	M0	IB	T1b, T2a	N0	M0
IIA	T2b, T3a	N0	M0	IIA	T2b, T3a	N0	M0
IIB	T3b, T4a	N0	M0	IIB	T3b, T4a	N0	M0
IIC	T4b	N0	M0	IIC	T4b	N0	M0
III	Any T	N>N0	M0	IIIA	T1-4a	N1a, N2a	M0
IV	Any T	Any N	M1	IIIB	T1-4b	N1a, N2a	M0
					T1-4a	N1b, N2b, N2c	M0
				IIIC	T1-4b	N1b, N2b, N2c	M0
					Any T	N3	M0
				IV	Any T	Any N	M1

From Balch CM, Gershenwald JE, Soong SJ, et al. Final version of 2009 AJCC melanoma staging and classification. J Clin Oncol 27:6199-6206, 2009.
TNM, Tumor-node-metastasis.

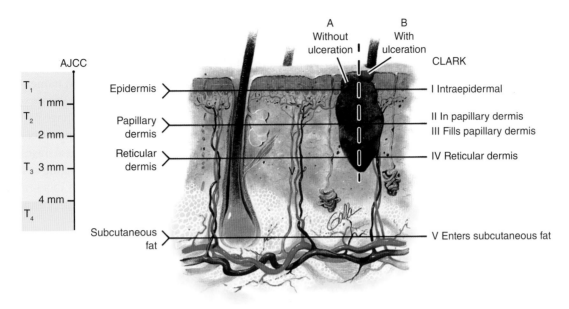

Fig. 39-2   The AJCC system compared with the Clark staging system.

THE AJCC SYSTEM

The AJCC system divides prognostic groups into four stages and is based on evaluations of the primary tumor (T), involvement of regional lymph nodes (N), and distant metastases (M). Staging for melanoma mirrors staging for other types of cancers; patients with localized disease are classified as stage I or II, involvement of regional lymph nodes are stage III, and distant metastatic disease is stage IV (Fig. 39-2).

STAGE I AND II: LOCALIZED MELANOMA

Primary tumor thickness, the presence of ulceration, and the primary tumor mitotic rate are the most powerful predictors of survival in localized melanoma. Tumor thickness was originally described by Breslow and remains an important prognostic factor in localized melanoma.[52] Modified now as even integers of 1.0, 2.0, and 4.0 mm in depth, the T category thresholds remain unchanged from the previous staging system.[53]

Tumor ulceration is defined as the histologic absence of intact epithelium over the melanoma. Ulceration remains an indicator of a biologically aggressive tumor,[54] and is considered one of the most reproducible histologic findings.[55] An ulcerative lesion has similar survival rates as nonulcerated lesions of the next highest T category and is staged accordingly. Primary tumor ulceration has also been shown to retain its prognostic value in patients with lymphatic involvement.[56]

A growing body of evidence points to the mitotic rate as an important prognostic feature,[57-59] prompting evaluation by the AJCC for inclusion in the current staging system. A multivariate analysis of 10,233 patients with stage I or II melanoma identified the mitotic rate of the primary tumor as the second most powerful predictor of survival, after tumor thickness.[51,60] After the mitotic rate and ulceration were included in the evaluation of T1 tumors the level of invasion was no longer statistically significant in predicting survival. Mitotic rate now replaces the level of invasion in defining T1a and T1b categories except in rare cases when mitotic rate is unavailable. First described by Clark in 1969,[57] the tumor's level of invasion has played an important role in melanoma risk stratification. The inclusion of mitotic rate in statistical analyses effectively antiquates Clark's levels of invasion, after 40 years of a prominent role in melanoma staging.[51]

Stage III: Regional Metastatic Melanoma

Sentinel lymph node biopsy has become standard in staging the regional nodal basin in patients with occult metastasis. Since its introduction by Morton in 1992,[61] it has been met with controversy, namely that immediate lymphadenectomy may not offer patients a significant overall survival benefit. Discourse has been especially vocal regarding its use in the head and neck, where complex lymphatic drainage patterns and difficult anatomy are often cited as barriers.[63,64] Despite some dispute, there is increasing agreement that sentinel lymph node biopsy does accurately stage regional nodal basins at risk for metastases and identifies patients who may benefit from total lymphadenectomy. In contrast to previous staging systems the majority of patients now included as stage III were identified as having micrometastasis in a sentinel lymph node. The AJCC Melanoma Staging Committee sought to reevaluate if the stage III inclusion criteria remained appropriate in this setting.

The most predictive independent factors for survival of patients with stage III disease included the number of tumor-bearing nodes, tumor burden, and the presence or absence of primary tumor ulceration.[51] Patients with intralymphatic metastasis continue to have prognoses similar to those with frank nodal metastasis and are included in stage III disease. Survival rates after 5 years vary widely, from 70% for patients with a thin melanoma with micrometastasis to one lymph node to 39% for patients with four or more involved lymph nodes. Patients identified with occult regional metastasis may have a survival benefit with immediate lymphadenectomy.[65]

Metastatic disease to a regional node is the single most important prognostic indicator in early stage melanoma[56] as both the primary predictor of disease recurrence and melanoma-specific death.[65] Given the drastic prognostic implications, accurate histologic staging of the sentinel lymph node is of paramount importance. Immunohistochemical (IHC) markers differ in sensitivity and specificity, and their use varies widely across institutions.[66] To define a positive specimen based on IHC alone, the AJCC Melanoma Staging Committee recommends at least one melanoma-associated marker in the presence of other malignant morphologic features.[51]

Patients with a positive sentinel lymph node will then undergo completion lymphadenectomy. Multiple studies have demonstrated considerably poorer prognosis in patients with additional positive nonsentinel lymph nodes.[67-69]

Stage IV: Distant Metastatic Melanoma

The site of distant metastases and the serum levels of LDH define the three categories of stage IV disease. Patients with metastasis in the skin, subcutaneous tissue, or distant lymph nodes have a 1-year survival rate of 62% and are categorized as M1a. Patients with lung metastasis are categorized as M1b with a 1-year survival rate of 53%. Distant metastasis to any other visceral organ is classified as M1c and has a dismal prognosis of 33% survival rate at 1 year.[51]

Significantly increased numbers of patients with stage IV disease made it possible to recognize elevated serum LDH as an independent and significant predictor of survival. Serum LDH should be measured at the first sign of distant metastatic disease; if this is elevated it delineates patients to the M1c category regardless of metastatic site.

OTHER PROGNOSTIC INDICATORS

Older age confers a poorer prognosis for melanoma survival. Although older patients present with thicker primary tumors, the negative impact remains even after correcting for tumor thickness.[56] Male sex has also been recognized as an independent risk for worse overall survival in some studies.[70]

Melanomas of the head and neck have a worse overall survival than those arising on the extremeties.[56,57,71] This fact holds true for patients with and without regional metastasis, although the site of the tumor was less important than other staging criteria.[56] Head and neck cutaneous melanoma also has a high local recurrence rate[72,73] possibly because of the surgeon's reluctance to violate critical structures in a narrow anatomic field.

Gene expression profiling holds much promise for the development of novel prognostic indicators. Current research suggests that overexpression of the *NCOA3* gene and osteopontin may serve as useful markers for involvement of the sentinel lymph node.[74,75] Future analysis of gene expression in tissue and serum samples may identify further prognostic indicators as we continue to improve our understanding of melanoma at a molecular level.

APPROACH TO STAGING PATIENTS WITH NEWLY DIAGNOSED MELANOMA

For the primary tumor to be staged accurately, patients with newly diagnosed melanoma should undergo complete excisional biopsy of the melanoma with narrow margins.[76] Pathologic examination will determine tumor depth, mitotic rate, and the presence of ulceration. Large lesions may warrant an incisional or punch biopsy, although sampling error may affect staging. Biopsies from multiple sites should be considered in very large lesions. Shave biopsies are discouraged because they obfuscate tumor thickness evaluation.[77]

In patients with clinically negative lymph nodes, performing a sentinel lymph node biopsy is recommended for T2 to T4 melanomas.[51] Sentinel lymph node biopsy may also be considered in patients with melanoma less than 1 mm in diameter, but with worrisome pathologic findings such as ulceration, extensive regression, or high mitotic rate.[78]

Most patients present without symptoms of distant metastasis. For localized melanoma no routine screening tests for metastatic disease are required, although the clinician may order specific tests based on patient history and physical examination.

Imaging is also optional for patients with occult nodal metastasis after a positive sentinel lymph node biopsy, although this may become important as a baseline for staging. Patients with clinically evident stage III disease with nodal or intralymphatic metastasis are at significant risk for distant metastasis. Fine needle aspiration of the node in question can confirm regional spread.[79] Historically, a chest radiograph and serum LDH were obtained routinely for patients with macrometastatic regional disease. PET-CT and brain MRI to assess for distant metastatic disease are now common practice in most institutions.

All patients with stage IV disease need evaluation for systemic disease to guide palliative treatment therapies. Further clinical guidelines for staging newly diagnosed melanoma are maintained by the National Comprehensive Cancer Network (NCCN) and can be found at *www.nccn.org*.[80] A brief algorithm[78] based on our institution's staging practice may be found in Table 39-2.

Table 39-2   Practical Guidelines for Initial Head and Neck Melanoma Evaluation

Stage	Evaluation
Stage 0	History and physical examination, no other tests
Stage I	History and physical examination, consider SLNB for patients with ulceration, high mitotic rate, or other aggressive pathologic features
Stage I-II	History and physical examination, SLNB
Stage III	History and physical examination, FNA neck mass, PET-CT (neck, chest, abdomen), brain MRI
Stage IV	History and physical examination, PET-CT (neck, chest, abdomen), brain MRI

CT, Computed tomography; *FNA,* fine needle aspiration; *MRI,* magnetic resonance imaging; *PET,* positron emission tomography; *SLNB,* sentinel lymph node biopsy.

UNKNOWN PRIMARY

Patients presenting with nodal disease in the absence of a primary tumor may be assumed to have regional metastatic disease. Local metastases to the skin or subcutaneous tissues should also be considered as regional stage III disease. Survival of patients is similar to or slightly better compared with those with known primary tumors of the same stage.[81,82]

HISTOLOGIC FEATURES

There are several different well-described histologic subtypes, although histologic subtype loses significance once one considers well-known prognostic variables such as thickness, ulceration, and sentinel lymph node biopsy status.[83]

COMMON HEAD AND NECK MELANOMA SUBTYPES

Superficial spreading melanoma is the most common melanoma type, accounting for approximately 70% of all cases. Superficial spreading melanoma frequently arises within a preexisting nevus and is recognized when an existing nevus that has been present for decades undergoes a change. It has a characteristic color variation that is often haphazard in appearance with areas of black, dark brown, tan, and blue-gray. Additionally, tumor regression can lead to areas of hypopigmentation that appear pink and white. These lesions are typically well circumscribed with scalloped and somewhat asymmetric borders.

Nodular melanoma is the second most common subtype in the head and neck, accounting for 15% to 30% of cases. These lesions have a characteristic blue-black or blue-red appearance. As the name nodular implies, they usually appear as a raised nodule. They are typically thick and even palpable, unlike most pigmented lesions. These lesions can be difficult to distinguish from a hemangioma, blue nevus, pyogenic granuloma, and pigmented basal cell carcinoma. Given such a differential it is important to biopsy these lesions to confirm diagnosis.

Lentigo maligna melanoma (LMM) is the final common type of melanoma seen in the head and neck. It is more common in older individuals and seems to occur in areas of chronic sun damage. LMM can present diagnostic and treatment challenges. LMM is thought to arise from lentigo maligna (LM), which is a precancerous lesion and for practical purposes is synonymous with melanoma in situ because it remains confined to the dermis. The percentage of LM lesions that will progress to LMM is unknown; however, most experts believe that given enough time, all LM would progress to LMM. Therefore LM lesions require excision. Determining the extent of the lesion can be challenging because this subtype is well known for is subclinical spread. A Woods light can often be helpful in detecting this subclinical spread to identify the borders of the lesion and ultimately achieve a clear margin. Additionally, atypical junctional melanocytic hyperplasia is often present extensively at the borders of these lesions. The malignant potential of this hyperplasia is less well defined, but to be cautious the surgeon should consider this to be precancerous and obtain a clear margin beyond this tissue.

Desmoplastic melanoma is a rare type of melanoma that warrants special attention. It is only 1% to 2% of all melanomas; however, 75% of these lesions occur in the head and neck region.[83] These lesions are typically firm, fibrous subcutaneous lesions that may not initially raise suspicion for melanoma. They typically lack the ABCDE (*a*symmetry, *b*order, *c*olor, *d*iameter, *e*volving) criteria for melanoma, and up to 75% of them are amelanotic and mistaken for a basal cell carcinoma. These lesions are known to be locally aggressive with an infiltrative pattern, which makes obtaining a clear margin difficult without the assistance of an experienced dermatopathologist. Histologically, they are composed of spindle cells and abundant collagen. Despite such an infiltrating nature and increased thickness at presentation they appear to have a lower propensity for regional lymphatic spread.[84] Another distinguishing feature is a subset called desmoplastic-neurotropic melanoma. Unlike all other melanomas, desmoplastic-neurotropic melanoma (as its name suggests) has a unique propensity for perineural spread. Therefore a large number of these will involve cranial nerves and potentially extend to the skull base. There is a local recurrence rate of approximately 50%. Such a high rate has numerous potential explanations, including (1) a delay in diagnosis because of the atypical appearance, allowing for increased subclinical spread, (2) a failure to achieve clear margins because of the challenging nature of identifying this tumor, and (3) neurotropism unique to this subtype, which leads to recurrence along nearby small caliber nerves.

MULTIDISCIPLINARY MANAGEMENT

The management of melanoma can range from very straightforward, requiring only wide local excision, to quite complex, as practitioners consider what margin should be used, the risk of occult disease, and the role of adjuvant treatments. Additionally, the management of melanoma has been evolving over the past several years with the addition of sentinel node biopsy and expanding systemic treatment options. A multidisciplinary team is optimal to best address these questions and to determine the best individualized treatment for each patient. This group should include dermatologists, head and neck surgical oncologists, medical oncologists, radiation oncologists, dermatopathologists, and reconstructive surgeons.

SURGICAL MANAGEMENT OF THE PRIMARY SITE

The standard of care for primary melanoma treatment continues to be surgical excision. Despite some recent advances and changes in the systemic treatments available, surgical excision continues to be the only curative modality. The purpose of wide local excision is twofold. The first goal is to achieve a clear margin around the primary tumor. The second goal is to identify and capture any early satellite lesions or intrinsic metastasis. Because of these considerations, wide margins are needed. Historically, a 4 to 5 cm margin was recommended.[84] However, in the head and neck region this was extremely challenging and not a realistic option in most cases. In the 1970s Breslow and Macht began to challenge this concept by using smaller margins. Since that time there have been several prospective randomized trials investigating appropriate surgical margins for cutaneous melanoma.[85]

The World Health Organization performed an international trial for patients with relatively thin melanomas, less than or equal to 2 mm thick. The patients were randomized to surgical margins of either 1 cm or 3 cm. At a mean follow-up of a year, the disease-free survival and overall survival rates reported between the two groups were equivalent,[86] justifying a 1 cm margin for melanomas 1 mm or less in thickness. A subset analysis of the WHO trial examined 245 patients with tumors measuring 1.1 to 2.0 mm in thickness. In this subgroup there did not appear to be a difference in disease-free survival and overall survival with respect to margins; however, there was a 3.3% local recurrence rate in patients undergoing a more narrow excision.

Based on this study, the Intergroup Melanoma Surgical Trial was initiated, in which 740 patients with intermediate thickness (1 to 4 mm) melanomas were randomized to wide local excision with 2 cm versus 4 cm margins. This study showed equivalent 10-year survival rates and local recurrence rates between these two groups. The recommendation was for a 2 cm margin for patients with intermediate thickness melanomas of 1.1 to 4 mm. However, this study did show that there was a slightly higher recurrence rate in a head and neck subgroup within the larger cohort.

A more recent prospective clinical trial randomized 900 patients with localized melanoma of at least 2 mm in thickness to either a 1 cm or 3 cm margin.[87] They found the survival between these groups to be identical, and there was no statistically significant difference identified between the two groups when considering local, regional, or distant recurrences separately. However, when all recurrences, including local and regional, were pooled together the 1 cm margin group had a statistically higher recurrence rate. Therefore there continues to be debate regarding whether a 1 cm or 2 cm margin should be performed in patients with 1 to 2 mm thick melanoma.

The recommended margin for a thick (greater than 4 mm) melanoma is 2 cm. Unlike other thicknesses, there are no prospective randomized trial data to provide further guidance. A retrospective study of 270 thick melanomas found that surgical margins greater than 2 cm did not lead to a difference in local recurrence rate, disease-free survival, or overall survival.[88]

Achieving clear margins and preventing local recurrence is a key first step in the management of melanoma. Although local recurrences from melanoma excision are typically very low, the consequences are significant. It has been estimated that if ideal margins were achieved 100% of the time, it would lead to a reduction in melanoma-related mortality and increased life expectancy of melanoma patients by 0.4 years. At first glance, this difference appears quite small; however, it equates to an estimated 11 additional years of life expectancy for those individuals who would have had a local recurrence following a 1 cm margin, but instead achieved a disease-free state after a wider surgical margin.

Current excision margin guidelines from the NCCN are summarized in Table 39-3, although there is a caveat for head and neck melanomas. These guidelines state that given the above data, functionally and cosmetically sensitive areas may be considered for a smaller margin. However, the decision to take a smaller margin should be very carefully considered and executed only when unacceptable functional consequences would result from full margins and after a comprehensive discussion with the patient. Additionally, not all margins are considered equal. If one area, such as close to the eyelid, requires a narrower margin the remainder of the circumference of the defect should still undergo the recommended wider margin, particularly if the direction of the expected path of lymphatic or satellite metastasis is in the surgically resectable margins.

The depth of excision should include full thickness of skin and all underlying subcutaneous fat. Ideally, the excision would be carried down to the next layer of underlying fascia, perichondrium, or periosteum. Additionally, these fascial layers should be resected if they were disturbed during a previous excision or biopsy or in the setting of direct invasion of a very thick tumor. In regions such as the scalp, it is straightfor-

Table 39-3   Guidelines for Melanoma Resection Margins

Tumor Thickness (mm)	Recommended Margin (cm)
In situ	0.5
≤1.0	1.0 cm
1.01-2.0	1-2
2.01-4.0	2.0
>4.0	2.0

Adapted from the NCCN 2010 Guidelines.

ward to remove the next fascial layer, the galea; however, in the medial cheek where this next fascial layer is over facial musculature, significant morbidity could arise from the acquisition of such a deep margin.

SURGICAL MANAGEMENT REGIONAL NODES

The surgical management of regional lymph nodes differs according to the patient's presenting lymph node status. When a patient presents with identifiable lymph node metastasis either on clinical examination or on radiographic study, the management of regional lymph nodes is fairly straightforward. However, when a patient presents without identifiable lymphadenopathy, the surgeon must depend on other prognostic information to help predict the risk of occult lymph node metastasis and guide management options, which include observation, sentinel lymph node biopsy, and elective lymphadenectomy.

THERAPEUTIC LYMPH NODE DISSECTION

When a patient presents with identifiable lymph node metastasis, that patient is also at very high risk of distant metastasis. Systemic metastatic staging workup should all be performed, including whole-body PET imaging with neck, chest and abdomen CT, and brain MRI. If there is no evidence of distant metastasis, therapeutic lymph node dissection is the treatment of choice. In this setting, the location of the primary melanoma should be considered. Dissection must include all potential draining lymph node basins and the intervening lymphatics between the primary tumor and the site of regional disease. The location of the primary tumor dictates the specific type of lymphadenectomy to be performed. It is uncommon for melanoma to involve critical structures such as facial nerve branches or other cranial nerves, thus these critical structures can routinely be preserved.

Fig. 39-3 illustrates the expected drainage patterns from different cutaneous areas of the head and neck. Whereas neck dissection for aerodigestive tract squamous cell carcinoma encompasses traditionally established lymph node basin levels 1, 2, 3, 4, and 5, in cutaneous malignancies one must consider additional lymphatic drainage basins, including the fascia encompassing the lateral aspect of the sternocleidomastoid muscle and the external jugular vein. Additionally, the parotid gland and postauricular and suboccipital lymph node basins are relevant areas for potential metastasis. Within level 5 it is common for lymph nodes to be present directly along the spinal accessory nerve, representing a spinal accessory chain.

If an imaginary plane is drawn coronal to the external auditory canal, the structures anterior to this, including the anterior scalp, temple, lateral forehead, lateral cheek, and anterior auricle, will commonly drain to the parotid lymph node basin. The anterior jugular chain, including levels 1, 2, 3, and 4, and the external jugular chain are at risk. When melanoma arises posterior to this coronal plane of the external auditory canal lymph node dissection should include the postauricular and suboccipital basins, and levels 2, 3, 4,

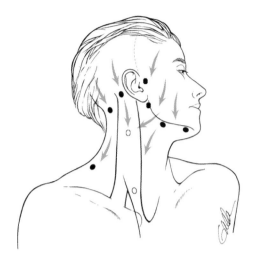

Fig. 39-3   Expected lymphatic drainage patterns from head and neck cutaneous malignancies.

Fig. 39-4   A comprehensive lymphadenectomy for a posterior scalp malignancy needs to include the postauricular nodes, suboccipital nodes, and external jugular vein nodes in lymph node basin levels 2 through 5.

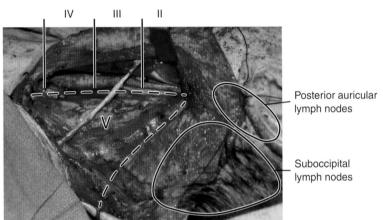

Posterior auricular lymph nodes

Suboccipital lymph nodes

and 5 lymph node basins (Fig. 39-4). Particular attention must be paid to these atypical basins, which are not routinely addressed during aerodigestive tract lymphadenectomy but are of paramount importance in the setting of melanoma. Primary lesions occurring in the most medial part of the cheek, upper and lower lip, and the neck do not routinely drain to the parotid, and dissection should focus on levels 1 through 4 and the perifacial lymph nodes, which run very close to the marginal mandibular nerve and carry a high risk of involvement.

Some current melanoma protocols require a complete lymphadenectomy before enrollment. Therefore comprehensive lymphadenectomy based on the at-risk lymph nodes should always be performed when considering adjuvant treatment.

ELECTIVE LYMPH NODE DISSECTION

Before the introduction of sentinel node biopsy, elective lymphadenectomy was routinely performed for patients without clinically evident disease. Historically, this has been a topic of controversy, because thin melanomas (less than 1 mm in thickness) have an excellent prognosis. Their 5-year survival rate is likely greater than 95% with wide local excision alone, so elective lymph node dissection in this setting is considered to be unnecessary. At the other end of the spectrum, thick melanomas (greater than 4 mm in thickness) have a very poor prognosis and a regional and distant metastasis rate of up to 70%.[89] Therefore there has been debate about the benefit of elective lymphadenectomy since it likely has little impact on survival. However, most feel that these patients will still benefit from elective node dissection by improvement of regional control and a decrease in painful, disfiguring, and uncontrolled regional tumor growth. The greatest controversy surrounds the decision to perform elective lymphadenectomy for patients with intermediate thickness melanomas (1.1 to 3.9 mm). In this population there is a 15% to 20% risk of occult lymph node metastasis, although current data suggest that there is likely limited benefit to elective lymph node dissection.

Between 1967 and 1974, the WHO Melanoma Group studied[90] 535 patients with stage 1 and 2 melanoma of the extremity. No difference in survival benefit was identified between patients who underwent wide local excision and observation compared to patients undergoing wide local excision and elective lymph node dissection. However, subsequent analysis incorporating tumor thickness and ulceration identified a subset of patients with a 22% improved 10-year survival rate with elective lymph node dissection. It is difficult to draw conclusions from this study for head and neck melanoma because there were very few patients with head and neck melanoma enrolled.

A subsequent study involving 740 patients with intermediate thickness tumor (1 to 4 mm)[91] identified ulceration, site, tumor thickness, and age as independent predictors of survival. The overall 5-year survival rates were not different between those undergoing wide local excision or wide local excision with lymph node dissection. However, subset analysis showed a significant survival benefit in patients 60 years of age and younger who underwent elective node dissection when their tumor was not ulcerated and was less than 2 mm in thickness.[92]

In another landmark study[93] of 240 patients with trunk melanomas measuring greater than 1.5 mm in thickness, no statistically significant difference was observed in survival rates between patients randomized to observation versus elective node dissection. Analysis identified only sex and tumor thickness to have a significant impact on survival. However, the study did identify a significant 5-year survival difference for patients with a micrometastasis identified during elective lymph node dissection compared with patients who were randomized to observation and who then developed regional metastasis requiring therapeutic lymph node dissection. This critical finding helped to highlight the potential benefit of identifying microscopic disease and ultimately became an important driver in the development of sentinel lymph node biopsy.

Only 20% of melanoma patients who present with localized disease harbor occult lymph node metastasis. These patients are the critical population to focus on, because they would potentially benefit from early removal of lymph node basins. Adjuvant melanoma therapy may impart a survival benefit in up to half the patients receiving treatment. Therefore detection of regional metastasis is important to help identify patients who should consider starting adjuvant treatment. However, when one considers the power calculations of these statistics, only 25% to 50% of the 20% of patients with occult disease would actually benefit from elective lymph node dissection. Ultimately only 5% to 10% of patients undergoing elective node dissection would have a survival advantage. To detect this small of a difference would require an extremely large clinical trial enrollment, likely numbering several thousand.

All of the studies mentioned here likely did not achieve adequate numbers to detect this difference. For this reason several groups have concluded that the 4% survival benefit observed in the elective lymph node dissection group is clinically significant although statistical significance was not reached.[94]

A last consideration for elective lymph node dissection is a practical one: in the head and neck region, an elective lymph node dissection yields 30 to 50 lymph nodes. The pathologist identifies all lymph nodes within the dissection specimen and assess each one with a single section in hematoxylin and eosin staining. This assessment is likely inadequate for detecting most cases of occult lymph node metastasis, so reports finding no evidence of lymph node metastasis are potentially inaccurate.

In summary, prospective randomized trials do not demonstrate an overall survival benefit for patients undergoing elective lymph node dissection. Therefore routine elective lymph node dissection is not part of current standard practice. Instead, the procedure has been replaced by sentinel node biopsy.

Sentinel Lymph Node Biopsy

Sentinel lymph node biopsy (SLNB) status has now been established as the single most important prognostic factor for melanoma patients.[95] This technique is a minimally invasive, cost effective, efficient, and accurate means of identifying the presence of occult lymph node metastasis in providing critical staging information. Among all melanoma patients 10% to 20% of individuals harbor occult microscopic lymph node metastasis. Morton et al[96] introduced SLNB for the evaluation of patients with trunk and extremity cutaneous melanoma in an attempt to identify the 20% of patients who may have occult microscopic regional spread, so that the other 80% of patients may be spared the morbidity of lymphadenectomy. An important aspect of this early work demonstrated that the sentinel lymph node accurately represents the status in the entire nodal basin from which it is obtained. Early experience with sentinel lymph node biopsy raised questions about the reliability of the procedure in the head and neck region. However, contemporary experience has shown that surgeons with an extensive background in head and neck lymphadenectomy are able to perform sentinel lymph node biopsy with the same sensitivity and specificity as other body sites.

The success of lymph node biopsy is highly dependent on selecting the appropriate patients. Patients presenting with palpable regional disease or distant metastasis should not undergo SLNB because additional prognostic information will not be gained. The SLNB technique has evolved significantly over the past few decades. This evolution has played an important role in increasing the sensitivity and specificity of head and neck SLNB in particular. Initially Morton and other early surgeons used only blue dye to identify the sentinel lymph node. Today, however, preoperative lymphoscintigraphy by nuclear medicine is considered a standard approach to identification of the relevant basins.[97]

Additionally, many institutions have incorporated single photon emission CT (SPECT) (Fig. 39-5). This provides additional anatomic information to plan appropriate incisions and the subsequent surgical course. The procedure begins approximately 2 to 4 hours before surgery; the patient undergoes an intradermal injection of a radioactive colloid into four quadrants surrounding the primary tumor. Lymphoscintigraphy and SPECT are then performed. These preoperative imaging studies can be particularly important in the

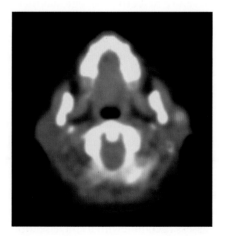

Fig. 39-5   Single photon emission CT helps define the expected three-dimensional location of the sentinel lymph nodes. This can provide important information beyond what can be ascertained from lymphoscintigraphy alone when a surgeon is working in the head and neck region. The node is visible as a red hue on this image.

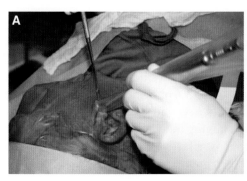
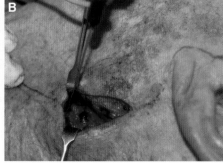

Fig. 39-6   Sentinel lymph node biopsy technique. **A,** Intraoperative use of the handheld probe to guide dissection. **B,** Blue dye can also provide a visual clue during the dissection.

head and neck region, where multiple potential lymph node basins are at risk, including the potential for bilateral drainage as lesions approach or potentially involve the midline.

After preoperative imaging studies, patients undergo intraoperative lymphatic mapping using isosulfan blue dye (Lymphazurin 1%). Dye is injected into the four quadrants of the intradermal layer surrounding the primary melanoma lesion. Most surgeons prefer to perform wide local excision of the primary tumor before performing the sentinel lymph node biopsy. This reduces the phenomenon of radioactive shine through, which can be problematic in the head and neck region because the lymph nodes are often in close proximity to the primary tumor in comparison with other body sites.

The development of the handheld gamma probe in coordination with the preoperative lymphoscintigraphy has contributed to improving the reliability of head and neck SLNB. After wide local excision the probe is used to identify the areas of increased activity (Fig. 39-6).

Information garnered from lymph node mapping, combined with SPECT, is used to plan incisions. One must consider the potential need for future lymph node dissection that may encompass a parotidectomy and anterior neck dissection or posterior neck dissection. Generally, the smallest incision possible should be performed without compromising visualization of critical cranial nerves or compromising the dissection. When working in the parotid region, facial nerve monitoring is routinely used, which is thought to improve safety. Sentinel lymph nodes are identified using a combination of a gamma probe and visual cues from the blue dye. The sentinel node is then dissected from the surrounding tissue, with care not to disrupt the capsule of the node. When a surgeon is working within the parotid gland or close to any cranial nerves, dissection should be performed in the direction of the expected course of the nerve. All lymph nodes registering greater than 10% of the hottest lymph node identified should be removed. The procedure is considered complete when all these nodes have been removed and the background radioactivity is less than 10% of the hottest sentinel node. In the head and neck region 2 or 3 lymph nodes are routinely identified. However, this number may range from a single node to as high as 6 or 7 nodes.

The histopathologic assessment of a sentinel lymph node is much more exhaustive than the assessment that is performed during a standard neck dissection. One standardized approach involves serial sectioning of approximately 5 μm thick sections followed by staining with hematoxylin and eosin.[98] All sentinel lymph nodes that are negative on hematoxylin and eosin staining are then subjected to melanoma-specific IHC staining for S100, melan-A, and MART1. Specific protocols for the IHC staining may vary between institutions and may be dermatopathologist-driven. The sensitivities for S100 and melan-A are greater than 95% and therefore are preferred over HMB45, which carries only 75% sensitivity. Microscopic melanoma would be very difficult to identify on frozen section hematoxylin and eosin staining alone, so frozen section analysis is not recommended. Once this tissue is frozen further IHC staining cannot be performed, and valuable tissue may be lost. Tumor cells may occupy less than 2% of the entire lymph node volume, so rigorous pathologic analysis and interpretation by experienced pathologists is important. The average volume of a positive sentinel lymph node is only 4.7 mm.[99] Several studies highlight the limitation of using hematoxylin and eosin staining alone. In one study only 73% of metastatic sentinel lymph nodes were identified using hematoxylin and eosin staining alone.[100] In a second study 21% of positive sentinel lymph nodes were negative on initial hematoxylin and eosin staining but were identified with further IHC. This type of rigorous histologic analysis is more thorough, cost effective, and complete compared with traditional pathologic assessment of a lymphadenectomy specimen.

Sentinel lymph node biopsy in the head and neck is best performed by a surgeon who is experienced in all head and neck lymphadenectomy techniques, including parotidectomy, neck dissection involving levels 1 through 5, and suboccipital and postauricular lymph node dissection. Several studies have highlighted the importance of surgical experience in the success of SLNB, demonstrating a higher false negative rate for less skilled surgeons. One important lesson from the Multicenter Selective Lymphadenectomy Trial (MSLT-I) was the identification of a 55-case learning curve that was required to achieve at least 95% accuracy with sentinel lymph node biopsy.[101]

Thorough communication with the nuclear medicine team is important. Reviewing the preoperative lymphoscintigraphy and SPECT provides valuable preoperative information to make appropriate incisions to access the at-risk lymph nodes. The corrected lesion must be identified for the nuclear medicine team, because many of these patients no longer have a pigmented lesion remaining after a punch biopsy or excisional biopsy. Other skin lesions and multiple scars can make identification of the primary site difficult for someone not familiar with the patient. Therefore meticulous communication between the surgeon and nuclear medicine team is critical.

Studies have found that the pathologic status of the SLN is the most important prognostic factor for both recurrence and overall survival.[102] For stage III melanoma there is an almost 20% survival benefit in patients with occult microscopic disease compared with a population of patients who, under observation, ultimately developed macroscopic palpable disease. Studies like this have shown a survival benefit to be so compelling that the AJCC has now incorporated SLNB into the staging system.[103]

As previously mentioned, SLNB has long held a defined role in evaluation of melanomas of the trunk and extremities. However, only recently has the same sensitivity and specificity been achieved in the head and neck region. The complexity of the lymphatic system has been repeatedly demonstrated; one study reported a 34% discordance between the clinical prediction of lymphatic drainage and the ultimate findings on lymphoscintigraphy.[104] In addition to this complexity the prospect of injuring important structures, such as the facial nerve or other cranial nerves, has factored into decisions about whether SLNB should be performed.

Regarding morbidity, the removal of head and neck lymph nodes does not cause the same level of lymphedema as it might cause in the axilla or groin. Facial nerve injury has been shown to be extremely low in patients undergoing parotid nodal basin SLNB.[105] In one cohort of 300 patients none sustained facial nerve injury. SPECT can provide preoperative guidance for determining if lymph nodes are adjacent to the parotid gland or if they are in the parotid gland itself; this information can assist in incision planning and appropriate facial nerve monitoring.

Some have suggested that sentinel lymph node biopsy may increase the risk of in-transit metastasis (ITM), a phenomenon that is thought to arise when melanoma cells detach from the primary lesion and become lodged in the dermal plexus of lymphatics.[106] Development of ITM presents a therapeutic challenge and carries a poor prognosis. Original studies suggesting this increased risk were flawed, and a more recent prospective study of more than 4400 patients undergoing wide local excision alone, wide local excision and sentinel lymph node biopsy, and elective neck dissection identified a correlation between ITM and increasing Breslow depth, Clark level, and T stage. It did not identify a statistically significant difference between ITM and tumor recurrence in these treatment groups. Additional studies have concluded that tumor biology, and not surgical procedures, dictates melanoma metastatic behavior.[107] Finally, in a large MSLT-1 study there was no correction identified between ITM and SLNB.

Although the prognostic role of SLNB is clear, its impact on overall survival remains to be determined. At present SLNB is considered the most reliable means of regional staging. It is more sensitive and specific than CT, MRI, PET, elective lymph node dissection, ultrasound, and clinical examination. For appropriately assessed patients SLNB provides important prognostic information to all parties and guides subsequent treatment options. SLNB helps identify patients harboring occult metastasis who may benefit from early therapeutic lymph node dissection and identifies patients who are candidates for adjuvant treatment such as interferon or adjuvant therapy protocols that are currently enrolling patients.

Nonsurgical Therapies
Radiotherapy

Melanoma is a radioresistant tumor. To date, most studies provide no evidence that adjuvant radiation to the primary or regional lymphatics improves survival. A phase II clinical trial found that large-dose hypofractionated radiation can be used as an adjuvant treatment to surgery for head and neck cutaneous melanoma for patients at high risk of local regional recurrence.[108,109] The study showed a local regional control rate of 88% compared with historical control of 50% to 70%. Improved regional control is important because of the significant morbidity that can be induced by uncontrolled local regional disease. Uncontrolled growth can affect quality of life by causing significant pain, complex wound breakdown that requires nursing care, and socially debilitating cosmetic disfiguration.

The most common application of radiotherapy to melanoma is adjuvant treatment after therapeutic lymphadenectomy. In this setting there is a 15% to 20% or greater risk of recurrence. Two recent randomized trials (RTOG93-02 and ECOG3697) performed in United States that examined this use of adjuvant radiotherapy were closed because of nonaccrual.[110] In a phase II study by the Trans Tasman Radiation Oncology Group (TROG)[111] examining adjuvant postoperative radiotherapy after nodal surgery, patients underwent 48 Gy in 20 fractions to the nodal basin. Regional infield relapse was observed in 6.8% of patients, and the overall survival was 36% at 5 years. The progression-free survival and regional control rates were 27% and 91%, respectively, at 5 years. Patients with more than two nodes involved had significantly worse relapse rates overall and for progression-free survival. Another recent study compared observation versus radiation in high-risk patients, as defined by a metastatic node involving the parotid gland, greater than two axillary nodes, greater than three groin nodes, the presence of extracapsular spread, and lymph node size greater than 3 cm. An interim analysis was recently presented and demonstrated no improvement in survival. The infield failure rate was 27% in the observation group and only 18% in the radiotherapy group, with a hazard ratio of 1.8. Current common practice at many academic institutions is that radiotherapy should be considered in patients with extracapsular spread, multiple lymph nodes involved, lymph nodes greater than 3 cm, or any recurrent disease after previous lymph node dissection.

Chemotherapy

Melanoma is a chemoresistant tumor. Historically chemotherapy has played a very limited role in the treatment of melanoma and is usually reserved for the palliative setting. Dacarbazine was the first chemotherapeutic agent to show significant activity against melanoma and is currently the only chemotherapy approved by the FDA for use in melanoma. Despite its approval, the response rate to dacarbazine is quite low, ranging from 10% to 20%. Overall, fewer than 5% of the individuals being treated have a complete response to dacarbazine.[112]

Immunotherapy has shown greater potential than traditional chemotherapeutic agents. Immunotherapy can be considered in two broad categories. The first is specific immunotherapeutic agents that regulate the antibody and cytotoxic T-cell and respond specifically to the patient's tumor or to known melanoma antigens. Most melanoma vaccines fall into this categorization. The other broad category is nonspecific immunotherapeutic agents that stimulate the host immune system without targeting melanoma tumor antigens. This includes interferon (IFN), interleukin, and microbacterial products such as Bacille Calmette-Guerin.

Interferon is the most commonly used agent today. High-dose IFN-alfa 2b is currently the only FDA-approved adjuvant treatment for stage III melanoma. Its mechanism of action includes direct antiproliferative effects, immune stimulation through enhancement of natural killer cells, increased histocompatibility antigen expression on melanoma cells, macrophage phagocytosis, and enhanced T-cell mediated cytotoxicity. Of the different types of IFN (IFN-alfa, IFN-beta, and IFN-gamma), IFN-alfa 2b is the only treatment currently approved for adjuvant treatment of melanoma after surgical treatment. Three large clinical trials involving IFN-alfa 2b have been conducted by the Eastern Cooperative Oncology Group (ECOG). ECOG trial E1684 was the first study to demonstrate the efficacy of IFN-alfa 2b.[113] The regimen consisted of high-dose interferon (20 million units/m^2/d) administered intravenously 5 days per week for 4 weeks. Maintenance treatment was then initiated consisting of 48 weeks of subcutaneous IFN-alfa 2b (10 million units/m^2/d) administered 3 days per week. The prolonged disease-free survival rate and overall survival rate in the treatment in E1684 ultimately led to FDA approval of adjuvant high-dose IFN-alfa 2b.

The follow-up trial, E1690, did not confirm the efficacy of IFN-alfa. However, close inspection of this study shows that there are clinical differences in patients involved in these studies.[114] E1690 did not require pathologic staging with elective lymph node dissection or sentinel node biopsy nor were the patients stratified by ulceration, which we now know are clinically important issues. The most recent ECOG study confirmed the efficacy of high-dose IFN-alfa. The relapse-free and overall survival rates were so significantly improved that the study was terminated early.

IFN-alfa 2b can be challenging to tolerate.[115] Treatment lasts 1 year and almost every individual reports flulike symptoms during the initial treatment course. Severe and intolerable fatigue is reported in 20% to 30% of patients, and an additional 2% to 10% of patients reported neurologic and psychiatric side effects, including depression, anxiety, suicidal ideation, and difficulty with cognition. Patients also require close monitoring for myelosuppression, thyroid dysfunction, and elevated liver enzymes. Almost half of the patients require dose reduction or delay in treatment because of these side effects.

There has been considerable interest in cutaneous melanomas that carry mutations in *BRAF*, which lead to constitutive activation through the MAP kinase pathway. Approximately 40% to 60% of cutaneous melanomas carry this mutation. Vemurafenib is a coinhibitor of mutated *BRAF* and has recently been studied in phase I and phase II trials.[116] These initial studies confirmed a response rate of 53%. More recently, a randomized phase III trial comparing dacarbazine to vemurafenib showed that overall survival was 84% in the vemurafenib group and 64% in the dacarbazine group. Vemurafenib was associated with a 63% relative reduction in the risk of death and 74% in the risk of either death or disease progression compared with dacarbazine.[117]

Subsequent studies have found resistance to therapy with *BRAF* kinase inhibitors. This has led to further investigations using a selective *BRAF* inhibitor and a selective MAP kinase inhibitor. A recent study showed that median progression-free survival in patients receiving combined treatment was 9.4 months compared with 5.8 months in patients receiving monotherapy.[118] In addition, 76% of patients had a complete or partial response compared with only 54% of the patients receiving monotherapy. This will be an area of future interest and investigation.

The second area of recent interest and advancement in systemic treatments has been the introduction of ipilimumab, which blocks the cytotoxic T-lymphocyte associated antigen to potentiate antitumor T-cell response. This drug is now FDA approved. Its initial phase III study examined patients with unresectable stage III or IV melanoma whose disease progressed while they were receiving therapy for metastatic disease.[119] The mean overall survival achieved was 10 months among patients receiving ipilimumab, compared with 6.4 months in patients receiving Gp100 alone. Grade 3 or 4 immune-related adverse events occurred in 10% to 15% of patients. In this study there was a death rate of 2.1%, with half of these attributed to immune-related adverse events. Subsequent studies have begun investigating ipilimumab's use in the adjuvant setting. These studies are reaching accrual and should be available in the near future.

SURVEILLANCE

The primary goals in follow-up of melanoma patients are (1) early detection of local-regional tumor recurrence, (2) early identification of second primary tumors including melanoma and other skin cancers, (3) continuing patient education, and (4) psychological support. Each follow-up visit should include an inquiry into new or changing skin lesions. A review of systems concerning distant metastasis should be performed. A thorough examination of the skin and mucosa is required with particular attention paid to the original melanoma site and associated draining nodal basins. Photo documentation and dermoscopy have proven helpful in monitoring change in patients who have a substantial number of nevi. This vigilant monitoring is particularly important among elderly patients, in whom a change in nevus appearance is more likely to be a melanoma than it is in younger patients. Each follow-up visit should be viewed as an opportunity to reeducate patients on the ABCDE melanoma warning signs and the importance of monthly skin self-examination. Studies have demonstrated that melanoma patients who practice monthly self-examination are diagnosed with thinner lesions at the time of recurrence. Sun education should be discussed, including the use of sunscreen and protective clothing and limiting the duration of exposure.

KEY POINTS

- Sentinel lymph node biopsy is the most important prognostic factor for melanoma outcome.
- Lymphatic drainage from head and neck skin can be complex and less predictable than other body sites.
- Appropriate and comprehensive lymphadenectomy is critical for regional control.
- Adjuvant radiation should be considered for high-risk regional adenopathy (in cases of multiple lymph nodes greater than 3 cm, extracapsular spread, or parotid involvement).
- IFN-alfa 2b is the current common practice for adjuvant treatment of regional metastatic melanoma.
- New agents such as BRAF inhibitors and ipilimumab offer the greatest promise for systemic treatments.

REFERENCES

1. Geller AC, Miller DR, Annas GD, et al. Melanoma incidence and mortality among US whites, 1969-1999. JAMA 288:1719-1720, 2002.
2. de Vries E, Bray FI, Coebergh JW, et al. Changing epidemiology of malignant cutaneous melanoma in Europe 1953-1997: rising trends in incidence and mortality but recent stabilizations in western Europe and decreases in Scandinavia. Int J Cancer 107:119-126, 2003.
3. Garbe C, Leiter U. Melanoma epidemiology and trends. Clin Dermatol 27:3-9, 2009.
4. MacLennan R, Green AC, McLeod GR, et al. Increasing incidence of cutaneous melanoma in Queensland, Australia. J Natl Cancer Inst 84:1427-1432, 1992.
5. Jemal A, Siegel R, Ward E, et al. Cancer statistics, 2009. CA Cancer J Clin 59:225-249, 2009.
6. Rigel DS, Carucci JA. Malignant melanoma: prevention, early detection, and treatment in the 21st century. CA Cancer J Clin 50:215-236; quiz 237-240, 2000.
7. Jemal A, Devesa SS, Hartge P, et al. Recent trends in cutaneous melanoma incidence among whites in the United States. J Natl Cancer Inst 93:678-683, 2001.
8. Dennis LK. Analysis of the melanoma epidemic, both apparent and real: data from the 1973 through 1994 surveillance, epidemiology, and end results program registry. Arch Dermatol 135:275-280, 1999.
9. Marrett LD, Nguyen HL, Armstrong BK. Trends in the incidence of cutaneous malignant melanoma in New South Wales, 1983-1996. Int J Cancer 92:457-462, 2001.
10. U.S. Department of Health and Human Services. Surveillance, Epidemiology and End Results. Bethesda, Maryland: National Cancer Institute, Surveillance Systems Branch, 2009.
11. Beddingfield FC III. The melanoma epidemic: res ipsa loquitur. Oncologist 8:459-465, 2003.
12. Moan J, Dahlback A. The relationship between skin cancers, solar radiation and ozone depletion. Br J Cancer 65:916-921, 1992.
13. Slaper H, Velders GJ, Daniel JS, et al. Estimates of ozone depletion and skin cancer incidence to examine the Vienna Convention achievements. Nature 384:256-258, 1996.
14. Robinson JK, Rigel DS, Amonette RA. Trends in sun exposure knowledge, attitudes, and behaviors: 1986 to 1996. J Am Acad Dermatol 37:179-186, 1997.
15. Robinson JK, Kim J, Rosenbaum S, et al. Indoor tanning knowledge, attitudes, and behavior among young adults from 1988-2007. Arch Dermatol 144:484-488, 2008.
16. Lamberg L. "Epidemic" of malignant melanoma: true increase or better detection? JAMA 287:2201, 2002.
17. Swerlick RA, Chen S. The melanoma epidemic. Is increased surveillance the solution or the problem? Arch Dermatol 132:881-884, 1996.
18. Linos E, Swetter SM, Cockburn MG, et al. Increasing burden of melanoma in the United States. J Invest Dermatol 129:1666-1674, 2009.
19. Welch HG, Woloshin S, Schwartz LM. Skin biopsy rates and incidence of melanoma: population based ecological study. BMJ 331:481, 2005.
20. Levell NJ, Beattie CC, Shuster S, et al. Melanoma epidemic: a midsummer night's dream? Br J Dermatol 161:630-634, 2009.
21. Bosetti C, La Vecchia C, Naldi L, et al. Mortality from cutaneous malignant melanoma in Europe. Has the epidemic levelled off? Melanoma Res 14:301-309, 2004.
22. Crocetti E, Carli P. Changes from mid-1980s to late 1990s among clinical and demographic correlates of melanoma thickness. Eur J Dermatol 13:72-75, 2003.
23. Clark WH Jr, Reimer RR, Greene M, et al. Origin of familial malignant melanomas from heritable melanocytic lesions. 'The B-K mole syndrome'. Arch Dermatol 114:732-738, 1978.
24. Lynch HT, Frichot BC III, Lynch JF. Familial atypical multiple mole-melanoma syndrome. J Med Genet 15:352-356, 1978.
25. Pho L, Grossman D, Leachman SA. Melanoma genetics: a review of genetic factors and clinical phenotypes in familial melanoma. Curr Opin Oncol 18:173-179, 2006.
26. Cleaver JE. Defective repair replication of DNA in xeroderma pigmentosum. Nature 218:652-656, 1968.
27. Kraemer KH, Levy DD, Parris CN, et al. Xeroderma pigmentosum and related disorders: examining the linkage between defective DNA repair and cancer. J Invest Dermatol 103(5 Suppl):96S-101S, 1994.
28. Freedberg IM, Eisen AZ, Wolff K, et al, eds. Fitzpatrick's Dermatology in General Medicine, ed 6. New York: McGraw-Hill, 2003.

29. Kobayashi N, Muramatsu T, Yamashina Y, et al. Melanin reduces ultraviolet-induced DNA damage formation and killing rate in cultured human melanoma cells. J Invest Dermatol 101:685-689, 1993.

30. Holman CD, Armstrong BK. Pigmentary traits, ethnic origin, benign nevi, and family history as risk factors for cutaneous malignant melanoma. J Natl Cancer Inst 72:257-266, 1984.

31. Armstrong BK, Kricker A. The epidemiology of UV induced skin cancer. J Photochem Photobiol B 63:8-18, 2001.

32. Bliss JM, Ford D, Swerdlow AJ, et al. Risk of cutaneous melanoma associated with pigmentation characteristics and freckling: systematic overview of 10 case-control studies. The International Melanoma Analysis Group (IMAGE). Int J Cancer 62:367-376, 1995.

33. Cho E, Rosner BA, Feskanich D, et al. Risk factors and individual probabilities of melanoma for whites. J Clin Oncol 23:2669-2675, 2005.

> *This article highlights the risk factors for developing melanoma. The study identifies older age, male sex, family history of melanoma, higher number of nevi, history of severe sunburn, and light hair color as each associated with a significantly elevated risk of melanoma.*

34. Tsao H, Bevona C, Goggins W, et al. The transformation rate of moles (melanocytic nevi) into cutaneous melanoma: a population-based estimate. Arch Dermatol 139:282-288, 2003.

35. Bataille V, Bishop JA, Sasieni P, et al. Risk of cutaneous melanoma in relation to the numbers, types and sites of naevi: a case-control study. Br J Cancer 73:1605-1611, 1996.

36. Olsen CM, Zens MS, Stukel TA, et al. Nevus density and melanoma risk in women: a pooled analysis to test the divergent pathway hypothesis. Int J Cancer 124:937-944, 2009.

37. Whiteman DC, Watt P, Purdie DM, et al. Melanocytic nevi, solar keratoses, and divergent pathways to cutaneous melanoma. J Natl Cancer Inst 95:806-812, 2003.

38. Cho E, Rosner BA, Colditz GA. Risk factors for melanoma by body site. Cancer Epidemiol Biomarkers Prev 14:1241-1244, 2005.

39. Ha L, Noonan FP, De Fabo EC, et al. Animal models of melanoma. J Investig Dermatol Symp Proc 10:86-88, 2005.

40. Bulliard JL, Cox B, Elwood JM. Latitude gradients in melanoma incidence and mortality in the non-Maori population of New Zealand. Cancer Causes Control 5:234-240, 1994.

41. Elwood JM, Jopson J. Melanoma and sun exposure: an overview of published studies. Int J Cancer 73:198-203, 1997.

42. Elwood JM, Gallagher RP. Body site distribution of cutaneous malignant melanoma in relationship to patterns of sun exposure. Int J Cancer 78:276-280, 1998.

43. Chang YM, Barrett JH, Bishop DT, et al. Sun exposure and melanoma risk at different latitudes: a pooled analysis of 5700 cases and 7216 controls. Int J Epidemiol 38:814-830, 2009.

44. Stern RS, Weinstein MC, Baker SG. Risk reduction for nonmelanoma skin cancer with childhood sunscreen use. Arch Dermatol 122:537-545, 1986.

45. Wolf P, Quehenberger F, Mullegger R, et al. Phenotypic markers, sunlight-related factors and sunscreen use in patients with cutaneous melanoma: an Austrian case-control study. Melanoma Res 8:370-378, 1998.

46. Rigel DS. The effect of sunscreen on melanoma risk. Dermatol Clin 20:601-606, 2002.

47. Autier P. Sunscreen abuse for intentional sun exposure. Br J Dermatol 161(Suppl 3):S40-S45, 2009.

48. Gallagher RP, Rivers JK, Lee TK, et al. Broad-spectrum sunscreen use and the development of new nevi in white children: A randomized controlled trial. JAMA 283:2955-2960, 2000.

49. Westerdahl J, Ingvar C, Masback A, et al. Sunscreen use and malignant melanoma. Int J Cancer 87:145-150, 2000.

50. Balch CM, Gershenwald JE, Soong SJ, et al. Final version of 2009 AJCC melanoma staging and classification. J Clin Oncol 27:6199-6206, 2009.

51. Eigentler TK, Buettner PG, Leiter U, et al. Impact of ulceration in stages I to III cutaneous melanoma as staged by the American Joint Committee on Cancer Staging System: an analysis of the German Central Malignant Melanoma Registry. J Clin Oncol 22:4376-4383, 2004.

52. Balch CM, Soong SJ, Gershenwald JE, et al. Prognostic factors analysis of 17,600 melanoma patients: validation of the American Joint Committee on Cancer Melanoma Staging System. J Clin Oncol 19:3622-3634, 2001.

53. Corona R, Mele A, Amini M, et al. Interobserver variability on the histopathologic diagnosis of cutaneous melanoma and other pigmented skin lesions. J Clin Oncol 14:1218-1223, 1996.

54. Paek SC, Griffith KA, Johnson TM, et al. The impact of factors beyond Breslow depth on predicting sentinel lymph node positivity in melanoma. Cancer 109:100-108, 2007.

55. Sondak VK, Taylor JM, Sabel MS, et al. Mitotic rate and younger age are predictors of sentinel lymph node positivity: lessons learned from the generation of a probabilistic model. Ann Surg Oncol 11:247-258, 2004.

56. Azzola MF, Shaw HM, Thompson JF, et al. Tumor mitotic rate is a more powerful prognostic indicator than ulceration in patients with primary cutaneous melanoma: an analysis of 3661 patients from a single center. Cancer 97:1488-1498, 2003.

57. Clark WH Jr, From L, Bernardino EA, et al. The histogenesis and biologic behavior of primary human malignant melanomas of the skin. Cancer Res 29:705-727, 1969.

58. Morton DL, Wen DR, Wong JH, et al. Technical details of intraoperative lymphatic mapping for early stage melanoma. Arch Surg 127:392-399, 1992.

59. Chao C, Wong SL, Edwards MJ, et al. Sentinel lymph node biopsy for head and neck melanomas. Ann Surg Oncol 10:21-26, 2003.

60. O'Brien CJ, Uren RF, Thompson JF, et al. Prediction of potential metastatic sites in cutaneous head and neck melanoma using lymphoscintigraphy. Am J Surg 170:461-466, 1995.

61. Morton DL, Thompson JF, Cochran AJ, et al. Sentinel-node biopsy or nodal observation in melanoma. N Engl J Med 355:1307-1317, 2006.

62. Ohsie SJ, Sarantopoulos GP, Cochran AJ, et al. Immunohistochemical characteristics of melanoma. J Cutan Pathol 35:433-444, 2008.

63. Roka F, Mastan P, Binder M, et al. Prediction of non-sentinel node status and outcome in sentinel node-positive melanoma patients. Eur J Surg Oncol 34:82-88, 2008.

64. Cascinelli N, Bombardieri E, Bufalino R, et al. Sentinel and nonsentinel node status in stage IB and II melanoma patients: two-step prognostic indicators of survival. J Clin Oncol 24:4464-4471, 2006.

65. Ariyan C, Brady MS, Gonen M, et al. Positive nonsentinel node status predicts mortality in patients with cutaneous melanoma. Ann Surg Oncol 16:186-190, 2009.

66. Scoggins CR, Ross MI, Reintgen DS, et al. Gender-related differences in outcome for melanoma patients. Ann Surg 243:693-698; discussion 698-700, 2006.

67. Lachiewicz AM, Berwick M, Wiggins CL, et al. Survival differences between patients with scalp or neck melanoma and those with melanoma of other sites in the Surveillance, Epidemiology, and End Results (SEER) program. Arch Dermatol 144:515-521, 2008.

68. Fisher SR. Cutaneous malignant melanoma of the head and neck. Laryngoscope 99:822-836, 1989.

69. Fisher SR, Seigler HF, George SL. Therapeutic and prognostic considerations of head and neck melanoma. Ann Plast Surg 28:78-80, 1992.

70. Haqq C, Nosrati M, Sudilovsky D, et al. The gene expression signatures of melanoma progression. Proc Natl Acad Sci U S A 102:6092-6097, 2005.

71. Rangel J, Nosrati M, Torabian S, et al. Osteopontin as a molecular prognostic marker for melanoma. Cancer 112:144-150, 2008.

72. Sober AJ, Chuang TY, Duvic M, et al. Guidelines of care for primary cutaneous melanoma. J Am Acad Dermatol 45:579-586, 2001.

73. Stell VH, Norton HJ, Smith KS, et al. Method of biopsy and incidence of positive margins in primary melanoma. Ann Surg Oncol 14:893-898, 2007.

74. Johnson TM, Bradford CR, Gruber SB, et al. Staging workup, sentinel node biopsy, and follow-up tests for melanoma: update of current concepts. Arch Dermatol 140:107-113, 2004.

75. Basler GC, Fader DJ, Yahanda A, et al. The utility of fine needle aspiration in the diagnosis of melanoma metastatic to lymph nodes. J Am Acad Dermatol 36:403-408, 1997.

76. National Comprehensive Cancer Network Clinical Practice Guidelines in Oncology, v.1. 2010.

77. Cormier JN, Xing Y, Feng L, et al. Metastatic melanoma to lymph nodes in patients with unknown primary sites. Cancer 106:2012-2020, 2006.

78. Lee CC, Faries MB, Wanek LA, et al. Improved survival after lymphadenectomy for nodal metastasis from an unknown primary melanoma. J Clin Oncol 26:535-541, 2008.

79. Soufir N, Ollivaud L, Bertrand G, et al. A French CDK4-positive melanoma family with a co-inherited EDNRB mutation. J Dermatol Sci 46:61-64, 2007.

80. Box NF, Duffy DL, Chen W, et al. MC1R genotype modifies risk of melanoma in families segregating CDKN2A mutations. Am J Hum Genet 69:765-773, 2001.

81. Duggleby WF, Stoll H, Priore RL, et al. A genetic analysis of melanoma—polygenic inheritance as a threshold trait. Am J Epidemiol 114:63-72, 1981.

82. Rhodes AR, Weinstock MA, Fitzpatrick TB, et al. Risk factors for cutaneous melanoma. A practical method of recognizing predisposed individuals. JAMA 258:3146-3154, 1987.

83. Carlson JA, Dickersin GR, Sober AJ, et al. Desmoplastic neurotropic melanoma. A clinicopathologic analysis of 28 cases. Cancer 75:478-494, 1995.

84. Handley WS. The pathology of melanotic growths in relation to their operative treatment. Lancet 1:996-1003, 1907.

85. Breslow A, Macht SD. Optimal size of resection for thin cutaneous melanoma. Surg Gynecol Obstet 145:691-692, 1997.

86. Balch CM, Soong SJ, Smith T, et al. Long-term results of a prospective surgical trial comparing 2 cm vs. 4 cm excision margins for 740 patients with 1-4 mm melanomas. Ann Surg Oncol 8:101-108, 2001.
    This key study was critical to decreasing the recommended margin for wide local excision. This is particularly important in the head and neck region where such a large margin is always nearly impossible.

87. Thomas JM, Newton-Bishop J, A'Hern R, et al. Excision margins in high-risk melanoma. N Engl J Med 350:757-766, 2004.

88. Heaton KM, Sussman JJ, Gershenwald JE, et al. Surgical margins and prognostic factors in patients with thick (>4mm) primary melanomas. Ann Surg Oncol 5:322-328, 1998.

89. Stadelmann WK, McMasters K, Digenis AG, et al. Cutaneous melanoma of the head and neck: advances in evaluation and treatment. Plast Reconstr Surg 105:2105-2126, 2000.

90. Veronesi U, Adamus J, Bandiera DC, et al. Inefficacy of immediate node dissection in stage I melanoma of the limbs. N Engl J Med 297:627-630, 1977.

91. Balch CM, Soong SJ, Bartolucci AA, et al. Efficacy of an elective regional lymph node dissection of 1 to 4 mm thick melanomas for patients 60 years of age and younger. Ann Surg 224:255-266, 1996.

92. Balch CM, Soong SJ, Ross MI, et al. Long-term results of a multi-institutional randomized trial comparing prognostic factors and surgical results for intermediate thickness melanomas (1.0 to 4.0 mm): Intergroup Melanoma Surgical Trial. Ann Surg Oncol 7:87-97, 2000.

93. Cascinelli N, Morabito A, Santinami M, et al. Immediate or delayed dissection of regional nodes in patients with melanoma of the trunk: a randomized trial. WHO Melanoma Programme. Lancet 351:793-796, 1998.

94. McMasters KM, Sondak VK, Lotze MT, et al. Recent advances in melanoma staging and therapy. Ann Surg Oncol 6:467-475, 1999.

95. Balch CM, Buzaid AC, Soong SJ, et al. Final version of the American Joint Committee on Cancer staging system for cutaneous melanoma. J Clin Oncol 19:3635-3648, 2001.

96. Morton DL, Wen DR, Wong JH, et al. Technical details of intraoperative lymphatic mapping for early stage melanoma. Ann Surg 127:392-399, 1992.
    This landmark study described Dr. Morton's early experience with developing the sentinel lymph node technique. This manuscript offers numerous lessons on the technique and helps provide perspective for the technique as it is applied today.

97. Morton DL, Thompson JF, Essner R, et al. Validation of the accuracy of intraoperative lymphatic mapping and sentinel lymphadenectomy for early-stage melanoma. Ann Surg 230:453-463, 1999.

98. Karimipour DJ, Lowe L, Su L, et al. Standard immunostains for melanoma in sentinel lymph node specimens: which ones are most useful? J Am Acad Dermatol 50:759-764, 2004.

99. Wagner JD, Davidson D, Coleman JJ III, et al. Lymph node tumor volumes in patients undergoing sentinel lymph node biopsy for cutaneous melanoma. Ann Surg Oncol 6:398-404, 1999.

100. Joseph E, Brobeil A, Glass F, et al. Results of complete lymph node dissection in 83 melanoma patients with positive sentinel nodes. Ann Surg Oncol 5:119-125, 1998.

101. Morton DL, Thompson JF, Cochran AJ, et al. Sentinel-node biopsy or nodal observation in melanoma. N Engl J Med 355:1307-1317, 2006.
     This landmark prospective trial firmly established sentinel lymph node biopsy as the most important prognostic factor for melanoma. It also provided data suggesting that identifying micrometastasis has a greater than 20% survival benefit compared with identifying disease at a macroscopic level.

102. Gershenwald JE, Colome MI, Lee JE, et al. Patterns of recurrence following a negative sentinel lymph node biopsy in 243 patients with stage I or II melanoma. J Clin Oncol 16:2253-2254, 1998.

103. Balch CM, Gershenwald JE, Soong SJ, et al. Update of the melanoma staging system: the importance of sentinel node staging and primary tumor mitotic rate. J Surg Onc 104:379-385, 2011.

104. O'Brien CJ, Uren RF, Thompson JF, et al. Prediction of potential metastatic sites in cutaneous head and neck melanoma using lymphoscintigraphy. Am J Surg 170:461-446, 1995.

105. Schmalbach CE, Nussenbaum B, Rees RS, et al. Reliability of sentinel lymph node mapping with biopsy for head and neck cutaneous melanoma. Arch Otolaryngol Head Neck Surg 129:61-65, 2003.

106. Thomas JM, Clark MA. Selective lymphadenectomy in sentinel node-positive patients may increase the risk of local/in-transit recurrence in malignant melanoma. Eur J Surg Oncol 30:686-691, 2004.

107. Pawlik TM, Ross MI, Thompson JF, et al. The risk of in-transit melanoma metastasis depends on tumor biology and not the surgical approach to regional lymph nodes. J Clin Ocol 23:4588-4590, 2005.

108. Ang KK, Byers RM, Peters LJ, et al. Regional radiotherapy as adjuvant treatment for head and neck malignant melanoma. Arch Otolaryngol Head Neck Surg 116:169-172, 1990.

109. Ang KK, Peters LJ, Weber RS, et al. Postoperative radiotherapy for cutaneous melanoma of the head and neck region. Int J Radiat Oncol 30:795-798, 1994.

110. Ridge JA. Adjuvant radiation after lymph node dissection for melanoma. Ann Surg Oncol 7:550-551, 2000.

111. Burmeister BH, Mark Smithers B, Burmeister E, et al. A prospective phase II study of adjuvant postoperative radiation therapy following nodal surgery in malignant melanoma-Trans Tasman Radiation Oncology Group (TROG) Study 96.06. Radiother Oncol 81:136-142, 2006.

112. Atkins MB, Buzaid AC, Houghton AN. Systemic chemotherapy and biochemotherapy. In Balch CM, Houghton AN, Sober AJ, et al, eds. Cutaneous Melanoma. St Louis: Quality Medical Publishing, 2003.

113. Kirkwood JM, Strawderman MH, Ernstoff MC, et al. Interferon alpha-2b adjuvant therapy of high-risk resected cutaneous melanoma: the Eastern Cooperative Oncology Group Trial EST 1684. J Clin Oncol 14:7-17, 1996.

114. Kirkwood JM, Ibrahim JG, Sondak VK, et al. High- and low-dose interferon alfa-2b in high-risk melanoma: first analysis of Intergroup Trial E1690/S9111/C9190. J Clin Oncol 18:2444-2459, 2000.

115. Kirkwood JM, Ibrahim JG, Sosman JA, et al. High-dose interferon alfa-2b significantly prolongs relapse-free and overall survival compared with the GM2-KLH/QS-21 vaccine in patients with resected stage IIB-III melanoma: results of Intergroup Trial E1694/S9512/C509801. J Clin Oncol 19:2370-2380, 2001.

116. Flaherty KT, Puzanov I, Kim KB, et al. Inhibition of mutated, activated BRAF in metastatic melanoma. N Engl J Med 363:809-819, 2010.

This study is a landmark for identifying the first targeted therapy in melanoma. This study describes the initial findings and potential implications of a BRAF inhibitor for the treatment of melanoma.

117. Sosman JA, Kim KB, Schuchter L, et al. Survival in BRAF V600-mutant advanced melanoma treated with vemurafenib. N Engl J Med 366:707-714, 2012.

118. Kim KB, Kefford R, Pavlick AC, et al. Phase II study of the MEK1/MEK2 inhibitor Trametinib in patients with metastatic BRAF-mutant cutaneous melanoma previously treated with or without a BRAF inhibitor. J Clin Oncol 31:482-489, 2013.

119. Hodi FS, O'Day SJ, McDermott DF, et al. Improved survival with ipilimumab in patients with metastatic melanoma. N Engl J Med 363:711-723, 2010.

40

Rhytidectomy

Garrett Griffin ▪ *Babak Azizzadeh*

The face lift, or *rhytidectomy,* has been the cornerstone of facial rejuvenation surgery for the past century. Traditional goals of face-lift surgery include tightening the jawline, improving the cervicomental angle, and removing excess skin. Rhytidectomy, which literally translates to "removal of wrinkles," has become an increasingly outdated term as our understanding of facial aging has improved. Today we better understand that facial aging is a result of differences in skin quality and elasticity, alterations in the volume and distribution of facial fat, and changes in the facial skeleton.[1-9] Together these changes alter the shape of the face over time. The youthful female face is heart shaped with a narrow, taut jawline and a wide orbitomalar complex that focuses attention around the eyes. This zone is referred to as the *triangle of youth.* With age, relative facial volume moves from the upper to lower third of the face and manifests as jowling and cervicofacial laxity. This phenomenon creates a more rectangular or pyramidal shape, sometimes called the *pyramid of age* (Fig. 40-1).

Facial aging is a three-dimensional process that is a result of *devolumization* as much as it is a result of *descent.* Thus rhytidectomy is increasingly used as a facial reshaping procedure. With these concepts in mind rhytidectomy has become just one, albeit powerful, tool among many that surgeons may use to reestablish a more youthful facial contour.

Over the past 40 years, aesthetic surgeons have developed increasingly invasive surgical techniques in an attempt to simultaneously efface the nasolabial fold while lifting the lower face and neck. The concept of aging during this evolutionary period was that the midface was ptotic. Now surgeons have come to understand that midface volume loss is a more important factor in the aging process, making the surgical

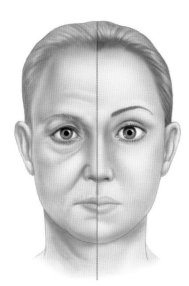

Fig. 40-1 The aging face has a pyramidal or rectangular shape with a wide, squared-off jawline and loss of upper facial volume *(left).* The youthful facial shape in both men and women is triangular, with a narrow jawline and a wide orbitomalar complex *(right).*

midface lift less of a necessity. More complicated face-lift techniques also require greater operating time and a more prolonged recovery and theoretically pose an increased risk to the facial nerve. An alternative philosophy is to perform a less-invasive face lift with autologous fat grafting or injectable fillers to address age-related changes in facial volume.

The original face lifts were likely performed by German surgeons in the first decade of the twentieth century.[10] These early procedures consisted of targeted skin excision only, with the tension of the lift supported by the skin itself. This resulted in significant tension on the suture line with short-lived results. No significant advancements were made in face-lift surgery until the 1960s when Aufricht,[11] Webster,[12] and others began plicating the deeper layers to improve their results. During the same period Skoog[13] reported using the platysma and superficial fascia of the face, as it was then known, to support the tension of the lift. Several years later Mitz and Peyronie[14] characterized the superficial fascia of the face as the cephalad extension of the platysma, calling it the *superficial musculoaponeurotic system,* or SMAS. Surgeons found the SMAS to be relatively inelastic, rendering their face lifts more long lasting. Furthermore because the SMAS supported the tension of the lift there was no tension on the suture line, which resulted in a finer scar. This class of face lift became known as the *SMAS rhytidectomy.* In general, SMAS face lifts produce substantial benefit in the neck and jowl but exert minimal effect on the midface or nasolabial fold. This is because the SMAS envelops the facial musculature, including the zygomaticus major, which is firmly fixed to the bone over the malar eminence. Thus superolateral tension on the SMAS is not transmitted medial to the zygomaticus major, where the midface and nasolabial fold are located.

In 1990 Hamra[15] reported the deep plane face lift as a procedure designed to achieve more significant improvement in the nasolabial fold and midface. As the name implies the major technical difference from SMAS rhytidectomy is that the primary plane of elevation is below the SMAS. The sub-SMAS dissection begins over the parotid gland at the lateral edge of the platysma muscle and proceeds medially just beyond the nasolabial fold. The most challenging maneuver is releasing the SMAS from the superficial surface of the orbicularis oculi and zygomaticus major muscles, which is what theoretically enables midface elevation and effacement of the nasolabial fold. The primary drawbacks of this technique are prolonged recovery time and a possible increase in facial nerve injury. The facial nerve is relatively exposed between the anterior edge of the parotid gland and lateral edge of the zygomaticus major where the sub-SMAS dissection takes place.

Proponents of the deep plane technique emphasize that the facial nerve branches are held down beneath the deeper parotideomasseteric fascia in this region, enabling a safe if somewhat tedious dissection. The tension of the lift in the deep plane technique is held by the SMAS, thereby reducing the tension on the skin and improving longevity of the lift. In analyzing his early results, Hamra reported that the deep plane lift failed to address laxity and descent of the orbicularis oculi muscle, which he considered an important sign of facial aging. He modified his deep plane technique to include elevation and suspension of a composite soft tissue flap containing the orbicularis oculi muscle, which he called a *composite face lift.*[16] These concepts predated our current understanding of facial volume loss as a key component of midface aging. Aesthetically, surgeons are now less concerned about nasolabial fold effacement and more focused on refilling the anterior and lateral midface.

In the 1990s Owsley[17,18] reported a face-lift technique that eventually came to be known as an *extended supra-SMAS rhytidectomy.* The purpose of this technique was to achieve the same improvement in the midface and nasolabial fold as the deep plane lift but in a way that limited risk to the facial nerve. In this procedure a traditional SMAS-type facial suspension is completed first to address the jowl and neck. The second stage of the procedure is completed before the skin is tailored or closed. A supra-SMAS dissection is begun at the orbicularis oculi and zygomaticus major muscles and continued medially beyond the nasolabial fold. The midface is then suspended superolaterally to the SMAS and temporalis fascia to achieve a midface lift and to efface the nasolabial fold.

In contrast to Owsley, who dissected the medial cheek in a more superficial plane to protect the facial nerve, another group of surgeons began dissecting the midface in the deeper subperiosteal plane. This movement was started by Tessier[19] to rejuvenate the brow region and was expanded in application by Psillakis et al[20] to include the entire maxilla and periorbital region. However, these authors reported unacceptably high rates of injury to the upper facial nerve branches. Ramirez et al[21] reported an improved, safer extended subperiosteal face lift in 1991 and later adapted Isse's endoscopic forehead lift[22] to create the *endoscopic full face lift* in 1994.[23] The endoscopic full face lift only modestly improves the lower face and neck, necessitating a separate SMAS-type face lift for patients with moderate to severe jowling.[24]

The 1990s also saw an increased emphasis on minimally invasive approaches across all medical disciplines. In response aesthetic surgeons developed *short-scar face lifts,* which require shorter incisions without a postauricular component. Saylan[25] was the first to describe a short-scar face lift, which he called the "S-lift" for the shape of the incision. However, Daniel Baker's SMASectomy[26] and Tonnard and Verpaele's minimal access cranial suspension (MACS) lift[27] are the short-scar face lifts that are most popular today. Short-scar face lifts necessitate a more vertical vector of lift than more traditional rhytidectomy approaches because there is no occipital incision to enable a lateral pull. Although this vertical lift can be an important tool for facial reshaping, short-scar face lifts may be less appropriate for patients who require a multivector approach.

ANATOMY

Facial anatomy is covered in detail in Chapter 1. A thorough understanding of facial nerve anatomy is critical to safely perform face-lift surgery. The facial nerve trunk exits the stylomastoid foramen and enters the body of the parotid gland before arborizing. Classic descriptions focus on five main facial nerve branches: the temporal, zygomatic, buccal, marginal mandibular, and cervical. More modern anatomic studies emphasize the variation in branching patterns among individuals.[28] For a surgeon performing face lifts, the most important anatomic principle is that the facial nerve branches are relatively unprotected between the anterior edge of the parotid gland and lateral edge of the intrinsic facial muscles. The muscles around the eye and central face receive innervation from numerous buccal and zygomatic facial nerve branches. In contrast, the temporal (also known as the frontal) and marginal mandibular nerve are typically terminal branches and serve as the only innervation to the frontalis muscle and lip depressors, respectively. Hence injury to one of these branches is more likely to cause noticeable facial asymmetry.

The temporal branch of the facial nerve is at risk during both SMAS and deep plane techniques because of its relatively superficial location. Typically 2 to 4 rami pass over the zygomatic arch. The "danger zone" differs between studies, but facial nerve branches have been found to cross the inferior edge of the zygomatic arch between 8 mm anterior to the anterior external acoustic meatus (bony landmark) and 17 mm posterior to the junction of the arch with the zygomatic body[29-31] (Fig. 40-2).

Over the arch these branches lie relatively deep beneath the parotideomasseteric fascia.[30] However, above the zygomatic arch the nerve branches become more superficial. One recent study identified a fascial transition zone beginning 15 mm superior to the zygomatic arch and 15 mm posterior to the lateral orbital rim, where the frontal branch enters the underside of the temporoparietal fascia. For this reason dissection in the temple should proceed either in the subperiosteal plane or just deep to hair follicles, splitting the subcutaneous fat, to help protect the nerve.

The marginal mandibular branch of the facial nerve emerges from the parotid gland near the angle of the mandible and travels deep to the platysma muscle and parotideomasseteric fascia over the surface of the masseter muscle. As its name implies, it proceeds anteriorly near the inferior border of the mandible and passes superficially to the facial artery and vein before innervating the lip depressors. A surgeon perform-

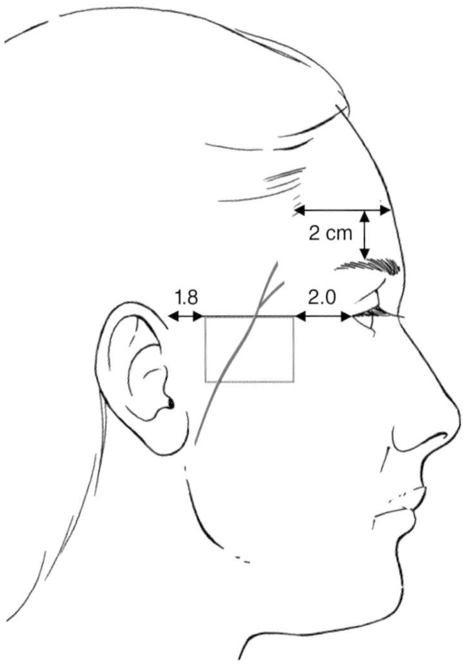

Fig. 40-2   The frontal branch of the facial nerve crosses the zygomatic arch between 1.8 cm in front of the helical root and 2 cm posterior to the lateral orbital rim. Directly over the arch the nerve is quite deep, running beneath the parotideomasseteric fascia. Thus sub-SMAS dissection over the arch itself is theoretically safe, as in a high-SMAS face lift. Starting approximately 15 mm above the arch the nerve enters the underside of the temporoparietal fascia (SMAS).[31] If dissection during face lift proceeds into this danger area, it is critical that the dissection remain in the subcutaneous fat superficial to the SMAS.

ing dissection deep to the platysma in this region should proceed with caution. The marginal nerve is long and thin and very susceptible to neuropraxia or inadvertent injury during cautery of small branches of the facial vessels.[32,33]

PATIENT EVALUATION AND PREOPERATIVE PLANNING

As with all aesthetic surgery consultations, the initial encounter must focus on the goals of the patient. A technically perfect face-lift result with no perioperative issues will not produce a satisfied patient if his or her objectives are not met. Patients differ in their ability to articulate their desired changes and in their sophistication regarding the range of interventions available for the aging face. It is extremely valuable to ask the patient to look in a mirror at the beginning of the consultation to help identify his or her concerns. Even very sophisticated patients are often interested in the opinion of the surgeon regarding which regions or characteristics are most amenable to facial rejuvenation. To ensure the patient and physician are communicating clearly the surgeon can point to these areas with a cotton-tipped applicator while the patient continues to look in the mirror. If the surgeon thinks that a face lift will benefit the patient, it is helpful to have the patient look in the mirror while the surgeon uses his or her hands to lift both sides of the face to create an appearance that resembles an achievable postoperative result. A variety of photomorphing packages are available, but they often do not demonstrate the result of a face lift as well as simply repositioning the facial tissues with one's hands.

The submentum deserves a careful visual and tactile analysis to identify the anatomic components that need alteration. An aging neck can be a result of any combination of lax skin, excess submental fat, poor hyoid position, platysmal banding, and microgenia.

Most patients have a moderate degree of facial asymmetry, which should be pointed out and discussed because even a very well-executed surgery cannot eliminate facial asymmetry. The surgeon must emphasize that the goal of aesthetic surgery is improvement not perfection.

A complete medical history must be obtained at the initial consultation to ensure that the patient is healthy enough for elective aesthetic surgery. Chronic medical problems such as asthma and diabetes should be optimally controlled before surgery. Any personal or family history of coagulopathy or problems with anesthesia must be carefully evaluated. All prior facial surgery must be discussed. In some cases it might be necessary to obtain past operative reports.

As injectable fillers have become more popular, it has become increasingly important to ask about any history of filler placement. Patients with a history of herpes labialis should be given 2 g of valacyclovir twice on the day before surgery to guard against reactivation. Chemotherapeutic and immunomodulatory drug regimens including oral steroids can affect healing and increase infection risk and will need to be discussed with the prescribing physician before surgery. It is essential to inquire about tobacco and drug use. Active smokers are at higher risk of skin slough and hematoma and should be asked to quit for at least 2 to 4 weeks before surgery.[33,34] Parikh and Jacono[35] examined complications in 183 deep plane face-lift patients, 15 (8%) of whom were smokers, and found no difference between smokers and nonsmokers. These authors concluded that the deep plane lift, with its minimal subcutaneous undermining and thick soft tissue flap, is a safe alternative in active smokers.

Any significant psychiatric history, including anxiety and depression, should be addressed. It is not uncommon for patients to seek aesthetic surgery after a significant life change, such as divorce. These individuals may be reasonable candidates for surgery if they are emotionally stable and have realistic expectations.

Box 40-1 contains a list of medications that should be discontinued 7 to 14 days before surgery. A full set of high-quality preoperative photographs without makeup should also be obtained.

Box 40-1   Medications to Be Discontinued Before Surgery

Advil	Cama Inlay Tabs	Fiorinal
Alka-Seltzer	Cheracol capsules	Four-Way Cold Tablets
Anadin	Congespirin	Garlic
Anaprox	Cope	Gingko beloba
Arthritis Pain Formula	Coricidin	Gingseng
Ascodeen-30	Darvon Compound	Indocin
Ascriptin	Doan's Pills	Measurin
Aspirin	Dristan	Midol
Aspirin suppositories (all brands)	Duragesic	Monacet with Codeine
Bayer Aspirin	Ecotrin	Motrin
Buff-A-Comp	Empirin	Naprosyn
Buffadyne	Emprazil	Norgesic
Butalbital	Equagesic	Nuprin
Cama Arthritis Pain Reliever	Excedrin	Pamprin

TECHNIQUES

INCISIONS

The placement of face-lift incisions and their ultimate appearance is an important determinant of the quality of the outcome. In women, the face-lift incision used for most SMAS and deep plane techniques begins in the temporal region. The placement of the temporal incision depends on the amount of skin that is likely to be removed. Older patients and patients with significant skin laxity typically require more skin excision. If significant skin removal is expected it is best to place the temporal incision below the temporal hair tuft so as not to elevate the temporal hairline to an unnatural level after skin excision (Fig. 40-3, A).

Temporal hairline incisions are better camouflaged if they are trichophytic. If relatively moderate skin excision is expected the incision can simply pass obliquely within the hair down to the helical root. From the helical root the incision proceeds inferiorly at the junction of the auricle with the face; sometimes there is a natural skin fold in this location that can be used. Incisions may be made either in front of or behind the tragal cartilage. The advantage of a pretragal incision is that it preserves the delicate contour of the tragus and pretragal notch. The advantage of a retrotragal incision is that it is more hidden and has better patient acceptance. Most female patients request a retrotragal incision. If a retrotragal incision is used the skin that is placed back onto the tragus must be thinned down to the dermis to prevent unnatural fullness of the tragus postoperatively. The incision then continues in between the auricle and face and passes just inferior to the lobule. In the postauricular region, the incision is made several millimeters onto the concha (Fig. 40-3, B), so that after healing the incision will lie in the postauricular sulcus. The incision then turns back toward the occipital hairline at the point of maximal width of the auricle. At this point the incision may be made along the hairline or may trail off at a roughly 45-degree angle. If the incision is made at the hairline it should be made in a trichophytic fashion allowing hair to grow through the scar. In our opinion incisions along the occipital hairline heal in a less satisfactory manner.

The face-lift incision in men must be different from that in women because of the presence of facial hair. There is no need to place the temporal incision below the temporal tuft, because the skin that is elevated following the lift will continue to grow hair and can become a new sideburn. The other major difference is in the preauricular incision. The incision should be placed approximately 8 mm in front of the auricular

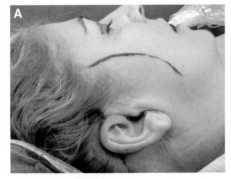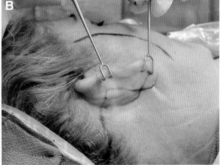

Fig. 40-3   **A,** In women, the incision is started in the temporal hairline, passing inferiorly in the preauricular crease and then retrotragally. **B,** Behind the ear, the incision passes onto the conchal bowl so that after healing it lies in the postauricular sulcus. The incision exits the concha at the auricle's widest point thereby maximizing camouflage of the incision. Finally, the incision enters the hairline and passes inferiorly at a 45-degree angle. This type of temple incision will minimally elevate the temporal hairline but we have not had issues with this. In patients requiring massive skin removal a temporal tuft incision might be more appropriate, although it is usually more conspicuous.

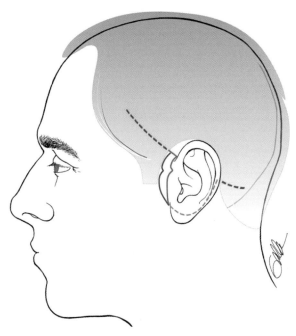

Fig. 40-4   In men, hair-bearing facial skin requires several incision modifications from the female face-lift incision (*blue,* male incision; *red,* female incision). The temporal incision can always be in the hairline because the elevated facial skin will continue to grow hair. The incision should pass 1 cm pretragally to avoid pulling facial hair too close to the auricle, which looks unnatural and is difficult to shave. Behind the ear the incision stays closer to the postauricular sulcus and jumps off the concha slightly more inferiorly to avoid pulling hair too high or onto the concha. The occipital hairline incision is basically the same as in women.

cartilage and should pass pretragally to avoid placing hair-bearing skin too close to the ear. The retroauricular incision does not require modification if the amount of planned skin removal is conservative. If significant skin removal is planned, the incision location for women risks pulling hair-bearing skin onto the back of the ear and high into the postauricular sulcus. In men requiring significant skin excision, the incision should be placed in the postauricular sulcus and should cross the postauricular skin more inferiorly (Fig. 40-4).

Submentoplasty

One of the primary goals of most patients undergoing face-lift surgery is improvement of the submentum and cervicomental angle. Ellenbogen and Karlin[36] described five visual criteria of a youthful neck profile: (1) distinct inferior mandibular border from mentum to angle with no jowl overhang, (2) slight subhyoid depression at the cervicomental angle, which gives the impression of a long neck, (3) visible thyroid cartilage contour, (4) distinct visible anterior border of the sternocleidomastoid muscle from the sternum to retromandibular region, and (5) cervicomental angle between 105 and 120 degrees. Anatomic factors, including a low hyoid, excess submental fat, skin laxity, platysmal banding, microgenia, and abnormal occlusion, can all contribute to an aged and unattractive appearing submental contour. The operative plan differs depending on which, if any, of these anatomic components is present.

In thin patients with submental skin laxity only, the skin removed with the rhytidectomy may be all that is needed. Excess submental fat can be either subcutaneous or subplatysmal. Subcutaneous fat can be excised with scissors under direct visualization or more commonly removed with suction-assisted lipectomy.

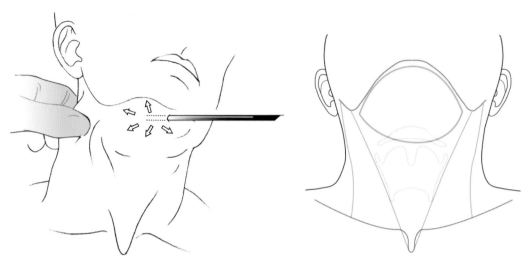

Fig. 40-5 Submental liposuction.

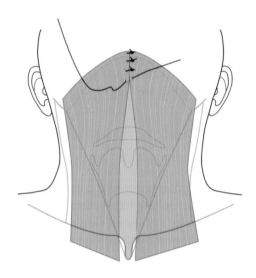

Fig. 40-6 Platysmaplasty is required in patients with prominent platysmal bands. If midline preplatysmal fat is removed, it is necessary to connect the medial platysmal edges to prevent a "cobra neck" deformity.

In either case the surgeon must be careful to leave a uniform layer of fat on the dermis to prevent contour irregularities. Direct excision of central subplatysmal fat can be a powerful technique, particularly in patients with poor hyoid position. Lateral subplatysmal liposuction carries a high risk of injury to the marginal mandibular nerve and is avoided by most surgeons (Fig. 40-5).

Medial platysmal banding is a result of age-related laxity and can be addressed with midline sutures, medial platysmal excision, lateral platysmal suspension, platysmal transection, or some combination of these. Most face lifts place lateral tension on the platysma muscle, but this technique may be insufficient in cases of moderate to severe banding. It is best to address midline platysmal banding directly at its origin. The goal of platysmal surgery is to create a taut muscular sling that supports a sharp cervicomental angle and has no visible banding. The platysmaplasty is typically performed after suction-assisted lipectomy but before the face lift and begins with a 2 to 3 cm incision placed within or just anterior to the submental crease (Fig. 40-6).

A mixture of blunt and sharp dissection is used to elevate the skin and soft tissue off the superficial surface of the platysma. The anterior edges of the platysma muscles are identified and dissected from the submentum to the superior edge of the thyroid cartilage. The anterior edges of the platysma muscles are then sutured together with interrupted 3-0 PDS sutures in buried fashion. Some authors perform a transverse incision or wedge excision of the muscle at the level of the hyoid before the midline suturing. The rationale for this maneuver is twofold: it may break the continuity of the anterior platysmal bands, helping to prevent their recurrence, and it allows the cephalad muscle to migrate superiorly thus creating an even sharper cervicomental angle. In older patients with significant platysmal laxity, a vertical excision of the anterior platysma may be necessary to achieve the desired tight muscular sling. Alternatively, a running 3-0 PDS suture can be placed from the submentum down to the thyroid cartilage, then up to the submentum and back down to the thyroid cartilage again. This "corset platysmaplasty" was described by Feldman.[37] It eliminates any free muscle edges that can return as platysmal bands while smoothing the contour where the muscles overlap. Some authors have criticized this technique for the recurrence of a single midline ridge or band over time. Guyuron has championed the "vest over pants" technique, wherein the medial edges of the platysmal muscles are overlapped, which should theoretically prevent a midline roll. He recently reported no recurrence of platysmal banding using this technique in 88 patients over 26 years with an average follow-up of 29 months.[37a] In any of these medial plication techniques if the platysma muscles are moved a significant distance toward the midline there is a tendency for the overlying skin to bunch medially. This can be remedied by completely separating the neck skin from the platysma muscles, allowing the skin to be redraped as necessary.

SMAS Rhytidectomy

There are multiple variations on the theme of SMAS rhytidectomy. A common approach is to perform what has been called a *short-flap SMAS rhytidectomy*, which is a modification of the technique originally popularized by Webster in the early 1980s.[38-39] Webster was the first to advocate rhytidectomy with conservative skin undermining to maintain the integrity of dermal-SMAS attachments. This concept was innovative for several reasons. First, Webster demonstrated that this technique combined with SMAS plication resulted in a better outcome than more aggressive surgical techniques.[40] Additionally, this method decreased tension on the incision and increased the amount of facial suspension from the procedure. A cadaveric study compared different SMAS face-lift techniques and found that wound tension increased significantly with increased skin undermining when compared with shorter skin flaps.[41] Webster's technique was further adapted by McCollough et al, who advocated maintaining the skin adipose-SMAS integrity for even better results and coined the procedure *suspension rhytidectomy*.[42]

The key components of the short-flap SMAS rhytidectomy are conservative undermining of the skin in the facial region and multivector SMAS imbrication. The midface is addressed with volume restoration (autologous fat grafting, injectable fillers, and implants) and the neck is addressed as needed based on the anatomic properties. The anterior dermal-SMAS attachments remain intact because of the conservative facial skin flap dissection, thereby allowing aggressive SMAS suspension while avoiding significant wound tension. The SMAS is an integral component of this procedure: it is the carrier of the rhytidectomy flap.

The short-flap SMAS rhytidectomy offers some distinct advantages over alternative rhytidectomy techniques. The procedure minimizes the risk for facial nerve injury by limiting the area of sub-SMAS dissection anterior to the parotid gland, and also minimizes the possibility for postoperative hematoma formation. Because of the limited elevation of the skin flap the likelihood of vascular compromise is also diminished, especially in smokers, diabetics, and elderly patients. Most patients undergoing this technique are able to resume normal activity within 7 to 10 days postoperatively.

In contrast to the short-flap SMAS rhytidectomy, long skin flaps separate the dermal-SMAS attachments, thereby negating the benefit of using the SMAS to support the lift. Mendelson and Muzaffar also demonstrated that releasing retaining ligaments in the prezygomatic space through extensive subcutaneous dissection can potentially cause nerve injury to the motor branch of the orbicularis oculi.[43-44]

To address facial volume deficiency, autologous fat grafting is frequently performed to the infraorbital, piriform, nasolabial, and buccal regions at the time of a short-flap SMAS rhytidectomy. Longer skin flaps can preclude the use of autologous fat grafting because of extensive undermining of the midface and lower facial tissue layers. Since the midface and prejowl regions are not dissected during the short-flap SMAS rhytidectomy, these areas can safely and accurately undergo fat grafting. Patients with significant skeletal deficiency may benefit from permanent midface implants, which will require a separate gingivobuccal sulcus incision. Patients may also use synthetic fillers postoperatively for volume restoration.

Patients may elect either general anesthesia or intravenous sedation. If general anesthesia is chosen the endotracheal tube is secured to the bottom teeth in the midline with dental floss or suture. Cefazolin and steroids are administered intravenously, and lower extremity intermittent compression devices are placed. If a submentoplasty is planned 1% lidocaine with 1:100,000 epinephrine is infiltrated into one side of the face and submental region before the patient is prepped and draped. This will maximize time for vasoconstriction to occur. Autoclave tape is placed circumferentially around the head 2 to 4 cm behind the hairline to properly secure the hair away from the surgical field. The entire face, anterior hairline, and autoclave tape are prepared with dilute Betadine. The endotracheal tube and circuit are wrapped in a clear plastic sheath typically used for endoscopic sinus surgery so that the tube can be freely manipulated during the case (Fig. 40-7).

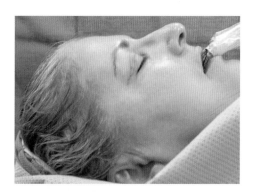

Fig. 40-7   The patient's hair is taped with autoclave tape, which keeps the hair out of the sterile field and enables the drapes to be stapled to the tape without leaving staple marks in the aesthetic patient's scalp. The endotracheal tube is secured to the midline mandibular teeth with dental floss or 2-0 silk suture. The endotracheal tube and circuit are covered in a camera bag and placed above the surgical drapes for easy manipulation.

Box 40-2   Recommended Order of Procedures

1. Transconjunctival lower blepharoplasty
2. Endoscopic brow lift
3. Endoscopic midface lift
4. Upper blepharoplasty
5. Lower blepharoplasty skin pinch
6. Submental liposuction
7. Platysmaplasty
8. Chin implant
9. Rhytidectomy

Some patients elect to undergo multiple procedures simultaneously; Box 40-2 outlines the recommended order. Before each portion of the procedure, a second round of local anesthetic using 1% lidocaine with 1:100,000 epinephrine can be considered, depending on the time since the initial injection, without exceeding the maximum dosage for lidocaine with epinephrine (7 mg/kg).

To address the neck region adequately, multiple procedures may be required in addition to the SMAS imbrication and lateral platysmal suspension. Depending on the preoperative diagnosis, chin augmentation, suction-assisted lipectomy, midline platysmaplasty, platysmal transection, and/or direct excision of subplatysmal fat are performed. Caution is used to avoid overzealous fat removal to prevent the potential complication of cobra neck deformity. Attention should be directed toward protecting the marginal mandibular nerves.

Once the adjunct procedures are completed, attention is directed toward performing the rhytidectomy. The skin anterior to the auricle is elevated first. The extent of facial skin undermining is only 4 to 6 cm in most patients. A ruler is used to mark out the planned distance of skin undermining before elevation to help achieve symmetry between the two sides (Fig. 40-8, *A*).

A gender-appropriate incision is made starting with a 2 to 3 cm incision in the anterior temporal hair tuft (see Fig. 40-4). The occipital incision is executed at a 45-degree angle and does not follow the hairline. A Brown Adson and No. 15 scalpel are used to begin the flap elevation in the subcutaneous plane at the temporal hair tuft and midface region. Once the correct plane is identified, the double-prong skin hook or four-prong rake is placed, and skin undermining proceeds with Metzenbaum scissors (Fig. 40-8, *B*). The surgeon retracts the already elevated flap posteriorly while the assistant exerts countertraction, which helps reveal the appropriate plane of dissection. A thick skin flap is dissected at the tragus just above the perichondrium. Aggressive thinning of the skin over the tragus down to the dermis at the end of the procedure significantly limits postoperative tragal fullness.

Dissection over the zygomatic arch and temple places the frontal branch of the facial nerve at risk; therefore elevation should be performed directly under the hair follicles. Transillumination may facilitate elevation of a flap of consistent thickness. Once the preauricular flap is elevated a moist surgical sponge is placed under the flap and attention is directed toward the postauricular elevation.

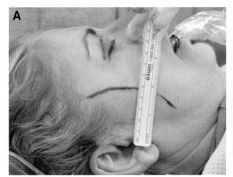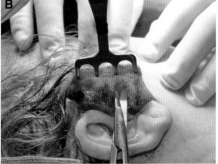

Fig. 40-8   **A,** The amount of planned skin undermining is marked using a ruler before making the incision. **B,** A gender-appropriate incision is made, and undermining begins anterior to the auricle. Initially the flap is elevated with forceps and a scalpel, and when there is enough room for a rake, the transition is made to scissor dissection. The assistant provides countertraction as the surgeon pulls the skin toward himself or herself. Transillumination can be used to help raise a flap of uniform thickness, as seen here.

Continued

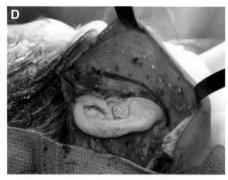

Fig. 40-8, cont'd   **C,** Once preauricular and postauricular elevation is complete, the area over the angle of the mandible is elevated. This helps protect the marginal nerve. **D,** The flap elevation is completed, and meticulous hemostasis is achieved with bipolar cautery. Transillumination demonstrates a uniform flap. The planned J-shaped SMAS excision has been marked. Xeroform has been placed in the ear canal to prevent blood from entering.

The posterior occipital flap is dissected initially with a No. 15 scalpel blade. Face-lift scissors are used to complete the postauricular dissection. The skin over the mastoid is thin and easy to tear or perforate. There is very little subcutaneous fat over the sternocleidomastoid muscle, and the skin is tightly adherent to the underlying muscle, making the dissection more difficult. The location of the sternocleidomastoid muscle fascia, external jugular vein, and great auricular nerve must be kept in mind to avoid injury. The inferior limit of the dissection lies 4 to 5 cm below the auricle. Complete cervical skin elevation connecting to the midline submental dissection is necessary to obtain good results in patients with significant skin laxity. A surgical sponge is placed under the postauricular flap.

The preauricular and postauricular dissections are then connected (Fig. 40-8, *C*). The dissection over the angle of the mandible is the most dangerous aspect of the dissection, because the marginal mandibular nerve is at risk. Doing this dissection last, with well-defined subcutaneous planes on either side, helps to raise a flap of uniform thickness and protect the nerve. Once the subcutaneous flap is completely raised, hemostasis is meticulously achieved with bipolar cautery (Fig. 40-8, *D*).

The SMAS imbrication is then initiated. Starting approximately 15 mm anterior to the auricle, a 1 cm-wide J-shaped strip of SMAS/platysma is excised anterior and inferior to the auricle with face-lift scissors (Fig. 40-9).

In this area the facial nerve is well protected deep within the parotid gland, making SMAS excision very safe. From this point sub-SMAS dissection can be performed if desired (Fig. 40-10).

The facial nerve branches are at increased risk as one passes anterior to the parotid gland. Extreme care is taken to stay superficial to the masseteric fascia if the sub-SMAS dissection is carried beyond the parotid gland. The facial nerve runs within and deep to this fascia. The edges of the SMAS are imbricated with multiple buried 3-0 PDS sutures to suspend the soft tissues in various vectors depending on the patient's aging process and desire to reshape the face (Fig. 40-11). The upper SMAS is typically secured in a more vertical fashion while the lower SMAS/platysma is secured to the mastoid fascia.

The vector of SMAS suspension is customized for each patient. Jacono and Ransom recently showed that the optimal angle of SMAS suspension depends on patient age.[45] Generally younger patients require a more superior vector, whereas older patients require a more lateral vector.

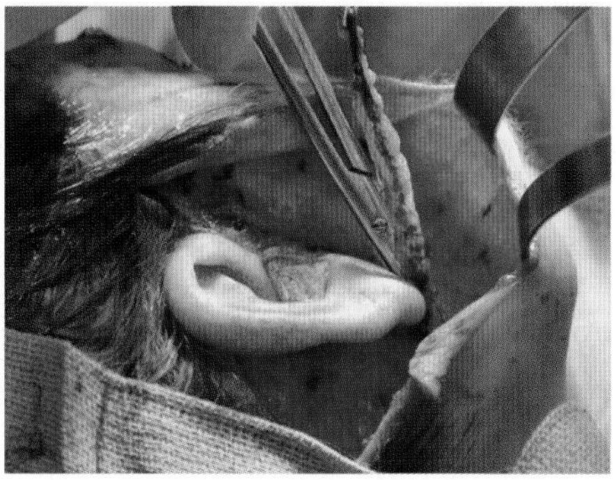

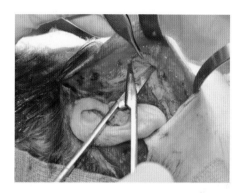

Fig. 40-9   A J-shaped strip of SMAS is removed from over the parotid gland, which helps protect the facial nerve. The exposed parotid capsule can be bipolared in patients with prominent parotid glands to help narrow the lower face.

Fig. 40-10   The medial cut edge of the SMAS can be used as the starting point for sub-SMAS (deep plane) elevation. Dissection beyond the anterior edge of the parotid puts the facial nerve at risk, but if it stays superficial to the masseteric fascia it can be performed safely.

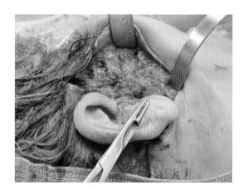

Fig. 40-11   The medial SMAS is imbricated to the lateral SMAS using 3-0 absorbable suture. Multiple sutures likely help maintain a long-lasting result.

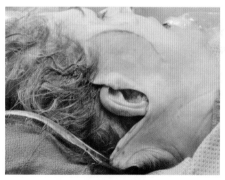

Fig. 40-12   Once SMAS imbrication is complete, the skin flap is redraped. This relatively conservative 5 cm subcutaneous elevation and 2 cm of SMAS undermining have yielded significant excess skin.

For individuals with cherubic faces and/or prominent parotid glands, the lower face may be narrowed by gently cauterizing the parotideomasseteric fascia just anterior to the auricle. The SMAS imbrication can be used to further taper the area, thereby decreasing its lateral projection. This subtle yet powerful technique can further restore the triangle of youth.

Additional subcutaneous undermining may be necessary if there is tethering of the anterior facial skin after SMAS suspension. At this point the excess skin is redraped and excised to complete the rhytidectomy (Fig. 40-12).

The goal of skin redraping is to minimize tension on the preauricular incision while distributing any potential tension on the postauricular incision. This portion of the procedure is critical for an optimal outcome of a nearly invisible scar. Skin suspension and excision is performed at four key anchor points. The helical root is the first anchor point (AP1). Adson forceps are used to determine the amount of excess skin, and a

No. 15 scalpel is used to create a slit in the flap (Fig. 40-13, *A*). The incision is closed to the base of the slit with a 4-0 PDS suture. A single hook is then placed at the superior aspect of the temporal incision, and the excess skin superior to AP1 is excised.

The antitragus serves as the second anchor point (AP2), which is placed in a similar fashion (Fig. 40-13, *B*). Once AP2 has been placed, the intervening skin between AP1 and AP2 is judiciously excised to avoid overexcision of the skin, which can lead to displacement of the tragus anteriorly. The skin that will be placed over the tragal cartilage is defatted to create a more delicate and natural-appearing tragus. The third anchor point (AP3) is placed toward the apex of the postauricular region (Fig. 40-13, *C*). Following this maneuver, a single hook places traction at the lateral apex of the occipital incision, and the excess skin is excised in a manner such that a straight occipital hairline is re-created. The tissue between AP2 and AP3 is draped over the ear lobule to assess the amount of skin to excise. Face-lift scissors are then used to excise the postauricular excess skin, because the apex will become the anchor point of the lobule attachment (AP4). One must be very conservative with skin excision under the lobule (Fig. 40-13, *D*). If there is any tension in this location, a "pixie ear" deformity may result.

Once skin tailoring is complete, additional 4-0 PDS deep dermal sutures are placed as necessary. A perforated 10 Fr drain is placed before closure. The preauricular incision is closed using a running locking 6-0 nylon or Prolene suture between AP1 and AP4. A 4-0 running plain gut suture is used to close the skin in

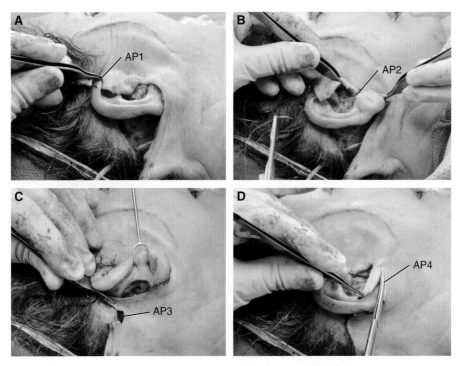

Fig. 40-13   Skin tailoring using four anchor points (APs), each secured with 4-0 PDS suture. Before tailoring is begun a 10 Fr drain is placed and put on wall suction. **A,** AP1 is at the helical root. A single-prong hook is then placed at the temporal apex and excess temporal skin is excised. **B,** AP2 is at the incisura. A small bite of cartilage is included for added stability. Excess skin is then excised between AP1 and AP2. It is important to have no tension on the flap in this location to prevent widening or an abnormal tragal contour. The flap over the tragus is thinned to mimic the native tragal skin. **C,** AP3 is high in the postauricular sulcus. A double-prong hook is placed in the occipital apex of the incision, and excess skin is removed. **D,** Finally, skin is conservatively trimmed from over the lobule. This should be done so that the skin flap rides under the lobule, which will support it during healing and prevent "pixie ear" deformity. This represents AP4. Skin is trimmed from over the concha to complete the tailoring.

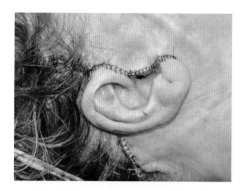

Fig. 40-14 Completed short-flap SMAS rhytidectomy. The incision has been closed with running locking 6-0 nylon in front of the ear, 4-0 plain gut behind the ear, and staples in the hairline. The drain can be seen running beneath the skin, which is a sign there is no fluid collection or hematoma. Ice in a sterile glove is applied while the second side is completed.

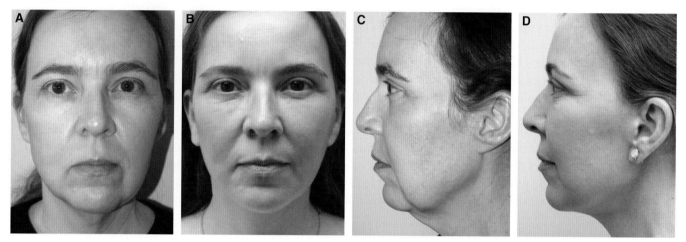

Fig. 40-15 Preoperative and postoperative views of a 54-year-old woman undergoing short-flap SMAS rhytidectomy with multilevel fat grafting to the infraorbit and midface. **A** and **C,** The patient before surgery. **B** and **D,** The patient 3 months after surgery. Her facial contour has been changed from rectangular to heart shaped. The lateral view shows significant improvement of jowling and neck laxity.

the postauricular region. Staples are used to close the incision in the temporal and occipital hairline (Fig. 40-14). If there is a submental incision it is closed in a single layer with running locking 6-0 nylon suture. Ice inside sterile gloves is placed on the first side while the face lift is performed on the second side. This promotes vasoconstriction and limits perioperative ecchymosis.

Volume restoration, a second key component of facial rejuvenation, is performed next in those who require it. Multilevel fat grafting is performed, most commonly in the infraorbit, piriform, buccal, and prejowl regions. At the conclusion of the procedures a light facial pressure dressing is applied. Fig. 40-15 displays a representative short-flap SMAS rhytidectomy result.

DEEP PLANE RHYTIDECTOMY

In 1990 Hamra published his technique[15] for deep plane rhytidectomy, which arose from a desire to achieve more effacement of the nasolabial fold than was possible with a SMAS face lift. In a follow-up paper[16] in 1992 he described the composite rhytidectomy. This added lower orbicularis oculi elevation and suspension to the deep plane technique, designed to more thoroughly address the nasojugal and palpebromalar grooves. The deep plane and composite rhytidectomies were developed based on the premise that facial aging was caused by descent of the platysma and orbicularis oculi muscles and the cheek fat. This concept is now heavily debated among aesthetic surgeons. Rohrich and Pessa have elegantly described the deep and superficial fat compartments in the midface,[7,46] and volume loss is now believed to be as important as tissue descent in causing the appearance of the nasolabial fold and palpebromalar grooves. Lambros[48] and others have shown that the lid-cheek junction and skin blemishes do not migrate inferiorly over time, and Rohrich et al[2] have demonstrated that adding volume to the midface fat compartments achieves significant facial rejuvenation. Thus the underlying basis of the deep plane and composite techniques may have been incomplete. In 2002 Hamra performed a retrospective analysis of his deep plane results 10 years after surgery and found that there was very little nasolabial fold effacement over the long term.[47] This further supports the conclusion that bone and deep fat loss are major contributors to nasolabial fold formation rather than tissue descent. However, there remain patient groups, such as older patients, who will obtain a better result with a deep plane face lift compared with other methods. Evidence-based outcomes and comparisons for the different types of face lift are discussed in a section later in this chapter.

The incision for the deep plane lift is similar to that for SFSR. Subcutaneous dissection is performed only 2 to 3 cm anterior to the auricle, ending inferiorly at the angle of the mandible. The SMAS is incised between the angle of the mandible and malar eminence, which is anterior to the frontal branch of the facial nerve. A mixture of sharp and blunt dissection in the sub-SMAS plane is carried anteriorly with the mandibular border as the inferior extent. Superiorly, the orbicularis oculi and zygomaticus musculature are identified, and the dissection transitions superficial to the zygomaticus muscle as one moves anteroinferiorly (Fig. 40-16).

The zygomaticus major muscle provides a landmark for dissection into the midface across the nasolabial fold without risk of injury to the terminal branches of the facial nerve, which course deep to the muscle. The SMAS becomes the platysma in the lower face and neck, and the dissection is continued either superficial or deep to the platysma, depending on surgeon preference. Beyond the anterior border of the parotid gland the facial nerve branches are stabilized by the masseteric fascia but can easily be transected if the surgeon is not in the correct plane. Some surgeons inject tumescent solution into the face before the face lift to help maintain hemostasis and to help hydrodissect the sub-SMAS plane. Submentoplasty with or without platysmaplasty is typically included, as described earlier in this chapter. When using the deep plane technique it is more common to completely dissect the neck skin from SCM to SCM. This is typically performed in the subcutaneous plane but can also be done bluntly just deep to the platysma[45]; the facial dissection is in a sub-SMAS plane, and the neck dissection is usually in a supraplatysmal plane. The SMAS and platysma are advanced superolaterally and attached to the tough preauricular and mastoid fascia to support the lift. The skin is redraped and tailored as necessary.

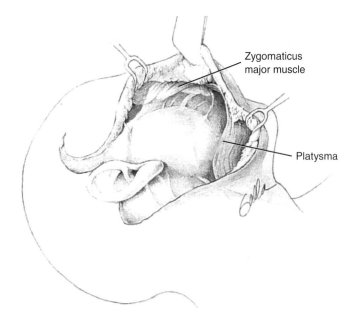

Zygomaticus
major muscle

Platysma

Fig. 40-16   Deep plane rhytidectomy. The zygomaticus major muscle is used as a marker to help safely carry the sub-SMAS dissection to the nasolabial fold. Supraplatysmal elevation in the neck is combined with subplatysmal elevation in the face. The masseteric fascia helps protect the facial nerve branches and parotid duct between the medial parotid gland and lateral zygomaticus major. When composite rhytidectomy technique is used, the orbicularis oculi muscle is elevated with the deep plane flap.

Theoretically, the deep plane face lift carries a higher risk of facial nerve injury as compared with other face-lift methods. Because it is a larger surgery the recovery time is often longer than that of the SFSR. Some well-designed studies do suggest that the deep plane allows excision of more skin and has a lower early revision (tuck-up) rate compared with SMAS face lifts.[48,49]

THE MINIMAL ACCESS CRANIAL SUSPENSION LIFT

The minimal access cranial suspension (MACS) lift is a type of short-scar face lift described by Tonnard and Verpaele in 2002,[27] whose goal was to achieve an effective, long-lasting face lift that could be completed relatively quickly under local anesthetic. Like all short-scar face lifts, the vector of facial lift is vertically oriented; there is no postauricular incision to permit a more lateral suspension. Extrapolating Jacono and Ransom's[45] findings with the deep plane lift to the MACS lift suggests that it is most appropriate for younger patients without significant neck skin laxity. Proponents of the MACS and other short-scar face lifts state that facial structures descend in a vertical plane and therefore should be elevated in a vertical plane. Short-scar and short-flap face lifts are different procedures and should not be confused with one another.

The SMAS plication technique in the MACS lift is somewhat unusual in that it uses purse-string sutures in and out of the SMAS to achieve the lift. This causes microplications throughout the SMAS but there is no excision or imbrication of the SMAS. Two or three sutures are used depending on whether midfacial elevation is desired. The first suture is called the *vertical loop* and primarily elevates the neck. The second suture is called the *oblique loop* and targets the jowl. The optional third suture is called the *malar loop* and targets the midface structures. The procedure is typically completed under local anesthesia. The incision begins at the auricular lobule and proceeds in the preauricular region in the standard, gender-appropriate fashion. The temporal incision is made 2 mm into the hairline in a trichophytic fashion, and it is zigzagged, which helps redrape the elevated facial skin at the end of the case. A subcutaneous flap is raised for 5 to 6 cm anterior to the auricle and inferior down to the mandibular angle. If the third midface suspension suture is planned, subcutaneous elevation proceeds over the malar eminence also. The purse-string sutures are anchored to the deep temporalis fascia above the zygomatic arch in a safe zone away from the course of the frontal branch of the facial nerve (Fig. 40-17).

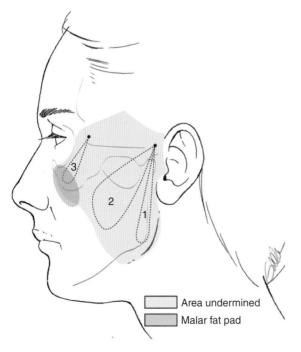

Area undermined
Malar fat pad

Fig. 40-17 The minimal access cranial suspension lift. Two or three purse-string sutures of 1-0 PDS are used to create microplications within the SMAS, which elevates the facial soft tissues. The lift is almost purely vertical, making it most appropriate for younger patients with mild to moderate aging in the neck.

Tonnard and Verpaele analyzed 1-year results of their first 450 patients and found that in 95% of cases the MACS lift with submental liposuction achieved the desired outcome. There was a 5% 1-year revision rate (with 7 patients requiring a secondary platysmaplasty and 16 patients requiring an occipital hairline incision to remove additional neck skin).[50]

EVIDENCE-BASED OUTCOMES AND COMPARISONS

There are relatively few well-designed studies comparing the efficacy of the various face-lift techniques. This paucity of outcomes information exists primarily because there is no universally accepted, validated, easy-to-perform outcome measure for facial rejuvenation surgery. A complete review of all outcomes studies is beyond the scope of this chapter and is well-covered in several recent evidence-based reviews,[51-53] although several relevant findings are summarized here.

In 1996 Ivy et al performed a prospective randomized study comparing the efficacy of the standard SMAS face lift with the composite and extended-SMAS techniques.[54] Subjects underwent conventional SMAS suspension on one side of the face and an extended SMAS or composite rhytidectomy on the other side of the face. Six surgeons, including three surgeons intimately involved with the study, scored improvement in the midface and nasolabial fold using photographs at 24 hours, 6 months, and 1 year postoperatively. The authors concluded that none of the techniques achieved any lasting improvement in the nasolabial fold or midface.

In 1998 Kamer and Frankel[48] retrospectively reviewed 279 SMAS suspension and 355 deep plane face lifts performed by the senior author. The primary outcome measure was the need for a *tuck-up procedure,* defined as any surgery within 18 months of the initial face lift designed to remove excess skin. There was a significantly lower tuck-up rate in the deep plane group (3.3% versus 11.4%, $p = 0.0001$).

In 2004 Becker and Bassichis[55] performed a retrospective review of 20 SMAS plication lifts and 20 deep plane face lifts performed by the senior author. Standard photographs taken between 6 and 18 months postoperatively were evaluated by four blinded facial plastic surgeons. Raters were asked to score the improvement at the melolabial fold, jowl, and cheek on an author-created 5-point scale between excellent (5) and poor (1). By means of a chi-square analysis the authors concluded that there was a trend toward better outcomes using SMAS-plication in younger patients and an improved result using the deep plane face lift in older patients.

In a fascinating 2006 study Litner and Adamson performed an intraoperative analysis of mean skin excess and movement of facial landmarks after three successive types of rhytidectomy in 32 patients.[49] All surgeries began with a subcutaneous elevation for 3 cm anterior and posterior to the auricle. First, a simple SMAS plication without any SMAS excision was completed. Second, a J-shaped SMAS excision was performed anterior and inferior to the auricle with SMAS imbrication. In the third and final successive procedure, a modified deep plane lift was executed. In the first 15 patients mean skin excess at the intertragal incisura was measured after each successive lift. The authors found an average of 10.4, 12.8, and 19.4 mm of excess skin after the SMAS plication, SMAS imbrication, and deep plane techniques. In the next 17 patients the authors measured the movement of facial landmarks in the midface, jawline, and neck after the three successive face lifts. Again the authors found that the deep plane technique achieved greater landmark movement in all three facial regions than SMAS imbrication, which in turn was more efficacious than the SMAS plication technique. None of the face lifts, including the deep plane technique, moved the midface landmark to any significant degree.

In 2006 Prado et al[56] retrospectively analyzed 82 patients undergoing short-scar face lifts, consisting of 41 MACS lifts and 41 lateral SMASectomy procedures. Two blinded plastic surgeons evaluated patient photographs 1 and 24 months postoperatively using the Strasser scale, which measures malposition, distortion, asymmetry, contour deformity, and scar. The surgeons also scored patient pain using a 10-point visual-analog scale at 24 hours after surgery (but the patients did not score their own pain). The authors found no difference in Strasser scores for the two different short-scar techniques. The MACS lift was significantly faster (165 versus 190 minutes, $p = 0.001$) but caused more pain (6 versus 4, $p = 0.0001$) than the lateral SMASectomy technique. The authors felt that more than 50% of the patients in each group needed a tuck-up procedure because of recurrent jowling, which suggests that short-scar face lifts may not be as long lasting as other techniques.

In 2010 Jacono and Stong[57] compared the movement of the nasolabial fold using a transtemporal midface lift versus the deep plane rhytidectomy in a cadaver model. They found that a transtemporal lift with a suture placed through the malar prominence achieved more lift than with standard deep plane lifting techniques (10.6 mm versus 7.4 mm, $p = 0.03$).

In 2011 Swanson performed an elegant assessment of subjective patient benefit after face lift. This parameter reflects an important method of analysis, particularly because rhytidectomy is an elective procedure designed to improve the patient's appearance and self-image. The author conducted an extensive interview with 93 patients at their 1-month postoperative visit after deep plane rhytidectomy, representing a response rate of 76% over the study period.[58] The average perceived age reduction was 11.9 years (range 0 to 28 years); 83% and 70% of patients noted improved self-image and quality of life, respectively; and 97% of patients reported a more youthful appearance. The study also yielded important data regarding postoperative recovery. Patients used narcotic pain medicine for an average of 5 days after surgery and returned to driving 7 days after surgery, although this was delayed an additional week on average in patients who were also undergoing blepharoplasty. Patients felt presentable in public 1 month after surgery, back to normal in 2.5 months, and noted that all postoperative edema had resolved by 80 days after surgery. In the future, comparing these data with patients after SMAS-imbrication face lift would confirm or refute the perceived faster recovery after less invasive face-lift techniques.

PERIOPERATIVE CARE

Elective facial surgery in general has a much higher risk of bleeding than deep venous thrombosisc (DVT). Chemoprophylaxis with heparin or low-molecular-weight heparin may increase the risk of bleeding, and the surgeon must carefully balance the risks of bleeding and thrombosis in each patient. There is a much higher risk of deep venous thrombosis in patients undergoing general anesthesia; intermittent compression devices significantly reduce this risk. Under conscious sedation[59] there are no reports of DVT after face lift, although this can be a silent complication if it does not progress to pulmonary embolism. The rate of bleeding complications has been reported to be much higher in patients receiving perioperative chemoprophylaxis compared with compression stockings alone (16.2% versus 1.1%, $p = 0.003$).

Several well-designed studies have examined the efficacy of tissue sealants and suction drains in reducing hematoma, bruising, and edema after rhytidectomy[60] and have shown no objective or patient-scored subjective difference in edema, hematoma, or pain at either 1 day or 1 week postoperatively. However, there appears to be a reduction in bruising on the drained side 1 week postoperatively. Fibrin glue applied under skin flaps appears to yield reduction in the incidence of hematoma and seroma and a significant reduction in prolonged edema and bruising. Some data suggest that fibrin glue may only be worthwhile to prevent hematoma in the higher-risk male population.

There are very few well-designed studies examining the effect of platelet gel after rhytidectomy, although some data suggest that its use results in less edema or bruising. Multiple small studies have examined the efficacy of platelet gels with mixed results. In a recently published commentary on the subject Farrior stated that he no longer uses autologous platelet gels because the benefit does not appear to outweigh the cost.[61]

There are no high-quality studies comparing the efficacy of tissue sealants to suction drains. The prevention of expanding hematomas is likely most dependent on surgical technique, and one should not depend on tissue sealants to prevent this potentially disastrous complication.

The effects of *Arnica montana* on postoperative bruising are equivocal, but there is likely no negative consequence to its use, and it is relatively inexpensive, although it is not FDA approved.

Most surgeons prescribe a week of oral antibiotics to cover gram positive organisms, whereas some surgeons prefer ciprofloxacin to cover *Pseudomonas* from the ear canal instead.

COMPLICATIONS

HEMATOMA

Hematoma is the most common perioperative complication after rhytidectomy. Large studies typically report a rate of 2% to 4%, and hematoma is more common in men because of the increased vascularity of their hair-bearing facial skin.[62,63] Hematomas can be classified into expanding and nonexpanding hematomas.

Expanding hematomas typically occur in the first 24 hours after surgery, heralded by frank blood in suction drains, increasing pain, and facial swelling. Swelling may not be immediately visible beneath compression dressings. Other possible findings on physical exam include a bluish discoloration to the buccal mucosa, eversion of the lips, and an unexpected amount of bruising. Expanding hematomas require prompt surgical drainage to prevent tissue necrosis and/or airway obstruction. All clots should be removed and the source of bleeding should be identified if possible. It is always necessary to place new suction drains. Some authors recommend placing fibrin glue in the wound because these patients are clearly in a high-risk group for bleeding. The patients should be seen with 24 hours after evacuation to check for reaccumulation.

The surgeon can evacuate smaller, *nonexpanding hematomas* at the bedside or in the office by taking out one or two sutures and passing a thin sterile Frazier suction into the area of blood accumulation. Small, nonexpanding hematomas will typically liquefy after 5 to 10 days and can also be aspirated with an 18-gauge needle.

SKIN LOSS

Skin flap necrosis can follow rhytidectomy for a variety of reasons. Hematoma is likely the most common cause. Surgical errors, including superficial dissection causing damage to the subdermal plexus, excess tension on the skin closure, and extensive cervicofacial dissection, can also cause skin slough. Tobacco use in the perioperative period is a modifiable risk factor. Skin loss is typically only partial thickness, and reepithelialization will occur with conservative wound care. Full-thickness skin loss may result in a hypertrophic scar, and large areas may require skin grafting. Hyperbaric oxygen may be beneficial in the management of these patients.

NERVE INJURY

The great auricular nerve is the most commonly injured nerve during rhytidectomy.[64] This is because of its superficial location on the surface of the SCM in the infraauricular region. The thick, fibrous attachment of the skin over the SCM and the minimal subcutaneous fat in this area also make it more difficult to establish a clear plane of dissection. Careful flap elevation under direct visualization is likely the best way to avoid injury to this nerve. If it is transected it should be repaired using a 9-0 nylon suture under magnification or with a nerve conduit.

Facial nerve injury is the most feared complication of rhytidectomy. The facial nerve is theoretically at more risk during deep plane, high SMAS, and endoscopic subperiosteal face lifts, but hard data confirming this hypothesis are elusive. Surgeons are understandably reticent to report permanent facial nerve injury data. After face-lift surgery, the facial function should be examined in the recovery area. Lidocaine can take up to 6 hours to wear off, so a region of dense paresis should be observed initially. A dense paresis lasting longer than 24 hours may be a result of a stretch, cautery, or transection injury. The best treatment for facial nerve transection involving the buccal and/or zygomatic branches is exploration with primary nerve repair. It is easier to find the injured nerve early, before significant scarring occurs. If a transection is believed to be unlikely, it is not unreasonable to observe the patient for 1 to 2 weeks for any sign of recovery, but exploration should occur within 30 days if possible. Most studies suggest that open and honest communication of medical errors helps to prevent and resolve malpractice claims.[65] If the face-lift surgeon is uncomfortable performing facial nerve exploration, the patient should be referred to a facial nerve expert.

SCARS

Rhytidectomy incisions usually heal well in the absence of significant tension on the closure line. The portion of the incision between the auricle and occipital hairline is probably most at risk of hypertrophic scarring. Hypertrophic scarring typically responds to serial injections of triamcinolone, although this does carry some risk of skin atrophy. There is some recent evidence that 5-fluorouracil (5-FU) injections are similarly efficacious with less risk of skin thinning and pigment change.[66,67] 5-FU is an antimetabolite that specifically targets synthetically active cells like fibroblasts and has been shown to specifically reduce type I collagen production in human fibroblasts.[68] Typical injections include 0.1 to 0.5 cc of 5-FU in a 9:1 mixture with triamcinolone (10 mg/cc) every 2 to 4 weeks, until an acceptable appearance is achieved.

Tension on the skin closure around the ear lobule can cause a variety of deformities, including inferior displacement of the earlobe, obliteration of the sulcus between the auricle and face, and "pixie ear" deformity. These deformities can typically be repaired at 6 to 12 months after surgery with scar excision and a tension-free closure. A retracted or pixie ear lobule can be released with a V-Y superior advancement of the earlobe.

HAIR LOSS

Hair loss is most common in the sideburn and temple. Permanent hair loss can occur with poor surgical technique after transecting or cauterizing hair follicles. However, even dissection in the proper subfollicular plane can cause telogen effluvium, in which case the hair should return within 6 months. As discussed earlier, when planning significant skin excision on a female patient it is important to use a trichophytic incision inferior to the temporal tuft to prevent excessive elevation of the preauricular hairline. It is also important to realign the occipital hairline after skin excision in the postauricular sulcus. In severe cases, micrograft hair transplantation is an option.

PAROTID INJURY

Sub-SMAS dissection risks injury to the parotid gland parenchyma and/or ductal system. This can result in a salivary accumulation beneath the superficial flap, which may delay healing. Furthermore, if the skin flap does not stick down, a persistent salivary leak can lead to a fistula or pseudocyst. If the parotid capsule is injured during a face-lift surgery it should be repaired as much as possible. The SMAS can then be used to reinforce this area during SMAS suspension. Salivary pseudocysts should be treated with light pressure dressings and intermittent needle aspiration until resolution. Larger pseudocysts and fistulas through the skin may require closed-suction drainage.

DEPRESSION

Short-term depression occurs in up to 50% of women undergoing rhytidectomy.[69] This symptom develops in the acute recovery period in response to edema, bruising, and overall unnatural appearance. It typically resolves once the patient's appearance normalizes. In rare cases, a short course of antidepressant medication is necessary. There is some association of selective serotonin reuptake inhibitors (SSRIs) with an increased risk of bleeding. However, a recent large retrospective analysis found no evidence that SSRI use increases the incidence of hematoma after rhytidectomy.[70]

CONCLUSION

Rhytidectomy continues to be one of the most powerful techniques in our armamentarium for facial rejuvenation. Most rhytidectomy techniques that employ SMAS suspension are very effective at improving the jaw line and repositioning ptotic tissues. Complementary techniques such as midface volume restoration, chin augmentation, and customized submentoplasty have allowed a more natural facial rejuvenation outcome.

KEY POINTS

- Modern concepts of facial aging emphasize deflation and the redistribution of facial volume from the upper to lower face. The youthful face has a narrow, sharp jawline with a wide orbitomalar complex that focuses attention around the eyes.
- Rhytidectomy should be thought of as a facial reshaping procedure.
- Short-flap SMAS rhytidectomy is a safe, relatively quick procedure that has a short recovery period but long-lasting results.
- The philosophical ideas that led to the development of the deep plane face lift are somewhat outdated. However, studies suggest that in patients with advanced facial aging and significant laxity, the deep plane lift can remove more skin and has a lower revision rate than SMAS rhytidectomy.
- The minimal access cranial suspension lift is a safe and effective short-scar rhytidectomy technique. It requires a vertical lift, making it most appropriate for younger patients who do not require a multivector approach.
- Patients who are having rhytidectomy under general anesthesia should have intermittent compression devices applied on the lower extremities to reduce the risk of deep venous thrombosis.
- Suction drains likely reduce the appearance of bruising after face-lift surgery. There is no evidence that tissue sealants or platelet gels reduce the risk of expanding hematoma or are cost effective.
- Patients with facial weakness after rhytidectomy should be followed carefully. Weakness in the frontal or marginal nerve distributions should be observed. Midface weakness should be explored, because this likely represents transection of a large buccal or zygomatic branch. Early exploration and primary repair gives the best chance for successful return of a spontaneous emotive smile.

REFERENCES

1. Uitto J. The role of elastin and collagen in cutaneous aging: intrinsic aging versus photoexposure. J Drugs Dermatol 7(2 Suppl):S12-S16, 2008.

2. Rohrich RJ, Pessa JE, Ristow B. The youthful cheek and the deep medial fat compartment. Plast Reconstr Surg 121:2107-2112, 2008.
   This landmark article began to delineate well-circumscribed fat compartments in the face and demonstrated how volume augmentation could significantly reverse age-related changes in the midface.

3. Zadoo VP, Pessa JE. Biological arches and changes to the curvilinear form of the aging maxilla. Plast Reconstr Surg 106:460-466, 2000.

4. Pessa JE, Zadoo VP, Yuan C, et al. Concertina effect and facial aging: nonlinear aspects of youthfulness and skeletal remodeling and why, perhaps, infants have jowls. Plast Reconstr Surg 103:635-644, 1999.

5. Pessa JE, Zadoo VP, Mutimer KL, et al. Relative maxillary retrusion as a natural consequence of aging: combining skeletal and soft-tissue changes into an integrated model of midfacial aging. Plast Reconstr Surg 102:205-212, 1998.

6. Pessa JE, Slice DE, Hanz KR, Broadbent TH, Rohrich RJ. Aging and the shape of the mandible. Plast Reconstr Surg 121:196-200, 2008.

7. Gierloff M, Stohring C, Buder T, et al. Aging changes in the midfacial fat compartments: a computed tomographic study. Plast Reconstr Surg 129:263-273, 2012.
   This groundbreaking study uses computed tomography to delineate the boundaries of the superficial and deep facial fat compartments, analyzes the changes that occur in these compartments with age, and proposes a theory for age-related facial volume changes.

8. Shaw RB, Katzel EB, Koltz PF, et al. Aging of the facial skeleton: Aesthetic implications and rejuvenation strategies. Plast Reconstr Surg 127:374-383, 2011.

9. Richard MJ, Morris C, Deen BF, et al. Analysis of the anatomic changes of the aging facial skeleton using computer-assisted tomography. Ophthal Plast Reconstr Surg 25:382-386, 2009.

10. Hollander E. Cosmetic surgery. In Joseph M, ed. Handbuch der Kosmetik. Leipzig, Germany: Veriag vot Velt, 1912.

11. Aufricht G. Surgery for excess skin of the face. Transactions of the Second International Congress of Plastic Surgery. Edinburgh: E & S Livingstone, 1960.

12. Webster RC, Smith RC, Papsidero MJ, et al. Comparison of SMAS plication with SMAS imbrication in face lifting. Laryngoscope 92:901-912, 1982.

13. Skoog T. Plastic Surgery: New Methods and Refinements. Philadelphia: Saunders, 1974.

14. Mitz V, Peyronie M. The superficial musculo-aponeurotic system (SMAS) in the parotid and cheek area. Plast Reconstr Surg 58:80-88, 1976.
    The first detailed description of the SMAS.

15. Hamra ST. The deep plane rhytidectomy. Plast Reconstr Surg 86:53-61, 1990.
    The first description of the deep plane face lift.

16. Hamra ST. Composite rhytidectomy. Plast Reconstr Surg 90:1-13, 1992.

17. Owsley JQ. Lifting the malar fat pad for correction of prominent nasolabial folds. Plast Reconstr Surg 91:463-474, 1993.

18. Owsley JQ, Fiala TG. Update: lifting the malar fat pad for correction of prominent nasolabial folds. Plast Reconstr Surg 100:715-722, 1997.

19. Tessier P. [Subperiosteal face-lift] Ann Chir Plast Esthet 34:193-197, 1989.

20. Psillakis JM, Rumley TO, Camargos A. Subperiosteal approach as an improved concept for correction of the aging face. Plast Reconstr Surg 82:383-394, 1988.

21. Ramirez OM, Mailard GF, Musolas A. The extended subperiosteal midface lift: a definitive soft tissue remodeling for facial rejuvenation. Plast Reconstr Surg 88:227-236, 1991.

22. Isse NG. Endoscopic facial rejuvenation: endoforehead, the functional lift. Case reports. Aesthetic Plast Surg 18:21-29, 1994.

23. Ramirez OM. Endoscopic full facelift. Aesthetic Plast Surg 18:363-371, 1994.

24. Baker SR. Triplane rhytidectomy: combining the best of all worlds. Arch Otolaryngol Head Neck Surg 123:1167-1172, 1997.

25. Saylan Z. The s-lift for facial rejuvenation. Int J Cosmet Surg 7:18-23, 1999.

26. Baker D. Minimal incision rhytidectomy (short scar facelift) with lateral SMASectomy. Aesthetic Surg J 21:68-79, 2001.

27. Tonnard P, Verpaele A, Monstrey S, et al. Minimal access cranial suspension lift: a modified S-lift. Plast Reconstr Surg 109:2074-2086, 2002.
    The first in-depth description of the MACS lift.

28. Tzafetta K, Terzis JK. Essays on the facial nerve: part I. Microanatomy. Plast Reconstr Surg 125:879-889, 2010.

29. Gosain AK, Sewall SR, Yousif NJ. The temporal branch of the facial nerve: how reliably can we predict its path? Plast Reconstr Surg 99:1223-1233, 1997.
    A careful, in-depth cadaver study of the anatomy of the temporal branch of the facial nerve in relation to the zygomatic arch.

30. Trussler AP, Stephan P, Hatef D, et al. The frontal branch of the facial nerve across the zygomatic arch: anatomical relevance of the high-SMAS technique. Plast Reconstr Surg 125:1221-1229, 2010.

31. Agarwal CA, Mendenhall SD, Foreman KB, et al. The course of the frontal branch of the facial nerve in relation to fascial planes: an anatomic study. Plast Reconstr Surg 125:532-537, 2010.
    A careful, in-depth cadaver study analyzing the location of the frontal branch of the facial nerve in relation to the SMAS and parotideomasseteric fascia over the zygomatic arch and in the temple.

32. Janfaza P, Cheney ML. Superficial structures of the face, head and parotid region. In Janfaza P, Nadol JB, Galla R, et al. Surgical Anatomy of the Head and Neck. Cambridge, MA: Harvard University Press, 2011.

33. Rees TD, Liverett DM, Guy CL. The effect of cigarette smoking on skin-flap survival in the face lift patient. Plast Reconstr Surg 73:911-915, 1984.

34. Grover R, Jones BM, Waterhouse N. The prevention of hematoma following rhytidectomy: a review of 1078 consecutive facelifts. Br J Plast Surg 54:481-486, 2001.

35. Parikh S, Jacono A. Deep plane face-lift as an alternative in the smoking patient. Arch Facial Plast Surg 13:283-285, 2011.

36. Ellenbogen R, Karlin JV. Visual criteria for success in restoring the youthful neck. Plast Reconstr Surg 66:826-837, 1980.
    An important historical paper identifying the aesthetic components of a youthful neckline.

37. Feldman JJ. Corset platysmaplasty. Plast Reconstr Surg 85:333-343, 1990.
    Initial description of a powerful, commonly practiced platysmaplasty method.

37a. Guyuron B, Sadek EY, Ahmadian R. A 26-year experience with vest-over-pants technique platysmarrhaphy. Plast Reconstr Surg 126:1027-1034, 2010.

38. Webster RC, Smith RC, Smith KF. Face lift, part I: extent of undermining of skin flaps. Head Neck Surg 5:525-534, 1983.

39. Webster RC, Hamdan U, Fuleihan N, et al. The considered and considerate facelift. Am J Cosmet Surg 2:1-5, 1985.

40. Webster RC, Smith RC, Papsidero MJ, et al. Comparison of SMAS plication with SMAS imbrication in face lifting. Laryngoscope 92:901-912, 1982.

41. Burgess LP, Casler JD, Kryzer TC. Wound tension in rhytidectomy. Effects of skin flap undermining and superficial musculoaponeurotic system suspension. Arch Otolaryngol Head Neck Surg 119:173-176, 1993.

42. McCollough EG, Perkins SW, Langsdon PR. SASMAS suspension rhytidectomy. Rationale and long-term experience. Arch Otolaryngol Head Neck Surg 115:228-234, 1989.

43. Mendelson BC, Muzaffar AR, Adams WP. Surgical anatomy of the midcheek and malar mounds. Plast Reconstr Surg 110:885-896, 2002.

44. Muzaffar AR, Mendelson BC, Adams WP. Surgical anatomy of the ligamentous attachments of the lower lid and lateral canthus. Plast Reconstr Surg 110:873-884, 2002.

45. Jacono AA, Ransom ER. Patient-specific rhytidectomy: finding the angle of maximal rejuvenation. Aesthetic Surg J 32:804-813, 2012.
    A fascinating study comparing the ideal angle of SMAS suspension during deep plane face lift performed in younger versus older patients.

46. Rohrich RJ, Pessa JE. The retaining system of the face: histologic evaluation of the septal boundaries of the subcutaneous fat compartments. Plast Reconstr Surg 121:1904-1909, 2008.
    A landmark within-subject chronologic analysis of what changes and what does not in periorbital and midfacial anatomy with aging. One of the first studies to emphasize deflation, not descent, as the primary cause of midfacial aging.

47. Hamra ST. A study of the long-term effect of malar fat repositioning in face lift surgery: short-term success but long-term failure. Plast Reconstr Surg 110:940-951, 2002.
   Hamra's own analysis of his 10-year results using the deep plane technique showing that nasolabial fold effacement did not last.

48. Kamer FM, Frankel AS. SMAS rhytidectomy versus deep plane rhytidectomy: an objective comparison. Plast Reconstr Surg 102:878-881, 1998.
   Single-surgeon comparison of more than 600 deep plane and SMAS face lifts.

49. Litner JA, Adamson PA. Limited vs. extended face-lift techniques: objective analysis of intraoperative results. Arch Facial Plast Surg 8:186-190, 2006.
   A fascinating analysis of facial landmark movement and skin excision achieved using SMAS and deep plane techniques.

50. Tonnard PL, Verpaele A, Gaia S. Optimizing results from minimal access cranial suspension lifting (MACS-lift). Aesth Plast Surg 29:213-220, 2005.

51. Marcus BC. Rhytidectomy: current concepts, controversies and the state of the art. Curr Opin Otolaryngol Head Neck Surg 20:262-266, 2012.

52. Stuzin JM. MOC-PS CME article: face lifting. Plast Reconstr Surg 121:1-19, 2008.

53. Chang S, Pusic A, Rohrich RJ. A systematic review of comparison of efficacy and complication rates among face-lift techniques. Plast Reconstr Surg 127:423-433, 2011.
   The most thorough review of evidence-based data regarding rhytidectomy.

54. Ivy EJ, Lorenc ZP, Aston SJ. Is there a difference? A prospective study comparing lateral and standard SMAS face lifts with extended SMAS and composite rhytidectomies. Plast Reconstr Surg 98:1135-1143, 1996.

55. Becker FF, Bassichis BA. Deep-plane face-lift vs. superficial musculoaponeurotic system plication face-lift: a comparative study. Arch Facial Plast Surg 6:8-13, 2004.

56. Prado A, Andrades P, Danilla S, et al. A clinical retrospective study comparing two short-scar face lifts: minimal access cranial suspension versus lateral SMASectomy. Plast Reconstr Surg 117:1413-1425, 2006.

57. Jacono AA, Stong BC. Anatomic comparison of the deep-plane face-lift and the transtemporal midface lift. Arch Facial Plast Surg 12:339-341, 2010.

58. Swanson E. Outcome analysis in 93 facial rejuvenation patients treated with a deep-plane face lift. Plast Reconstr Surg 127:823-834, 2011.

59. Durnig P, Jungwirth W. Low-molecular-weight heparin and postoperative bleeding in rhytidectomy. Plast Reconstr Surg 118:502-507, 2006.

60. Jones BM, Grover R, Hamilton S. The efficacy of surgical drainage in cervicofacial rhytidectomy: a prospective, randomized, controlled trial. Plast Reconstr Surg 120:263-270, 2007.

61. Farrior E, Ladner K. A retrospective review of the use of autologous platelet gels for rhytidectomy. Arch Facial Plast Surg 14:83-84, 2012.

62. Pitanguy I, Machado BH. Facial rejuvenation surgery: a retrospective study of 8788 cases. Aesthetic Surg J 32:393-412, 2012.

63. Warren RJ, Aston SJ, Mendelson BC. Face lift. Plast Reconstr Surg 128:747e-764e, 2011.

64. Baker SR. Rhytidectomy. In Cummings CW, Flint PW, Haughey BH, et al. Otolaryngology Head and Neck Surgery. St Louis: Mosby, 2005.

65. Robbennolt JK. Apologies and legal settlement: an empirical examination. Mich Law Rev 102:460-516, 2003.

66. Fitzpatrick RE. Treatment of inflamed hypertrophic scars using intralesional 5-FU. Dermatol Surg 25:224-232, 1999.

67. Manuskiatti W, Fitzpatrick RE. Treatment response of keloidal and hypertrophic sternotomy scars: comparison among intralesional corticosteroid, 5-fluorouracil, and 585-nm flashlamp-pumped pulsed-dye laser treatments. Arch Dermatol 138:1149-1155, 2002.

68. Bulstrode NW, Mudera V, McGrouther DA, et al. 5-fluorouracil selectively inhibits collagen synthesis. Plast Reconstr Surg 116:209-221, 2005.

69. Goin MK, Burgoyne RW, Goin JM, et al. A prospective psychological study of 50 female face-lift patients. Plast Reconstr Surg 65:436-442, 1980.

70. Harirchian S, Zoumalan RA, Rosenberg DB. Antidepressants and bleeding risk after face-lift surgery. Arch Facial Plast Surg 14:248-252, 2012.

41

Skin Resurfacing: Laser, Chemical Peels, and Mechanical Dermabrasion

Lori A. Brightman ▪ *Kavitha K. Reddy*
Caitlyn D. Clark ▪ *Oon Tian Tan*

Anumber of various techniques to improve the appearance of aging skin have been the focus of intense activity within the field of aesthetic surgery. The public has increasingly sought interventions that will preserve a youthful appearance and camouflage aging skin. This demand has expanded the market and driven innovations that address the classic signs of skin aging. Such demands have led to the evolution of several skin-resurfacing methods to address the wrinkles and blemishes that arise from photoaged skin, as well as to address other disfiguring skin conditions such as scars and cutaneous discoloration (such as lentigines). These methods employ lasers, chemical peels, and mechanical dermabrasion; all methods are designed to induce controlled injury to the skin. The rationale is that the injury heals by regeneration with new collagen, thereby altering the effects of photoaging.[1]

HISTORICAL PERSPECTIVE: CHEMICAL EXFOLIATION

The desire to improve skin texture using chemical exfoliation dates to ancient Egypt. This was achieved by the application of a variety of animal oils and alabaster (Fig. 41-1). The use of other chemicals evolved over time, including sulphur, mustards, and limestone.[2] In the Middle Ages wine was used as a chemical exfoliant, with tartaric acid as the active agent. However, it was not until the early twentieth century that modern chemical exfoliation was introduced by George MacKee, who applied phenol (carbolic acid) to treat acne scars in 1903.[3] He recommended superficial peels in which phenol was applied to the skin for 30 to 60 seconds, then washed off immediately with ethanol; this required four to six treatments at 2-month intervals.[4,5] Phenol peels continued to be used for cosmetic treatment in the 1930s to treat laxity of the

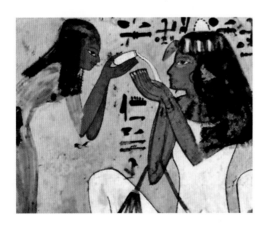

Fig. 41-1 Painting depicting chemical exfoliation in ancient Egypt.

lower eyelids by Sir Harold Gillies, and by others to remove wrinkles, including those in the cervical area.[6] However, this technique soon fell out of favor because of the scarring that resulted in a significant percentage of cases.

It was not until 1941 that Eller and Wolff[7] reintroduced the use of phenol in a combination paste with resorcinol in conjunction with carbon dioxide cryotherapy to desquamate and resurface the skin. In 1941 salicylic acid under occlusion was introduced by Urkov[8] for skin resurfacing. Detailed histologic changes following topical application of phenol to actinically damaged skin were documented by Ayres in 1960 in dermal collagen.[4,5,8] He demonstrated that following this injury, repair resulted in the formation of parallel bundles of horizontally arranged new collagen, 0.3 to 0.4 mm thick, in the subepidermal layer of the dermis. He noted that these histologic changes were very similar to those observed following dermabrasion. From these findings, in 1961 Baker and Gordon advocated the use of a 50% phenol solution occluded with a waterproof tape-mask.[5] This technique was further modified by McCullough and Hillman[6] in 1980, who demonstrated that patients were more comfortable and achieved similar results when the phenol was applied to the skin without occlusion. Litton in 1962 was one of the first investigators to demonstrate histologically that the papillary dermis was widened after phenol peeling. These histologic findings were further substantiated by Stegman in 1980 following phenol peeling in both sun-damaged and nondamaged skin.[4,5]

In the 1980s interest focused on finding alternatives to the standard phenol peels. In 1989 Stagnone[9] reported that the skin appeared refreshed with superficial peels. Trichloracetic acid (TCA) was advocated for light and medium depth peels by Brody in 1986. Weiss, in 1988, demonstrated that the topical use of retinoic acid (retin A) for 6 months or longer would effectively improve wrinkling of the skin and at the same time remove actinic and pigmented solar keratosis. Resurgance of combination substances followed for different depth peels. Stagnone and Brody advocated the use of Jessner's solution (resorcinol, salicylic acid and lactic acid), a modified Unna's resorcinol paste, alpha-hydroxy acids and retinoic acid for light peels. TCA, 5-fluorouracil (5FU) and carbon dioxide cryotherapy were also discussed by Brody who proposed that these agents used alone or in combination could be used for light, medium, or deeper-depth peels.

HISTORICAL PERSPECTIVE: LASERS

LASER is the acronym for *l*ight *a*mplification by *s*timulated *e*mission of *r*adiation. The theorectical basis for lasers was formulated by Albert Einstein in 1917, who first explained the theory of stimulated emission. However, it was in the late 1940s and 1950s that scientists and engineers, including Charles Townes, Joseph Weber, Alexander Prokohorov and Nikolai G. Basov, applied this principal and pioneered the device that amplified microwaves for application in microwave communications systems; that is, MASER (*m*icrowave *a*mplification by the *s*timulated *e*mission of *r*adiation).[10] It was Townes and other engineers who created an optical MASER, a device for creating powerful beams of light using higher frequency energy to stimulate what was later known as the lasing medium. Despite such progress, it was Theodore Maiman, at the Hughes Research Laboratory in California, who made the first functional ruby laser in 1960 by shining a high-powered xenon flashlamp on a ruby rod with silver-coated surface at 693.7 nm of 1 ms duration and a power output of a billion watts per pulse.[11]

One year after Maiman published his paper on the ruby laser, ophthalmologists who were already using xenon lamps for retinal photocoagulation described studies using the laser for treating retinal tears, flat detachments, angiomas, and tumors.[12]

In dermatology, there was already a long tradition of using light for the treatment of cutaneous conditions, such as the Finsen lamp in 1899 for lupus vulgaris; artificial UV light sources to treat rickets and promote wound healing in 1901; and the combination of light and tar for psoriasis in 1925. Laser technology was embraced by Leon Goldman in 1961. He and his coworkers published their first study on the effects of lasers on selective destruction of pigmented lesions of the skin in 1963.[13] They described the highly selective injury of pigmented structures in the skin, including hair follicles, with no damage to adjacent or underlying uninvolved skin. He went on to report use of the laser for the removal of tattoos, nevi, and melanomas with the Q-switched ruby laser.[14] As new lasers developed, Goldman and his coworkers began to treat new cutaneous lesions such as vascular malformations with the argon laser, and later with the continuous neodymium:yttrium-aluminium garnet (Nd:YAG) laser.

Advances in the use of chemical peels and various laser applications have been continuous since these early efforts. These will be discussed later in this chapter.

PATIENT SELECTION AND ASSESSMENT

To achieve optimal results from skin rejuvenation procedures, careful patient selection and assessment are critical (Box 41-1). Selection of patients is based on certain criteria including, skin color and sunburn history (Fitzpatrick skin type) (Table 41-1), history of sun exposure, condition of photoaged skin (Glogau classification) (Table 41-2), general medical condition, smoking history, as well as history of scarring and response to previous cosmetic procedures. All of these variables help to assess how the skin will react to the induced injury and thus determine the best rejuvenation procedure appropriate for that individual. Together, they contribute to optimizing a good skin rejuvenation result. Pertinent past medical history includes noting a tendency toward postinflammatory hypopigmentation or hyperpigmentation, a history of radiation exposure, history of prior skin procedures including type; and timing of each; history of skin disease including conditions with risk of koebnerization (vitiligo, psoriasis, and others) or melasma, history of HSV; and medication history including history of isotretinoin use. With particular attention to any retinoids, immunosuppressants, photosensitizing medications, or anticoagulants. Physical examination of the affected site as well as the background skin provides valuable information such as amount and type of epidermal and dermal melanin, thickness and elasticity of the dermis, and the type and sites of the patient's cutaneous concern (hypopigmentation, hyperpigmentation, dermal or epidermal atrophy or hypertrophy) to be corrected.

Box 41-1   Criteria Used to Assess and Select Patients for Skin Rejuvenation Procedures

Fitzpatrick skin type: Skin types I to III should be ideal
Skin types IV to VI may produce postinflammatory hyperpigmentation
Glogau's classification of photoaging
General medical evaluation, including cardiac status
History of drug allergies
History of herpes simplex
History of recent isotretinoin is contraindicated
History of sun exposure
History of smoking
History of previous cosmetic procedures
History of scarring
Pregnancy history
Discussion of patient expectations

Table 41-1 Fitzpatrick Classification

Skin Type	Skin Color	Characteristics
I	White, very fair, red or blond hair, freckles, blue eyes	Always burns Never tans
II	White, fair, red or blond hair, blue, hazel or green eyes	Usually burns, tans with difficulty
III	Cream/beige, fair, with any eye or hair color very common	Sometimes mild burn, gradually tans to light brown
IV	Beige with a brown tint Typical Mediterranean white	Rarely burns, tans with ease to moderate brown
V	Dark brown	Very rarely burns, tans very easily
VI	Black	Never burns, tans easily, deeply pigmented

Data from Fitzpatrick TB. The validity and practicality of sun reactive skin types I through VI. Arch Dermatol 124:869-871, 1988.

Table 41-2 Glogau's Classification of Photoaging Groups

Group Characteristics	Classification	Age (yr)	Typical	Description of Skin
I	Mild	28-35	No wrinkles	Early photoaging: Mild pigment changes, no keratosis, minimal wrinkles, women wear minimal or no makeup
II	Moderate	35-50	Wrinkles in motion (during animation)	Early to moderate photoaging: Early brown spots visible, keratosis palpable but not visible, parallel smile lines begin to appear, women wear some foundation
III	Advanced	50-65	Wrinkles at rest	Advanced photoaging: Obvious visible capillaries (telangiectasias), visible keratosis, women wear heavier foundation always
IV	Severe	60-75	Only wrinkles	Severe photoaging: Yellow-gray skin color, skin malignancies, wrinkles throughout, no normal skin, cannot wear makeup because it cakes and cracks

Data from Glogau RG, Matarasso SL. Chemical face peeling: patient and peeling agent selection. Facial Plast Surg 11:1-8, 1995.

The Fitzpatrick skin type, which classifies the skin (types I through VI) according to its color and sun-burn history (see Table 41-1), will help the physician determine the type of skin rejuvenation technique most useful for a given individual. The Fitzpatrick skin-typing system ranges from a classification of I for extremely fair white skin, progressing to VI for dark black skin.[15] Patients with skin types I through III are ideal candidates for all the procedures discussed in this chapter. Patients with skin types IV to VI, by contrast, should be treated with caution, if at all, because of such adverse effects as postinflammatory hy-perpigmentation or hypopigmentation.

Diverse skin phototypes may be treated with resurfacing though caution is important, as risks of dyspig-mentation increase in darker skin types. Hyperpigmentation or hypopigmentation may occur with ab-lative or with nonablative resurfacing. Delayed hypopigmentation has been observed, particularly after nonfractional ablative treatments. Postinflammatory hyperpigmentation risk is dependent in part on skin type, sun exposure, history of melasma or prior postinflammatory hyperpigmentation, and density and energy of treatment.[16] Additional risks associated with resurfacing include poor reepithelialization in pa-tients with a history of radiation exposure, morphea (localized scleroderma), or other conditions affecting follicular stem cells. In addition, isotretinoin or systemic retinoid treatment within 6 to 12 months before treatment may increase the tendency to scarring, so skin procedures are typically deferred until 6 to 12 months after exposure, although the literature suggests these risks may be somewhat exaggerated.[17-19] Face lifts and blepharoplasty may alter blood supply and increase the risk of scarring; therefore skin procedures should also generally be deferred until several months after surgery.[20] There are greater risks of scarring at certain anatomic sites, including the neck and chest, so sites are usually not treated with nonfractional ablative lasers. If treatment is performed, conservative application of fractional ablative or nonablative lasers presents a safer alternative.

Once the appropriate options have been presented, the following patient factors influence the surgeon's decision to use a particular ablative or nonablative laser or energy-based treatment:

- A desire for fewer treatment sessions
- Tolerance for the required recovery time and potential side effects
- The patient's ability to comply with postoperative care
- His or her desired rate of achieving the desired resurfacing
- The likely efficacy of the technique to achieve the patient's goals

For the treating physician, all of the above factors, as well as the desired depths and pattern of injury, should be considered when selecting the appropriate device, settings, and placement of the device.

The Glogau system ranges from I to IV[21] (see Table 41-2) and classifies the severity of photodamage based on the degree of epidermal and dermal degeneration; category I is classified as mild, where there is a mini-mal degree of photodamage, and wrinkles are not readily evident. As rhytids become progressively more severe, the categories progress upward to category IV. The most severe photoaging, with the skin covered with rhytids and yellowish-gray skin discoloration, is classified as Glogau's category IV. Such extensive in-jury requires a deep peel or resurfacing procedure[22] to make any significant improvement.

LASER SKIN RESURFACING
Laser and Energy-Based Resurfacing
Epidermal and dermal irregularities resulting from photodamage and other environmental insults, from chronologic aging, or from scars have all been successfully improved or resolved with laser, light, ultra-sound, and/or radiofrequency technologies. Lasers and energy-based devices have a distinct advantage over chemical peels or mechanical dermabrasion in that the dermis may be targeted, with partial or complete sparing of the epidermis. In addition, more selective targeting of particular cutaneous sites or structures

is possible, providing safer, more effective results when the treatment is performed with optimal settings and delivery technique. Laser, light, and other energy-based technologies provide an array of effective options for cutaneous tightening and resurfacing (Table 41-3).

Ablative Lasers

Ablative lasers, including the carbon dioxide (CO_2) (10,600 nm) and erbium-doped yttrium-aluminum garnet (Er:YAG) (2940 nm) lasers (Fig. 41-2), create thermal damage sufficient to produce tissue ablation or destruction; the targeted chromophore is water, though depth of destruction is dictated by laser type (see Fig. 41-2). Nonfractional ablative lasers destroy the entire epidermis in the treated area along with

Table 41-3   Ablative and Nonablative Resurfacing Devices*

Ablative Resurfacing Devices						
Device	**Category**	**Manufacturer**	**Wavelength (nm)**	**Fluence**	**Pulse Width**	**Comments**
Fraxel Repair	Ablative laser	Solta Medical	10,600; fractional	≤70 mJ/ MTZ	NA	Roller tip with intelligent optical tracking system, built-in air evacuator
SmartSkin	Ablative laser	Cynosure	10,600; fractional	≤30 W	150-20,000 ms	Scanning patterns
SmartXide DOT	Ablative laser	DEKA Medical	10,600; fractional	150 W	0.2-80 ms	Three scanning modes
UltraPulse	Ablative laser	Lumenis	10,600; fractional	1-225 mJ	<1 ms	CoolScan and DeepFX handpieces
Icon 2940	Ablative laser	Palomar	2940; fractional	2-5.5 mJ/ 0.1 mm	0.25-5 ms	
ProFractional	Ablative laser	Sciton	2940; fractional	≤400 J/cm²	Variable	Expandable module
Harmony Pixel 2940	Ablative laser	Alma Lasers	2940; fractional	300-2500 mJ/ pulse	Short, medium, or long	
Xeo Pearl	Ablative laser	Cutera	2790; available pearl fractional	60-320 mJ/ microspot	600 ms	Combination ablation and coagulation
ePrime/ Evolastin	Radiofrequency	Syneron/ Candela	Radiofrequency	Max voltage 84 VRMS	NA	Bipolar paired microneedles
Aluma	Radiofrequency	Lumenis	Radiofrequency, bipolar	2-20 W	1-5 sec	6 × 25 mm and 3 × 18 mm tips
eMatrix/ Sublative	Radiofrequency	Syneron/ Candela	Radiofrequency, bipolar, fractional	≤62 mJ/pin	NA	Spot size 12 × 12 mm, 64 or 144 pins
Thermage	Radiofrequency	Solta Medical	Radiofrequency, monopolar	≤400 W	200 ms	CPT and NXT systems
Ultherapy	Ultrasound	Ulthera	Fractional focused ultrasound	4 MHz and 7 MHz	NA	3 transducers available for different depths of penetration; 1.5, 3.0, or 4.5 mm

*This list is not comprehensive; verify all information with each device's manufacturer.
J, Joule; *MHz,* megahertz; *mJ,* millijoules; *mm,* millimeters; *ms,* microseconds; *MTZ,* microthermal zones; *nm,* nanometers; *sec,* seconds; *VRMS,* voltage root-mean-square; *W,* watts.

Nonablative Resurfacing Devices

Device	Category	Manufacturer	Wavelength (nm)	Fluence	Pulse Width	Comments
Fraxel Dual	Nonablative laser	Solta Medical	1550/1927	≤70 mJ/MTZ/≤20 mJ/MTZ	NA	Integrated Zimmer cooling; Intelligent optical tracking system
Icon 1540	Nonablative laser	Palomar	1540; fractional	≤70 mJ/microbeam	10 and 15 ms	
ARAMIS	Nonablative laser	Quantel Derma	1540	≤126 J/cm²	3.3 ms	Has skin cooling
Affirm	Nonablative laser	Cynosure	1440, 1320	≤14 J/cm²	3 ms	Air cooling
MOSAIC	Nonablative laser	Lutronic	1550 nm	4-70 mJ	NA	Hair and skin treatment tips
Clear and Brilliant	Nonablative laser	Solta Medical	1440	≤9 mJ/MTZ	NA	Low, medium, and high settings; 1927 nm and 1440 nm
Portrait PSR	Nonablative laser	Energist Group	Plasma Energy	1-10 W	NA	

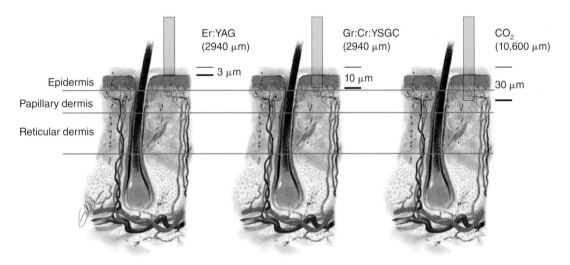

Fig. 41-2   Cutaneous layers with the penetration depth of three common ablative lasers.

the superficial dermis, destroying epidermal and superficial dermal cells or deposits. A number of conditions improve with such destruction and subsequent reepithelialization, including photodamage, atrophic scarring, rhinophyma, xanthelasma, angiofibromas, adnexal tumors, and epidermal nevi. There are often substantial improvements in texture and tone, though these methods also carry significant risks of hyperpigmentation or hypopigmentation, prolonged erythema (in particular, when treating the face), healing times lasting several weeks, and risks of scarring, especially when used over large surface areas.[17]

Fractional photothermolysis (FP) is a technique designed to reduce the risks associated with ablative laser therapy. Rather than affecting the entire surface, the laser is delivered in a gridded pattern leaving islands of undamaged skin throughout the treated area. Fractional ablative laser techniques provide continued efficacy with great improvements in safety compared to nonfractional laser treatments, and have become a valuable and widely utilized treatment option.[23] Fractional photothermolysis allows untreated intervening skin to provide follicular stem cells for rapid reepithelialization of nearby damaged skin, resulting in faster healing and reduced risks of dyspigmentation or scarring. Reepithelialization occurs in 2 to 3 days, and extrusion of microepidermal necrotic debris (MENDS) produces small brown flakes on the skin.[24] Histologic evaluation of skin treated by FP shows regular microthermal zones (MTZ), each of which consists of a tapered ablative zone, surrounded by an eschar and zone of thermal coagulation.[24] Injury depth reaches 1 to 1.5 mm with higher energy levels (70 mJ).[25]

Carbon dioxide (CO_2) lasers produce a wavelength of 10,600 nm, absorbed by water. Ablation is produced at fluencies (energy density) of 5 J/cm^2 or higher (see Fig. 41-2).[26-28] Below this threshold, coagulation and tissue dessication predominate.[29] With adjusted settings, the CO_2 laser penetration may reach 20 to 30 μm with thermal damage extending to 100 to 150 μm.[26-28]

Er:YAG lasers (2940 nm) deliver light at a wavelength readily absorbed by water, which allows limited ablation, with less surrounding thermal damage. Variable pulse Er:YAG lasers vary the pulse duration to achieve more ablation or more thermal damage.[30] The shorter Er:YAG wavelength achieves less penetration depth, reaching only 10 to 40 μm of thermal injury[17] (see Fig. 41-2).

Nonablative Lasers

Nonablative lasers encompass a wide variety of wavelengths in a large array of devices (Table 41-4) and produce less thermal damage than ablative lasers, causing injury without tissue vaporization and leaving the epidermis intact. Although there is often reduced efficacy per session (and sometimes overall) compared with ablative treatments, safety is increased and downtime reduced with nonablative lasers. Multiple treatments are often required to achieve optimal results.

Clinical Efficacy Lasers have demonstrated efficacy in improving myriad epidermal and dermal abnormalities. Photodamaged aged skin shows reduced rhytids and pigmentation as well as mild tightening after fractional and nonfractional CO_2 laser treatment, with fractional treatments having an improved safety profile.[31-36] Nonablative resurfacing also significantly improves photodamage, rhytids, skin texture, and scarring, and improvements increase over a treatment series. Improvements in texture, photodamage-

Table 41-4 Nonablative Lasers (Fractional)

Laser	Wavelength (nm)
Fraxel Dual (Solta Medical)	1927 thalium 1550 erbium-doped
Lux 1540 Handpiece (Palomar)	1540
Clear and Brilliant (Solta Medical)	1440
"Generic" Fractional Nonablative Lasers	
Diode laser	532
Infrared laser	1350
Erbium YAG (Er:YAG)	1064
Yttrium-scandium-gallium-garnet (YSAGG)	2790

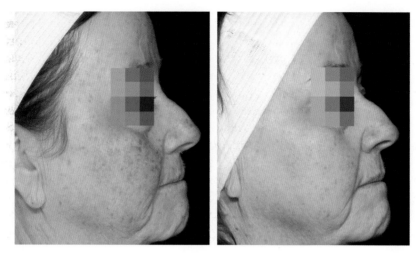

Fig. 41-3   Preoperative and postoperative photographs demonstrating the effectiveness of laser treatments on actinic keratosis and solar damage.

associated hyperpigmentation, and rhytids have also been demonstrated, with superficial to moderate rhytids responding more than deep rhytids.[37] Nonfacial sites have also shown substantial improvement in photodamaged skin, with an excellent safety profile after nonablative treatments.[38,39]

Lower-energy nonablative fractional devices have also produced improvements in texture and tone. While efficacy appears lower, side effects including erythema, edema, hyperpigmentation, and hypopigmentation are also comparatively reduced, making these excellent options for patients desiring reduced to no downtime, those seeking more frequent or adjunctive options, and those who want to minimize irritation or pigmentary risks. A low-energy device primarily for home use, a fractional nonablative 1410 nm diode laser (PaloVia Skin Renewing Laser), has been reported to produce microthermal zones of injury extending to 250 μm[40] and has a manufacturer-recommended treatment regimen of daily use for 1 month, followed by twice-weekly maintenance treatments.[41] Two prospective studies each showed improvement in periorbital rhytids after the initial 4-week treatment phase[40] and ongoing improvement after another 4 to 12 weeks of twice-weekly maintenance treatments.

Actinic keratoses, a marker of photodamage and abnormal cellular proliferation, are reduced after laser treatments[42-44] (Fig. 41-3), although histologic changes of actinic keratoses persist in posttreatment biopsy specimens.[43] Actinic cheilitis has also been treated successfully using the 1927 nm fractional nonablative laser.[45]

Scars, including hypertrophic and atrophic scars, also improve with laser treatment.[25] Atrophic scars, including surgical, traumatic, and acne scars, have shown significant improvement after fractional ablative treatments in multiple studies, including objective improvements in depth using three-dimensional imaging.[46-48]

A study of 15 subjects with skin phototypes I through IV and moderate to severe acne scarring showed a mean 67% improvement in acne scar depth and 26% to 50% improvement in texture, reduction of atrophy, and overall improvement after a series of two or three full-face fractional CO_2 laser treatments[35] (Fig. 41-4). Acne scarring also responds well to nonablative FP after a series of treatments in a variety of skin types, showing 22% to 75% improvement in depth in a variety of studies.[37,46,49] In addition, scarlike tissue resulting from hemangioma improves in appearance and texture with fractional ablative laser treatments.[50] Scars often respond despite being mature or long-standing; however, optimal results are achieved when scars are treated early—6 to 10 weeks after the causative injury.[17]

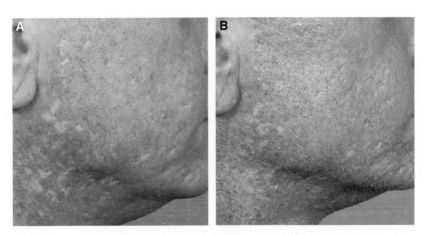

Fig. 41-4   Acne scars treated with functional CO_2 laser. **A,** Baseline. **B,** Three months after treatment.

Dyspigmentation may be cautiously addressed using laser treatments. Hypopigmentation from various causes, including prior nonfractional ablative treatment, frequently improves with the use of fractional ablative treatments.[22] Melasma has shown 75% to 100% clearance in some reports,[51] yet moderate to poor response in many others.[52,53] Darker skin types with melasma often show less improvement, and patients with dark skin have a greater risk of dyspigmentation after resurfacing treatments.[52]

Genetically based dermatoses, including epidermal nevi,[54] and angiofibroma, found in the setting of tuberous sclerosis, are often addressed with ablative laser treatment. Although a single session may result in lasting improvement, recurrence is common because of the ongoing behavior of genetically mutated cells, and repeat treatments may be required for optimal control.

Radiofrequency Devices   *Radiofrequency,* or electrical energy, produces thermal injury as a result of tissue impedance of current flow,[55] promoting neocollagenesis and elastogenesis.[55] Clinically, treated skin shows lifting, tightening, and increased elasticity.[56] A variation of radiofrequency technology, plasma radiofrequency, involves the reaction of high-energy radiofrequency with nitrogen to produce nitrogen plasma, which is applied to produce thermal damage at various cutaneous levels. The effects vary from superficial sloughing to dermal heating, with subsequent neocollagenesis.[57] Radiofrequency action is chromophore independent; epidermal cooling technology and/or careful monitoring of dermal and surface temperature helps to reduce the risks of bulk heating and epidermal damage.[58] Monopolar, bipolar, and tripolar devices are available, and the pulse pattern may be fixed or modified. The depth and pattern of injury depends on the position and distance of the treatment tip and/or needles, the amount of current applied, the tissue resistance, and the duration of current application.[58]

Clinical Efficacy   Radiofrequency treatment significantly reduces rhytids and laxity, with results that increase over the 3- to 6-month period after treatment; improvements are dependent largely on treatment settings and number of passes performed.[59-61] Patient may return to normal activities within 24 hours after treatment and have shown no scarring or adverse effects[61] (Fig. 41-5).

The cheeks and periorbital skin appear to respond most to RF treatments, whereas the neck demonstrates less significant improvements.[58,62,63] In a study using a nonablative monopolar RF device (ThermaCool TC), for 50 patients with phototypes I through IV with mild to moderate cheek or neck laxity receiving a single treatment, 28 of 30 patients showed significant improvement in the nasolabial and melolabial folds, and 17 of 20 patients showed improvement in neck laxity.[58] Cheek laxity continued to decrease at each visit over 6 months of follow-up. Periorbital skin has also shown reduced rhytids and laxity in these study participants, again improving over 6 months after treatment.

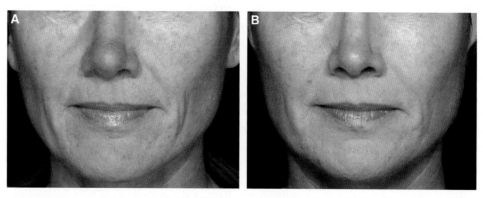

Fig. 41-5   This patient underwent bipolar fractional radiofrequency treatment. **A,** Before treatment. **B,** Three months after the last of three treatments.

A prospective multicenter study of 72 patients with eyelid laxity receiving a single treatment using a 0.25 cm² monopolar RF tip (ThermaCool, Thermage) showed that 88% of subjects demonstrated upper eyelid tightening, 86% showed reduction of hooding, and 71% to 74% showed lower eyelid tightening.[63,64] Results are somewhat variable, with some patients experiencing no improvement after treatment.[64] Hsu and Kaminer[65] and Alster and Tanzi[58] suggested that younger patients respond more optimally to RF and that patients over age 62 with significant photodamage may not respond as well. Higher-energy treatments appear to produce more significant results, but multiple passes or lower-fluence treatments also result in improvement.

In plasma RF technology, multiple low- and mid-energy treatments have yielded improvement in superficial rhytids, skin texture, scars, and discoloration; however, single or few high-energy treatments have been found to be most effective, particularly in skin tightening.[66-70] Lower-energy treatments are recommended for nonfacial sites: Alster and Konda[57] showed improvement of moderate photodamage after treatment (1.0 to 1.8 J) of the neck, chest, and hands.

Candidate Selection

Radiofrequency treatment should be avoided in individuals with pacemakers or implantable cardiac defibrillators; alternatively, cardiology clearance should be obtained before treatment. A history of metal implants or other permanent implants (such as permanent fillers or silicone) in the treatment area is also a contraindication to radiofrequency treatment.

Perioperative Care   Infection prophylaxis should be considered when performing dermal resurfacing. Ablative treatments break the skin barrier, allowing an entry route for pathogens, leading to increased risks of infection, scarring, and sepsis if inadequate postoperative care is provided or carried out by the patient. Although nonablative treatments have a lower risk of infection, some risk remains due to an altered skin barrier. In addition, any type of resurfacing can trigger HSV activation. Oral antiherpetic prophylaxis is advised for all patients undergoing full-face or perioral resurfacing regardless of clinical HSV history, beginning one day preoperatively and continuing for 7 to 10 days, or until complete reepithelialization.[71] Patients who cannot take or who decline antiviral prophylaxis should be treated cautiously or not at all. In ablative procedures, oral antibiotic prophylaxis against common skin flora using cephalosporins, penicillin derivatives, or macrolides is advised during the same time period.[71] Antifungals are generally not prescribed but can be considered.[72]

Ocular protection is a primary safety consideration. External goggles, with the appropriate protection specified by the device manufacturer, suffice when the periorbital area is avoided, but if the periorbital area is to be treated, appropriate intraocular shields may be placed.

Preoperatively, gentle bland skin care is advised. Most active-ingredient topicals such as glycolic acids or scrubs should be discontinued several weeks before the procedure, though topical tretinoin may be continued and may even improve outcomes.[17,73] Postoperative wound care varies according to the type of resurfacing performed. After ablative procedures, distilled water soaks, application of petrolatum ointment, and placement of a sterile protective face mask is recommended. Continued wound care by the patient using frequent soaks of distilled water and moist wound care using petrolatum ointment are critical to achieving optimal reepithelialization and reducing the risk of scarring. After reepithelialization or after nonablative treatments, gentle cleansing is indicated, followed by application of light moisturizers. Makeup may be lightly applied on reepithelialized skin. Photoprotection for several weeks is critical to reducing risks of prolonged erythema and dyspigmentation.

Anesthesia Requirements   Topical anesthesia is typically sufficient for nonablative treatments, although an occasional patient requires an injected local anesthetic or other measures, depending on the individual's pain threshold. Ablative treatment is more likely to produce significant pain and adequate injected local anesthesia and/or nerve blocks are recommended. Microneedle-based radiofrequency treatment usually requires at least topical anesthesia, with an injected or a tumescent local anesthetic often recommended. Cold air cooling during the resurfacing procedures often aids in improving comfort.[17]

Adjunctive agents such as anxiolytics, mild sedatives, or nonsteroidal antiinflammatory agents are frequently helpful in cases of full-face ablative procedures. General anesthesia is rarely required for any resurfacing unless the patient is unable to tolerate treatment under local anesthesia or prefers to be treated under general anesthesia.

Side Effects and Complications   Erythema develops during and after nonablative treatments, and erythema, crusting, oozing, and bleeding develop during and after ablative treatments. Petechiae and purpura may arise from resurfacing procedures. Reepithelialization occurs over a period of up to several weeks in nonfractional ablation, and in 2 or 3 days after fractional ablative treatments. Erythema persists for several months after nonfractional ablative treatment and gradually decreases over 1 to 3 months in fractional ablative treatment. After nonablative treatments, erythema and edema generally last 2 or 3 days, but the erythema can persist for weeks in some patients. Erythema is often followed by areas of desquamation for 1 or 2 days. After radiofrequency treatments, erythema is often shorter lived, lasting 2 to 12 hours.[58] Slight scaling may appear for 3 to 5 days after treatment. For all resurfacing treatments, intensity and duration of side effects may often be predicted based on the type of energy, density, fluence, and number of passes delivered.

To minimize postoperative side effects, 590 nm yellow LED (light-emitting diode, a semiconductor light source) treatment has been shown to reduce the duration of erythema following fractional nonablative laser treatment.[74] Edema may be reduced with use of oral or topical corticosteroids. Crusting may be avoided with frequent soaks and moist wound care. Postoperative pain should be minimal; significant pain suggests possible infection or another cause. Self-limited acneiform eruptions are common after resurfacing and can be managed with noncomedogenic products and 2.5% benzoyl peroxide.

Long-term risks of resurfacing include hyperpigmentation, hypopigmentation, and/or scarring. Scarring is fortunately uncommon, but does occur, and may be attributed to high fluences, excessive passes or pulse stacking, inadequate preoperative or postoperative care, aggressive treatment of scar-prone sites, or other factors,[17,75,76] although scarring does occasionally occur when none of those factors is present. Early scarring should be promptly treated using appropriate skin care, possible laser treatment, and, for hypertrophic scars, consideration of the use of intralesional 5FU and/or intralesional triamcinolone, pulsed-dye laser, or silicone gel sheeting. Hyperpigmentation is managed with aggressive photoprotection and topical antipigmentation agents. Fractional laser, excimer laser, and/or topical repigmentation-promoting drugs (such as bimatoprost) may be considered in cases of hypopigmentation. Suspected infections should be investigated with prompt appropriate cultures and empiric treatment, with close evaluation for resolution.

Radiofrequency treatments heat the deep dermis including nerves and temporary dysesthesias have been rarely reported.[58] Subcutaneous fat atrophy has also been reported and in many cases resolves over several months.[77]

CHEMICAL PEELS AND MECHANICAL DERMABRASION

CHEMICAL PEELS

Chemical peels have been used to successfully resurface sun-damaged skin, rhytids, lentigines, superficial keratoses and acne scars. The technique compromises the application of caustic agents to the skin, down to the dermis, which leads to sloughing of the epidermis and parts of the dermis and finally, reepithelialization of the skin. The different combinations of acidic and basic compounds create a controlled skin injury to the desired depth for the condition being treated, as summarized in Table 41-5. There are different chemical peel procedures, depending on the depth of the desired peel: superficial, medium-depth, and deep (Fig. 41-6).

As soon as the chemicals are applied to the skin, blistering and sloughing of the superficial layers occur. This is followed by coagulation and inflammation of the treated sites which then progresses to healing and reepithelialization of the peeled area. Once reepithelialization is complete, granulation tissue formation ensues, followed by angiogenesis and finally collagen remodeling.

Table 41-5   Chemical Components Based on Depth of Procedure

Superficial Peel: Very Light	Superficial Peel: Light	Medium-Depth Peel	Deep Peel
Glogau I/skin types I-III	Glogau I/skin types I-III	Glogau III/skin types I-III	Glogau III/skin types I-III
Stratum corneum to stratum granulosum	Basal layer or upper papillary dermal depth	Papillary dermis to the upper reticular dermis	To midreticular dermis
Low-potency formulations of glycolic acid or other alpha hydroxy acids	70% glycolic acid	Combination peels, single or multiple applications of 88% phenol	Unoccluded or occluded Baker-Gordon phenol-croton oil peel
10%-20% TCA	25%-35% TCA	CO_2 laser + 35%-40% TCA	TCA concentration >50%
Jessner's solution, tretinoin Resorcinol	Jessner's solution	Jessner's solution and 35% TCA	
Salicylic acid		70% glycolic acid and 35% TCA	
Alpha hydroxy acids		Full-strength phenol, 88% unoccluded	

Continued

Table 41-5　Chemical Components Based on Depth of Procedure—cont'd

Superficial Peel: Very Light	Superficial Peel: Light	Medium-Depth Peel	Deep Peel
Solid carbon dioxide		Peeling complete: 7-8 days	
Peeling complete: 0-3 days	Peeling complete: 3-7 days	Can be repeated in 6-8 weeks	Peeling complete: 8-10 days, up to 3 weeks
Can usually be done as often as once a week	Can be repeated in 4 weeks		Should be done by physician

Superficial peels are indicated for the management of acne and postinflammatory erythema, fine rhytids, mild photoaging, epidermal growths including lentigines and keratoses, melasma and other pigmentary dyschromias.[78] The intent of superficial peels is to exfoliate the stratum corneum or entire epidermis, with the goal of encouraging regrowth of epidermis with a more youthful appearance. These superficial peels produce minimal discomfort, and recovery time is short. The healing time is usually one to 10 days depending on the strength of the chemical. Because of the superficial depth of the peels, best results are achieved with multiple treatments. A benefit of the shallow effects of superficial peels is that they are safe for all skin types (see Table 41-6).

Within the category of superficial peels, they can be further divided into very light and light treatments. A *very light peel* results in injury of the stratum corneum down to the stratum granulosum (see Fig. 41- 6). This injury is usually achieved using low potency formulations of glycolic acid or other alpha hydroxy acids, 10% to 20% trichloracetic acid (TCA), Jessner's solution (resorcinol, salicylic acid and lactic acid), resorcinol, tretinoin, salicylic acid, or even solid carbon dioxide. Healing occurs in usually 1 to 3 days. Because the peel is intentionally superficial, it may be repeated as often as once per week.

By contrast, in a *light peel,* where more potent chemicals are applied to the skin, the induced injury penetrates the epidermis down to the basal layer (see Fig. 41-6). Chemicals used to produce this level of injury include 70% glycolic acid, 25% to 35% TCA, and Jessner's solution. Peeling of the skin in this instance is usually complete in 3 to 7 days, and the procedure may be safely repeated in 4 weeks.

Chemical peeling produces a series of wound-healing stages, governed somewhat by the anatomical location of the peel, the thickness of the epidermis and dermis, and the number of adnexal structures present.

In general, patients with a Glogau I classification (see Table 41-2) have early photoaging in the sun-exposed skin, but are absent or have minimal wrinkles and mild pigmentary changes, respond best to superficial chemical peels or microdermabrasion in conjunction with medical or cosmeceutical therapy.[22]

By contrast, patients with a Glogau II classification (see Table 41-2), exhibiting early to moderate photoaging, wrinkles present on motion, visible brown spots, and palpable but not visible keratoses, would best benefit from a *medium-depth chemical peel.* They will also benefit from long-term medical therapy including a retinoid and/or an alpha hydroxy acid. Medium-depth peels damage the skin through the papillary dermis, creating epidermal necrosis as well as necrosis of part or all of the papillary dermis. An inflammatory reaction ensues in the upper reticular dermis. The medium-depth peel is also indicated for

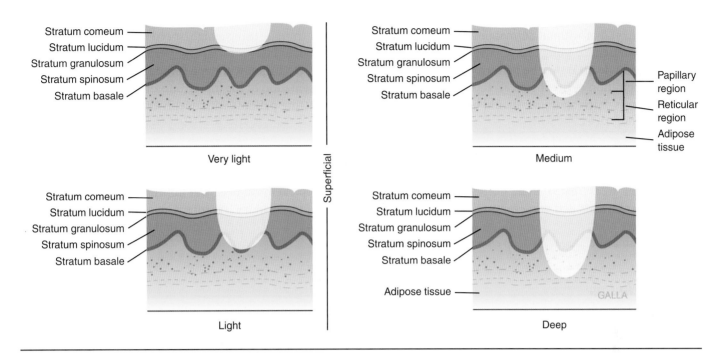

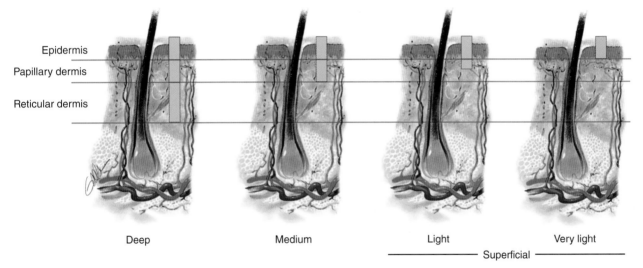

Fig. 41-6   Cutaneous layers, with depth of penetration of superficial, medium, and deep chemical peelings.

actinic keratoses, mild photoaging of the skin including rhytides, pigmentary dyschromias and improving depressed scars. Medium-depth chemical peels are ideal for moderate, nondynamic wrinkles because of the depth of induced injury. They may also be used for blending purposes following other procedures; for example, a patient with advanced photoaging changes in the periorbital area could have deep peels or laser resurfacing performed in these areas, and the medium-depth peel could be used for the rest of the face, where the photoaging rhytids are less severe.

Patients with Glogau III classification of photoaged skin (see Table 41-3), where wrinkles are present at rest, typically benefit from prolonged medical treatment in conjunction with a medium-depth chemical peel, with or without dermasanding (a surgical skin-planing technique using a high-speed rotary abrasive instrument or sandpaper), a deep chemical peel, dermabrasion, or laser resurfacing. *Deep chemical peels* (see Table 41-5) may be performed occluded or unoccluded.[78] Occlusion with tape is thought to increase penetration of the chemicals into the dermis, and extend presentation of the injury into the midreticular dermis. Such an injury should be especially beneficial for treating patients with deeply lined, "weather-beaten" faces.

Unoccluded treatments, by contrast, allow more vigorous cleansing of the skin as well as the application of more peel solution to the area. Thus, the applied solution will penetrate less deeply into the skin compared to the areas treated under occlusion. The main goal of the deep chemical peel is to improve or eliminate deep furrows and other textural changes, as well as eliminate pigmentary irregularities associated with severe photoaging. It should be noted that there are significant risks of complications and increased morbidity associated with deep chemical peels.

Technique

Anatomic areas of the face are peeled sequentially, from forehead to temple to cheeks, then lips and eyelids. Before the chemical peel is performed, the skin to be treated should be properly defatted with acetone. Such delicate areas as inside the nose, lips, and medial canthus should be protected with topical petrolatum jelly. The peeling agent should be applied and left for the appropriate time. At the end of the required period, the peeled area should be neutralized and the solution removed.

Chemical peeling of the eyelids is particularly beneficial for patients with laxity, loss of texture, and fine wrinkling of the eyelid skin, most commonly from aging. The best results are achieved in those with Fitzpatrick skin types I, II, and III. Those individuals with skin types IV, V, and VI are more likely to develop pigmentary problems and are not good candidates for this technique. Both upper and lower eyelids as well as periorbital skin may be treated. Depending on the skin texture, TCA has been the peeling agent most commonly used for these areas. The concentration of TCA used will dictate the response desired, for example, a 20% TCA peel will yield a refreshing effect whereas a medium-depth 35% peel produces a more dramatic result. Eyelid chemical peels can be standalone procedures or performed in combination with blepharoplasty or after surgery.

Preoperative Considerations

Many patients would benefit from botulinum toxin injections to alleviate dynamic wrinkles before chemical peeling, because they enhance results of resurfacing procedures by immobilizing the muscles implicated in the development of rhytids during the critical time of postoperative collagen remodeling.[78] All patients undergoing medium-depth or deep resurfacing should also be treated prophylactically with an antiviral agent, regardless of whether or not there is a history of herpes simplex virus. Therapy may be considered in conjunction with superficial resurfacing in patients with a strong history of recurrent herpes simplex. Recommended prophylaxis is acyclovir 400 mg three times a day or valacyclovir 500 mg twice a day, beginning on the day of the procedure, for at least 10 to 14 days.[79] Topical tretinoin applied nightly before the procedure is suggested, with a milder formulation of tretinoin given to patients with sensitive skin because of the tendency for retinoids to cause irritation within 1 to 2 weeks of starting therapy.[79]

On the day of the surgery, the patient should wash his or her face with a gentle cleanser and not apply cosmetics. It must also be verified that the patient has been compliant with antimicrobial prophylaxis.

Postchemical Peel Expectations

A reaction similar to sunburn can be expected following a chemical peel involving redness and scaling for 3 to 7 days. Medium-depth and deep peels may result in blistering for 7 to 14 days and swelling. If the area was bandaged, the bandage may improve the effectiveness of treatment, and is usually removed within several days. Sun exposure should be avoided for several months after a chemical peel, as the new skin is vulnerable to solar damage.

Contraindications

Absolute contraindications to chemical peeling include a poor physician-patient relationship, lack of psychological stability and mental preparedness, unrealistic expectations, poor general health and nutritional status, complete absence of intact pilosebaceous units on the face and active infection or open wounds,[80] including herpes simplex, and open acne cysts. Relative indications include history of abnormal scar formation or delayed wound healing, history of therapeutic radiation exposure, a history of certain skin diseases such as rosacea, seborrheic dermatitis, psoriasis and vitiligo, or active retinoid dermatitis. Fitzpatrick skin types IV, V, and VI are also relative contraindications.[81] There are also some contraindications that only apply to medium-depth and deep peels but not to superficial peels; those include isotretinoin therapy within the past 6 months, a medium-depth or deep resurfacing procedure within the last 3 to 12 months, or recent facial surgery involving extensive undermining, such as a rhytidectomy.

Comparative Effectiveness

Repetitive superficial peels are generally less effective than single medium or deep peels.[22] Fractional nonablative lasers are about as effective as light chemical peels. Medium-depth chemical peels are reliable, efficacious and safe. Deep and very deep phenol peels where the chemical penetrates to the intermediate reticular dermis and upper to midreticular dermis, respectively, have been largely replaced by lasers. These latter techniques have reduced the adverse effects specific to the deeper peels.

Mechanical Dermabrasion
Dermabrasion, Dermasanding, and Microdermabrasion

Dermabrasion is a mechanical skin-resurfacing method in which the epidermis and superficial dermis are removed in an attempt to smooth irregularities and promote normal wound healing that leads to rejuvenation.[82-84] This "cold steel" method is highly technique specific in terms of outcome but may avoid the complications of scarring and pigmentary changes that plague other resurfacing techniques. The goal of treatment is to remove a controlled thickness of damaged skin without disturbing the reticular dermis and thereby avoid scarring. Dermabrasion is especially useful for the treatment of scars (acne scars in particular) but also benefits patients with moderate wrinkles, uneven skin surfaces, local facial rhytids, premalignant solar keratoses, rhinophyma, and unwanted tattoos.[22]

Preoperative Preparations

Antiviral therapy is prescribed preoperatively if the patient has a history of herpes infection.[85-87] Preoperative testing for HIV and hepatitis are required due to the airborne and aerosolized particles produced in surgery. Preoperative application of petroleum jelly to the hairline will minimize entanglement of the hair with the spinning tip.

Dermabrasion Procedure

Proper skin tumescence helps maintain a uniform depth of dermabrasion and maximizes the surgeon's control of the dermabrader.[88] Gentian violet stains the epidermis and can therefore help to ensure that the surgeon achieves an appropriate depth.[89]

The strokes of the dermabrader are made 45 degrees to the axis of the scar on the first pass and then perpendicular to the axis of the initial dermabrasion on subsequent passes.[90] The direction of motion should be perpendicular to the rotation of the fraise drill tip to maximize control. A yellow color marks the reticular dermis, and the superficial reticular dermis is characterized by parallel-oriented strands, whereas the deeper dermis characteristically consists of frayed white strands.[89] The depth of the abrasion is controlled by the pressure of the handpiece and the speed of the pass. Dermabrasion of the face generally requires two passes. The affected area is treated in 1 to 2 square inch segments by stabilizing the area with the nondominant hand and applying several short bursts of the freezing agent.[88] The handpiece is kept in motion at all times to avoid heat conduction to underlying tissue and to produce more uniform wound depth. To produce the feathering effect, the pressure and number of strokes are decreased between the treated and nontreated areas. Generally, dermabrasion is performed according to facial subunits to avoid conspicuous lines of demarcation. Dermabrasion may be performed in a stepwise procedure in which the surgeon is able to freeze and abrade one area at a time, moving from the outermost and dependent areas to central and superior areas.

As the epidermis is removed, no bleeding occurs because of the absence of blood vessels. When the papillary dermis is reached, a uniform bleeding over a smooth, shiny surface occurs. Once the reticular dermis is entered, the bleeding becomes brisk and confluent. Active bleeding stops after 1 to 2 minutes, and the abraded surface becomes a glistening red that reflects the vascular phase and early vasoconstriction.

The wire brush and diamond fraise are the most common methods of dermabrasion. Wire brush dermabraders may only be rotated clockwise. The skin must be held taut to prevent the instrument from skipping and gouging the skin.[90] Diamond fraise dermabraders can be used with speeds up to 60,000 rpm.[89] Diamond fraise dermabraders are more adaptable, because they vary in width and textures. Both wire brush and diamond fraise dermabrasions involve the same indications, consultations, and preoperative preparations. The custom shapes of the diamond fraises improve their usefulness over the wire brush for feathering scars and abrading concave anatomical locations. The diamond fraise technique requires multiple passes, with heavy downward pressure, which does lead to a higher risk of thermal injury than with the wire brush, though they may be used without spray refrigerant, required when using the wire brush.

Pitfalls of dermabrasion include the need for significant protective wear due to the airborne and aerosolized particles, and the high correlation between technique and results; results of dermarbrasion are highly operator dependant.

Postoperative Care

The patient's head should be elevated while sleeping for at least 48 hours after dermabrasion in order to minimize swelling. Alcohol, smoking, and aspirin products should be avoided. Antiviral agents should be continued after the procedure, and strenuous activities should be avoided for 4 to 6 weeks after dermabrasion.[85-87] Sun should be avoided for at least 12 months, but if that is not possible, a sun block of at least 30 SPF should be worn at all times.

The treated area may be covered with a silicone mesh dressing after the procedure, which is left in place for 1 to 2 days. The patient may apply a cold compress over the mesh dressing to relieve burning and itching, and absorb any wound drainage. Clean gauze should be soaked in ice and water and wrung out before application over the mesh dressing, and the gauze should be replaced as it becomes soiled. Once the dressing is removed, the face may be washed gently 2 to 4 times a day with a gentle soap-free cleanser. The face should then be dried and a thin layer of healing ointment should be applied. The area may be covered with a bandage to avoid air sensitivity. Ointment applications continue several times a day until crusting has subsided (7-10 days). Once the crusting resolves, the patient begins using a moisturizer and wearing makeup. Pigmentation will return to the area in 6-12 months, after which light sun exposure may be tolerated. Pinkness or redness may persist for up to six months.

Comparative Effectiveness

When compared with other skin resurfacing procedures, dermabrasion is still a desirable method. In a study that compared dermabrasion with CO_2 laser treatment of perioral wrinkles, laser treatment had a significantly higher erythema score at one month, and small but significantly greater improvement in perioral wrinkles at 6 months.[27] Biomechanical measurements suggested that the laser treatment resulted in a skin condition more similar to skin in younger patients with higher levels of neocollagenesis. Dermabrasion was found to enable more controllable planing of the area of concern to yield with less bleaching of the skin as compared with peels. Laser appeared to produce more consistent vaporization of the skin with minimal unwanted thermal damage, and to produce a more precise control of depth. Both laser and dermabrasion are useful techniques for resurfacing, with the laser resulting in better overall elasticity but more postoperative pain and dermabrasion, resulting in shorter healing time and less postoperative erythema and morbidity than the CO_2 laser treatment.[91]

Contraindications

Dermabrasion is not suited for certain anatomic structures prone to wrinkling, such as the periorbital area and the lower lip above the chin, because of mechanical limitations.[92] Erythema, telangiectasiae, milia, acne flares, postinflammatory hyperpigmentation are normal postoperative sequelae.[88] There is a long learning curve because it is so highly technique specific. Patients who are immunosuppressed or have a history of koebnerizing conditions such as lichen planus or psoriasis, a tendency towards hyperpigmentation or hypopigmentation or keloid or hypertrophic scar formation are at higher risk for postoperative complications. Precautions for AIDS and hepatitis patients must be taken due to the production of aerosolized particles from the procedure. There is potential for scarring with herpes reactivation during the reepithelialization phase. Hypertrophic scars may result from dermabrasion performed on a patient with ongoing or recent use of isotretinoin.[93] There is an increased risk of hyperpigmentation for patients with Fitzpatrick type III or IV skin. Permanent hypopigmentation is seen in 20% to 30% of patients and is more common in individuals with Fitzpatrick types III and IV. Acne flares from the occlusive nature of the postoperative dressing may be managed with oral antibiotics and routine topical acne medications. Postoperative scarring results from many factors, such as hereditary predisposition, time interval between multiple surgical procedures, depth of wounding, surgical site and possibility of poor postoperative care or infection, exposure to isotretinoin.[93] Dermabrasion is not recommended for patients with herpes simplex virus, those who are hypopigmentation or hyperpigmentation susceptible, or those with chronic radiodermatitis, pyoderma, psychosis, severe psychoneurosis, alcoholism, xeroderma pigmentosum, verrucae planae, and burn scars.

Less-Invasive Options

Dermasanding and microdermabrasion are less-invasive mechanical techniques that require more frequent treatments to obtain the desired results, but typically have fewer negative side effects. Microdermabrasion involves removal of the stratum corneum only, with little disruption of the lower dermis or basal cell layer. It is considered the superficial form of mechanical treatment. The most aggressive microdermabrasion may involve penetration to the basal cell layer and is classified as a very light resurfacing technique or superficial method of disrupting the upper epidermis. The removal of the stratum corneum and surface debris stimulate more rapid epidermal proliferation. The handpiece for the microdermabrasion is a closed system that emits aluminum oxide crystals that are directed toward the skin at high speeds and simultaneously removes them with suction. The procedure is indicated for acne with open and closed comedones; improving the texture of photoaging skin, especially in the early phases of development; and for stimulating epidermal regeneration for conditions such as pigmentary dyschromias, melasma, and superficial epidermal lesions. Microdermabrasion is considered a lunchtime procedure with little to no downtime, after which the patient can return to work and almost immediately use makeup and daily cleansing. The few postoperative complications from microdermabrasion are erythema, edema, and occasionally skin sensitivity for a number of hours after the procedure. Medium-depth procedures result in destruction of the epidermis and entrance into the papillary dermis, and are achievable with microdermabrasion equipment. Microdermabrasion equipment, however, is not often used for this depth because the injury produced is not well controlled at this deeper level and may produce undesirable sequelae.

Medium-depth injury is generally achieved by light diamond fraise dermabrasion and dermasanding. Manual dermasanding involves abrading the skin by hand power using silicone carbide sandpaper or wall screen, commercially available at hardware stores. The depth of penetration is dependent upon the type of paper or grit used, the force applied by the surgeon, and the duration of contact with the skin. Gauze pads, 1½ by 2 inches, are moistened with saline and wrapped with sandpaper that is always kept moist; these are moved back and forth across the desired area in circular motions. The advantages of manual dermasanding include greater control over the depth of injury, particularly on localized areas such as the lips and orbital rims; a better ability to blend with untreated skin; lower cost; greater simplicity of instrumentation and setup; the fact that there is no risk of aerosolization of infectious particles during the procedure; and reduced risk of intraoperative injury.

Manual dermasanding can be performed without the use of refrigerant to blend traumatic scars, acne scars, and postsurgical scars using fine grit paper. The fine grit can also remove necrotic debris after laser resurfacing and blend demarcation zones of other procedures. Dermasanding may also remove thick epidermal lesions that medium-depth chemical peeling cannot remove.

LASER HAIR REMOVAL

Removal of unwanted facial and body hair can be accomplished using several modalities, including waxing, electrolysis,[94] chemical epilation, electroepilation,[95] and most recently, lasers.[96,97] Most of these treatments do not permanently remove hair. In addition, adverse effects, including scarring and pigmentary changes, have also resulted from many of these procedures.

MECHANISM OF ACTION

The principle underlying laser hair removal is termed *selective photothermolysis,* where the combination of laser wavelength, pulse duration, and exposure time are calculated to optimize damage to a selected target (chromophore) in the tissue, with minimal damage to adjacent healthy structures such as collagen.[98]

Each hair has four distinct anatomic regions (Fig. 41-7), the bulb; the lower portion extending from the base of the follicle to the insertion of the arrector pili muscle; the isthmus, extending from the insertion of the arrector pili to the entrance of the sebaceous duct; and the upper portion, or infundibulum, extending from the entrance of the sebaceous gland to the follicular orifice. The papilla, which is an extremely vascular part of the follicle, provides nutrients to the hair. The bulge is responsible for the cycling and regeneration of the hair. Therefore both these areas must be destroyed to achieve permanent suppression or destruction of the hair follicle.

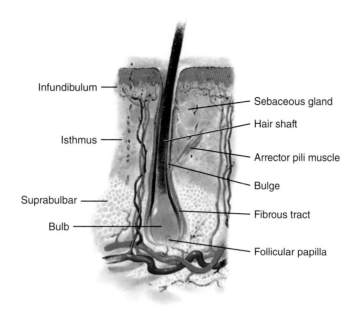

Fig. 41-7   Anatomy of the hair follicle.

Table 41-6   Hair Growth Cycle

Body Area	Anagen (%)	Telogen (%)
Scalp	84	14[89]
Beard (chin)	70	30
Upper lip	65	35
Axilla	30	70
Bikini	30	70

Melanin is the primary chromophore in the hair, targeted by the laser beam for selective destruction. There are two types of melanin in hair, eumelanin, giving hair a brown or black color and pheomelanin, producing a blonde or red color. Because light from the laser beam is best absorbed by dark color, individuals with light skin and dark hair are the best candidates and are most likely to have superior results.

The selective absorption of the laser light by the melanin pigment in the hair shaft leads to heating of the unit and transfer of the heat to the follicular unit (see Fig. 41-7). Heating of the follicular unit and transfer of this heat to adjacent cellular structures will lead to the destruction of the bulge and papilla.

There are three phases in hair growth: anagen, catagen, and telogen. The distribution of each of the different hair cycle growth phases will vary with the anatomic sites on the body (Table 41-6). Because anagen is the active hair growth phase, it is the phase targeted by and most responsive to the laser; multiple laser treatments will be needed to remove the hair in any given anatomic area.

Table 41-7   Lasers Used for Laser Hair Removal

Laser	Wavelength (nm)	Pulse Duration	Comment
Ruby	694	Q-switched	No longer used for hair removal
Nd:YAG[91]	1064	Q-switched	Most effective on skin types II-VI
Alexandrite[92]	755	10-50 msec	Most effective on skin types I-IV
Diode	810	15-40 msec	Most effective on skin types I-IV
Intense pulsed light (not a laser)	600-1200		Most effective on skin types I-IV

Laser Parameters

The common laser systems used for hair removal include the alexandrite and Nd:YAG lasers (Table 41-7). For laser hair removal to be effective, the laser beam must penetrate 1 to 2 mm into the dermis. The depth of penetration of the laser light is controlled by its wavelength, the Nd:YAG at 1064 nm penetrating more deeply than the ruby laser at 694 nm. The alexandrite laser at 755 nm, a wavelength between the ruby and the Nd:YAG, has been reported to penetrate 3 to 4 mm into the dermis.[99] Thus the Nd:YAG, because of its depth of penetration, makes it safer for treating a wider range of skin types, including Fitzpatrick skin types V and VI. Other laser parameters of pulse duration, spot size, and fluence all contribute to confining the targeted melanin injury in the hair follicle. A long pulse duration or exposure time will heat the tissue more slowly compared with shorter pulse durations. The longer pulse durations are more suitable for treating darker skin types, whereas the shorter pulse durations are more effective for treating light-colored hair. *Spot size,* or the diameter of the laser beam, is another laser parameter that will control the effectiveness of laser hair removal. The diameter of the laser beam will also control the depth of penetration of the laser beam—the larger the diameter, the deeper the penetration depth. It has been calculated that spot sizes of between 3-5 mm diameter are required for effective hair removal.

A certain level of fluence, or energy, is required to effectively destroy the hair follicle. Two important factors controlling the appropriate energy level to be used are the confinement of thermal injury and the amount of available laser energy per spot size. Thus the longer the pulse duration, the wider the dissipation of thermal injury to adjacent tissues. By contrast, the smaller the spot size (1 mm diameter spot size) the more superficial the depth of penetration.[100] However, a larger spot size, provided there is sufficient energy being delivered from the laser system, will penetrate more deeply. Another advantage of using a larger spot size is that it permits efficient treatment of larger areas of the body.

INTENSE PULSED LIGHT

Intense pulsed light (IPL), a nonlaser light source, uses incoherent light (xenon flash lamp) in the broadband spectrum (600 to 1200 nm). Filters are used to fine-tune the wavelength to optimize the treatment parameters to the patient's skin type.

Cooling Systems

Cooling systems are used in combination with all laser hair removal systems. A variety of cooling systems have been used including air cooling, cooling gel, and cryogen spray (-30 to $-50°$ C). The cooling system is aimed at minimizing thermal diffusion and injury to the epidermis and protecting healthy tissues adjacent to the hair follicle. At the same time, cooling of the treated site also promotes confinement of the laser beam to the targeted hair follicle melanin.

While air cooling has been shown to be effective, an important disadvantage is that this system comes as a freestanding unit. Cooling gels are generally not as effective as the cryogen sprays or air cooling systems. The cooled gel is applied to the skin surface to be treated; the cooling effect is superficial, transient, and untidy. Most of the current laser systems for laser hair removal are now sold with built-in cooling systems.

Preoperative Considerations

The choice of the appropriate laser is critical to achieving successful laser hair removal with minimal adverse affects to the treated areas; one must take into consideration the patient's skin color, color of hair, and the anatomic location of hairs to be removed (see Table 41-7).

Before laser hair removal, the patient is instructed to minimize ultraviolet light exposure to the treatment area and refrain from epilating, waxing, or tweezing the hairs for at least 4 weeks before the laser hair removal procedure and throughout the duration of the multiple-session treatment period. Shaving is permitted.

Side Effects

Side effects may occur after laser hair removal. Mild side effects include erythema, pruritus, and edema (particularly perifollicular swelling). These adverse effects are rare, transient and often clear within 2-3 days. More serious side effects may occur, including hypopigmentation or hyperpigmentation, or in extreme cases, burning of the skin. Such severe reactions often lead to blistering of the treated area, scabbing, possible infection, and scar formation. Many of these severe adverse effects can be avoided by use of the appropriate laser and correct laser parameters.

Laser Safety

Protective eyewear specific for the laser being used must be worn by all individuals in the laser treatment room. Protective eyewear should be worn by all personnel throughout the treatment and must not be removed during the procedure. Treatment room doors should remain closed during the treatment and warning signs must be posted in prominent places in the clinic. In the room, reflective surfaces such as mirrors and metallic surfaces should either be removed or covered.

Periorbital areas, including eyebrows should be avoided. Fig. 41-8 shows typical preoperative and postoperative appearance of oral laser hair removal following several sessions.

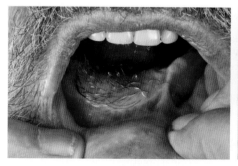 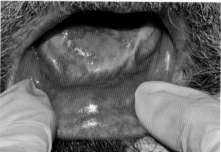

Fig. 41-8   Before and after laser hair removal.

KEY POINTS

- Ablative lasers, including CO_2 and erbium, target water and create thermal damage.
- Fractional photothermocysis ablates some areas while leaving adjacent areas undamaged, and permits more rapid healing.
- Nonablative lasers produce less damage, and preserve the epidermis.
- Lasers may cause dyspigmentation.
- Radiofrequency treatment involves creating thermal injury via delivering electrical energy.
- Chemical peels may be superficial (10% to 20% TCA), medium (CO_2 plus 35% to 40% TCA), or deep (TCA concentration greater than 50%).
- Occluded peels penetrate more deeply.
- Mechanical dermabrasion may be performed with wire brush or diamond fraise, but carries a risk of scarring if performed too deeply.
- Laser hair removal requires multiple treatments, and is most effective on darker, melanocyte-rich hair.

REFERENCES

1. Hirsch RJ, Dayan SH, Shah AR. Superficial skin resurfacing. Facial Plast Surg Clin North Am 12:311-321, v-vi, 2004.
2. Brody HJ, Alt TH. Cosmetic surgery of the skin: principles and techniques. In Coleman WP, ed. Chemical Peeling. Philadelphia: BC Decker, 1991.
3. MacKee GM, Karp FL. The treatment of post-acne scars with phenol. Br J Dermatol 64:456-459, 1952.
4. Brody HJ, Hailey CW. Medium-depth chemical peeling of the skin: a variation of superficial chemosurgery. J Dermatol Surg Oncol 12:1268-1275, 1986.
5. Kligman AM, Baker TJ, Gordon HL. Long-term histologic follow-up of phenol peels. Plast Reconstr Surg 75:652-659, 1985.
    A histologic study describing the effects of phenol peels on severe actinic damaged skin.
6. Symposium on the aging face. Otolaryngol Clin North Am 13:207-397, 1980.
7. Eller J, Wolff S. Skin peeling and scarification in the treatment of pitted scars, pigmentations and certain facial blemishes. JAMA 116:934-938, 1941.
8. Urkov JC. Surface defects of the skin; treatment by controlled exfoliation. Ill Med J 89:75-81, 1946.
9. Stagnone JJ. Chemabrasion, a combined technique of chemical-peeling and dermabrasion. J Dermatol Surg Oncol 3:217-219, 1977.
10. Basov NG, Prokhorov AM. Application of molecular beams to the radio spectroscopic study of the rotation spectra of molecules. Zh Eksp Theo Fiz 27:431, 1954.
11. Maiman TH. Stimulated optical radiation in ruby. Nature 187:493-494, 1960.
    This author was the first investigator, at Hughes Research Laboratories, to build the first laser system.
12. Campbell CJ, Noyori KS, Rittler MC, et al. Retinal coagulation: clinical studies. Ann N Y Acad Sci 122:780-782, 1965.
13. Goldman L, Blaney DJ, Kindel DJ Jr, et al. Effect of the laser beam on the skin. Preliminary Report. J Invest Dermatol 40:121-122, 1963.
    One of the first publications, over 50 years ago, describing the effect of laser energy on hair removal.
14. Goldman L, Blaney DJ, Kindel DJ Jr, et al. Pathology of the effect of the laser beam on the skin. Nature 197:912-914, 1963.
15. Fitzpatrick TB, Eisen AZ, Wolff K, et al, eds. Dermatology in General Medicine, vol 2, ed 3. New York: McGraw-Hill, 1987.
16. Chan HH, Manstein D, Yu CS, et al. The prevalence and risk factors of post-inflammatory hyperpigmentation after fractional resurfacing in Asians. Lasers Surg Med 39:381-385, 2007.
17. Brightman LA, Brauer JA, Anolik R, et al. Ablative and fractional ablative lasers. Dermatol Clin 27:479-489, vi-vii, 2009.

18. Zachariae H. Delayed wound healing and keloid formation following argon laser treatment or dermabrasion during isotretinoin treatment. Br J Dermatol 118:703-706, 1988.

19. Bernestein LJ, Geronemus RG. Keloid formation with the 585-nm pulsed dye laser during isotretinoin treatment. Arch Dermatol 133:111-112, 1997.

20. Hayes DK, Berkland ME, Stambaugh KI. Dermal healing after local skin flaps and chemical peel. Arch Otolaryngol Head Neck Surg 116:794-797, 1990.

21. Glogau RG, Matarasso SL. Chemical facial peeling: patient and peeling agent selection. Facial Plast Surg 11:1-8, 1995.

22. Monheit G. Chemical peels. Skin Ther Lett 9:6-11, 2004.

23. Manstein D, Herron GS, Sink RK, et al. Fractional photothermolysis: a new concept for cutaneous remodeling using microscopic patterns of thermal injury. Lasers Surg Med 34:426-438, 2004.

24. Hantash BM, Bedi VP, Kapadia B, et al. In vivo histological evaluation of a novel ablative fractional resurfacing device. Lasers Surg Med 39:96-107, 2007.

25. Hunzeker CM, Weiss ET, Geronemus RG. Fractionated CO_2 laser resurfacing: our experience with more than 2000 treatments. Aesthet Surg J 29:317-322, 2009.

26. Walsh JT Jr, Flotte TJ, Anderson RR, et al. Pulsed CO_2 laser tissue ablation: effect of tissue type and pulse duration on thermal damage. Lasers Surg Med 8:108-118, 1988.

27. Kauvar AN, Waldorf HA, Geronemus RG. A histopathological comparison of "char-free" carbon dioxide lasers. Dermatol Surg 22:343-348, 1996.

28. Green HA, Domankevitz Y, Nishioka NS. Pulsed carbon dioxide laser ablation of burned skin: in vitro and in vivo analysis. Lasers Surg Med 10:476-484, 1990.

29. Kauvar AN, Geronemus RG. Histology of laser resurfacing. Dermatol Clin 15:459-467, 1997.

30. Newman JB, Lord JL, Ash K, et al. Variable pulse erbium:YAG laser skin resurfacing of perioral rhytides and side-by-side comparison with carbon dioxide laser. Lasers Surg Med 26:208-214, 2000.

31. Alexiades-Armenakas M, Sarnoff D, Gotkin R, et al. Multi-center clinical study and review of fractional ablative CO_2 laser resurfacing for the treatment of rhytides, photoaging, scars and striae. J Drugs Dermatol 10:352-362, 2011.

32. Haedersdal M, Moreau KE, Beyer DM, et al. Fractional nonablative 1540 nm laser resurfacing for thermal burn scars: a randomized controlled trial. Lasers Surg Med 41:189-195, 2009.

33. Waldorf HA, Kauvar AN, Geronemus RG. Skin resurfacing of fine to deep rhytides using a char-free carbon dioxide laser in 47 patients. Dermatol Surg 21:940-946, 1995.

34. Fitzpatrick RE, Goldman MP, Satur NM, et al. Pulsed carbon dioxide laser resurfacing of photo-aged facial skin. Arch Dermatol 132:395-402, 1996.

    These authors describe the use of the high-energy short pulsed carbon dioxide (ultrapulse) laser to rejuvenate photodamaged skin.

35. Chapas AM, Brightman L, Sukal S, et al. Successful treatment of acneiform scarring with CO_2 ablative fractional resurfacing. Lasers Surg Med 40:381-386, 2008.

36. Gotkin RH, Sarnoff DS, Cannarozzo G, et al. Ablative skin resurfacing with a novel microablative CO_2 laser. J Drugs Dermatol 8:138-144, 2009.

37. Geronemus RG. Fractional photothermolysis: current and future applications. Lasers Surg Med 38:169-176, 2006.

38. Jih MH, Goldberg LH, Kimyai-Asadi A. Fractional photothermolysis for photoaging of hands. Dermatol Surg 34:73-78, 2008.

39. Wanner M, Tanzi EL, Alster TS. Fractional photothermolysis: treatment of facial and nonfacial cutaneous photodamage with a 1,550-nm erbium-doped fiber laser. Dermatol Surg 33:23-28, 2007.

40. Metelitsa AI, Green JB. Home-use laser and light devices for the skin: an update. Semin Cutan Med Surg 30:144-147, 2011.

41. Palomar Medical Technologies. Manufacturer website. Available at *www.palovia.com.*

42. Prens SP, de Vries K, Neumann HA, et al. Nonablative fractional resurfacing in combination with topical tretinoin cream as a field treatment modality for multiple actinic keratosis: a pilot study and a review of other field treatment modalities. J Dermatolog Treat 24:227-231, 2013.

43. Katz TM, Goldberg LH, Marquez D, et al. Nonablative fractional photothermolysis for facial actinic keratoses: 6-month follow-up with histologic evaluation. J Am Acad Dermatol 65:349-356, 2011.

44. Weiss ET, Brauer JA, Anolik R, et al. 1927-nm fractional resurfacing of facial actinic keratoses: a promising new therapeutic option. J Am Acad Dermatol 68:98-102, 2013.

45. Ghasri P, Admani S, Petelin A, et al. Treatment of actinic cheilitis using a 1,927-nm thulium fractional laser. Dermatol Surg 38:504-507, 2012.

46. Alster TS, Tanzi EL, Lazarus M. The use of fractional laser photothermolysis for the treatment of atrophic scars. Dermatol Surg 33:295-299, 2007.

47. Alster TS, West TB. Resurfacing of atrophic facial acne scars with a high-energy, pulsed carbon dioxide laser. Dermatol Surg 22:151-154; discussion 154-155, 1996.

48. Weiss ET, Chapas A, Brightman L, et al. Successful treatment of atrophic postoperative and traumatic scarring with carbon dioxide ablative fractional resurfacing: quantitative volumetric scar improvement. Arch Dermatol 146:133-140, 2010.

49. Lee HS, Lee JH, Ahn GY, et al. Fractional photothermolysis for the treatment of acne scars: a report of 27 Korean patients. J Dermatolog Treat 19:45-49, 2008.

50. Brightman LA, Brauer JA, Terushkin V, et al. Ablative fractional resurfacing for involuted hemangioma residuum. Arch Dermatol 148:1294-1298, 2012.

51. Rokhsar CK, Fitzpatrick RE. The treatment of melasma with fractional photothermolysis: a pilot study. Dermatol Surg 31:1645-1650, 2005.

52. Goldberg DJ, Berlin AL, Phelps R. Histologic and ultrastructural analysis of melasma after fractional resurfacing. Lasers Surg Med 40:134-138, 2008.

53. Naito SK. Fractional photothermolysis treatment for resistant melasma in Chinese females. J Cosmet Laser Ther 9:161-163, 2007.

54. Michel JL, Has C, Has V. Resurfacing CO2 laser treatment of linear verrucous epidermal nevus. Eur J Dermatol 11:436-469, 2001.

55. Alexiades-Armenakas M, Rosenberg D, Renton B, et al. Blinded, randomized, quantitative grading comparison of minimally invasive, fractional radiofrequency and surgical face-lift to treat skin laxity. Arch Dermatol 146:396-405, 2010.

56. Willey A, Kilmer S, Newman J, et al. Elastometry and clinical results after bipolar radiofrequency treatment of skin. Dermatol Surg 36:877-884, 2010.

57. Alster TS, Konda S. Plasma skin resurfacing for regeneration of neck, chest, and hands: investigation of a novel device. Dermatol Surg 33:1315-1321, 2007.

58. Alster TS, Tanzi E. Improvement of neck and cheek laxity with a nonablative radiofrequency device: a lifting experience. Dermatol Surg 30(4 Pt 1):503-507; discussion 507, 2004.

59. Alexiades-Armenakas M, Dover JS, Arndt KA. Unipolar versus bipolar radiofrequency treatment of rhytides and laxity using a mobile painless delivery method. Lasers Surg Med 40:446-453, 2008.

60. Levenberg A. Clinical experience with a TriPollar radiofrequency system for facial and body aesthetic treatments. Eur J Dermatol 20:615-619, 2010.

61. Lee HS, Lee DH, Won CH, et al. Fractional rejuvenation using a novel bipolar radiofrequency system in Asian skin. Dermatol Surg 37:1611-1619, 2011.

62. Yu CS, Yeung CK, Shek SY, et al. Combined infrared light and bipolar radiofrequency for skin tightening in Asians. Lasers Surg Med 39:471-475, 2007.

63. Carruthers J, Carruthers A. Shrinking upper and lower eyelid skin with a novel radiofrequency tip. Dermatol Surg 33:802-809, 2007.

64. Biesman BS, Baker SS, Carruthers J, et al. Monopolar radiofrequency treatment of human eyelids: a prospective, multicenter, efficacy trial. Lasers Surg Med 38:890-898, 2006.

65. Hsu TS, Kaminer MS. The use of nonablative radiofrequency technology to tighten the lower face and neck. Semin Cutan Med Surg 22:115-123, 2003.

66. Bogle MA, Arndt KA, Dover JS. Plasma skin regeneration technology. J Drugs Dermatol 6:1110-1112, 2007.

67. Kono T, Groff WF, Sakurai H, et al. Treatment of traumatic scars using plasma skin regeneration (PSR) system. Lasers Surg Med 41:128-130, 2009.

68. Kilmer S, Semchyshyn N, Shah G, et al. A pilot study on the use of a plasma skin regeneration device (Portrait PSR3) in full facial rejuvenation procedures. Lasers Med Sci 22:101-109, 2007.

69. Potter MJ, Harrison R, Ramsden A, et al. Facial acne and fine lines: transforming patient outcomes with plasma skin regeneration. Ann Plast Surg 58:608-613, 2007.

70. Bogle MA, Arndt KA, Dover JS. Evaluation of plasma skin regeneration technology in low-energy full-facial rejuvenation. Arch Dermatol 143:168-174, 2007.

71. Nestor MS. Prophylaxis for and treatment of uncomplicated skin and skin structure infections in laser and cosmetic surgery. J Drugs Dermatol 4(6 Suppl):s20-s25, 2005.

72. Conn H, Nanda VS. Prophylactic fluconazole promotes reepithelialization in full-face carbon dioxide laser skin resurfacing. Lasers Surg Med 26:201-207, 2000.
73. Alt TH. Technical aids for dermabrasion. J Dermatol Surg Oncol 13:638-648, 1987.
74. Alster TS, Wanitphakdeedecha R. Improvement of postfractional laser erythema with light-emitting diode photomodulation. Dermatol Surg 35:813-815, 2009.
75. Ross RB, Spencer J. Scarring and persistent erythema after fractionated ablative CO2 laser resurfacing. J Drugs Dermatol 7:1072-1073, 2008.
76. Fife DJ, Fitzpatrick RE, Zachary CB. Complications of fractional CO2 laser resurfacing: four cases. Lasers Surg Med 41:179-184, 2009.
77. Weiss RA, Weiss MA, Munavalli G, et al. Monopolar radiofrequency facial tightening: a retrospective analysis of efficacy and safety in over 600 treatments. J Drugs Dermatol 5:707-712, 2006.
78. Stegman, SJ. A comparative histologic study of the effect of three peeling agents and dermabrasion on normal and sundamaged skin. Aesthetic Plast Surg 6:123-135, 1982.
    This paper describes the histologic findings, in normal and sundamaged skin, following treatment using 60% trichloracetic acid, 100% phenol, Baker's phenol mixture, and dermabrasion.
79. Sadick NS. Overview of complications of nonsurgical facial rejuvenation procedures. Clin Plast Surg 28:163-176, 2001.
80. Brody HJ, ed. Chemical Peeling and Resurfacing, ed 2. St Louis: Mosby–Year Book, 1997.
81. Humphrey TR, Werth V, Dzubow L, et al. Treatment of photodamaged skin with trichloracetic acid and topical tretinoin. J Am Acad Dermatol 34:638-644, 1996.
82. Kurtin A. Corrective surgical planing of skin; new technique for treatment of acne scars and other skin defects. AMA Arch Derm Syphilol 68:389-397, 1953.
83. McEvitt WG. Treatment of acne pits by abrasion with sandpaper. J Am Med Assoc 142:647, 1950.
84. Davis EC, Callender VD. Aesthetic dermatology for aging ethnic skin. Dermatol Surg 37:901-917, 2011.
85. Gilbert S. Improving the outcome of facial resurfacing—prevention of herpes simplex virus type 1 reactivation. J Antimicrob Chemother 47(Suppl T1):29-34, 2001.
86. Beeson WH, Rachel JD. Valacyclovir prophylaxis for herpes simplex virus infection recurrence following laser skin refurfacing. Dermatol Surg 28:331-336, 2002.
87. Gilbert S, McBurney E. Use of valacyclovir for herpes simplex virus-1 (HSV-1) prophylaxis after facial resurfacing: a randomized clinical trial of dosing regimens. Dermatol Surg 26:50-54, 2000.
88. Yarborough JM Jr. Dermabrasive surgery. State of the art. Clin Dermatol 5:75-80, 1987.
89. Surowitz JB, Shockley WW. Enhancement of facial scars with dermabrasion. Facial Plast Surg Clin North Am 19:517-525, 2011.
90. Bradley DT, Park SS. Scar revision via resurfacing. Facial Plast Surg 17:253-262, 2001.
91. Jared Christophel J, Elm C, Endrizzi BT, et al. A randomized controlled trial of fractional laser therapy and dermabrasion for scar resurfacing. Dermatol Surg 38:595-602, 2012.
92. Kitzmiller WJ, Visscher M, Page DA, et al. A controlled evaluation of dermabrasion versus CO2 laser resurfacing for the treatment of perioral wrinkles. Plast Reconstr Surg 106:1366-1372; discussion 1373-1374, 2000.
93. Rubenstein R, Roenigk HH Jr, Stegman SJ, et al. Atypical keloids after dermabrasion of patients taking isotretinoin. J Am Acad Dermatol 15(2 Pt 1):280-285, 1986.
94. Richards RN, Uy M, Meharg, G. Temporary hair removal in patients with hirsuitism: a clinical study. Cutis 45:199-202, 1990.
95. Ellis FA. Electrolysis versus high frequency currents in the treatment of hypertrichosis: a comparative histologic and clinical study. Arch Derm Syphilol 56:291-305, 1947.
96. Wheeland RG. Lasers for removing unwanted hair and rejuvenating skin. West J Med 169:228-229, 1998.
97. Lask G, Elman M, Slatkine M, et al. Laser-assisted hair removal by selective photothermolysis. Preliminary results. Dermatol Surg 23:737-739, 1997.
98. Anderson RR, Parrish JA. Selective photothermolysis: precise microsurgery by selective absorption of pulsed radiation. Science 220:524-527, 1983.
99. El-Badawi AS, Shaheen MA, Maher HM, et al. A comparative study between alexandrite laser and intense pulsed light in axillary hair removal. Egypt J Plast Reconstr Surg 28:125-132, 2004.
100. Tan OT, Motemedi M, Welch AJ, et al. Spotsize effects on guinea pig skin following pulsed irradiation. J Invest Dermatol 90:877-881, 1988.

42

Volume Replacement and Chemodenervation in the Aging Face

Roxana Cobo

The development of injectable treatments for contouring and adding volume to the face and the judicious use of botulinum toxins for the treatment of exaggerated facial rhytids have been a significant revolution in the specialty of facial plastic surgery. These minimally invasive techniques were initially popularized by dermatology, and in the last decade have become an important tool for all specialists who perform cosmetic procedures. Patients now have a wider range of options in facial rejuvenation, from traditional surgical techniques to those that can easily be performed in an office setting with minimal discomfort, reduced morbidity, and minimal expense.

CHEMODENERVATION IN THE AGING FACE

HISTORICAL BACKGROUND

Botulinum A toxin, recognized as one of the most acutely toxic substances known, was originally known as "sausage poison" because it was identified in poorly preserved meat products. Its ability to immobilize muscles was first theorized to have potential medical application in the late nineteenth century, and it was first purified in 1928.[1] Alan Scott,[2] in 1973, was the first to report the use of botulinum A toxin (BTX-A) for the treatment of strabismus. Subsequently, it was used for other ophthalmologic pathology, including nystagmus, lateral rectus palsy, and blepharospasm. The toxin is also administered for dystonia, spasticity, hemifacial spasm, tension headaches, tics, tremors of different causes, hyperhidrosis, and an expanding list of other conditions.[3]

Cosmetic uses for BTX-A were first reported by Blitzer et al[4] and Carruthers et al.[5] They recognized that hyperfunctional facial lines were dramatically improved, especially in the glabella, the forehead, periorbit (crow's-feet), and neck. Early on, a distinction was made between responsive lines and facial lines that were the result of actinic damage and would not improve with BTX-A injections. Cosmetic improvement was attained by injecting hyperfunctional lines that resulted from contraction of the subcutaneous facial muscles.[5]

Physiology/Mechanism of Action

Botulinum toxin is an exotoxin that is produced by the obligate anaerobic bacterium *Clostridium botulinum*. Eight subunits have been described; of these, types A, B, and E have been associated with botulism in humans. The neurotoxin produces a flaccid paralysis of striate muscles by inhibiting the release of acetylcholine at the neuromuscular junction (NMJ). Paralysis of the muscle appears 2 to 5 days after injection and endures for 3 to 4 months. The toxin binds irreversibly at the NMJ, but reinnervation is produced by neurogenesis and formation of new axonal sprouts.[6]

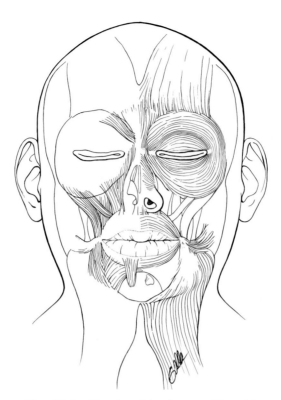

Fig. 42-1   Muscles of the face (see Fig. 1-21).

Table 42-1   Facial Cosmetic Injection Sites for BTX-A

Site	Muscle Involved
Upper Face	
Forehead	Frontalis
Glabella	Procerus
	Corrugator
	Depressor supercilii
Crow's-feet	Orbicularis oculi
Lower lid lines	
Tail of brow	Orbicularis oculi
Midface	
Bunny lines	Nasalis
Lower Face and Neck	
Lip lines	Orbicularis oris
Downturn line of oral commissure	Depressor anguli oris
Chin dimpling	Mentalis
Masseter hypertrophy	Masseter
Platysmal bands/neck lines	Platysma

Today the cosmetic applications of BTX-A are widespread and well accepted and tolerated by patients. The application technique is straightforward and uncomplicated, but it requires precise knowledge of the targeted anatomic structures (Fig. 42-1). Best results are achieved when these injections are carefully titrated and injection is tailored to the specific needs of each patient (Table 42-1).

Products

BTX-A is available commercially as Botox, Dysport, and Xeomin. The FDA approved Botox (onabotulinumtoxinA) for cosmetic use in 2002. Dysport (abobotulinumtoxinA) has been available for cosmetic use in Europe and other countries worldwide since 2001. It was approved by the FDA for cosmetic use in the United States in 2009. Botox is available in 100 U per vial of frozen lyophilized toxin. The toxin is shipped from the distributor on dry ice and must be stored in a freezer at −5° C until reconstitution. Dysport is available in 300 U per vial (in the United States) and 500 U per vial and is stored at 2° to 8° C.[7,8] Xeomin (incobotulinumtoxinA) is available in 50 U/vial aliquots.

RECONSTITUTION METHOD

BTX is an unstable toxin, and if not treated properly, can denature easily. The diluent used is 0.9% sterile nonpreserved saline solution. The inherent vacuum of the vial should draw the solution into the vial without forceful injection. The vial may then be gently inverted, without shaking, to complete reconstitution. Reconstituted toxin must be kept refrigerated—not frozen—until injection, and ideally should be used in the first hour after reconstitution, although this is controversial and many authors feel that it can be refrigerated for several weeks and maintain efficacy.[9,10] Long-term storage of solubilized toxin is not a relevant concern to most practitioners.

A tuberculin syringe with a 27-gauge needle is used for injection. The doses of toxin are usually calculated in 0.1 ml aliquots, so the more saline added to the vial, the smaller the dose per 0.1 ml. Most authors agree that high dilutions have the disadvantages of short duration of action and diffusion to adjacent muscles. Although the units of Botox and Dysport are not considered equivalent, for practical purposes only, 1 unit of Botox is approximately equal to 3 to 4 units of Dysport.[7,8] This ratio is obtained by diluting each vial of Botox to 2 ml and Dysport to 2.5 ml of unpreserved saline solution, which gives a concentration of 5 U:0.1 ml of Botox and 20 U:0.1 ml of Dysport. One common dilution method involves reconstituting each vial of Botox with 2.5 ml (0.1 ml = 4 units) and each 500 U vial of Dysport in 3.3 ml (0.1 ml = 15 units), with comparable results.

PATIENT EVALUATION AND INJECTION TECHNIQUE

A standard medical history should be obtained, and the patient's face should be evaluated to define areas to be treated. Ideally, standard photographs should be taken with the patient's face at rest and with animation. The procedure and its possible complications are thoroughly discussed with the patient before the procedure and an informed consent is obtained. The patient's face is then cleaned with an alcohol swab and the treatment areas marked. Although most treating clinicians do not use an injected local anesthetic or nerve blocks, the area may be iced or prepared with a topical anesthetic. Injections are not usually performed under EMG guidance.

The patient is seated upright and asked to frown, smile, and pucker to activate the muscles to be treated. The area is marked and the site is injected using a tuberculin syringe with a 27- or 30-gauge needle. Mild pressure is applied on the sites after injection, and ice may be used to decrease swelling and ecchymosis. After the injections have been completed, the patient should avoid rubbing or massaging the injected area and should stay upright for the next 4 hours to avoid migration of the toxin into the orbital septum. Active use of injected muscles (such as smiling, frowning, squinting, and puckering) should be encouraged after injection, because this will facilitate absorption of the toxin.

Table 42-2   Botox and Dysport Dose Range for Each Site

	Botox 100 U/Vial	**Dysport 500 U/Vial**
Dilution with unpreserved saline 0.9%	2 ml 0.1 ml = 5 U	2.5 ml 0.1 ml = 20 U
Glabella	20-25 women 30-35 men	80-100 women 120-135 men
Horizontal forehead lines	8-15 U	30-60 U
Crow's-feet	12-15 U	48-60 U
Bunny lines	4-8 U	16-32 U
Marionette lines	4-8 U	16-32 U
Platysmal bands	12-30 U	50-200 U
Mentalis muscle	5 U	20 U

1 unit of Botox = Approximately 4 units of Dysport.

SPECIFIC INJECTION SITES

BTX-A should be injected directly into the muscle that was targeted as problematic before treatment.[11-14] Precise knowledge of the different anatomic structures is required to avoid complications. The dosages of BTX-A described in Table 42-2 are in Botox units, and the standard conversion between Botox units and Dysport units is given. No studies to date have established the superiority of one product over the other.

Glabella
- Target muscles: Brow depressors
  - Procerus: 4 to 5 U
  - Corrugator + depressor supercilii: 16 to 20 U
- Important injection landmarks (Fig. 42-2)
  - Procerus: Midway between medial ends of both eyebrows.
  - Corrugator: Vertical line above the inner canthus and the superior margin of the bony orbital rim. A second injection is placed 5 mm lateral to the first injection and all of the extension of the muscle is treated in this way.

The area of the procerus can be localized by staying in the midline. To avoid diffusion into the orbital septum, adjacent musculature should not be massaged. Excellent resolution of glabellar rhytids can be expected with effective treatment (Fig. 42-3).
- Cautions
  - Do not inject under the eyebrows at the level of the midpupillary line (this may result in ptosis of the eyebrow).
  - Avoid directing an injection toward the medial canthus.

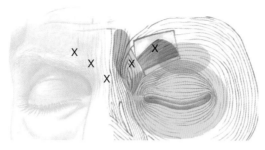

Fig. 42-2   Injection in the glabellar area. Five sites are marked *(X)*. The first one is placed in the midline between the heads of the eyebrows. The lateral marks treat the corrugators. The first mark is placed following a vertical line that crosses the medial canthus and ends in the superior edge of the bony orbit. A second mark is placed 5 mm lateral, slightly above the orbital rim, to treat the lateral portion of the muscle. The shaded blue areas represent the zones to be avoided.

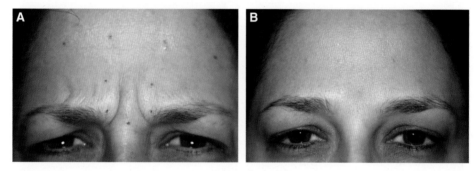

Fig. 42-3   **A,** Preinjection and **B,** postinjection views of a patient who received glabellar BTX-A injections. Note how her frown lines have been attenuated.

Horizontal Forehead Lines

- Target muscles: Frontalis
  - Frontalis: 8 to 15 U
- Important injection landmarks (Fig. 42-4)
  - Horizontal lines across the forehead midway between the patient's eyebrows and hairline are an important landmark. The injection sites are evenly spaced across forehead.
  - Lateral injections should be placed 1 cm medial to the lateral end of the forehead wrinkle and at a minimum 1.5 cm above the lateral portion of the brow.
- Recommendations
  - Do not inject the frontalis muscle in the area that supports the ptotic brow (older patients).
  - Do not inject more than 1 cm lateral to the lateral end of the forehead wrinkle; this can produce an expressionless forehead.
  - Do not inject in proximity to the brow; ptosis of the lateral aspect of the brow can result.

Excellent resolution of forehead rhytids can be expected with effective treatment (Fig. 42-5).

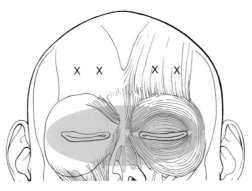

Fig. 42-4   Forehead injection sites. Marks are placed midway between the hairline and eyebrows. No marks are placed in the midline, because the frontalis muscle diverges laterally. The shaded blue area represents the zone to be avoided.

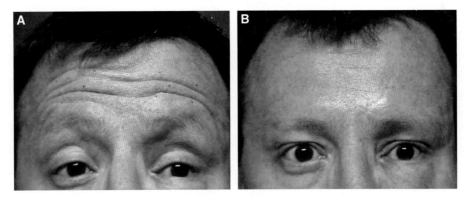

Fig. 42-5   **A,** Preinjection and **B,** postinjection views of a patient receiving BTX-A in the forehead.

Crow's-Feet

- Target muscles: Orbicularis oculi
  - Orbicularis oculi: 12 to 15 U per side
- Important injection landmarks (Fig. 42-6)
  - The first injection point is marked 1 cm lateral to the bony orbital rim.
  - The second and third marks are placed 1 cm superiorly and inferiorly.
  - The muscle is directly under the skin. The injection should be placed superficially.
- Recommendations
  - Do not inject close to margin of zygoma. This will result in an asymmetric smile.
  - Do not inject medial to a vertical line drawn through the lateral canthus, because ectropion or ptotic lateral lower eyelid may result.
  - Inject at least 1 cm lateral to the orbital rim.

Excellent resolution of lateral canthal rhytids can be expected with effective treatment (Fig. 42-7).

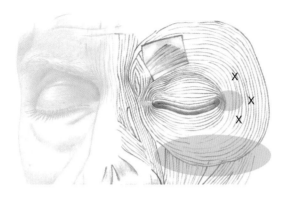

Fig. 42-6   Injection of crow's-feet. Marks are placed 1 cm lateral to the bony orbital rim. Injection sites are marked *(X)*. The first mark is at the level of the lateral canthus. Second and third sites are marked 1 cm superior and inferior to first site. Injections should not be placed toward the zygoma or near the lateral canthus, which is indicated in blue.

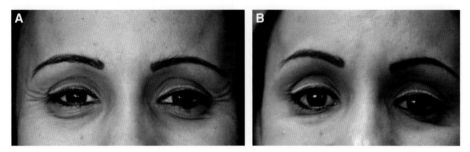

Fig. 42-7   **A,** Preinjection and **B,** postinjection views of patient with BTX-A treatment of crow's-feet.

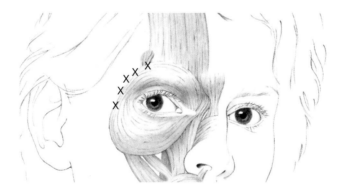

Fig. 42-8   Brow elevation. Sites are marked in superolateral portion of the orbicularis oculi, taking care not to inject the lateral portion of the frontalis muscle. Although the existence of an independent lateral brow depressor muscle is not established, a segment of muscle is depicted here, based on the observation that BTX-A treatment in this area results in elevation of the resting position of the lateral brow ("chemical brow lift").

Brow Elevation

- Target muscles: Frontalis and orbicularis oculi
  - Create an open eye look: inject the glabellar muscles at the inferior aspect of the medial brow without injecting the frontalis.
  - To elevate the lateral brow, inject the lateral-superior portion of the orbicularis oculi muscle.
- Important injection landmarks (Fig. 42-8)
  - Elevation of the medial portion of the brow: Do not inject the medial portion of the frontalis muscle.
  - Elevation of the tail of the brow: Do not inject the lateral portion of the frontalis. Inject the lateral portion of the orbicularis following the orbital rim just below the lateral brow.
  - Do not massage the injected area.

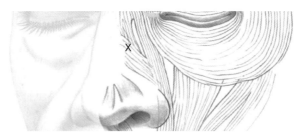

Fig. 42-9   Injection of "bunny lines." Site is marked directly over the nasalis muscle on the nasal dorsum. Contralateral injection site is not shown.

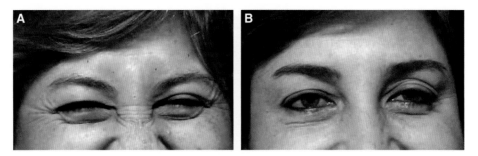

Fig. 42-10   **A,** Preinjection and **B,** postinjection views of patient who received BTX-A treatment of bunny lines and crow's-feet.

"Bunny Lines" or Nasal Scrunch
- Target muscles: Nasalis
  - Nasalis muscle: 2 to 4 U per side
- Important injection landmarks (Fig. 42-9)
  - The injection site is directly over the horizontal nasal rhytids at the lateral sidewalls of the nasal dorsum.
- Recommendations
  - Avoid injection into the nasofacial groove.
  - Inadvertent injection of the levator anguli oris or levator labii superioris alaeque nasi muscle can result in lip ptosis or lip asymmetries.

Excellent resolution of bunny lines can be expected with effective treatment (Fig. 42-10).

MARIONETTE LINES
- Target muscles: Depressor anguli oris
  - Depressor anguli oris: 2 to 4 U per side
- Important injection landmarks (Fig. 42-11)
  - To identify the injection sites a line is drawn 7 to 10 mm lateral to oral commissure and 8 to 10 mm inferior.
- Recommendation
  - Avoid injecting near the orbicularis oris; oral incompetence and the inability to pucker the lips may result.

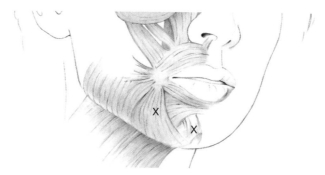

Fig. 42-11   Injection of lip depressors (lateral *X*) and mentalis muscle (medial *X*). Depressor site is marked 7 to 10 mm lateral and 8 to 10 mm inferior to the oral commissure; 2 to 5 U are injected on each side. The mentalis site is marked at a point midway between the lower vermilion border and the mandibular symphysis; 2 to 5 U are injected on each side.

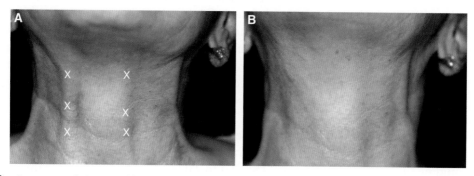

Fig. 42-12   Injection of platysmal bands. **A,** Sites are marked following the most prominent platysmal bands and placed approximately 2 cm apart. **B,** View of the patient after injection with BTX-A.

Mentalis Muscle: Peau d'Orange

- Target muscles: Mentalis muscle
  - Mentalis muscle: 5 U
- Important injection landmarks (see Fig. 42-11)
  - The injection is placed at a point halfway between lower vermilion border and the edge of the chin (symphysis).
- Recommendation
  - Do not inject in close proximity to the lip: Weakening of the orbicularis oris can result in oral incompetence.

Platysmal Bands

  - Target muscles: Platysma muscles (neck banding)
  - Platysma muscle: 12 to 30 U (2 U per injection site following the platysmal bands)
- Important injection landmarks (Fig. 42-12)
  - The injection site should be initiated 2 cm below the angle of the mandible.
  - The injection points should follow the platysmal band inferiorly, placing each injection at least 2 cm apart.
- Recommendations
  - The patient is asked to contract the muscles of the neck, and the band is identified and manually secured.

- The toxin should be injected at 2 cm intervals.
- The toxin should not be injected below the muscle. This can diffuse into the neck and result in dysphagia (weakness of sternohyoid muscle), alterations in voice (compromise of the cricothyroid muscle), and neck weakness (compromise of the sternocleidomastoid muscle).

Excellent resolution of platysmal banding can be expected with effective treatment (see Fig. 42-12).

Side Effects and Complications

Patients with NMJ disorders (such myasthenia gravis, Eaton-Lambert disease, and neurologic degenerative diseases) should not be injected with BTX-A. Concomitant use of penicillamine, quinine, aminoglycosides, and calcium channel blockers can potentiate the effect of BTX-A and should be avoided.

Complications with BTX-A injections are not common. Generalized reactions include nausea, malaise, fatigue, and flulike symptoms. Reactions can also be seen at the injection site. These include pain, edema, erythema, and bruising. Headaches can be exacerbated after injection. Localized reactions can be treated by preparing the area to be injected with a topical anesthetic (EMLA) and/or the use of ice packs. Aspirin and NSAIDs should be avoided for 10 days before injection. Patients receiving anticoagulation therapy should not be injected. Transient weakness of untreated neighboring muscles or asymmetrical paralysis can occur. Paralysis can be treated by injecting the contralateral muscle group. Weakness is usually transient and resolves relatively quickly.

Ptosis is probably the most important complication seen with BTX-A injections. It can last for 3 to 5 weeks, but it is reversible. Treatment involves the administration of eye drops containing alpha-adrenergic agonists (apraclonidine [0.5%] or phenylephrine [2.5%]), 1 to 2 drops on the affected side three times a day. These are midriatic agents that stimulate Müller's muscle, resulting in a 1 to 2 mm elevation of the upper eyelid. Ideally, the treatment should continue until the problematic ptosis is resolved.

Immunity to repeated BTX-A has been reported, but no systematic clinical studies have been formally conducted. Patients with reported immunity are characterized by the absence of response to treatment and lack of muscle atrophy in the injected area. The general recommendation is to use the smallest dose possible, avoid frequent reinjections, and extend the interval between treatments.[13]

FOLLOW-UP

Patients are asked to return to the office 1 to 2 weeks after injection so the effectiveness of treatment can be evaluated. Photographs are taken, and if persistent hyperfunctional muscles are present, small amounts of toxin can be injected in specific areas to augment the treatment effect. Patients are typically retreated every 4 to 6 months, or when patient reports a recurrence of bothersome muscle activity. Chemical peels, lasers, and injections of filler agents can complement BTX-A treatment.

VOLUME REPLACEMENT IN THE AGING FACE

It is now well established that aging is a process that is affected by intrinsic and extrinsic factors (see Chapter 6). With the aging process, the skeletal framework is reduced, production of collagen is diminished, and the skin and muscle lose elasticity. These intrinsic factors are exacerbated by environmental factors

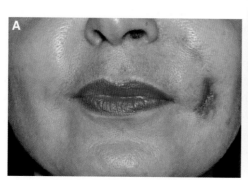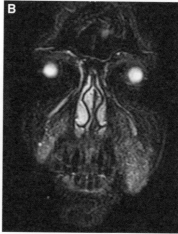

Fig. 42-13   Example of silicone granuloma resulting from nasolabial and melolabial fold injection. **A,** Clinical photograph. **B,** MRI scan demonstrates the presence of silicone granuloma bilaterally.

such as sun exposure, smoking, alcohol intake, and underlying chronic illnesses. The final result is a face that appears volume depleted, with loss of elasticity of its structures. Volume replenishment has become a crucial part of facial rejuvenation procedures. Historically, myriad substances have been used to replace facial volume, including paraffin, silicone, and the bovine collagens, some with unfavorable outcomes.[14] The unacceptably high rate of granuloma formation resulting from the use of injectable silicone formulations (Fig. 42-13) has led to its removal from most international markets. The ideal substance would be one that could easily be removed, would not produce any allergic reactions, is durable, and is completely integrated by the body. Three approaches to volume replacement include direct volume replacement into rhytids with hyaluronic acid and/or hydroxyapatite, indirect volume augmentation through volume-restoring agents that promote collagen formation, and lipofilling with autologous fat.

DIRECT VOLUME REPLACEMENT
Hyaluronic Acids

Hyaluronic acid (HA) is a natural complex sugar found in all living organisms. It is found in multiple human tissues, including skin, dermis, connective tissues, and synovial tissues and fluid.[15,16] It hydrates the skin by binding to water and providing the tissues with volume, turgor, and elasticity. The sources for commercial HA are vitreous humor, tendons, skin, umbilical cord, and bacterial cultures. Naturally occurring HA is too unstable to be injected into the skin. Most of it will be degraded within a few days. For this reason, and to produce a HA filler that lasts longer and resists the effects of degradation, the molecules must be cross-linked to each other to develop a molecule that is larger and more resistant. There are several ways of doing this, but the products that are most commonly used today contain no animal protein and are produced with recombinant bacterial technology (through a bacterial streptococcal fermentation process). The result is a three-dimensional molecular structure that is stable and elastic. The injected gel is slowly absorbed by surrounding tissues and finally disappears by degradation. The complete process can last more than 6 months, depending on where the gel was injected. For this reason, many consider HA to be the ideal filler. It contains very little or no protein, is not degraded quickly, and the effect is subtle and incorporated well by surrounding tissues. The substance can be injected at different skin levels and can be safely combined with other injectables, even those that are permanent.

Products

These products are cross-linked bacteria-derived HA:

- Juvéderm: Approved in 2006 by the FDA as a dermal filler for the treatment of facial rhytids and contour defects. The difference between the different products is the size of the molecule.
  - Juvéderm Ultra: Regular filler
  - Juvéderm Ultra Plus: Used to treat deeper facial folds
- Restylane family: Approved in 2003 by the FDA as a filler for treatment of facial wrinkles and folds. The product is 1% crosslinked HA that is based on nonanimal stabilized hyaluronic acid (NASHA) produced by a streptococcal fermentation process.
  - Restylane Fine Lines
  - Restylane Touch
  - Restylane Lipp
  - Restylane SubQ
  - Restylane Vital

There are multiple uses for HA in clinical facial practice. Its main uses are correction of nasolabial folds (Fig. 42-14), marionette lines, lip contouring (Fig. 42-15), and augmentation. Today, with the different molecules available, its uses have increased dramatically. Larger molecules are used for restoration of facial volume, such as cheek contouring and mandibular augmentation. Smaller-sized molecules are used to fill in hollow lower lids and tear trough deformities (Fig. 42-16) and to elevate the lateral brow. These substances are also used to correct postrhinoplasty deformities (Fig. 42-17), acne scars, and traumatic scars (Box 42-1). Myriad other products are under development; some have already reached the market, and a great number of products are likely to become available over the next decade.

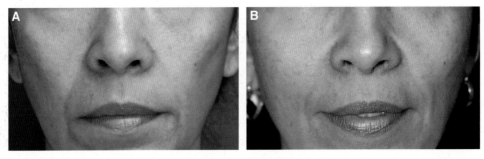

Fig. 42-14 **A,** Pretreatment and **B,** posttreatment views of a patient with nasolabial area treated with 1.0 cc of Perlane. Material was administered in a deeper plane using a threading technique.

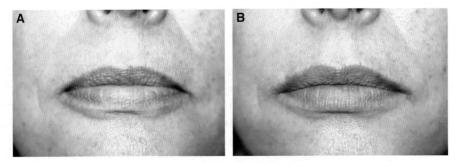

Fig. 42-15 **A,** Preinjection and **B,** postinjection views of a patient's lips treated with Restylane and Perlane. Restylane Fine Lines was used to delineate lips and Perlane was used to increase volume.

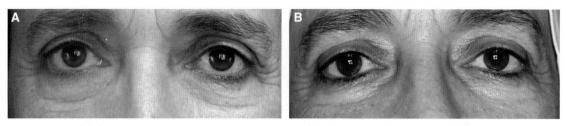

Fig. 42-16   **A,** Preinjection and **B,** postinjection views of a patient treated with Restylane in the infraorbital rim area. Injections were placed as deep as possible, depositing small quantities of gel following the inferior orbital rim and extending slightly into the tear trough area. Although the defect was not completely corrected, there is improvement of this area.

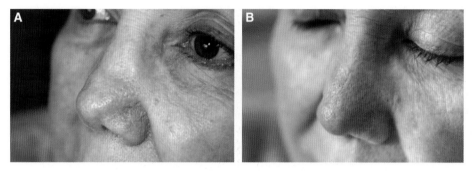

Fig. 42-17   **A,** Preinjection and **B,** postinjection views of a patient with a marked depression of the left middle third of the nose that was treated with a subdermal injection of Perlane. It is important not to overcorrect in this area.

Box 42-1   Clinical Applications of Hyaluronic Acid in the Face

- Correction of deep rhytids
- Correction of periocular rhytids
- Correction of hollow in infraorbital rim
- Cheek augmentation
- Correction of nasolabial folds
- Correction of mental fold
- Correction of marionette lines
- Correction of nasal deformities
- Correction of acne scars/traumatic scars
- Lip contouring and enhancement

TECHNIQUE

Informed consent should be obtained and standard photographs taken. The area to be injected should be covered with a topical anesthetic, then cleaned accordingly. The targeted areas for treatment are marked with the patient sitting upright. The patient is then reclined to a 45-degree supine position. Occasionally, nerve blocks are used with 1% lidocaine. In some practices, injection with needles has recently been replaced by injection with microcannulas. These cannulas have a blunt tip, are flexible, fit on any Luer-Lok syringe, and come in different sizes. There are several advantages of these cannulas over hypodermic needles[17] (Fig. 42-18):

- Less bleeding and bruising
- Less risk of intravascular injection
- Less discomfort during injection

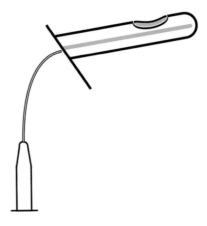

Fig. 42-18 Microcannula design. Magnified schematic shows a hole in the wall of the microcannula.

Several points should be considered when using cannulas:

- An entry port in the skin should be made with a needle before use of a cannula. The entry puncture should be performed with a needle of the same gauge or similar gauge as the cannula to be used.
- The cannula is inserted its full length or as needed. It is normal to feel some resistance to the advancement of the cannula.
- Caution must be exercised with the amount injected. The plunger pressure decreases and the filler flow increases with use of a cannula as compared with a needle.
- Filling is performed from superior to inferior and from deep to superficial. The same injection techniques performed with needles can be accomplished with cannulas (linear threading and multiple microdeposits of gel). Material should be injected while the cannula is being withdrawn.
- Less posttreatment massage is necessary when using cannulas.

COMPLICATIONS

Adverse events can occur with any of the facial fillers commercially available today, and must be recognized and corrected.[18,19] The most common adverse events are:

- Erythema
- Swelling
- Pain
- Ecchymosis
- Infection
- Formation of nodules
- Intravascular injection
- Tyndall effect

Most of these reactions can easily be treated with ice packs and pain medications. Infections should be diagnosed quickly and treated with the appropriate antibiotics. The Tyndall effect (blue bump formation) and formation of nodules is more commonly seen in the periorbital area and is a result of too-superficial injections of HA. Treatment involves injection of hyaluronidase into the lesion. The visible bump usually resolves after several days.

Intravascular injections, although rare, can become a major complication if they are not diagnosed and treated accordingly. An intraarterial occlusion is usually immediate, producing severe pain associated with skin blanching or violet coloration. It is more commonly seen in the glabellar area. Injection should be stopped immediately and the area should be massaged vigorously. If the filler agent used was HA, hy-

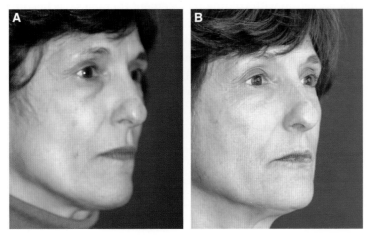

Fig. 42-19   Example of volume augmentation using Sculptra. **A,** Preoperative view. **B,** Postoperative view.

aluronidase should be injected. In addition, 2% nitroglycerin paste should be applied, aspirin should be given, and warm compresses should be placed on the affected area. Close follow-up of the patient is essential to ensure an optimal outcome.

INDIRECT VOLUME REPLACEMENT

Sculptra (poly-L-lactic acid) is an injectable polyester that is delivered in microspheres; it is indicated for attenuation of shallow to deep facial rhytids. Unlike hyaluronic acid and calcium hydroxyapatite fillers, Sculptra is a synthetic material that does not serve as a filler, but rather as a volume restorative agent. After injection, the poly-L-lactic acid stimulates the body to lay down collagen adjacent to the polymer molecules, resulting in recruitment of one's own collagen to the region over time (Fig. 42-19). Typically, two to three injections spaced 4 to 6 weeks apart are required. The effect lasts approximately 2 years. In addition, unlike with other fillers, the patient does not experience the final result immediately after injection.

LIPOFILLING

Lipoinjection (fat grafting) can restore long-lasting volume in the face. There is debate, however, regarding the exact mechanism of action. Some purport that lipoinjection restores volume by delivering healthy adipocytes from a distant site. Others feel that during harvest, some adipocytes undergo necrosis, stimulating replacement by cystic or fibrotic autologous material after injection. Fat can be harvested from multiple sites through a blunt-tipped cannula using a tumescent anesthetic solution. Typically, absorption occurs to a modest degree after injection, requiring approximately 30% to 50% overcorrection with injection. Lipofilling is indicated for attenuation of nasolabial folds, marionette lines, and glabellar furrows. It can also be used to augment volume in the lips and for correction of hemifacial atrophy.

CONCLUSION

Botulinum A toxin injections and hyaluronic acid filler agents have become a valuable tool in facial cosmetic surgery. BTX-A injections are safe and effective in the treatment of dynamic hyperfunctional facial rhytids. Volume replacement is being performed with filler agents with very good results. HA in its different preparations has become a straightforward and effective method for volume replacement in the face. More and more frequently, patients are seeking nonsurgical alternatives to facial rejuvenation. The combination of chemodenervation with volume replacement therapies has become an excellent option, and is attractive to many patients because of its minimal risk and minimal interferance with normal daily activities. The existence of these various nonsurgical options has opened an interesting window in facial rejuvenation (Table 42-3). It is the specialist's responsibility to offer patients a wide range of options for facial rejuvenation. Patients must be educated about all existing treatment choices and must understand the advantages and limitations of current therapy so that they have realistic expectations.

Table 42-3   Commercially Available Injectables and Filler Agents

Product Name	Component	Manufacturer	Duration (months)
Injectables			
Botox	OnabotulinumtoxinA	Allergan	3-6
Dysport	AbobotulinumtoxinA	Medicis/Ipsen	3-6
Xeomin	IncobotulinumtoxinA	Merz	3-6
Lantox (Russia) Prosigne (Brazil) Redux (Peru)	OnabotulinumtoxinA	Lanzhou Institute (China)	3-6
Neuronox Siax	OnabotulinumtoxinA	South Korea	3-6
NeuroBloc Myobloc	RimabotulinumtoxinB	Solstice	2
Fillers			
Short-Term Fillers			
Collagen Products			
Zyderm/Zyplast	Bovine collagen	Allergan	3-6
CosmoDerm-CosmoPlast	Human collagen	Allergan	3-6
Hyaluronic Acids			
Restylane	Hyaluronic acid	Medicis	3-6
Perlane	Hyaluronic acid	Medicis	6-9
Juvéderm	Hyaluronic acid	Allergan	6-9
Belotero	Hyaluronic acid	Merz	6-12
Hylaform	Hyaluronic acid	Genzyme	6-9
Puragen	Hyaluronic acid	Mentor	6-9
Prevelle	Hyaluronic acid	Mentor	6-9
Long-Term Fillers (Semipermanent)			
Radiesse	Calcium hydroxylapatite	Merz	12-18
Sculptra	Poly-L-lactic acid	Dermik	12-24
Permanent Fillers			
Artefill	Polymethylmethacrylate plus bovine collagen	Artes	Permanent

KEY POINTS

- Trends toward more minimally invasive interventions for the aging face have increased the popularity of injectable therapy for facial aging.
- Botulinum toxin has enjoyed decades of use as a temporary muscle paralytic agent in the treatment of movement disorders, and is now FDA approved for the treatment of age-related rhytids.
- Age-related volume loss in the face can be addressed with direct volume replacement, indirect volume replacement with collagen recruitment, and lipofilling.

REFERENCES

1. Tessmer Snipe P, Sommer H. Studies on botulinus toxin. 3. Acid precipitation of botulinus toxin. J Infect Dis 43:152-160, 1928.
2. Scott AB. Botulinum toxin injection into extraocular muscles as an alternative to strabismus surgery. Ophthalmology 87:1044-1049, 1980.
   The author explains how strabismus can be treated by injecting botulinum toxin in specific muscles of the orbital region without having to perform surgery.
3. Carruthers A, Kiene K, Carruthers J. Botulinum A exotoxin use in clinical dermatology. J Am Acad Dermatol 34:788-797, 1996.
4. Blitzer A, Brin AF, Keen MF, et al. Botulinum toxin for the treatment of hyperfunctional lines of the face. Arch Otolaryngol Head Neck Surg 119:1018-1023, 1993.
5. Carruthers A, Carruthers JD. The use of botulinum toxin to treat glabellar frown lines and other facial wrinkles. Cosmet Dermatol 7:11-15, 1994.
6. Brin MF. Botulinum toxin therapy: basic science and overview of other therapeutics. In Blitzer A, Binder WJ, Carruthers A, eds. Management of Facial Lines and Wrinkles. Philadelphia: Lippincott Williams & Wilkins, 2000.
7. Lowe NJ. Botulinum toxin type A for facial rejuvenation. United States and United Kingdom perspectives. Dermatol Surg 24:1216-1218, 1998.
8. Nettar KD, Yu KC, Bapna S, et al. An internally controlled, double-blind comparison of the efficacy of onabotulinumtoxinA and abobotulinumtoxinA. Arch Facial Plast Surg 13:380-386, 2011.
9. Klein A. Dilution and storage of botulinum toxin. Dermatol Surg 24:1179-1180, 1998.
10. Hexsal DM, de Almeida AT, Rutowitsch M, et al. Multicenter, double-blind study of the efficacy of injections with botulinum toxin type A reconstituted up to six consecutive weeks before application. Dermatol Surg 29:523-529, 2003.
11. Cobo R, Roy D. Botulinum toxin A: treatment of hyperfunctional facial lines. In Vuyk HD, Lohuis PJ. Facial Plastic and Reconstructive Surgery. London: Edward Arnold, 2006.
12. Cobo R. Botulinum exotoxin A injections. In Thomas JR, ed. Advanced Therapy in Facial Plastic and Reconstructive Surgery. Shelton, CT: PMPH-USA, 2010.
13. Petrus G, Lewis D, Maas C. Anatomic considerations for treatment with botulinum toxin. Facial Plast Surg Clin N Am 15:1-9, 2007.
    The authors present a revision on vectors of contraction of different facial muscle that can be treated with botulinum toxin.
14. Kontis TC, Rivkin A. The history of injectable fillers. Facial Plast Surg 25:67-72, 2009.
15. Brandt FS, Cazzaniga A. Hyaluronic acid fillers: Restylane and Perlane. Facial Plast Surg Clin N Am 15:63-76, 2007.
16. Born T. Hyaluronic acids. Clin Plastic Surg 33:525-538, 2006.
17. DeJoseph LM. Cannulas for facial filler placement. Facial Plast Surg Clin N Am 20:215-220, 2012.
18. Lowe NJ, Maxwell CA, Patnaik R. Adverse reactions to dermal fillers: review. Dermatol Surg 31(11 Pt 2):1616-1625, 2005.
19. Sclafani A, Fagien S. Treatment of injectable soft tissue filler complications. Dermatol Surg 35:1672-1680, 2009.
    The authors present different treatment options for complications that can be produced when injecting soft tissue fillers in the face.

PART III

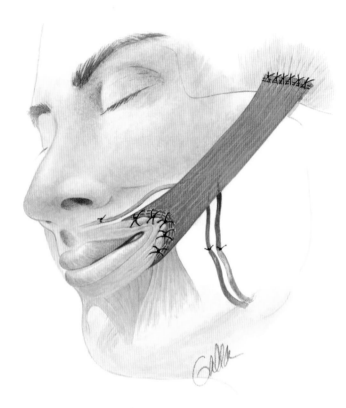

We restore, repair and make whole those parts . . . which nature
has given but which fortune has taken away, not so much
that they may delight the eye but that they may buoy up
the spirit and help the mind of the afflicted.
—Gaspare Tagliacozzi (1545-1599)

Conditions Affecting Multiple
Facial Zones or Tissues

43

Impaired Facial Movement: Paralysis, Synkinesis, and Spasm

Tessa A. Hadlock ▪ Mack L. Cheney

Facial expression is the cornerstone of nonverbal communication. Throughout mammalian evolution, facial expression has been critical in intraspecies interactions, and across human history has served as a primary mechanism for the expression of emotions.[1] Fascination with the twisted nature of the face in human facial paralysis has been depicted in ancient artifacts, masks, and sculpture from Greek, Roman, pre-Colombian, and African cultures[2-5] (Fig. 43-1); and a thorough description of unilateral and bilateral paralysis appears in the ninth century writings of Persian physician Razi.[6,7]

The establishment of the modern era of facial nerve anatomy and physiology is credited to Sir Charles Bell, a Scottish surgeon who presented a paper to the Royal Society in London in 1821 describing the trajectory of the facial nerve and a thorough description of the condition of acute unilateral facial paralysis that still bears his name.[8] The classic electrophysiologic studies of the muscles of facial expression (Fig. 43-2) performed by the French neurologist Guillaume Duchenne[9] set the stage for generations of surgeons to work toward developing reconstructive options for the paralyzed face.

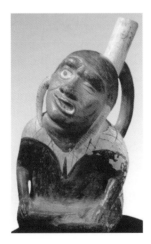

Fig. 43-1   Ancient Peruvian sculpture depicting an individual with facial paralysis.

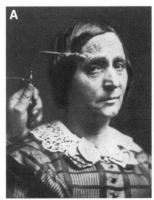
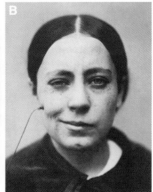

Fig. 43-2   Examples of Duchenne's seminal experiments with facial nerve stimulation and the resulting expressions. **A,** Stimulation of the frontal branch causing lateral brow movement. **B,** Stimulation of the zygomaticus major causing smiling. (Reprinted from Guillaume Duchenne. Mécanisme de la Physionomie Humaine, 1861.)

The role of facial expression in humans has been the subject of an extensive body of contemporary literature pioneered by Paul Ekman.[10-14] Over the past several decades, renewed interest has developed in the psychology of facial paralysis and the fascinating relationship between facial expression and affect, behavior, and emotions. The finding that the act of smiling may actually produce more benevolent behaviors and optimistic feelings within an individual[15-18] has provided additional impetus for the facial reanimation surgeon interested in restoring this critical and underappreciated function to the face.

In addition to its role in producing expressions, the facial musculature is responsible for myriad other important functions that lead to significant morbidity when impaired. Among the most relevant movements that may be individually or collectively impaired are brow elevation, blinking (eye closure), inspiratory nostril dilation, smiling, manipulation of the food bolus, movement of the lips with eating and speaking, and lower lip movement. The goal of modern facial reanimation surgery is to restore both static facial landmark positions and symmetry, and to restore dynamic facial movements and spontaneous facial expressions.

ANATOMY AND PHYSIOLOGY

Detailed descriptions of facial nerve anatomy in the soft tissues of the face are provided in Chapter 1 (see Fig. 1-21). Beginning centrally, nerve fibers responsible for voluntary motor action originate in the lower portion of the precentral gyrus. These fibers cross in the caudal pontine region and reach the facial nerve nucleus, located in the contralateral pons, and innervate the upper facial muscles. The frontotemporal cerebral cortex and parts of the limbic and basal ganglion provide central connections for involuntary expression. The facial nerve nucleus is located dorsolaterally in the pons. The nerve exits the nucleus, passes around the abducens nucleus, and exits the brainstem close to the cerebellopontine junction. The nervus intermedius and vestibulocochlear nerve join the facial nerve in the cerebellopontine angle. These nerves together, void of epineurium, span the 17 to 24 mm gap between the brainstem and the porus acusticus, after which they enter the internal auditory canal (IAC). The facial nerve occupies the anterosuperior quadrant of the IAC before entering the fallopian canal. The entrance of the fallopian canal, the meatal foramen, is the narrowest segment of the intratemporal bony channel; it is in this location that the nerve is most susceptible to impairment caused by inflammation.

The course of the facial nerve within the temporal bone is divided into three segments: the labyrinthine segment (4 mm, meatal foramen to geniculate ganglion), the tympanic segment (11 mm, geniculate ganglion to second genu), and the mastoid segment (13 mm, second genu to stylomastoid foramen). The greater superficial petrosal nerve branches at the geniculate ganglion, bringing parasympathetic fibers to the nose, lacrimal gland, and palate (Fig. 43-3). Stapedius muscle innervation arises from the proximal tympanic segment. The chorda tympani nerve exits from the facial nerve between the lateral semicircular canal and stylomastoid foramen, carrying parasympathetic fibers to the submandibular and sublingual glands and sensory taste fibers from the anterior two thirds of the tongue. Whereas proximally the nerve is surrounded only by cerebrospinal fluid and pia mater, as it travels distally through the bone it becomes progressively encased by a layer of epineurium (Fig. 43-4).

Extratemporally, the facial nerve has five general divisions: temporal, zygomatic, buccal, mandibular, and cervical. There is significant variation and overlap within these zones (Fig. 43-5, *A*), although generally the temporal branch alone innervates the frontalis and corrugator supercilii, and the marginal mandibular branch alone innervates the lip depressors (Fig. 43-5, *B*). Isolated branch injuries in these areas thus produce characteristic functional deficits (Fig. 43-6).

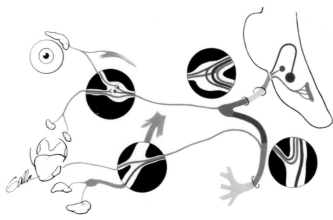

Fig. 43-3 The facial nerve. The nerve exits the pons *(orange)* and traverses the cerebellopontine angle. It then spans the IAC *(yellow)* and forms its first turn at the geniculate ganglion *(purple)* to enter the middle ear *(dark green)*. The nerve enters the mastoid at its second genu *(brown)* and runs vertically to exit the temporal bone at the stylomastoid foramen *(pink)*. Extratemporally the motor segment divides at the pes anserinus into the distinct branches. Within the pons, the motor nucleus *(blue)*, superior salivatory nucleus *(brown)*, and nucleus fascicularis solitarius *(light green)* give rise to motor, autonomic, and special sensory divisions of the facial nerve, respectively. At the geniculate ganglion, the greater superficial petrosal nerve (GSPN) branches off the main trunk with preganglionic, parasympathetic afferents *(brown)* destined to synapse at the pterygopalatine ganglion and provide input to the lacrimal, nasal, and palatine glands. Special sensory afferents traveling with the GSPN provide sensation to the palatine taste buds *(green)*. The chorda tympani branches from the vertical segment of the facial nerve, carrying special sensory afferents *(green)* and preganglionic parasympathetic fibers *(brown)*. This branch joins the lingual nerve and synapses, and gives rise to postganglionic, parasympathetic fibers at the submandibular ganglion that innervate the sublingual and submandibular glands. Special sensory afferent fibers also travel in the chorda tympani and provide taste to the anterior two thirds of the tongue *(green)* that travel to the nucleus solitarius *(light green)*.

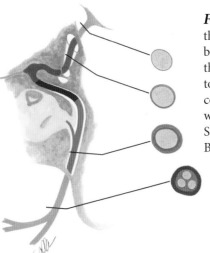

Fig. 43-4 Topographic arrangement of the cornerstone tissue components of the facial nerve. In the cerebellopontine angle the nerve is monofascicular and bound by only the perineurium that arises from pia and arachnoid tissue. Within the IAC the nerve gains epineurium. As the nerve enters the middle ear and mastoid segments, the perineurium and epineurium become thicker. The nerve becomes polyfascicular upon exiting the stylomastoid foramen, and is enclosed within a dense nerve sheath. (Modified from Nadol JB, Schuknecht HF, eds. Surgery of the Ear and Temporal Bone. Philadelphia: Raven Press, 1993.)

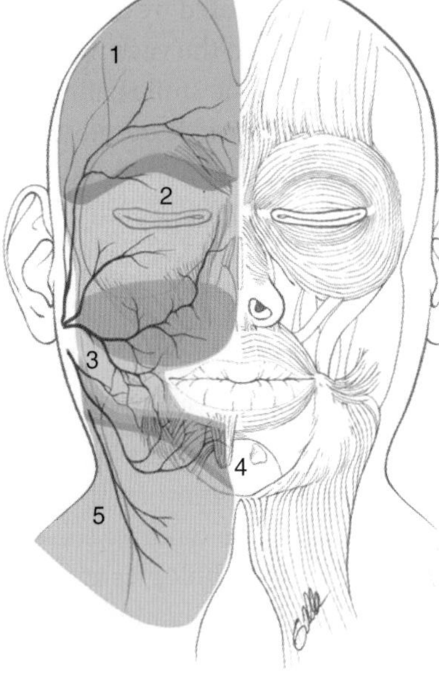

Fig. 43-5 Peripheral distribution of the facial nerve, showing the zone innervated by each division. After the nerve bifurcates at the pes anserinus, the upper division gives rise to the temporal *(pink)* and zygomatic *(blue)* branches whereas the lower division gives rise to the buccal *(yellow)*, marginal mandibular *(purple)*, and cervical *(green)* branches. There is significant overlap between the zygomatic and buccal distributions, depicted by the green overlap in blue and yellow zones.

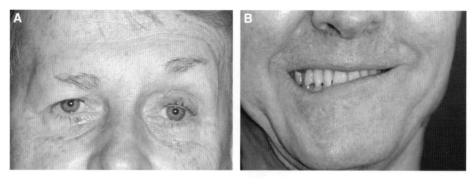

Fig. 43-6 Examples of isolated branch injuries. **A,** Isolated frontal branch injury after temporomandibular joint replacement. **B,** Isolated marginal mandibular branch injury after face lift.

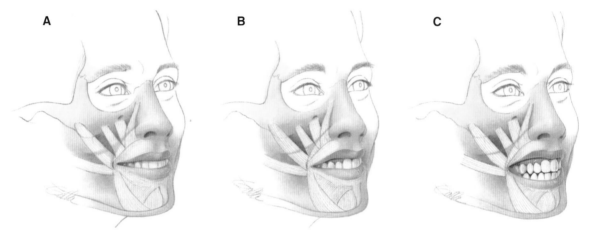

Fig. 43-7 Smile types, with dominant smiling musculature depicted in green. **A,** The zygomaticus major smile, produced by a dominant zygomaticus major muscle and the buccinators, resulting in the corners of the mouth being elevated first. **B,** The canine smile results from a codominant levator labii superioris, which contracts first on initiation of a smile, followed by activation of the zygomaticus major and buccinator for elevation of the corners of the mouth. **C,** The full denture smile results from full activation of elevators and depressors of the lips and angles of the mouth, thus displaying both maxillary and mandibular teeth.

SMILE ANATOMY

A smile is created by the muscles of the lips and midface. Smiles differ in their line of contracture, point of insertion, and the varying strengths of each muscle group.[19] The interaction of these three components creates three basic smile patterns: the zygomaticus major smile, dominated by the zygomaticus major muscle (occurring in 67% of individuals); the canine smile, dominated by the levator labii superioris (occurring in 31% of individuals); and the full-denture smile, codominated by the lip elevators and the lip depressors (occurring in 2% of individuals) (Fig. 43-7).

EPIDEMIOLOGIC FACTORS

Facial nerve dysfunction may arise from a variety of clinical conditions (Box 43-1), although most common etiologic factors are viruses, Lyme disease, temporal bone fracture, postsurgical causes, and benign or malignant tumors. Bilateral facial paralysis has a shorter differential diagnosis, with Lyme disease, Guillain-Barré syndrome, congenital Mobius syndrome, and cavernous brainstem hemangiomas and other brainstem pathologies at the top of the list (Box 43-2). Meticulous history-taking, clinical examination, hematologic evaluation, and detailed imaging studies will usually yield a diagnosis.

Box 43-1   Differential Diagnosis of Facial Paralysis

Birth
Mobius syndrome
Molding
Forceps delivery
Dystrophic myotonica

Trauma
Basal skull fractures
Facial injuries
Penetrating middle ear injury
Slag injury to middle ear
Altitude paralysis (barotrauma)
Scuba diving (barotrauma)
Lightning injury
Nose-blowing palsy
Reactive neuroma
Welder's spark

Neurologic
Opercular syndrome (cortical
    lesion in facial motor area)
Millard-Gubler syndrome
    (abducens palsy with contralat-
    eral hemiplegia caused by lesion
    in base of pons)
Cephalic tetanus
Wernicke-Korsakoff syndrome
Pseudotumor cerebri
Lacunar syndrome

Infection
External otitis
Otitis media
Mastoiditis
Chicken pox
Herpes zoster cephalicus
Encephalitis
Poliomyelitis (type 1)
Mumps
Mononucleosis
Leprosy
Influenza
Coxsackie virus
Malaria
Syphilis
Scleroma

Tuberculosis
Botulism
Acute hemorrhagic conjunctivitis
Gnathostomiasis
Mucormycosis
Lyme disease
Cat scratch disease
Acquired immunodeficiency
    syndrome
Sinus thrombosis
Acute suppurative parotitis

Toxic
Thalidomide
Tetanus
Diphtheria
Carbon monoxide
Ethylene glycol
Arsenic intoxication
Alcoholism

Iatrogenic
Mandibular block anesthesia
Antitetanus serum
Vaccine for rabies
Postimmunization
Parotid surgery
Temporal bone surgery
Posttonsillectomy and
    adenoidectomy
Iontophoresis
Embolization
Dental
Sagittal split osteotomy

Idiopathic
Bell's
Inherited Bell's palsy
Melkersson-Rosenthal syndrome
Hereditary hypertrophic neuropa-
    thy (Charcot-Marie-Tooth dis-
    ease, Dejerine-Sottas disease)
Autoimmune syndrome
Temporal arteritis
Thrombotic thrombocytopenic
    purpura

Periarteritis nodosa
Landry-Guillain-Barré syndrome
Multiple sclerosis
Myasthenia gravis
Amyloidosis
Sarcoidosis
Osteoporosis
Osteogenesis imperfect
Cleidocranial dysostosis

Metabolic
Diabetes mellitus
Hyperthyroidism
Hypothyroidism
Pregnancy
Hypertension
Acute porphyria
Vitamin A deficiency

Neoplastic
Cholesteatoma
Seventh nerve tumor
Glomus jugulare tumor
Leukemia
Meningioma
Hemangioblastoma
Sarcoma
Carcinoma (invading or metastatic)
Anomalous sigmoid sinus
Carotid artery aneurysm
Hemangioma of tympanum
Hydradenoma
Schwannoma
Teratoma
Histiocytosis
Fibrous dysplasia
Von Recklinghausen disease
Benign parotid gland lesions
Temporal bone myeloma
Endolymphatic sac tumors
Malignant parotid lesions
Fibrosarcoma
Ossifying hemangioma
Granular cell myoblastoma
Seventh nerve tumor (cylindroma)

Box 43-2   Causes of Bilateral Facial Paralysis

Lyme disease	Syphilis
Mononucleosis	Leprosy
Varicella zoster	Bilateral temporal bone fracture
Landry-Guillain-Barré syndrome	Mobius syndrome
Leukemia	Brainstem stroke
Sarcoidosis	Bell's palsy
Meningitis	Chemotherapy agent side effect

VIRAL PARALYSIS

Viral reactivation is the most common cause of facial paralysis and presents as a rapidly evolving unilateral paralysis of all branches, with a fully evolved clinical picture within 72 hours of onset. Bell's palsy is thought to represent reactivation of dormant herpes simplex virus in the geniculate ganglion,[20-22] and reactivation of herpes zoster is called *herpes zoster oticus* or Ramsey Hunt syndrome. Both may be preceded by periauricular pain, dysgeusia, and the perception of facial numbness, although the latter is further characterized by vestibular symptoms and a vesicular outbreak on the pinna or in the external auditory canal or tympanic membrane. Occasionally, vesicles will be absent despite severe pain and vestibular symptoms; this condition is called *zoster sine herpete.*

The early treatment of viral facial paralysis involves oral corticosteroids and antiviral agents, although some controversy remains regarding the efficacy of the latter.[23-25] Meticulous eye care, with drops, ointment, and nightly eye taping, is critical for corneal protection; and it appears that early facial nerve decompression may lead to improved outcomes for patients with Bell's palsy, with electroneuronography results showing less than 10% compound action potential amplitudes and no voluntary motor units on needle EMG examination on the affected side within 12 days of the onset of the weakness.[26]

LYME-ASSOCIATED PARALYSIS

Lyme-associated facial paralysis, resulting from neuroborreliosis, is a rapid onset weakness involving all branches, and may involve both sides of the face. It predictably occurs in conjunction with other symptoms of Lyme disease, such as headache, arthralgias, rash, fatigue, and fevers. Although the mechanism is not well understood, it is treated with antibiotics against *Borrelia burgdorferi,* and tends to recover in a pattern similar to viral facial paralysis.

TEMPORAL BONE FRACTURES

Blunt head trauma may result in fracture of the temporal bone, either longitudinal or transverse, depending on the orientation of the force with respect to the long axis of the temporal bone (Fig. 43-8). Transverse fractures are associated with complete sensorineural hearing loss and a 50% likelihood of yielding facial paralysis, whereas longitudinal fractures carry a 15% incidence of facial paralysis. When the facial nerve is damaged, most often the fracture impinges on its labyrinthine and perigeniculate segment. Generally, a patient presenting with a temporal bone fracture and immediate onset facial paralysis warrants exploration as soon as medically feasible, whereas in cases of delayed onset facial paralysis, observation with an expectation of spontaneous improvement is warranted.[27]

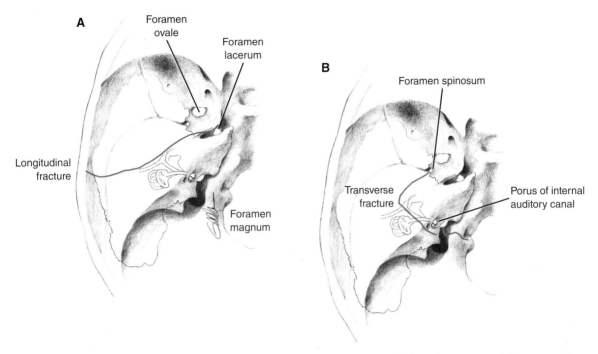

Fig. 43-8   Axial view of the temporal bone demonstrating longitudinal (**A**) and transverse (**B**) temporal bone fractures. Red lines depict the course of the fracture lines.

Table 43-1   Sunderland Classification of Nerve Injury

Sunderland	Injury	Neurosensory Impairment
I (Neuropraxia)	Intrafascicular edema, conduction block, possible segmental demyelination	Neuritis Paresthesia
II (Axonotmesis)	Axons severed, endoneurial tube intact	Paresthesia Episodic dysesthesia
III (Axonotmesis)	Endoneurial tube torn	Paresthesia, dysesthesia
IV (Axonotmesis)	Only epineurium intact	Hypoesthesia, dysesthesia, neuroma formation
V (Neurotmesis)	Loss of continuity	Anesthetic, intractable pain, neuroma formation

Data from Sunderland S. A classification of peripheral nerve injuries producing loss of function. Brain 74:491-516, 1951.

POSTSURGICAL PARALYSIS

Postoperative iatrogenic facial weakness arises unexpectedly from skull base surgery, otologic surgery, parotid surgery, mandibular surgery, and facial plastic surgery.[28,29] When weakness occurs, the anatomic status of the nerve is either known (intact, discontinuous without repair or grafting, or discontinuous but repaired or grafted), or unknown. If the status is unknown, the Sunderland nerve injury classification system becomes relevant (Table 43-1). This scale describes the degree of injury based on level of anatomic

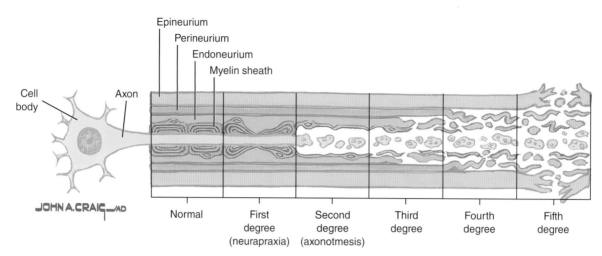

Classification of nerve injury by degree of involvement of various neural layers

Fig. 43-9　Five degrees of nerve injury as described by Sunderland. (Netter medical illustration, used with permission of Elsevier. All rights reserved.)

disruption (Fig. 43-9); levels I-III ordinarily enjoy a meaningful degree of spontaneous recovery, although levels IV and V generally yield poorer outcomes than that expected through excising the damaged area and repairing or cable grafting the area. Electroneuronography (EnOG) can only distinguish level I from all other levels, thus unless testing reveals level I injury (establishing continuity and portending a good prognosis), the data may not help in clinical decision-making regarding exploring the facial nerve after potential injury. Generally, if the facial nerve was not directly visualized during an operation that results in persistent postoperative paralysis, direct surgical exploration is warranted unless neurapraxia is established by EnOG.[29] If a transection is identified, a tensionless primary epineurial repair is executed (Fig. 43-10), or if necessary, a cable graft repair is performed (Fig. 43-11). If neural repair is executed within several months of injury, acceptable functional recovery is expected.

TUMORS

Benign facial nerve tumors give rise to characteristic patterns of facial weakness. Patients may report Bell's palsy-type episodes, which are recurrent on a single side, with each episode resulting in potentially more severe sequelae. When carefully examined between episodes, these patients usually demonstrate elements of facial flaccidity mixed with elements of hypertonicity, synkinesis, and spasm; a mixed picture suggests a benign facial nerve tumor (Fig. 43-12). Alternatively, patients may report gradual onset facial weakness over several years to decades, without evidence of malignancy, and often with negative radiographic and neurologic workups. High-resolution temporal bone CT or MRI scans generally reveal a facial nerve schwannoma or geniculate ganglion hemangioma (a misnomer for an osseous vascular malformation arising in the vicinity of the geniculate ganglion) (Fig. 43-13). Treatment involves possible facial nerve decompression,[30] and tumor resection only when hearing is endangered or when facial function has declined to the point that equivalent results could be expected through cable grafting.

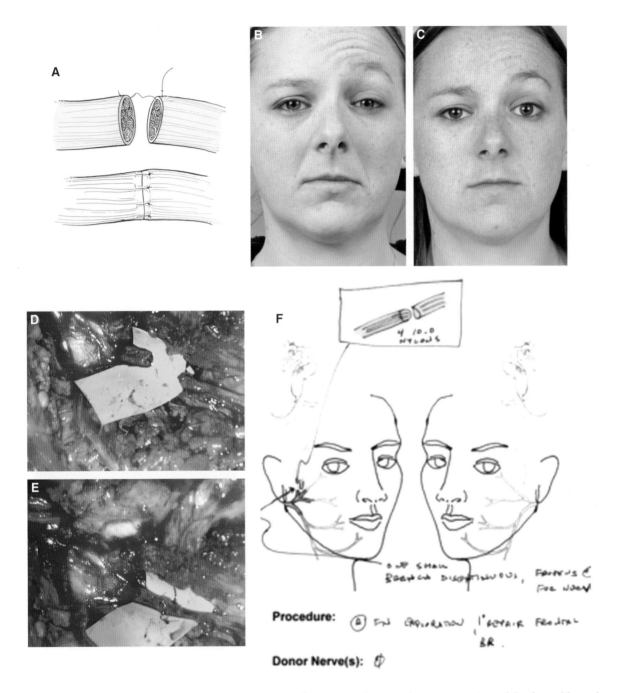

Fig. 43-10   Epineurial repair technique. **A,** Epineurial repair. **B,** Case involving transection of the frontal branch of the facial nerve. Preexploration view, showing lack of brow elevation during attempts at brow raising. **C,** Patient at 4 months after surgery, demonstrating the return of mild brow elevation. **D** and **E,** Intraoperative view showing two nerve endings with precoaptation and postcoaptation. **F,** Drawing of epineurial repair.

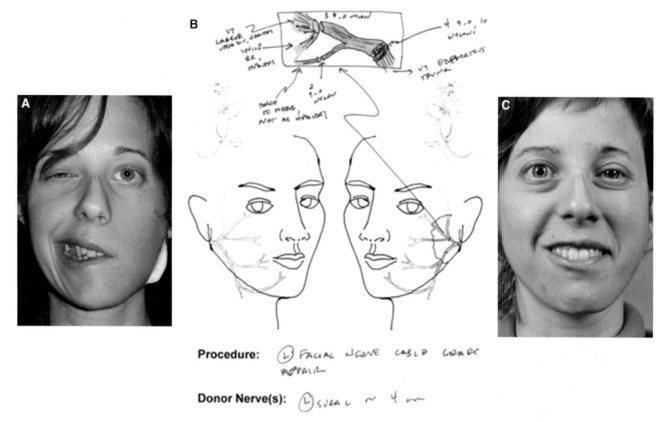

Procedure: ⓛ FACIAL NERVE CABLE GRAFT REPAIR

Donor Nerve(s): ⓛ SURAL ~ 4 cm

Fig. 43-11   Results of cable graft repair of a complete facial nerve transection injury. **A,** Preoperative smile after iatrogenic facial nerve transection during mandibular ramus fracture reduction. **B,** Drawing of graft placement and details. **C,** Final result after 10 months, with patient showing excellent tone and meaningful smile, but significant ocular synkinesis.

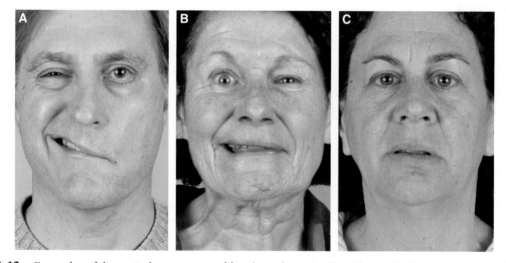

Fig. 43-12   Examples of the typical appearance of facial paralysis. **A,** Flaccid state. **B,** Hypertonic state. **C,** Mixed picture on the left side, with a widened palpebral fissure, hyperprominent nasolabial fold, and platysmal banding.

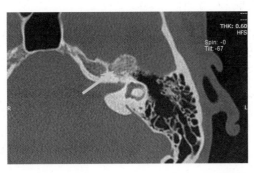

Fig. 43-13   Axial CT scan demonstrating a geniculate ganglion hemangioma *(arrow)*.

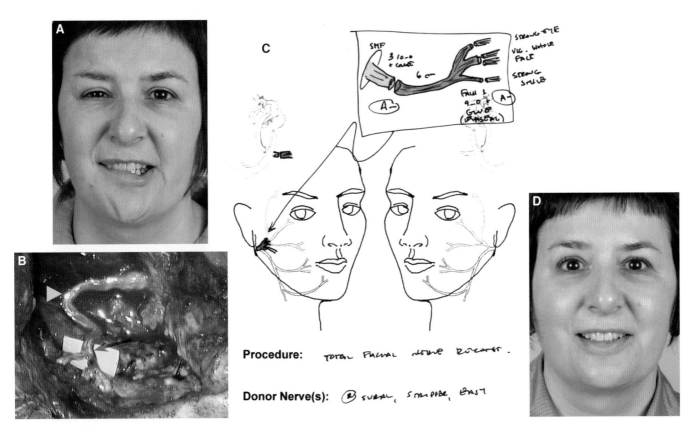

Fig. 43-14   Example of intentional total facial nerve sacrifice with cable grafting, for malignancy extirpation. **A,** Preoperative normal smile. **B,** Sural nerve cable graft *(yellow arrowhead),* with interfascicular dissection to accommodate four distal neurorrhaphies *(green arrow).* **C,** Drawing of graft placement and details. **D,** Patient's smile 6 months after surgery.

Malignant tumors yield facial paralysis by direct invasion, with certain malignancies possessing exceptionally high neurotrophic tendencies, including adenoid cystic carcinomas and metastatic squamous cell carcinomas from cutaneous lesions. The clinical presentation is classically described as slow onset facial paralysis, progressing insidiously over weeks to months, and accompanied by dull and progressing pain. Very rarely, acute facial paralysis that does not recover spontaneously is attributed to malignancy.[31] Treatment involves malignancy extirpation, with cable graft reconstruction of the nerve if clean margins are obtained proximally and distally (Figs. 43-14 and 43-15). Most commonly, the sural or great auricular

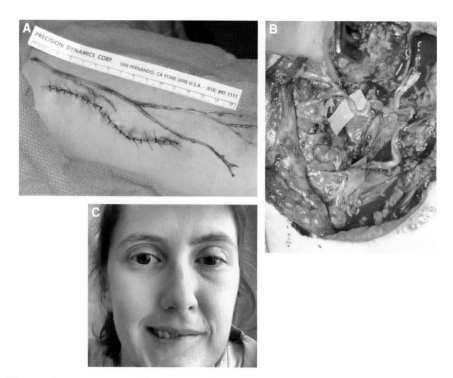

Fig. 43-15   The patient is a 33-year-old woman with biopsy-proven mucoepidermoid carcinoma of the left parotid gland with perineural invasion. **A,** Nerve harvested in the upper arm. **B,** Inset with proximal coaptation at the geniculate ganglion, and four distal coaptation sites *(arrows)*. **C,** Patient's smile 10 months after surgery. Note meaningful smile but significant ocular synkinesis.

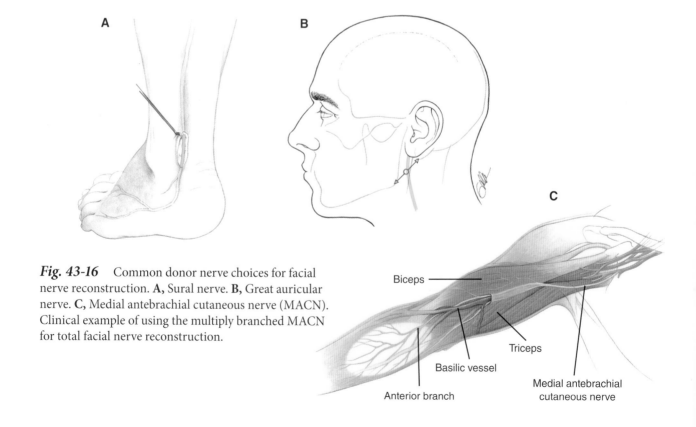

Fig. 43-16   Common donor nerve choices for facial nerve reconstruction. **A,** Sural nerve. **B,** Great auricular nerve. **C,** Medial antebrachial cutaneous nerve (MACN). Clinical example of using the multiply branched MACN for total facial nerve reconstruction.

Biceps

Triceps

Basilic vessel

Anterior branch

Medial antebrachial cutaneous nerve

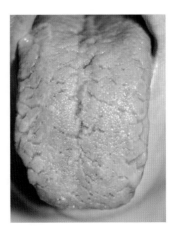

Fig. 43-17   Tongue fissuring in Melkersson-Rosenthal syndrome.

nerve is used as a donor, although the medial antebrachial cutaneous nerve is a multiply branched donor nerve harvested with minimal morbidity, which permits total facial nerve replacement from skull base to multiple distal branches (Fig. 43-16). Some surgeons advocate grafting even in the absence of clean margins,[32] and most agree that postoperative radiotherapy does not preclude cable grafting in these settings.[33]

OTHER CAUSES OF FACIAL WEAKNESS

Although the list of causes of facial paralysis is exhaustive, several conditions warrant special mention. Melkersson-Rosenthal syndrome is a condition characterized by recurrent facial paralysis, which may alternate sides. Patients with this syndrome report noninflammatory facial edema and congenital tongue fissuring (Fig. 43-17). Surgical nerve decompression is indicated to prevent end-stage synkinesis. Deposition diseases (sarcoidosis, amyloidosis) may affect facial nerve function, acute otitis media, malignant otitis externa, cholesteatoma, multiple sclerosis, and other systemic neurologic and neuromuscular conditions. Underlying conditions must be identified and treated as part of a comprehensive plan to improve facial function outcomes.

CLASSIFICATION

Facial paralysis may be considered in terms of whether it is flaccid, hypertonic/synkinetic, or mixed, and by the function of each facial zone. For several decades, the House-Brackmann scale (Table 43-2) has been widely used to describe facial function in many different clinical situations, although its original purpose was specifically to describe facial recovery after vestibular schwannoma treatment.[34] Because the scale lacks both zonal information and the ability to quantify synkinesis, it was recently modified to address these shortcomings.[35] Several automated assessments of facial function and programs are emerging in the facial reanimation literature that offer quantitative assessment of digital photographs and video clips,

Table 43-2   House-Brackmann Facial Nerve Recovery Scale

Grade	Description	Characteristics
I	Normal	Normal facial function in all areas
II	Mild dysfunction	Slight weakness noticeable on close inspection; may have very slight synkinesis
III	Moderate dysfunction	Obvious, but not disfiguring, difference between 2 sides; noticeable, but not severe, synkinesis, contracture, or hemifacial spasm; complete eye closure with effort
IV	Moderately severe dysfunction	Obvious weakness or disfiguring asymmetry; normal symmetry and tone at rest; incomplete eye closure
V	Severe dysfunction	Only barely perceptible motion; asymmetry at rest
VI	Total paralysis	No movement

Data from House JW, Brackmann DE. Facial nerve grading system. Otolaryngol Head Neck Surg 93:146-147, 1985.

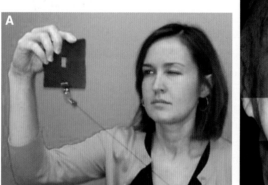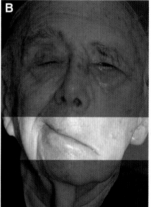

Fig. 43-18   Meticulous zonal assessment of the facial nerve. **A,** Clinician examines the patient through a view-finder, permitting square or rectangular view of each facial zone in isolation. **B,** Photograph with all but the perioral zone greyed out, analogous to the view through the viewfinder.

so that comparative assessments may be made of outcome after recovery and intervention.[36-39] A facial nerve-specific quality of life instrument has been developed and popularized to gauge the effect of different interventions on quality of life in this population.[37-40]

A rigorous zonal approach to facial function analysis is critical to developing an appropriate individualized treatment plan (Fig. 43-18). Patients must undergo photography of the eight standard expressions (Fig. 43-19), videography, and have documented recordings of the resting position and movement of facial landmarks on a worksheet (Fig. 43-20). To isolate the function of each facial zone, the clinician may examine the face through a viewfinder that excludes the healthy side of the face and the other facial zones during formal assessment (see Fig. 43-18, *B*). Once the clinician has developed a good understanding of the static and dynamic issues in each zone, and the likelihood of spontaneous change, a comprehensive treatment algorithm may be generated.

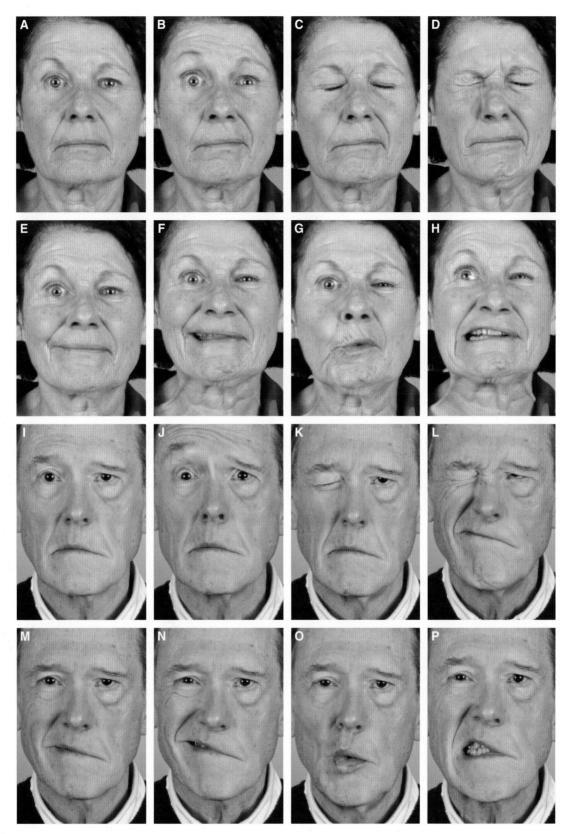

Fig. 43-19   Examples of the eight standard views in facial paralysis, illustrating the difference between the frozen, hypertonic state **(A-H),** and the flaccid state **(I-P).** *From left to right:* At rest, brows elevated, gentle eye closure, tight eye closure, small smile, large smile, saying "oo," and saying "ee."

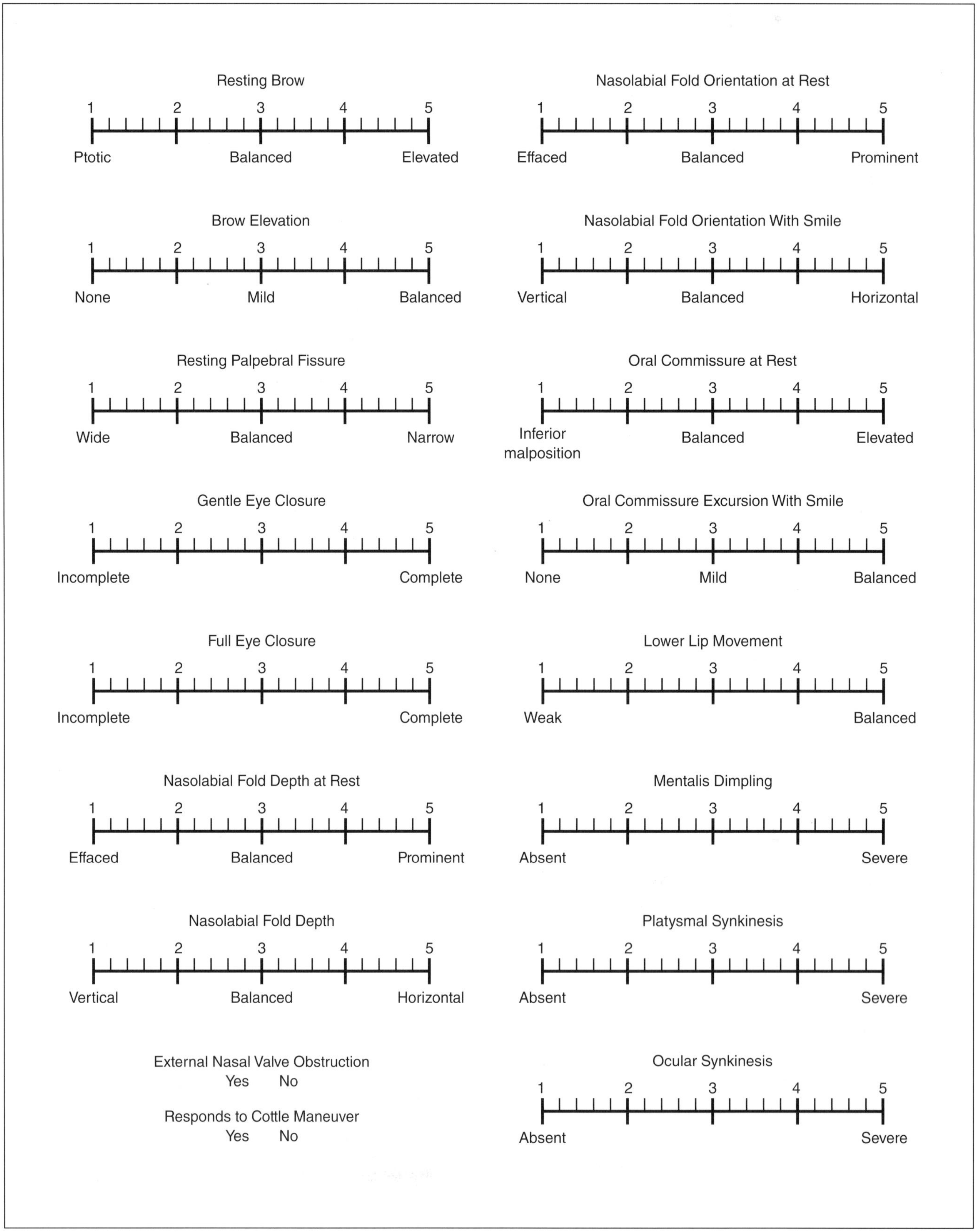

Resting Brow

```
1        2        3        4        5
```
Ptotic   Balanced   Elevated

Nasolabial Fold Orientation at Rest

```
1        2        3        4        5
```
Effaced   Balanced   Prominent

Brow Elevation

```
1        2        3        4        5
```
None   Mild   Balanced

Nasolabial Fold Orientation With Smile

```
1        2        3        4        5
```
Vertical   Balanced   Horizontal

Resting Palpebral Fissure

```
1        2        3        4        5
```
Wide   Balanced   Narrow

Oral Commissure at Rest

```
1        2        3        4        5
```
Inferior   Balanced   Elevated
malposition

Gentle Eye Closure

```
1        2        3        4        5
```
Incomplete   Complete

Oral Commissure Excursion With Smile

```
1        2        3        4        5
```
None   Mild   Balanced

Full Eye Closure

```
1        2        3        4        5
```
Incomplete   Complete

Lower Lip Movement

```
1        2        3        4        5
```
Weak   Balanced

Nasolabial Fold Depth at Rest

```
1        2        3        4        5
```
Effaced   Balanced   Prominent

Mentalis Dimpling

```
1        2        3        4        5
```
Absent   Severe

Nasolabial Fold Depth

```
1        2        3        4        5
```
Vertical   Balanced   Horizontal

Platysmal Synkinesis

```
1        2        3        4        5
```
Absent   Severe

External Nasal Valve Obstruction
Yes   No

Responds to Cottle Maneuver
Yes   No

Ocular Synkinesis

```
1        2        3        4        5
```
Absent   Severe

Fig. 43-20   Standard worksheet for assessing the facial zones in facial paralysis, which encourages documentation of facial landmarks both at rest and with volitional movements.

ZONE-BASED SURGERY FOR THE PARALYZED FACE

BROW PTOSIS CORRECTION

For brow ptosis correction, surgery is most often performed in the office setting. The brow may be secured into appropriate anatomic position with a subperiosteal dissection followed by soft tissue fixation using biodegradable polymeric devices (Fig. 43-21), or by use of suture-bearing bone pins. Direct brow lifting, midforehead brow lifting, and suture-based techniques are also reasonable options (Fig. 43-22).

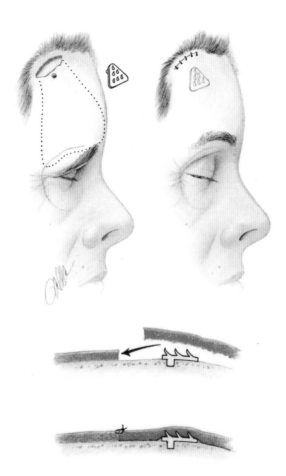

Fig. 43-21   Brow ptosis correction. *Top:* Note an elliptical incision at or behind the hairline, with subperiosteal dissection indicated by the dotted lines, with subsequent elevation of the brow secured by polymer device. *Bottom:* The subcutaneous and dermal tissues are pressed onto the tines of the polymer device to secure the brow at the appropriate height. Note the device is secured to the calvarium through hand drilling of a well into the bone.

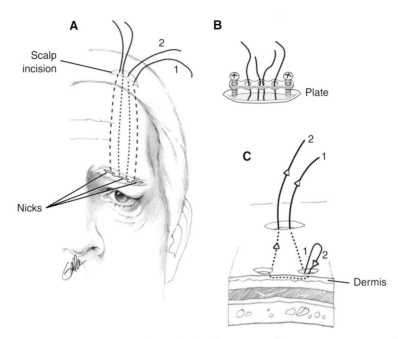

Fig. 43-22   "Power" brow lifting. **A,** Three nicks in the hair-bearing eyebrow permit passage of two 2-0 monofilament sutures subdermally from the brow to the hairline incision, each in loop fashion. **B,** Sutures are secured to a reconstruction plate. **C,** Passage of the suture from one nick subdermally to the adjacent nick, permitting reorientation of the long straight needle for passage superiorly out the hairline incision.

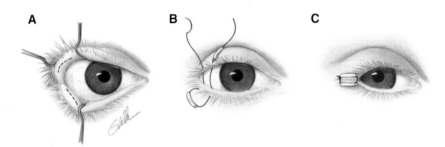

Fig. 43-23   Tarsorrhaphy. **A,** Area to be denuded. **B,** Suture passed over thin tubing. **C,** Final inset of suture. Note good apposition of the denuded areas.

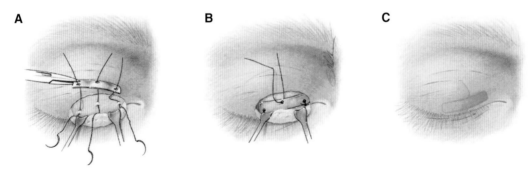

Fig. 43-24   Eyelid weight placement. **A** and **B,** Incision in supratarsal crease, with exposure of superficial surface of tarsal plate. Sutures penetrate partial-thickness through the tarsal plate and are secured to predrilled holes in the eyelid weight. **C,** Inset of the weight, with the inferior edge parallel to and 2 mm above the free lid margin.

SURGERY FOR THE FLACCID UPPER EYELID

Eyelid weighting techniques, eyelid spring placement, and tarsorrhaphy are all approaches to the paralyzed eye. The most predictable of these approaches is tarsorrhaphy (Fig. 43-23), which is extremely effective at protecting the cornea, but yields the least favorable aesthetic result. Preservation of the native lateral canthus is critical to prevent permanent rounding of the canthus on tarsorrhaphy takedown.

Placement of a gold or platinum weight is extremely useful in the treatment of lagophthalmos (Fig. 43-24). The thin profile platinum weight is thinner compared with gold, because of its higher density, and possesses a more favorable hypoallergenic profile. The procedure is performed under local anesthesia. An incision is made in the supratarsal crease, and a plane is developed deep to the orbicularis oculi, exposing the superficial surface of the tarsal plate. The implant is centered between the pupil and the medial limbus, and secured to the tarsal plate with 6-0 clear nylon sutures. In cases of spontaneous recovery, the eyelid weight may be easily removed.

Eyelid spring implantation involves placing a magnetized thin-wire implant into the upper lid. Although the procedure was designed to achieve a more natural blink, it carries a high revision rate (nearly 100%), and thus lacks the reliability of eyelid weighting.

SURGERY FOR THE FLACCID LOWER EYELID

The paralyzed lower lid may be repositioned using a tarsal strip procedure, in which a canthotomy and cantholysis are performed, and a small segment of the lateral tarsus is removed. The tarsus is then deepithelialized and secured to the lateral orbital rim to tighten the lower lid (Fig. 43-25); although recurrent laxity and lateralization of the lacrimal punctum may occur. Alternative approaches include placement of an autologous sling (Fig. 43-26) from the nasal bone medially, through the lower eyelid, to the superolateral orbital rim. Fascia lata harvested from the thigh is fashioned into a thin strip, secured to the nasal bone with a single bone anchor, and tunneled subcutaneously with a fascia needle. An incision is made in the lateral brow, exposing the superolateral orbital rim, and a hole is drilled in the lateral orbital rim through which a suture attached to the fascia lata is secured. Tension on the lower lid can be precisely set to achieve the appropriate height.

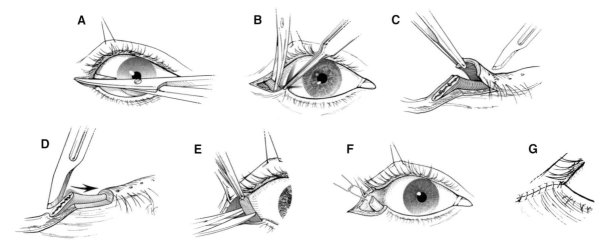

Fig. 43-25   Lower lid elevation in the paralyzed eye. **A,** Canthotomy. **B,** Inferior cantholysis. **C,** Denuding the gray line. **D,** Sharp deepithelialization of the conjunctival covering of the tarsal plate. **E,** Amputation of a segment of the tarsal plate. **F,** Suture resuspension of the tarsal plate to the periosteum of the superolateral orbital rim. **G,** Final closure.

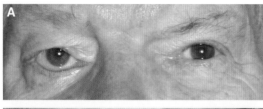

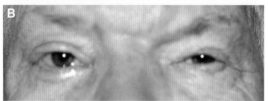

Fig. 43-26   Example of result after fascia lata resuspension of the lower eyelid. **A,** Preoperative view. **B,** View one year postoperatively, with excellent medial canthal position maintained.

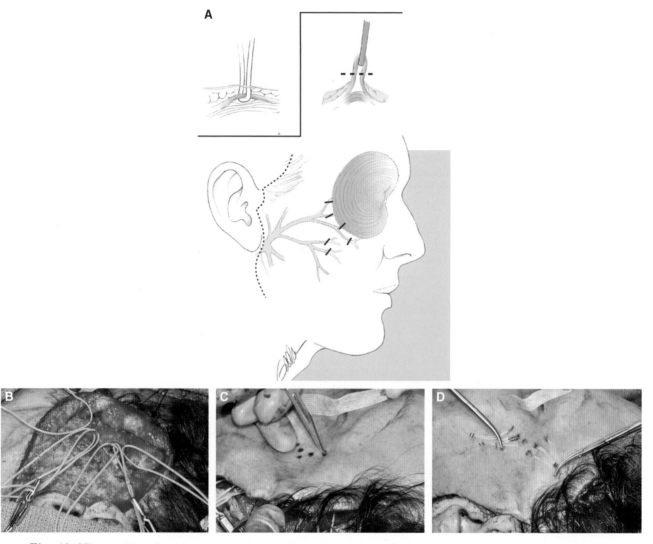

Fig. 43-27   Highly selective neurectomy procedure. **A,** Location of ocular branches and their intact delivery through the skin using vessel loops. **B-D,** Operative views demonstrating tagged ocular branches and their delivery through the skin with small stabs made with a No. 11 blade.

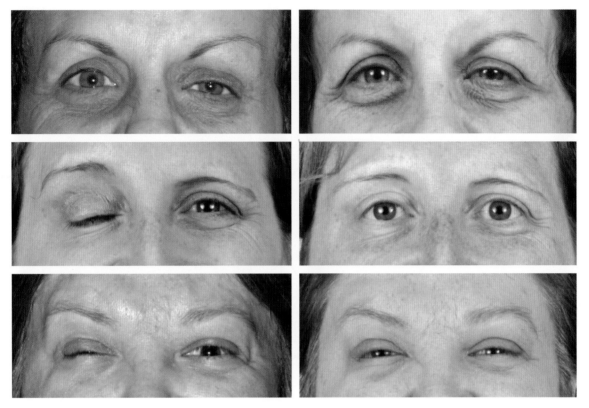

Fig. 43-28   Results after highly selective neurectomy. *Left column:* Preoperative views of three different patients, with significant eye closure during smiling. *Right column:* Long-term result with smiling, showing maintenance of balanced palpebral fissure width with smiling.

SURGERY FOR REFRACTORY SYNKINESIS

When patients become refractory to chemodenervation for ocular synkinesis treatment (see later section on adjunctive procedures), permanent orbicularis oculi partial denervation may be performed through a two-step, highly selective neurectomy (Fig. 43-27).

During the first step, facial nerve branches are identified through a preauricular incision that continues along the parotideomasseteric fascia to the anterior border of the gland. Using a nerve stimulator, branches innervating the orbicularis oculi are isolated with vessel loops and delivered in continuity through the skin, through stab incisions oriented parallel to the relaxed skin tension lines. The preauricular incision is closed and the patient awakened from anesthesia. In the second step, performed the same day in the clinic setting, the patient repeatedly smiles on command, and each nerve branch is divided in turn, until there is a suitable decrease in synkinetic closure of the eye during smiling, without lagophthalmos (Fig. 43-28). The remaining branches are released into the wound, in continuity.

NASAL BASE CORRECTION

External nasal valve collapse may be corrected using a static fascia lata sling technique.[41] Fascia lata is harvested from the lateral thigh and tunneled subcutaneously from a temporal and preauricular incision to an incision in the alar crease. The fascia is secured medially to the nasal ala, and laterally to the temporalis fascia (Fig. 43-29). Additional lower lateral cartilage batten grafting may help in cases of persistent valve collapse caused by lower lateral cartilage incompetence during inspiration.

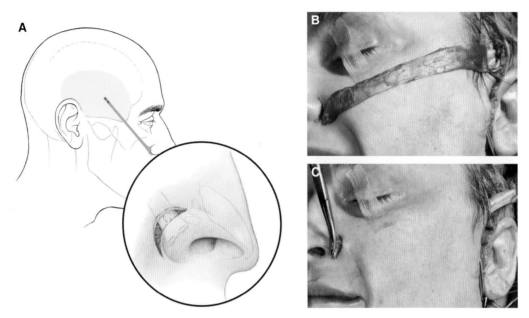

Fig. 43-29   External nasal valve suspension in the paralyzed face. **A,** Placement of the fascia lata onto the accessory cartilages of the ala through an alar crease incision. **B** and **C,** Intraoperative view of fascia lata placement through a subcutaneous tunnel. Note the alar crease incision and the preauricular incision.

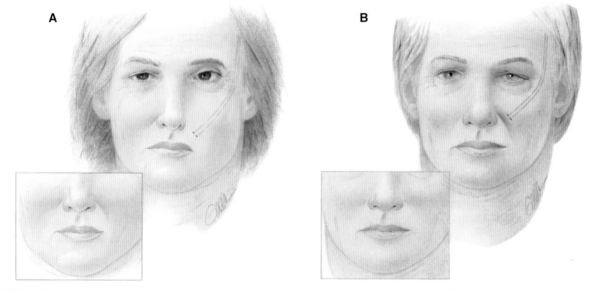

Fig. 43-30   Nasolabial fold modifications. **A,** Technique of introducing a nasolabial fold. Note the lack of a nasolabial fold on the left, and the position of the nicks required for passage of the sutures. The location of the incisions for passage of the sutures is *medial* to the desired position of the neonasolabial fold. Inset shows postoperative result. **B,** Technique of effacement of a hyperprominent nasolabial fold. Note midfacial hypertonicity and hyperprominence of the nasolabial fold on the left. The location of the incisions for passage of the sutures is *lateral* to the nasolabial fold, as it would be in cosmetic midface lifting. Inset illustrates expected result.

ADJUSTING THE NASOLABIAL FOLD

Nasolabial fold (NLF) abnormalities are addressed according to whether there is flaccid or hypertonic facial paralysis. Suture suspension techniques analogous to those used during face lifting[42] are placed either medial to the fold (to define an effaced NLF), or lateral to the fold (to soften a hyperprominent NLF)[43] (Fig. 43-30).

SURGERY FOR SMILE RESTORATION

Restoration of the smile is one of the most important goals of the facial reanimation surgeon. Options for smile reanimation include static suspension or muscle transfer for dynamic reanimation. Static suspension is usually reserved for patients with a poor prognosis, the very elderly, or patients who report dynamic reanimation failures. Regional muscle options include the temporalis, masseter, and digastric muscles, although nearly all reanimation surgeons have abandoned masseter muscle transfer because of its unfavorable vector pull and its characteristic facial contour deficit. The temporalis muscle remains popular because of its surgical simplicity, fan-shaped vascular and muscular architecture, and low morbidity (Fig. 43-31).

TEMPORALIS TRANSFER

The procedure is performed through an incision extending from the preauricular area to the attachment point of the lobule, and may extend several centimeters below the angle of the mandible. Temporalis transposition procedures involve elevating a temporoparietal fascia flap (TPFF) from the muscular fascia of the temporalis muscle, on its vascular pedicle, and rotating it posteriorly to expose the underlying muscle. A 1.5 cm strip of temporalis muscle is elevated off the calvarium to the level of the zygomatic arch, reflected over the arch, and secured to the modiolus (Fig. 43-32). Orthodromic temporalis transfer, which has be-

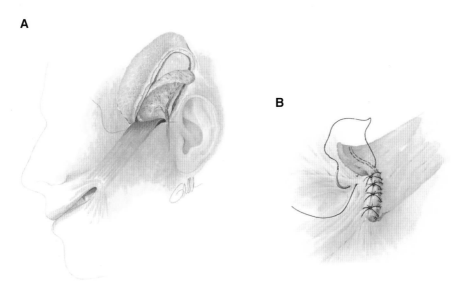

Fig. 43-31   **A,** Temporalis muscle transposition. **B,** Coaptation of the edge of the temporalis muscle to the lateral border of the orbicularis oris, at the modiolus.

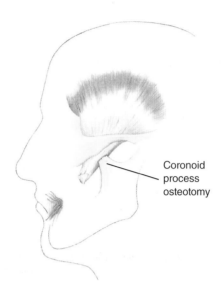

Coronoid
process
osteotomy

Fig. 43-32   Temporalis tendon transfer technique. The temporalis tendon is transferred to the modiolus.

come more popular in the past decade, involves exposing the temporalis tendon as it attaches to the coronoid process, removing it from the bone, and securing it to the modiolus (Fig. 43-32). This procedure may be performed through a lateral incision, a nasolabial crease incision, or intraorally.

Potential pitfalls that may arise after temporalis transposition include a muscular prominence overlying the zygomatic arch, excess midfacial bulk, hollowing and/or alopecia in the temporalis fossa, and inadequate excursion of the transferred muscle. These issues may be avoided with meticulous surgical technique and precise inset of the TPFF to obliterate the donor site deficit. Edentulous patients who are likely to have disuse atrophy of the muscle and patients with preoperative wasting or trigeminal dysfunction are not good surgical candidates.

FREE MUSCLE TRANSFER

Patients under 70 years of age, in whom life expectancy is reasonable, are appropriate candidates for free muscle transfer. A critical advantage of this approach over regional muscle is that when it is driven by a cross face nerve graft, it leads to both a voluntary and an involuntary, emotive smile, and excursion is often greater than that seen using temporalis transfer. Because microvascular anastomoses are required, patients with vascular disease or other significant comorbidities may not be appropriate candidates. Free muscle may also be driven by the ipsilateral motor branch to the masseter muscle in a single-stage operation; this approach results in higher success rates and greater excursion, but does not provide a completely involuntary, emotionally driven smile.

FIRST-STAGE CROSS-FACE NERVE GRAFTING

A preauricular incision is made on the nonparalyzed side of the face, and a skin flap is raised on the parotideomasseteric fascia until the masseter fascia is reached. Dissection within the fascia isolates several facial nerve branches; the branches yielding isolated smile movement are selected as the donor branches and transected sharply (Fig. 43-33). The sural nerve is harvested from the leg, secured to the donor facial nerve branches, and tunneled subcutaneously across the upper lip to the gingivobuccal sulcus on the paralyzed side, where the tip is marked with a 4-0 nylon suture and banked for later exposure (Fig. 43-34, *A*).

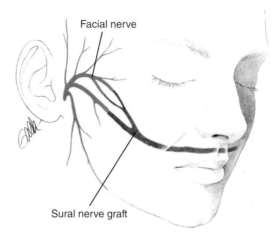

Facial nerve

Sural nerve graft

Fig. 43-33   First-stage cross-face nerve grafting. Facial nerve branches *(orange)* yielding isolated smile are transected and coapted to the sural nerve *(purple),* which travels subcutaneously in the lip to the paralyzed gingivobuccal sulcus.

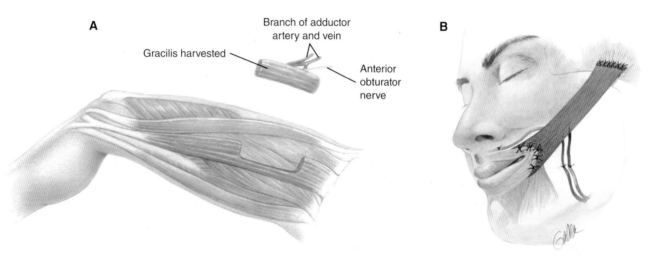

A

Gracilis harvested

Branch of adductor artery and vein

Anterior obturator nerve

B

Fig. 43-34   Free gracilis muscle transfer. **A,** Donor segment harvested from the medial thigh. **B,** Inset from the modiolus to the temporalis fascia. Note facial vessel anastomoses to the pedicle and neurorrhaphy to the tip of the sural nerve graft in the upper lip.

Axon growth across the graft is followed clinically by tapping on the graft (Tinel's sign); tingling in the zygomaticus muscle groups on the donor side indicates the presence of regenerating axons. Second-stage free muscle transfer takes place 6 to 9 months later.

FREE MUSCLE TRANSFER

The gracilis muscle was the first muscle used in successful facial reanimation[44] and remains the most popular choice for this purpose, although pectoralis minor and latissimus dorsi are favored by some centers.[45-47] The muscle is harvested from the medial aspect of the thigh through an incision 1.5 cm posterior and parallel to a line connecting the pubic tubercle and the medial tibial condyle (Fig. 43-35, *A*). The belly of the gracilis muscle is identified by locating the neurovascular pedicle entering its deep surface, 8 to 10 cm distal to the pubic tubercle. The obturator nerve is identified immediately proximal to the vascular pedicle and similarly traced, and the flap is harvested by removing approximately 40% of its width. For inset, a preauricular incision is extended below the mandible, and a thick skin flap is raised, extending medially to expose the orbicularis oris (Fig. 43-35, *B*). In the two-stage procedure, the stump of the cross face nerve graft is identified in the gingivobuccal sulcus, whereas in the single-stage procedure the masseteric nerve is identified by dissecting through the masseter muscle to its deep surface. The gracilis muscle is secured to the modiolus, stretched to its resting length, and secured to the temporalis fascia, taking into account the patient's smile vector. The microvascular anastomoses and the neurorrhaphy are performed and the incisions are closed over a Penrose drain. Movement is expected 3 to 6 months after transfer of a trigemi-nally driven muscle (Fig. 43-35), and 8 to 10 months after the two-stage muscle transfer (Fig. 43-36). Draw-backs include an 8% to 30% failure rate, excessive facial bulk, incorrect vector pull, and coactivation of the transferred muscle with chewing. Lack of excursion constitutes failure, and is thought to result from in-adequate ingrowth of the donor nerve fibers into the transferred muscle. Less commonly, microvascular failure or improper resting tension of the muscle may result in an unsatisfactory outcome.

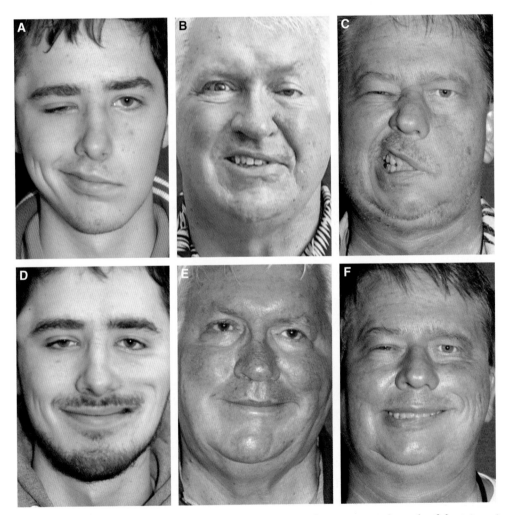

Fig. 43-35   Typical results after one-stage gracilis transfer using the masseteric branch of the trigeminal nerve. **A-C,** Preoperative smiles. **D-F,** Postoperative smiles.

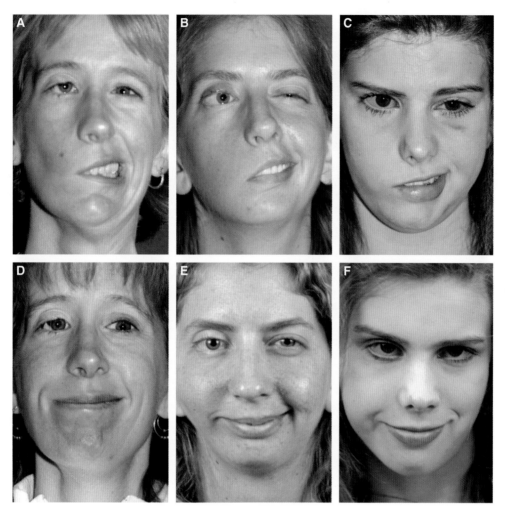

Fig. 43-36   Typical results after two-stage gracilis transfer using a cross face nerve graft. **A-C,** Preoperative smiles. **D-F,** Postoperative smiles.

Lip and Neck Surgery

In facial movement disorders, the lower lip is most commonly superiorly malpositioned, based on lack of depressor labii inferioris function. Lower lip malposition may be managed by camouflaging the asymmetry using contralateral lower lip weakening techniques, including chemodenervation with botulinum toxin and transection of fibers of the contralateral depressor labii inferioris[48] (Fig. 43-37). This procedure is performed under local anesthesia in the office setting, through a 1 cm incision in the lip mucosa and exposure and removal of a segment of the belly of the depressor labii inferioris. Dynamic reanimation to the affected lower lip has been described, using digastric muscle transfer (Fig. 43-38) and platysma transfer to the lower lip,[49] although the high success rate of contralateral lower lip weakening has diminished the focus on dynamic lower lip techniques.

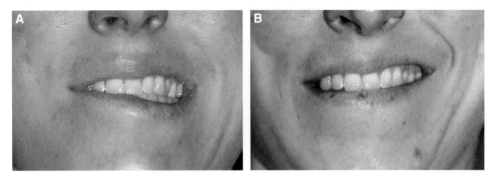

Fig. 43-37   Example of a depressor labii inferioris resection. **A,** Preoperative view, with superior malposition of the right lower lip. **B,** Postoperative view, demonstrating symmetry of lower lip position.

Fig. 43-38   Transfer of the anterior belly of the digastric muscle to introduce movement to the lower lip.

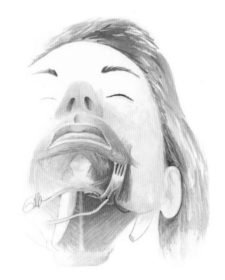

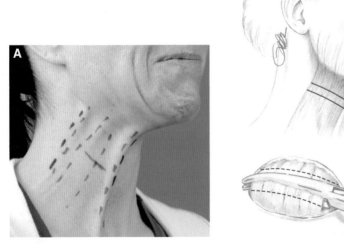

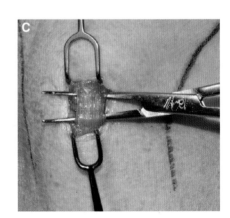

Fig. 43-39   Platysmectomy. **A,** Preoperative view showing extensive platysmal synkinesis. **B,** Location of the strip of muscle to be excised. **C,** Delivery of platysma through incision for removal.

Platysmal synkinesis is eliminated either using botulinum toxin, or through office-based platysmectomy,[50] which involves exposing the fibers of the muscle through a natural skin crease, and removing a 1 cm strip of the muscle to detach the superior from the inferior segments (Fig. 43-39).

ADJUNCTIVE PROCEDURES

The mainstays of adjunctive therapy in facial movement disorders include botulinum toxin administration and focused facial nerve physical therapy. Botulinum toxin is useful in the hypertonic, synkinetic face to prevent involuntary motion, particularly in the orbicularis oculi, the mentalis, and the platysma muscle (Fig. 43-40).

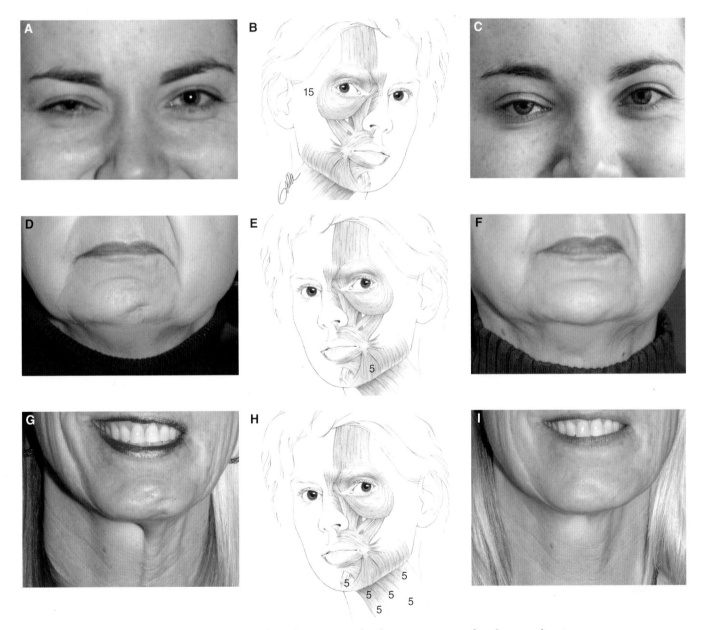

Fig. 43-40   Examples of the utility of botulinum toxin for the management of synkinesis, showing pretreatment state, injection map with number of units administered, and postchemodenervation view. **A-C,** Ocular synkinesis with smiling. **D-F,** Mentalis dimpling. **G-I,** Platysmal synkinesis.

In the contralateral healthy face, toxin administration is extremely effective in the brow and lower lip regions to establish improved facial balance (Fig. 43-41). The toxin may also be administered into the lacrimal gland as an antiautonomic agent to eliminate the syndrome of crocodile tears (Bogorad's syndrome), and to treat hypertonicity in a successfully innervated gracilis muscle if it cocontracts with chewing.

The four tenets of a comprehensive physical therapy program include patient education, soft tissue massage, neuromuscular retraining, and biofeedback.[51-54] Emphasis is placed on controlling the compensatory hyperactivity of the contralateral facial musculature, deliberately controlling synkinetic movement, and preventing the symptoms of facial fatigue (Fig. 43-42). Specific protocols assist in optimizing function after muscle transfer and in partial congenital cases, whose function falls in the gray zone between requiring facial reanimation surgery and avoiding it.

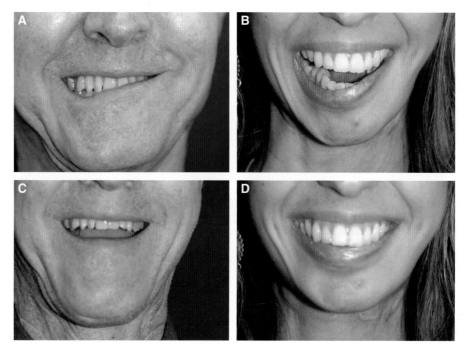

Fig. 43-41   Management of lower lip asymmetry by contralateral botulinum toxin administration. **A** and **B,** Predenervation. **C** and **D,** Postdenervation.

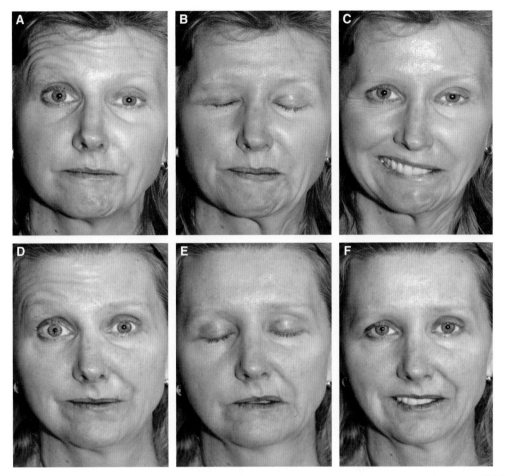

Fig. 43-42   Example of the effectiveness of physical therapy for facial synkinesis. **A-C,** Pretreatment. **D-F,** Post-physical therapy. Note improvements in balance in the brow *(left),* neck *(middle),* and smile *(right).*

SPECIAL CIRCUMSTANCES

Bilateral Facial Paralysis

The causes of bilateral facial paralysis are listed in Box 43-2. After posterior fossa surgery, cavernous brainstem hemangioma bleeding or surgery, brainstem stroke, or amyloidosis, bilateral paralysis is typically flaccid. Patients report lower lip flaccidity with oral incompetence, drooling, articulation difficulties, and masked facies. After bilateral synkinetic recovery from paralysis related to viral insults (HIV related), Guillain-Barré syndrome, Lyme disease, and Melkersson-Rosenthal syndrome, patients report frozen, hypertonic, and spastic paralysis, with speech impediments to the plosives, oral incompetence, and lack of meaningful smile (Fig. 43-43). Flaccid cases require the restoration of lower lip competence either through the introduction of muscle into both sides of the upper and lower lips, securing them in the midline during bilateral free muscle transfer[55] (Fig. 43-44); or with static suspension that traverses the whole of the lower lip. Frozen cases require chemodenervation, aggressive physical therapy, bilateral platysmectomy, and ultimately may also require free muscle transfer for smile restoration.

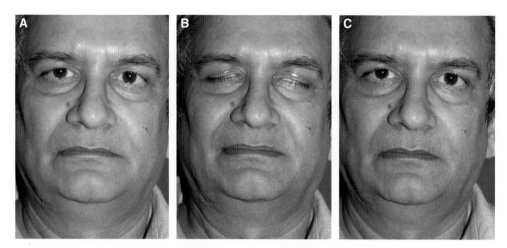

Fig. 43-43 Bilateral frozen face after Guillain-Barré syndrome. **A,** At rest. **B,** Eye closure. **C,** Big smile. Note the similarity in the patient's appearance in the photographs, despite attempts at different facial movements.

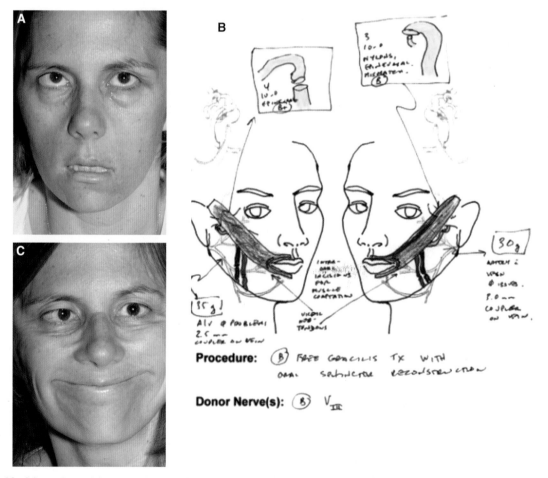

Fig. 43-44 Bilateral free gracilis transfer in flaccid facial paralysis after cavernous brainstem hemangioma extirpation. **A,** Preoperative smile. **B,** Drawing of gracilis transfer. **C,** Smile result after 4 months. Note volitional movement and lower lip competence.

LOSS OF PROXIMAL FACIAL NERVE WITH INTACT DISTAL NERVE AND MUSCULATURE

Neurootologists and neurosurgeons are occasionally faced with a situation in which there is no likelihood of spontaneous facial nerve recovery, because there is an inadequate proximal facial nerve stump for grafting after tumor extirpation. In these cases, providing an alternative source of axons from a different motor nerve will establish the return of tone and movement to the facial musculature. The procedure, referred to as a reinnervation procedure or a nerve substitution technique, may also be relevant when spontaneous recovery was expected but did not materialize within the first 12 months after skull base surgery. Hypoglossal facial transfer (Fig. 43-45) has been popular as a donor in reinnervation procedures for the past three decades, although many modifications have been described to reduce the resulting tongue morbid-

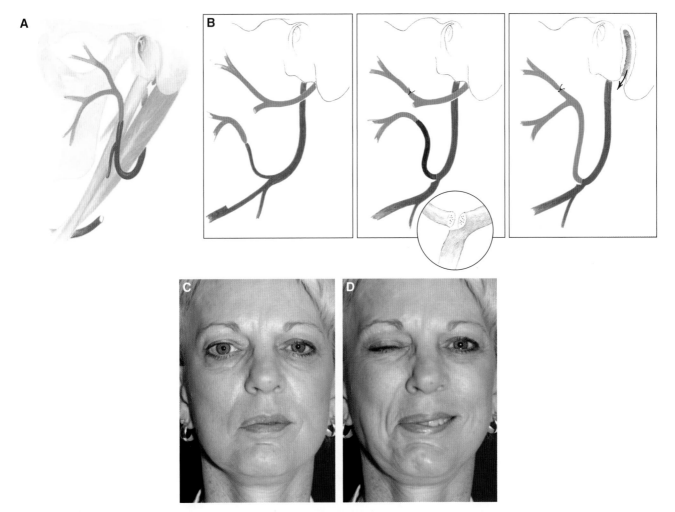

Fig. 43-45   Hypoglossal facial transfer. **A,** Classic operation. **B,** Modifications. **C,** Patient at rest. **D,** Patient with tongue movement. Note the mass movement, with hypertonicity, involuntary eye closure, and lack of meaningful commissure excursion.

ity and to diminish the degree of mass movement that arises after regeneration. Because the operation has significant shortcomings, there has been increasing interest in alternative sources of motor axons for reinnervation procedures,[56-58] with the masseteric branch of the trigeminal nerve gaining popularity based on its minimal donor morbidity and excellent provision of controllable input.[59]

HEMIFACIAL SPASM

Hemifacial spasm is a condition characterized by involuntary spasm of the orbicularis oculi muscle, which may progress to involve the entire hemiface. Attacks last seconds to minutes, may be associated with pain, and over time may increase in frequency, severity, and duration. The condition is thought to arise from

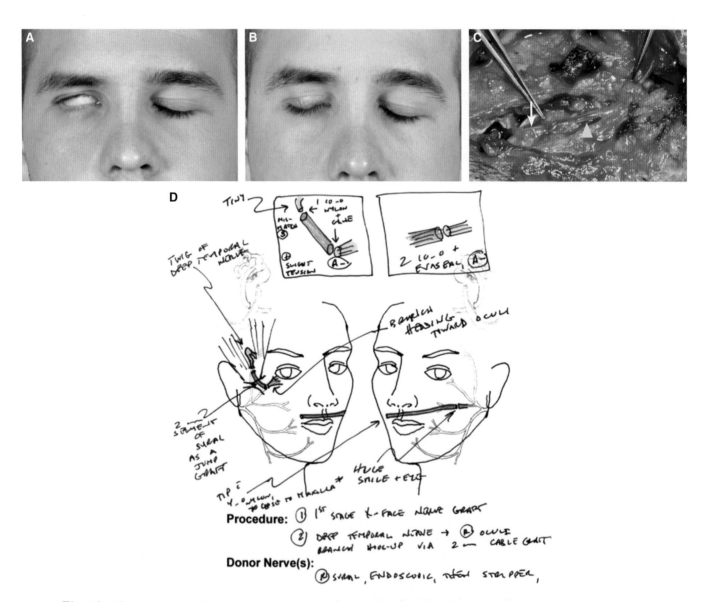

Fig. 43-46   Innervating the orbicularis to prevent chronic atrophy. **A,** Preoperative view of eye closure. **B,** Postoperative view of eye closure 6 months after procedure. **C,** Intraoperative view of the deep temporal nerve *(white arrow),* coapted through a short cable graft *(yellow arrowhead)* to a branch leading to the orbicularis oculi *(green arrow).* **D,** Drawing of the procedure. Note that in addition to the nerve transfer, an eyelid weight was placed that also contributes to eye closure.

vascular impingement on the root exit zone of the facial nerve in the cerebellopontine angle, and in severe cases may be treated with microvascular decompression (Fig. 43-46). Symptomatic relief may be afforded by botulinum toxin injection directly into the lower lamella of the orbicularis oculi muscle in doses higher than those required for synkinesis control.

CONCLUSION

Impaired facial movement is a devastating condition with functional, aesthetic, and communication deficits. Etiologic factors are varied, and treatment plans differ according to the natural history of each condition, patient goals and factors, and prognosis. Comprehensive management is most effectively delivered at specialized centers where a team of facial and plastic surgeons, neuro-otologists, oculoplastic surgeons, and physical therapists works together to deliver comprehensive rehabilitation.[43] Periodic systematic zonal reassessments of facial function are critical to assuring that the care plan addresses the changing examination.

KEY POINTS

- Facial paralysis leads to functional, aesthetic, and communication issues.
- The facial nerve has motor, sensory, and autonomic fibers, and there is significant arborization of the branches in the midface.
- Facial paralysis may be caused by hundreds of different conditions; the most common etiologic factors are viruses, Lyme disease, temporal bone fracture, postsurgical causes, and tumors.
- The House-Brackman score is used to grade facial function, although quantitative and automated programs are emerging that provide less subjective grades of facial function; Quality of Life instrument has been validated for the condition.
- The paralyzed face must be assessed and treated by zone.
- Surgical treatment options range from office-based periocular maneuvers to free tissue transfer for smile.
- Botulinum toxin chemodenervation and physical therapy are critical to optimizing outcome in facial nerve dysfunction.

REFERENCES

1. Darwin C. The Expression of the Emotions in Man and Animals. Minneapolis: Filiquarian, 2007.
2. Resende LA, Weber S. Peripheral facial palsy in the past. Arq Neuropsiquiatr 66:765-769, 2008.
3. Goldman L, Schechter CG. Art in medicine. New York J Med 67:1331-1334, 1967.
4. Canalis RF, Cino L. Ceramic representations of facial paralysis in ancient Peru. Otol Neurotol 24:828-831, 2003.
5. Steiner CB, El-Mallakh RS. Depiction of facial paralysis on an African mask. Neurology 38:822-823, 1988.
6. Razi al-Hawi al-Kabirfi al-Tib (Continens Liber): Hyderabad version (1955). Tabatabaie SM, trans. Tehran: al-Hawi Pharmaceutical Company, 1990.
7. Sajadi MM, Sajadi MR, Tabatabaie SM. The history of facial palsy and spasm: Hippocrates to Razi. Neurology 77:174-178, 2011.
8. Bell C. Essays on the Anatomy and Philosophy of Expression, ed 2. London: John Murray, 1824.
9. Duchenne G. Mécanisme de la Physionomie Humaine, ed 2. Paris: Librairie J.-B. Baillière et Fils, 1876.
     Landmark publication in which photographs depict the isolated activities of the muscles of facial expression. This work also includes an elegant description of the emotions tied to each muscle, referring, for example, to the zygomaticus major as the "muscle of joy," and the frontalis as the "muscle of attention."
10. Ekman P, Friesen WV. Unmasking the Face: A Guide to Recognizing Emotions from Facial Expressions. Los Altos, CA: Malor Books, 2003.

11. Ekman P, Rosenberg EL. What the Face Reveals: Basic and Applied Studies of Spontaneous Expression Using the Facial Action Coding System. New York: Oxford University Press, 2005.

12. Ekman, P. Darwin and Facial Expression: A Century of Research in Review. Los Altos, CA: Malor Books, 2006.

13. Ekman, P. The Face of Man: Expressions of Universal Emotions in a New Guinea Village. New York: Garland STPM Press, 1980.
    Cornerstone publication establishing the universality of facial expression in human emotion.

14. Ekman P, Friesen WV, Ellsworth P. Emotion in the Human Face: Guidelines for Research and an Integration of Findings. Oxford: Pergamon Press, 1972.

15. Niedenthal PM, Mermillod M, Maringer M, et al. The simulation of smiles (SMS) model: embodied simulation and the meaning of facial expression. Behav Brain Sci 33:417-433; discussion 433-480, 2010.

16. Halberstadt JB, Niedenthal PM. Emotional state and the use of stimulus dimensions in judgment. J Pers Soc Psychol 75:1017-1033, 1997.

17. Halberstadt JB, Niedenthal PM. Effects of emotion concepts on perceptual memory for emotional expressions. J Pers Soc Psychol 81:587-598, 2001.

18. Barrett LF, Niedenthal PM. Valence focus and the perception of facial affect. Emotion 4:266-274, 2004.

19. Rubin LR. The anatomy of a smile: its importance in the treatment of facial paralysis. Plast Reconstr Surg 53:384-387, 1974.
    Detailed description of different human smile types and their relevance to facial reanimation.

20. McCormick DP. Herpes-simplex virus as a cause of Bell's palsy. Lancet 299:937-939, 1972.

21. Furuta Y, Fukuda S, Chida E, et al. Reactivation of herpes simplex virus type 1 in patients with Bell's palsy. Med Virol 54:162-166, 1998.

22. Musani MA, Farooqui AN, Usman A, et al. Association of herpes simplex virus infection and Bell's palsy. J Pakistan Med Assoc 59:823-825, 2009.

23. Hato N, Yamada H, Kohno H, et al. Valacyclovir and prednisolone treatment for Bell's palsy: a multicenter, randomized, placebo-controlled study. Otol Neurotol 28:409-413, 2007.

24. Sullivan FM, Swan IR, Donnan PT, et al. Early treatment with prednisolone or acyclovir in Bell's palsy. New Engl J Med 357:1598-1607, 2007.

25. Hato N, Matsumoto S, Kisaki H, et al. Efficacy of early treatment of Bell's palsy with oral acyclovir and prednisolone. Otol Neurotol 24:948-951, 2003.

26. Gants, BJ, Rubinstein JT, Gidley P, et al. Surgical management of Bell's palsy. Laryngoscope 109:1177-1188, 1999.

27. Darrouzet V, Duclos JY, Liguoro D, et al. Management of facial paralysis resulting from temporal bone fractures: our experience in 115 cases. Otolaryngol Head Neck Surg 125:77-84, 2001.

28. Hohman MH, Hadlock TA. Epidemiology of Iatrogenic Facial Nerve Injury: A Decade of Experience. Laryngoscope 124:260-265, 2014.

29. Hadlock T. Evaluation and management of the patient with postoperative facial paralysis. Arch Otolaryngol Head Neck Surg 138:505-508, 2012.

30. Wilkinson EP, Hoa M, Slattery WH, et al. Evolution in the management of facial nerve schwannoma. Laryngoscope 121:2065-2074, 2011.

31. Quesnel AM, Lindsay RW, Hadlock TA. When the bell tolls on Bell's palsy: finding occult malignancy in acute-onset facial paralysis. Am J Otolaryngol 31:339-342, 2010.

32. Wax MK, Kaylie DM. Does a positive neural margin affect outcome in facial nerve grafting? Head Neck 29:546-549, 2007.

33. Brown PD, Eshleman JS, Foote RL, et al. An analysis of facial nerve function in irradiated and unirradiated facial nerve grafts. Int J Radiat Onc 48:737-743, 2000.

34. House JW, Brackmann DE. Facial nerve grading system. Otolaryngol Head Neck Surg 93:146-147, 1985.

35. Vrabec JT, Backous DD, Djalilian HR, et al. Facial nerve grading system 2.0. Otolaryngol Head Neck Surg 140:445-450, 2009.

36. Hadlock TA, Urban LS. Toward a universal, automated facial measurement tool in facial reanimation. Arch Facial Plast Surg 14:277-282, 2012.

37. Kleiss I, Hohman M, Quatela O, et al. Computer-assisted assessment of ocular synkinesis: a comparison of methods. Laryngoscope 123: 879-883, 2013.

38. Kahn JB, Gliklich RE, Boyev KP, et al. Validation of a patient-graded instrument for facial nerve paralysis: the FaCE scale. Laryngoscope 111:387-398, 2001.
    Validation manuscript for quality of life related to facial function.

39. Henstrom D, Malo J, Cheney M, et al. Platysmectomy benefits quality of life in patients with hypertonic facial paralysis. Arch Facial Plast Surg 13:239-243, 2011.

40. Hadlock T, Malo J, Cheney M, et al. Free gracilis transfer for smile in children: the MEEI experience in excursion and quality of life changes. Arch Facial Plast Surg 13:190-194, 2011.

41. Lindsay R, Smitson C, Edwards C, et al. Correction of the nasal base in the flaccidly paralyzed face: an orphaned problem in facial paralysis. Plast Reconstr Surg 126:185e-186e, 2010.

42. Keller GS, Namazie A, Blackwell K, et al. Elevation of the malar fat pad with a percutaneous technique. Arch Facial Plast Surg 4:20-22, 2002.

43. Hadlock T, Greenfield L, Robinson M, et al. Multimodality approach to management of the paralyzed face. Laryngoscope 116:1385-1389, 2006.

44. Harii K, Ohmori K, Torii S. Free gracilis muscle transplantation, with microneurovascular anastomoses for the treatment of facial paralysis. A preliminary report. Plast Reconstr Surg 57:133-143, 1976.
    Original description of gracilis transfer procedure for facial reanimation.

45. Harii K, Asato H, Yoshimura K, et al. One-stage transfer of the latissimus dorsi muscle for reanimation of a paralyzed face: a new alternative. Plast Reconstr Surg 103:941-951, 1998.

46. Koshima I, Moriguchi T, Soeda S, et al. Free rectus femoris muscle transfer for one-stage reconstruction of established facial paralysis. Plast Reconstr Surg 94:421-430, 1994.

47. Terzis JK. Pectoralis minor: a unique muscle for correction of facial palsy. Plast Reconstr Surg 83:767-776, 1989.

48. Lindsay R, Smitson C, Cheney M, et al. A systematic algorithm for the management of lower lip asymmetry. Am J Otolaryngol 32:1-7, 2011.

49. Terzis JK, Kalantarian B. Microsurgical strategies in 74 patients for restoration of dynamic depressor muscle mechanism: a neglected target in facial reanimation. Plast Reconstr Surg 105:1917-1931, 2000.

50. Henstrom D, Malo J, Cheney M, et al. Plastysmectomy: an effective intervention for facial synkinesis and hypertonicity. Arch Facial Plast Surg 13:239-243, 2011.

51. Lindsay R, Robinson M, Hadlock T. Comprehensive facial muscle retraining improves facial function in patients with chronic facial paralysis: the MEEI five year experience. Phys Ther 90:391-397, 2010.

52. Robinson M, Baiungo J, Hohman M, et al. Facial rehabilitation. Oper Techn Otolaryngol Head Neck Surg 23:288-296, 2012.

53. Brach JS, VanSwearingen JM. Physical therapy for facial paralysis: a tailored treatment approach. Phys Ther 79:397-404, 1999.

54. Diels HJ. Facial paralysis: is there a role for a therapist? Facial Plast Surg 16:361-364, 2000.

55. Lindsay R, Hadlock T, Cheney M. Bilateral simultaneous free gracilis muscle transfer: a realistic option in management of bilateral facial paralysis. Otolaryngol Head Neck Surg 141:139-141, 2009.

56. May M, Sobol SM, Mester SJ. Hypoglossal-facial nerve interpositional-jump graft for facial reanimation without tongue atrophy. Otolaryngol Head Neck Surg 104:818-825, 1991.

57. Terzis JK, Konofaos P. Nerve transfers in facial palsy. Facial Plast Surg 24:177-193, 2008.

58. Coleman CC, Walker JC. Technic of anastomosis of the branches of the facial nerve with the spinal accessory for facial paralysis. Ann Surg 131:960-966, 1950.

59. Manktelow R, Tomat L, Zuker R, et al. Smile reconstruction in adults with free muscle transfer innervated by the masseter motor nerve: effectiveness and cerebral adaptation. Plast Reconstr Surg 118:885-899, 2006.
    Large gracilis transfer series by leaders in facial reanimation, describing results and cerebral adaptation to trigeminally driven smile.

44

Craniofacial Surgery

David C. Kim ▪ *Anthony D. Holmes* ▪ *John G. Meara*

Patients with craniofacial anomalies have a complex array of medical and surgical issues that manifest within a large number of medical diagnoses, ranging from craniosynostosis to syndactyly. Before the pioneering work of Dr. Paul Tessier in the 1950s through the 1970s, the surgical correction of congenital and acquired deformities of the cranium, orbit, and facial skeleton was a feared endeavor. Only a few decades after Tessier's groundbreaking contributions, highly skilled craniofacial teams around the world have begun to routinely correct these deformities. As the procedures have become more widespread, the complexities of these patients' medical problems have been more thoroughly illuminated, and an interdisciplinary medical team is currently considered the standard of care. Multidisciplinary craniofacial centers exist worldwide, comprising representatives from anesthesiology, audiology, craniofacial surgery, dentistry, genetics, internal medicine, neurology, neurosurgery, nursing, ophthalmology, oral surgery, orthodontics, otolaryngology, pediatrics, physical anthropology, prosthodontics, psychiatry, radiology, social services, and speech pathology. It is critical for facial reconstructive surgeons to be able to recognize craniofacial anomalies and common craniofacial syndromes and to understand the essential treatment modalities and philosophies.

CRANIOFACIAL EMBRYOLOGY

Craniofacial development in the human embryo occurs during weeks 4 through 8 of gestation (Fig. 44-1). At the end of week 4, the stomodeum emerges. The frontonasal prominence descends from above as the precursor to the upper face and forebrain to meet the stomodeum. The two maxillary processes flank the stomodeum laterally, as the mandibular process develops inferiorly. The primitive nose and eyes are represented by the nasal and lens placodes that begin lateral to their final position and slowly migrate medially. The pharyngeal arches start to develop as the neural crest cells migrate to the head and neck. Each arch contains an artery, nerve, muscle, and cartilage. The arches are separated by pharyngeal grooves externally and pharyngeal pouches internally. Only the first four arches are visible at the end of week 4. The first arch, the mandibular arch, forms the mandibular prominence and the smaller maxillary prominence, and eventually the upper and lower jaw. The second arch, the hyoid arch, forms the hyoid bone. The third and fourth pharyngeal arches also begin to develop.

At the end of week 5, the medial and lateral nasal prominences of the frontonasal prominence develop between the laterally set eyes and begin their journey toward the midline, creating the nose. Inferiorly, at the junction of the head and neck, the external ear is emerging from the first and second pharyngeal arches. The second pharyngeal arch overgrows the third and fourth arches and forms the cervical sinus.

At week 6, upper eyelids are identifiable, and the eyes begin to take shape. The six hillocks of the auricle adjoin one other. The three anterior hillocks are derived from the first pharyngeal arch and the three posterior hillocks are derived from the second pharyngeal arch. The first pharyngeal pouch expands to become the tubotympanic recess, and eventually meets the first pharyngeal groove to form the tympanic membrane. The tubotympanic recess, in migrating away from the pharynx, forms the Eustachian tube. By the end of

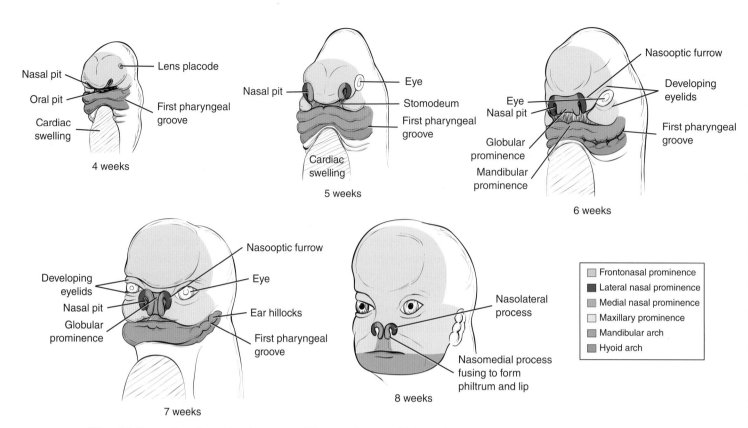

Fig. 44-1 Embryologic development of the maxilla, mandible, and ear. (From Bentz ML, Bauer BS, Zuker RM. Principles & Practice of Pediatric Plastic Surgery. St Louis: Quality Medical Publishing, 2008.)

week 6, the parathyroid glands begin to develop from the epithelium of the third and fourth pharyngeal arches. Eventually, the parathyroid glands from the third pharyngeal arch migrate caudally and lie inferior to the parathyroid glands from the fourth pharyngeal arch.

In week 7, the maxillary prominences merge medially with the lateral aspects of the medial nasal prominences, as the medial edges of the medial nasal prominences merge together in the center. During week 8, a recognizable face emerges with distinguishable ears, forward-facing eyes, eyelids, upper and lower lips, and a nose and chin with some noticeable projection. Between 6 and 8 weeks, the maxilla and mandible develop, establishing the basic structure of the face by the end of week 8. Coincident with the last few weeks of craniofacial development, the digits of the hands and feet become notched, webbed, and finally completely separated between weeks 6 and 8.[1,2]

NONSYNDROMIC CRANIOSYNOSTOSIS

Craniosynostosis refers to the premature fusion of the calvarial sutures, which occurs in 1:2000 births.[3] The sutures serve two main functions: first, as zones of compression during passage through the birth canal; and second, as zones of expansion, allowing the brain to grow freely until it reaches adult size and shape. Craniosynostosis limits growth perpendicular to the affected suture, creating recognizable patterns of deformity (Table 44-1). Sagittal synostosis is most common, followed by coronal, metopic, and lambdoid synostoses, in descending order. Premature fusion limits calvarial growth and can cause increased intra-

Table 44-1 Clinical Examination Findings in Craniosynostosis

Suture		Findings	Resultant Head Shape
Sagittal Normal		Bitemporal narrowing Biparietal narrowing Frontal bossing Occipital bossing Anterior advancement of vertex	Scaphocephaly
Metopic		Vertical forehead keel Bitemporal narrowing Superolateral orbital rim retraction Biparietal widening Orbital hypotelorism	Trigonocephaly
Unilateral coronal		Recessed ipsilateral forehead Elevation of ipsilateral orbit Deviation of nasal root to affected side Deviation of chin away from affected side Advancement/elevation of ipsilateral ear	Frontal plagiocephaly
Bilateral coronal		Recessed supraorbital rims Biparietal widening Shortened AP dimension Increased calvarial height Exorbitism	Turribrachycephaly
Lambdoid		Windswept appearance Ipsilateral mastoid bossing Ipsilateral cranial base flattening ± Ipsilateral ear deviation, posteriorly or inferiorly	Posterior plagiocephaly

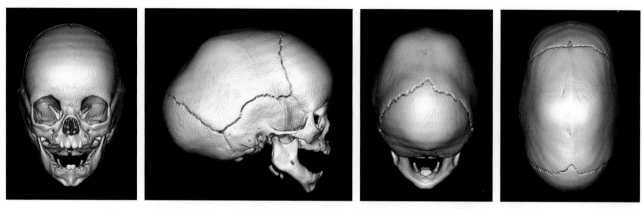

Fig. 44-2   Three-dimensional CT scan of sagittal synostosis.

cranial pressure.[4] This phenomenon occurs in both simple and complex craniosynostosis, affecting one or more sutures, respectively. In general, the more sutures involved, the greater the risk of increased pressure.

SAGITTAL CRANIOSYNOSTOSIS

Sagittal synostosis is the most common form of craniosynostosis. Involvement of the sagittal suture in nonsyndromic simple craniosynostosis reaches up to 57%.[5,6] Growth is limited in the coronal dimension, and elongated in the sagittal dimension, resulting in *scaphocephaly,* a term derived from the Greek, meaning "boatlike head." Patients demonstrate bitemporal/biparietal narrowing and frontal/occipital bossing. A ridge may be palpated along the sagittal suture, and the anterior and posterior fontanelles may be prematurely closed (Fig. 44-2).

UNILATERAL CORONAL CRANIOSYNOSTOSIS

Unilateral coronal craniosynostosis affects 14% of patients who have simple craniosynostosis.[3] Limited growth perpendicular to the coronal suture results in anterior plagiocephaly. Clinical exam findings include flattening of the ipsilateral forehead, elevation of the ipsilateral orbit, deviation of the nasal root toward the affected suture, deviation of the chin away from the suture, and advancement/elevation of the ipsilateral ear (Fig. 44-3). Asymmetry in the bony structure of the orbit usually causes a degree of strabismus as a result of ocular muscle imbalance.[7,8] Approximately one third of patients eventually require surgical strabismus correction. On an anteroposterior radiograph, the greater wing of the sphenoid is elevated, causing a *Harlequin deformity.*

BILATERAL CORONAL CRANIOSYNOSTOSIS

Bilateral coronal synostosis has an incidence of 6%. This finding is most commonly familial, and carries a risk for increased intracranial pressure.[3] Common facial findings in bilateral coronal synostosis include a flattened, retruded forehead and proptosis caused by a recessed supraorbital rim. Because of the lack of expansion anteriorly, compensatory growth in a superior and lateral direction usually results in a wider, taller head (turribrachycephaly). Patients may report strabismus; ophthalmologic evaluation is essential.

METOPIC CRANIOSYNOSTOSIS

Metopic synostosis makes up 5% to 27% of nonsyndromic craniosynostoses.[9-10] Premature fusion of the metopic suture results in trigonocephaly, characterized by bitemporal narrowing, a vertical keel at the metopic suture with retrusion of the superolateral orbital rims and orbital hypotelorism. Metopic ridging without any of these orbital findings is occasionally seen in infants in whom the metopic suture begins to fuse around the time of birth. This will slowly disappear without surgical treatment. Ordinarily, the metopic suture fuses sometime between birth and two years of age. True trigonocephaly is the result of earlier, in utero metopic fusion. The distinction should be made clinically and a radiograph or CT scan can be helpful in making the diagnosis (Fig. 44-4).

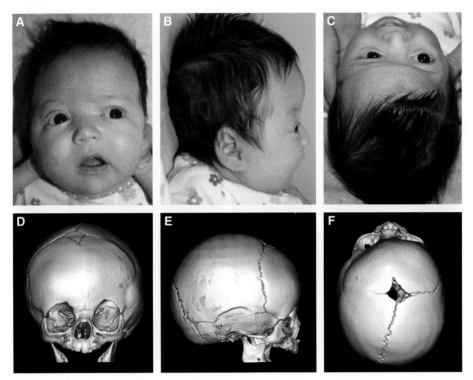

Fig. 44-3   Infant with right unilateral coronal synostosis in **A,** frontal, **B,** lateral, and **C,** vertex view. Three-dimensional CT scan images in **D,** AP, **E,** lateral, and **F,** vertex views. Note the elevation of the left orbit, flattening of the ipsilateral forehead, and deviation of the midface and lower face toward the affected suture.

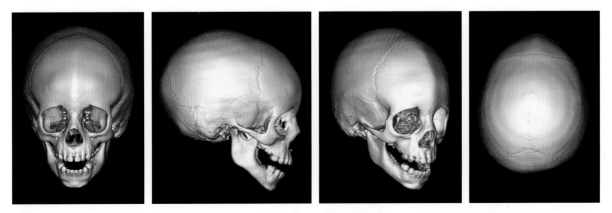

Fig. 44-4   Three-dimensional CT scans of metopic synostosis. Note the vertical frontal keel. The vertex view shows trigonocephaly, with bitemporal narrowing and biparietal widening. Orbital hypotelorism is difficult to identify here.

LAMBDOID CRANIOSYNOSTOSIS

Lambdoid synostosis is the rarest of the craniosynostoses, making up 3% to 5% of nonsyndromic cranio-synostoses.[3,5,11] The typical findings characteristic of lambdoid synostosis are ipsilateral occipital mastoid bulging, leading to a windswept appearance of the occiput. Traditionally, the ipsilateral ear is thought to be retracted toward the fused suture, but recent literature suggests that ear position is not consistently misplaced.[5] In one study, only mastoid bossing, inferior positioning of the ipsilateral ear, and skull base cant were consistent with clinical findings[12] (Fig. 44-5).

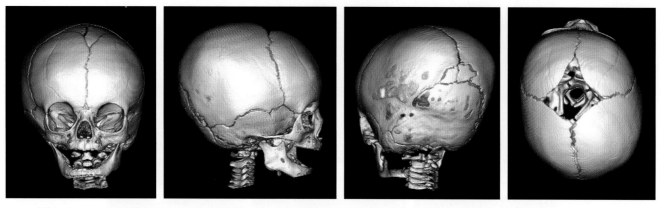

Fig. 44-5 Three-dimensional CT scans of left lambdoid synostosis. Note the posterior windswept appearance, with flattening of the occiput on the left side.

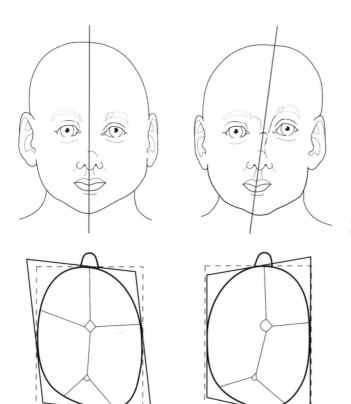

Fig. 44-6 Left unilateral coronal synostosis versus deformational plagiocephaly.

Table 44-2 Clinical Examination Findings in Deformational Plagiocephaly Versus Unilateral Coronal and Lambdoid Craniosynostosis

Frontal Bone Flattened on One Side	Deformational Plagiocephaly	Unilateral Coronal Craniosynostosis
Shape (vertex view)	Parallelogram	Trapezoidal
Ipsilateral ear (relation to contralateral ear)	Posterior	Anterior/superior
Occiput	Contralateral flattening	Variable
Orbit	Normal	Ipsilateral elevation
Palpebral fissure	Contralateral narrowing	Ipsilateral widening
Nasal root	Normal	Toward ipsilateral
Chin cant	Normal	Deviated away
Occiput Flattened on One Side	**Deformational Plagiocephaly**	**Lambdoid Craniosynostosis**
Shape (vertex view)	Parallelogram	Trapezoidal
Mastoid	Normal	Ipsilateral bossing
Ipsilateral ear (relation to contralateral ear)	Anterior	Variable
Forehead	Ipsilateral bossing	Normal
Malar region	Ipsilateral bossing	Normal/ipsilateral recessed
Cranial base	Ipsilateral flattening	Ipsilateral flattening

Deformational Plagiocephaly

Children with craniosynostosis can be identified at birth, or more commonly, in early infancy. Referral to a craniofacial surgeon should be made to differentiate between true craniosynostosis and abnormal head shape as a result of deformational changes (Fig. 44-6). Since the "Back to Sleep" campaign was instituted by the American Association of Pediatrics in 1992 to lessen the chance of sudden infant death syndrome,[13] the incidence of deformational plagiocephaly and deformational brachycephaly has increased significantly. In some regions it increased sixfold.[14] Screening for single-suture craniosynostosis in a sea of deformational plagiocephaly can be challenging, but seasoned clinicians can identify the key features for the correct diagnosis by direct examination. If necessary, radiographs and CT may be required. Radiographs can demonstrate the patency of sutures with minimal radiation exposure. CT with three-dimensional reconstruction can be useful in visualizing the extent of fusion, and is helpful in surgical planning (Table 44-2).

Deformational plagiocephaly is important to understand in discussion of craniosynostosis. Many key findings differentiate these conditions in frontal and vertex views. Deformational plagiocephaly is the consequence of spending a disproportionate amount of time on one side of the head, which results in insidious flattening of that side of the occiput, anterior advancement of the ipsilateral ear, bossing on the ipsilateral side of the forehead, bossing of the ipsilateral malar region, and contralateral parietal widening.[15] The position of the ears, orbits, brows, nasal root, and forehead distinguish craniosynostosis from deformational plagiocephaly (see Table 44-2). Treatment for deformational plagiocephaly involves repositioning strategies, "tummy time," and sometimes orthotic helmet therapy, which is usually instituted between 4 and 9 months (Fig. 44-7). Craniosynostosis requires surgical intervention.

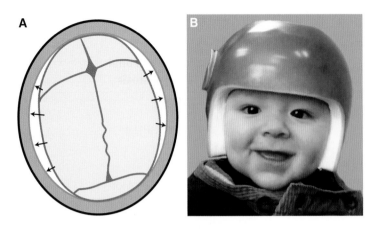

Fig. 44-7   Orthotic helmet for deformational plagiocephaly. **A,** Schematic diagram of a helmet. **B,** Child wearing an othotic helmet.

Deformational plagiocephaly has a strong association with congenital muscular torticollis.[16] Resolution of congenital torticollis plays a key role in improvement of the deformity. Surgical correction of torticollis is almost never necessary.

Increased Intracranial Pressure and Neurodevelopmental Delays

Hirsch et al[4] measured intracranial pressure (ICP) with epidural sensors and found that one third of patients with craniosynostosis have elevated ICP. After release of the affected sutures, ICP returned to normal levels. Numerous studies have demonstrated a risk for increased ICP in patients with craniosynostosis.[17-19]

Ultimately, the long-term concern for craniosynostosis is neurodevelopmental delay. Da Costa et al examined mental and motor aptitude in simple craniosynostosis patients and identified a general deficit in motor skills and a lack of accelerated mental function. In the sagittal synostosis subgroup, deficits were statistically significant in both motor and mental function. In the metopic subgroup, a delay in motor function was significant.[20]

CORRECTION OF CRANIOSYNOSTOSIS

The two major goals for craniosynostosis correction are to decrease ICP and to restore craniofacial anatomy. Numerous techniques for repair have been developed to achieve these goals. Initial attempts to treat this disorder involved simple suturectomy, but these procedures were relatively unsuccessful because of the high recurrence of sutural fusion. Subsequently, craniosynostosis procedures evolved into a plethora of calvarial remodeling operations that target specific aspects of abnormal head shape. Although techniques for each surgical problem are evolving rapidly, the basis of synostosis surgery has involved two principles: release or removal of the affected sutures and reestablishing the normal position of the affected bones.

Frontoorbital Advancement

One well-established technique for the treatment of craniosynostosis is frontoorbital advancement. This procedure corrects the position of the supraorbital rim and forehead while increasing intracranial volume (Fig. 44-8). Children with craniosynostosis of metopic, unilateral coronal, or bilateral coronal sutures have recessed supraorbital rims, leaving the eyes unprotected, and resulting in an abnormally shaped forehead. Using a coronal incision, the frontal bone and supraorbital rims are accessed. With the assistance of neuro-

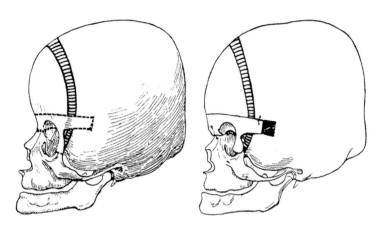

Fig. 44-8   Frontoorbital advancement. (From Katzen JT, McCarthy JG. Syndromes involving craniosynostosis and midface hypoplasia. Otolaryngol Clin North Am 33:1257-1284, 2000.)

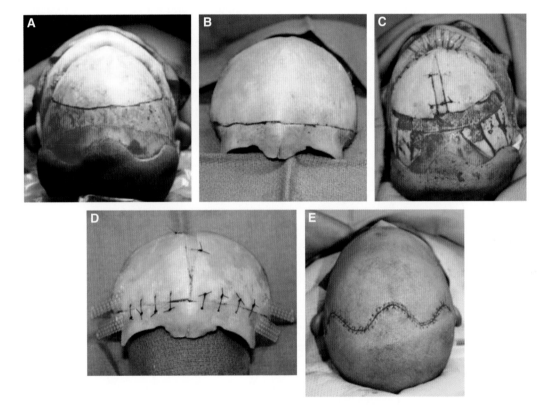

Fig. 44-9   **A,** Vertex view of infant with trigonocephaly from metopic craniosynostosis. The anterior scalp flap elevated after coronal incision and pre-operative marking demonstrates the superior aspect of the frontal osteotomy. **B,** Anterior view after ostectomy of frontal bone and supraorbital rim. **C,** Anterior view after vertex keel of frontal bone widened with wedge of bone graft secured with 2-0 PDS suture. Resorbable plates placed laterally allow for differential movement in anterior-posterior and superior-inferior planes. **D,** Vertex view after bony segments secured to the calvarium. Note the rounded forehead, anterior advancement of the bony segments, and barrel-stave osteotomies to increase cranial volume. **E,** Vertex view after scalp closure.

surgery, the frontal bone is removed 1.5 cm above a supraorbital bandeau. Next, the supraorbital bandeau is carefully extracted, taking care to protect the periorbita and brain. Both bony segments are then reshaped, advanced, and fixed. Fixation usually employs resorbable plates, screws, and sutures. The advanced bone is frequently slightly overcorrected to account for possible relapse and lessened growth potential in the areas of potential refusion (Fig. 44-9).

Pi Procedure for Sagittal Synostosis

The Pi procedure addresses two major issues of scaphocephaly: the elongated sagittal dimension and the narrowed transverse dimension. Osteotomies in the shape of the Greek symbol π were oriented transversely along the bilateral coronal sutures with parasagittal osteotomies on either side of the sagittal suture. This maneuver functionally decreases the length of the head, while widening the coronal dimension[21] (Fig. 44-10).

Melbourne Method for Total Vault Remodeling in Sagittal Synostosis

The Melbourne method introduces a third dimension to correction of sagittal synostosis. Like the Pi procedure, it shortens the elongated calvarium in the sagittal dimension and widens the narrowed head in the coronal direction, but it also elevates the vertex of the head, which is inferiorly displaced. A key component of this technique is removing a coronal band of bone and transferring it to the occiput, increasing the height and shortening the length of the head. Barrel stave osteotomies and lateral displacement of the parietal bony segments result in widening of the lateral dimension of a once-narrow head[22] (Fig. 44-11). This technique reshapes the fused sagittal suture and sets it in its final adult position (Fig. 44-12). The procedure increases the cranial vault volume and puts no pressure on the brain intraoperatively.

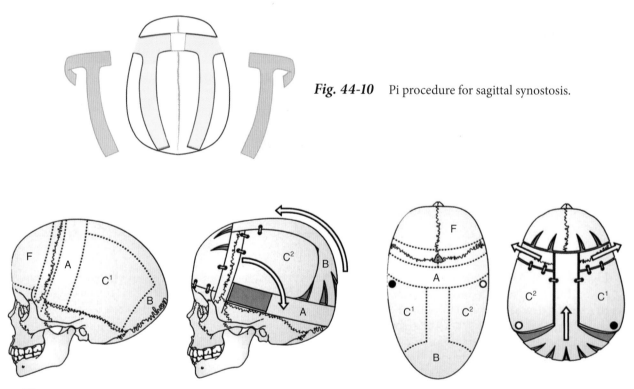

Fig. 44-10   Pi procedure for sagittal synostosis.

Fig. 44-11   Melbourne method for total vault remodeling. The frontal bone *(F)* is removed and widened. The coronal suture is undermined, split centrally and separated. Behind this, a coronal *A* bar is removed along with parasagittal, parietal areas *(C^1 and C^2)*. The fused sagittal suture, together with the protruding occiput is then removed and reshaped. The *A* bar is moved to the occipital area. The reshaped occiput is replaced on this bar, thus moving the sagittal suture anteriorly and elevating the vertex of the cranium. The *C* parietal areas are replaced and reconnected to the coronal suture bones allowing for biparietal expansion. The head shape is normalized and the cranial space increased. (From Greensmith AL, Holmes AD, Lo P, Maxiner W, Heggie AA, Meara JG. Complete correction of severe scaphocephaly: the Melbourne method of total vault remodeling. Plast Reconstr Surg 121:1300-1310, 2008.)

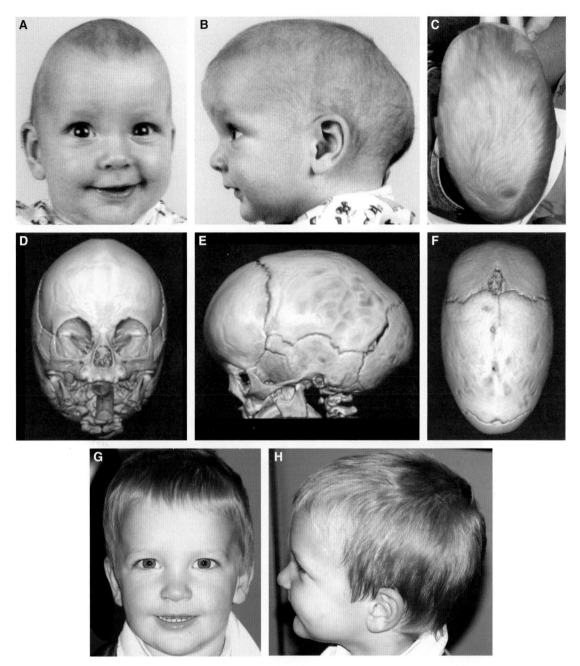

Fig. 44-12   **A-C,** Infant with classic scaphocephaly from sagittal synostosis. **D-F,** Three-dimensional scans show synostosis and skull shape. **G** and **H,** Photos 1 year postoperatively show normal growth and appearance, with total cranial vault reshaping and expansion.

Springs

To address the complication of refusion and relapse of the affected sutures in craniosynostosis, Persing and Lauritzen popularized the use of 1 to 1.3 mm steel wire springs that provide a constant pressure of 4 to 10 N of force against the edges of the released suture. The springs may expand up to 5 to 7 cm over a period of several weeks. Insertion of springs has become an adjunct maneuver to help treat craniosynostoses of all types.[23-25] The springs have to be removed when the expansion is completed (Fig. 44-13).

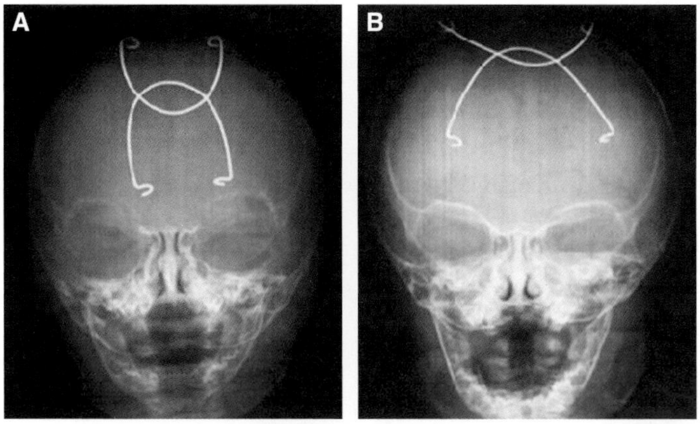

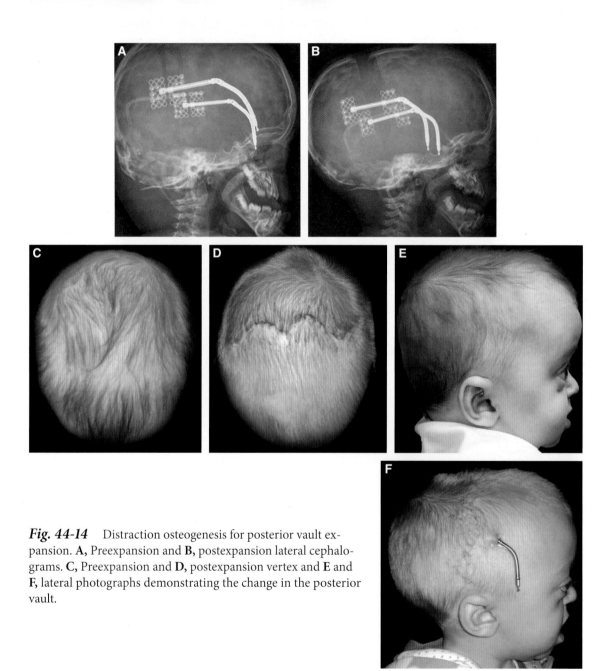

Fig. 44-13   Spring-mediated cranial reshaping for sagittal synostosis. **A,** Anterior view after sagittal suture ostectomy and initial spring placement. **B,** After spring expansion of the sagitttal suture.

Fig. 44-14   Distraction osteogenesis for posterior vault expansion. **A,** Preexpansion and **B,** postexpansion lateral cephalograms. **C,** Preexpansion and **D,** postexpansion vertex and **E** and **F,** lateral photographs demonstrating the change in the posterior vault.

DISTRACTION OSTEOGENESIS

In the 1950 and 1960s, Gavril Ilizarov introduced distraction osteogenesis as a surgical concept. The finding was serendipitous when nuts on the rods of the external fixator device used to compress bony nonunions were mistakenly turned backward, resulting in limb lengthening with the formation of new bone between the ostetomies.[26] The Ilizarov device has been modified and used extensively throughout the body. In craniofacial surgery, distraction osteogenesis is used frequently in the expansion of the mandible and midface, and now the calvarium. The protocol for distraction remains the same when used for craniosynostosis. After appropriate osteotomies are made, distractors are placed, and after a latency period of 3 to 5 days, the bony edges are distracted at a rate of 1 mm/day. When desired growth is achieved, the bone is allowed to consolidate for a time twice as long as the period of distraction. Technically, this concept can be implemented to treat any craniosynostosis, but it is particularly useful in posterior vault expansion in patients with venous outflow restrictions and Chiari malformation[27] (Fig. 44-14). The slow advancement with distraction is also useful in preventing surgical dead space (and hence infection) in major frontofacial movements, such as the Monobloc procedure.

ENDOSCOPIC RELEASE

In patients younger than 6 months, simple craniosynostoses can be treated endoscopically with a strip craniectomy of the affected suture and postoperative helmet therapy. Pioneering work performed by Barone and Jimenez[28] demonstrated that this approach is safe and effective. This technique is most commonly used for sagittal craniosynostosis, but can also be implemented to treat metopic, coronal, and lambdoid craniosynostosis. Recent studies have shown that endoscopic release for sagittal synostosis can be more cost-effective in the first year than open calvarial remodeling.[29]

SYNDROMIC CRANIOSYNOSTOSES

The list of syndromes that manifest craniosynostoses is extensive. Select syndromes of particular clinical relevance include Apert syndrome, Crouzon syndrome, Crouzon with acanthosis nigricans, Pfeiffer syndrome, Muenke syndrome, and Saethre-Chotzen syndrome.

Recently, an inundation of genetic information has enlightened the scientific community on some of the molecular causes of these disease processes. All of these syndromes are related to mutations in fibroblastic growth factor receptor *(FGFR)* genes. The only non-*FGFR*-related gene mutations are *TWIST* for Saethre-Chotzen syndrome and *MSX2* (5q35.2) for Boston-type craniosynostosis.[30] More than 98% of patients with Apert syndrome are associated with two gain-of-function mutations in the *FGFR2* gene (10q26-Ser252Trp or Pro253Arg).[31] Crouzon syndrome is caused by mutations on *FGFR2*,[32] but Crouzon with acanthosis nigricans is *FGFR3*-related.[33] Pfeiffer syndrome can be separated into three types. Type 1 mutations are 5% *FGFR1* (Pro252Arg mutation) and 95% *FGFR2*.[34,35] Types 2 and 3 are 100% *FGFR2*-related. *FGFR3* mutations are responsible for Muenke syndrome.[36] Although primarily related to *TWIST,* Saethre-Chotzen has also been identified with mutations of *FGFR2* and *FGFR3*[37] (Table 44-3).

As the genetic map is expanding, the well-established clinical similarities in these syndromes are being verified. Not only do these patients have complex craniosynostosis, but they also report midfacial hypoplasia, airway obstruction, hearing difficulties, and strabismus.

AIRWAY

Airway compromise is common in patients with craniofacial syndromes. In one study, 20% of all craniofacial patients and 48% of syndromic craniosynostosis patients were found to require tracheostomy. In addition, 7.6% of these patients had either choanal atresia or choanal stenosis.[38] Piriform aperture stenosis, although rare, is seen more frequently in craniofacial patients.[39]

Table 44-3 Molecular Basis of *FGFR*-Related Craniosynostosis Syndromes

Syndrome	Gene	Inheritance Pattern	Prevalence
Apert	*FGFR2* (10q26.13)	AD	15 in 1,000,000
Crouzon	*FGFR2* (10q26.13)	AD	15 in 1,000,000
Crouzon with acanthosis nigricans	*FGFR3* (4p16.3)	AD	NA
Pfeiffer	Type 1: *FGFR1* (5%) (8p11.23-p11.22), *FGFR2* (95%) Types 2 and 3: *FGFR2* only (10q26.13)	AD	10 in 1,000,000
Muenke	*FGFR3* (4p16.3)	AD	33 in 1,000,000
Saethre-Chotzen	*TWIST* (7p21.1), some *FGFR2/FGFR3*[1]	AD	20 in 1,000,000

Table 44-4 Disordered Breathing in Syndromic Patients

Syndrome	Airway Compromise
Apert	OSA midface, choanal stenosis, choanal atresia
Crouzon	OSA midface
Pfeiffer	OSA midface
Muenke	Usually none
Saethre-Chotzen	OSA midface

OSA, Obstructive sleep apnea.

Table 44-5 Hearing Loss in Syndromic Craniosynostosis

Syndrome	Hearing Loss (%)	Types of Hearing Loss			
		Sensorineural	Conductive	Mixed	Not Specified
Apert	44-80	2	93	5	0
Crouzon	28.5-74	26	60	14	0
Pfeiffer	85-92	4	81	15	0
Muenke	62.1	79	9	5	8
Saethre-Chotzen	28.6-59	NA	NA	NA	NA

If there is potential for airway compromise, diagnostic testing through nasal endoscopy, direct laryngoscopy, or video endoscopy/fluoroscopy must be employed for thorough evaluation. Sleep studies are helpful in determining severity of obstructive sleep apnea, identifying and categorizing the causes of apneic and hypoxic episodes into upper airway obstruction, lower airway obstruction, and central apnea.

Treatment options are diverse. Conservative interventions include prone/lateral positioning, nasopharyngeal or oropharyngeal airways, respiratory support with positive pressure ventilation, and intubation. Surgical interventions for airway compromise include release of choanal stenosis or atresia, tracheostomy, tonsillectomy and adenoidectomy, and midfacial advancement. Intubation should be performed by an experienced anesthesiologist or an otolaryngologist[40] (Table 44-4).

HEARING LOSS

Hearing loss in craniofacial syndromes is increasingly recognized, and treating physicians should have a high level of suspicion. Both conductive and sensorineural hearing loss have been noted.[41] In general hearing loss data are variable, but there are some notable trends. Pfeiffer syndrome, for example, has a high correlation with hearing loss, ranging from 85% to 92%.[42] Apert, Crouzon, Muenke, and Saethre-Chotzen syndromes follow in descending order of prevalence[43-45] (Table 44-5).

STRABISMUS

Premature sutural fusion affects not only cranial shape, but also facial and orbital anatomy in many cases. Structural changes of the orbit can lead to imbalance in tension and relaxation of the extraocular muscles and frank strabismus. Ocular problems are common with craniofacial anomalies. A recent meta-analysis revealed that 43% to 91% of syndromic craniosynostoses patients manifested some form of strabismus.[7]

DIFFERENTIATING FEATURES

APERT SYNDROME

Apert syndrome is a classic craniosynostotic syndrome with multisuture craniosynostosis, midfacial hypoplasia, symphalangism, and syndactyly of the upper and lower extremities (Fig. 44-15).

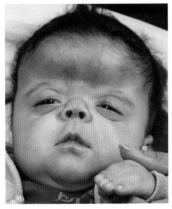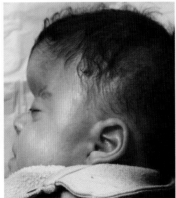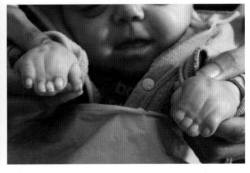

Fig. 44-15   Patient with Apert syndrome and bilateral coronal craniosynostosis. Note the recessed supraorbital rims, proptotic eyes, hypoplastic midface, and bilateral hand syndactyly, mitten hand deformity.

Upton[44] classified syndactyly of the fingers and toes into three groups:
1. "Mitten" hand: The thumb is fused to the index/middle/ring finger group.
2. "Spade" hand: Index, middle, and ring fingers are fused but the thumb is free.
3. "Rosebud" hand: All digits are fused together in a configuration that makes it difficult to identify any fingers.

Children with Apert syndrome are also noted to have cleft uvulas (26.5%), soft palatal clefts (23.5%), and Chiari malformations (29%).[45] Intellectual disability may be present in up to 50% of these children.[46-48]

CROUZON SYNDROME

Patients with Crouzon syndrome are unique among patients with syndromic craniosynostoses in that they do not have associated digital anomalies. Risk of intracranial hypertension is especially high in Crouzon syndrome, with a frequency of 62.5%, as opposed to 45% in Apert syndrome and 29% in other craniosynostotic syndromes[46,47] (Fig. 44-16).

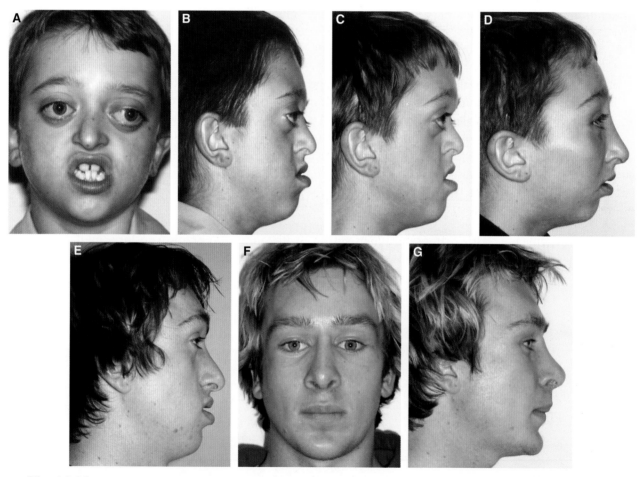

Fig. 44-16   **A** and **B,** Untreated Crouzon in patient at age 6. **C,** At age 7, a forehead and supraorbital correction were performed after bifrontoorbital advancement. **D,** At age 10, a LeFort III orbitomaxillary advancement and nasal bone graft was done. **E,** At age 16, after pubertal growth; note that mandibular growth has exceeded the maxilla. **F** and **G,** At age 19, final correction after bimaxillary surgery, genioplasty, and rhinoplasty.

CROUZON SYNDROME WITH ACANTHOSIS NIGRICANS

The findings in Crouzon syndrome with acanthosis nigricans are similar to those of Crouzon patients, but they also have uniquely associated acanthosis nigricans in the neck, axillae, groin, and antecubital fossae. This finding is not functionally consequential, but may help differentiate them from Crouzon patients during preparation for an intracranial operation. Crouzon patients with acanthosis nigricans have an increased risk for jugular foraminal stenosis, leading to intracranial venous hypertension and increased blood loss during intracranial procedures[49] (Fig. 44-17).

PFEIFFER SYNDROME

Nearly all patients with Pfeiffer syndrome have broad thumbs and broad great toes. This syndrome can also be associated with choanal stenosis and cleft palate.[50] Pfeiffer syndrome is subcategorized into three types.[51] Type 1 is less common and less severe; patients have normal intellect. Types 2 and 3 are associated with more intellectual disability. Type 2 is more often associated with *kleeblattschädel,* or cloverleaf-shaped head, in which most of the cranial sutures are fused. These patients usually have extreme proptosis. Type 3 carries a higher risk for early death[50] (Fig. 44-18).

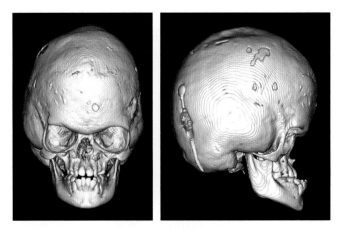

Fig. 44-17   Three-dimensional CT scans of a patient with Crouzonoid features, with acanthosis nigricans after frontoorbital advancement. Note the severe midfacial hypoplasia.

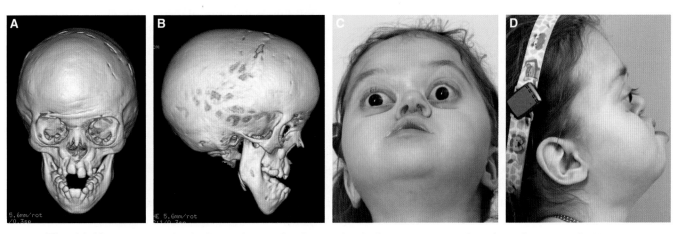

Fig. 44-18   Patient with Pfeiffer syndrome after frontoorbital advancement. **A** and **B,** Three-dimensional CT scans. **C** and **D,** Basal and lateral views. Note midfacial hypoplasia and the need for a tracheostomy. She has a bone-anchored hearing aid for conductive hearing loss.

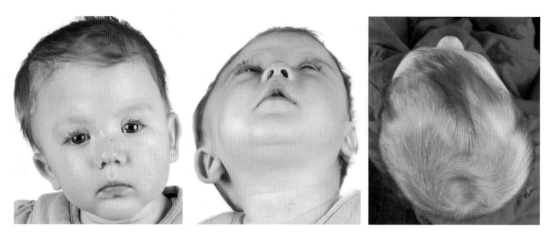

Fig. 44-19   Patient with Saethre-Chotzen syndrome with metopic and left unilateral coronal synostosis. Note bilateral eyelid ptosis and minor midfacial hypoplasia.

Muenke Syndrome

Muenke syndrome usually involves unilateral or bilateral coronal craniosynostosis, although findings are generally more subtle than in other syndromes. Maxillary hypoplasia is minimal, leading to less airway obstruction. Hearing loss is common. Hand/foot anomalies differ from Apert and Pfeiffer syndromes, and often manifest as carpal/tarsal fusions.[52] Megalencephaly without craniosynostosis has also been associated with Muenke syndrome.[49,53]

Saethre-Chotzen Syndrome

Saethre-Chotzen syndrome (Fig. 44-19) is characterized by upper eyelid ptosis, auricular anomalies (including prominent helical root, a low hairline, and hearing loss), and cutaneous syndactyly of the second and third digits of the hand. Maxillary hypoplasia is not as common with Saethre-Chotzen as it is with Apert and Crouzon syndromes. Intellectual development is frequently normal; however, severe mental retardation has been reported (Table 44-6).

Correction of Syndromic Craniosynostosis

Treatment for this complex group of patients can be a lifelong process. For example, treatment for a child with Apert syndrome starts immediately at birth and extends into adulthood. At birth, children are evaluated by geneticists, otolaryngologists, neonatologists, hand surgeons, and craniofacial surgeons.[53] A tracheostomy is performed if the upper airway is obstructed. Hand surgeons correct upper extremity syndactylies when the child is between 3 and 18 months. Calvarial remodeling occurs at age 9 months or later (Table 44-7).

In all syndromic synostosis, calvarial remodeling is similar to that described in the nonsyndromic section of this chapter, but the complexity of the multisuture synostosis may require a combination of techniques to restore a normal calvarial shape. Unfortunately, relapse is frequent in syndromic patients. Results of craniofacial procedures can be classified into four groups, according to the Whitaker classification[54] (Box 44-1). Among infants who had primary frontoorbital advancement procedures, reoperation for either supraorbital retrusion or frontal deformity can be as high as 100% in Apert patients, 26% in Crouzon, 38% in Pfeiffer, 65% in Saethre-Chotzen, and 65% in Muenke patients.[55,56]

Table 44-6   Unique Differences in Syndromic Craniosynostosis

Syndrome	Secondary Findings
Apert	Symphalangism and syndactyly of fingers and toes
Crouzon	No hand/foot anomalies
Crouzon with acanthosis nigricans	No hand/foot anomalies, acanthosis nigricans
Pfeiffer	Broad thumbs and great toes, brachysyndactyly, types 2 and 3 have neurologic disorders
Muenke	Flattened cheekbones but minimal midfacial hypoplasia, 5% with megalencephaly, carpal/tarsal fusions
Saethre-Chotzen	Small, malformed ears, broad thumbs/toes, syndactyly of digits 2 and 3 in the hand, low frontal hairline, prominent helical crus, minimal maxillary hypoplasia

Table 44-7   Apert Syndrome Timeline for Care

Age	Treatment
Birth	Evaluation by craniofacial surgeon, geneticist, neonatologist, and hand surgeon; tracheostomy if there is an airway obstruction
1-3 mo	Evaluation by audiologist
3-6 mo	Thumb separation (if needed)
6-12 mo	Border digit separation (if needed)
9-12 mo	Calvarial vault remodeling, cleft palate repair
12-18 mo	Inner digit separation (if needed)
<2-3 yr	Evaluation by pediatric dentist
5-7 yr	Toe separation (if needed)
6-10 yr	LeFort III advancement by distraction if: • A tracheostomy is in place • There is obstructive sleep apnea requiring continuous positive airway pressure • There are strong psychological grounds for aesthetic improvement
8-11 yr	Orthodontic intervention
Adulthood	LeFort III advancement or orthognathic surgery, frontal cranioplasty, rhinoplasty

---

Box 44-1   Whitaker Classification for Craniofacial Surgery Results

I   Excellent, no revisions necessary
II   Satisfactory, soft tissue revision only
III   Marginal, bony irregularities present, requiring structural revision procedure
IV   Unacceptable, repeat original procedure

LeFort III Advancement

One of the most acutely threatening problems with syndromic craniosynostoses is airway obstruction caused by midfacial hypoplasia. This is a common finding in patients with Apert, Crouzon, Crouzon with acanthosis nigricans, and Pfeiffer syndromes. Many of these patients require tracheostomies early in life, which is associated with high morbidity and an increased burden of care; it is also costly. In selected patients with tracheostomies, advancing the midface can open the airway and lead to earlier decannulation.

LeFort III advancement also corrects the concave facial profile and the proptosis. It improves the dental occlusion and the relationship between the upper and lower jaws. LeFort III procedures performed earlier in life substitute for the absent or inadequate growth in these syndromic patients. Therefore repeat advancement procedures are common until maturity. Bony distraction with either internal or rigid external distraction devices allows advancement of the midface in multiple directions and for an indefinite distance.

Technique for LeFort III Advancement

The periosteum overlying the maxilla and zygoma is elevated through an intraoral upper vestibular incision. The maxilla is released from the pterygoid muscle posteriorly. The orbits are dissected through a coronal approach to allow osteotomies of the zygomaticofrontal suture, lateral orbital wall, orbital floor, medial orbital wall, and nasofrontal junction. After the attachments of the masseter muscle are dissected, the zygomatic arches are osteotomized. A forked osteotome is used to separate the septum from the cranial base. With careful manipulation the entire LeFort III is then mobilized (Fig. 44-20).

For rigid external distraction devices, distracting plates are secured to the maxillae and connected to transoral extensions to apply anterior pull through an external frame. Alternatively, specialized transnasal hooks can be attached to the nasal vestibule region of the maxilla for distraction, thus keeping the mouth free of apparatus. A cranial halo or frame is secured to the skull and attached to the maxillary distraction connections with wires (Fig. 44-21). Specific protocols are followed for latency, distraction, and consolidation, resulting in adequate correction (Fig. 44-22).

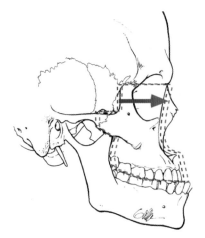

Fig. 44-20   LeFort III advancement.

Monobloc

Sometimes simultaneous advancement of the midface, supraorbital rim, and forehead is desired. Advancement of these facial features in one operation is called a monobloc advancement (Fig. 44-23).[57] There is controversy over monobloc advancement because the intracranial space is exposed to the nonsterile nasopharynx, mouth, and external environment, which markedly increases the infection rate. However, the risks are reduced if slow distraction is used. The expansion of the brain follows the distraction, eliminating the potential intracranial space that is prone to infection.[58]

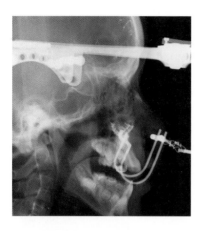

Fig. 44-21　Lateral cephalogram of patient with Apert syndrome with a rigid external distraction device for LeFort III advancement.

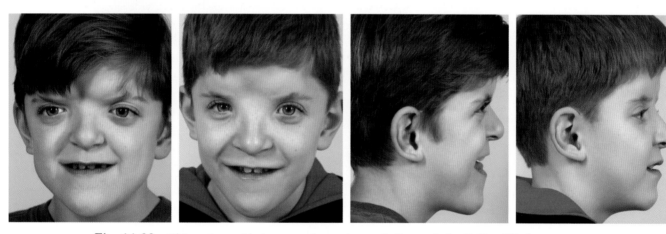

Fig. 44-22　This patient with Apert syndrome is seen before and after LeFort III advancement.

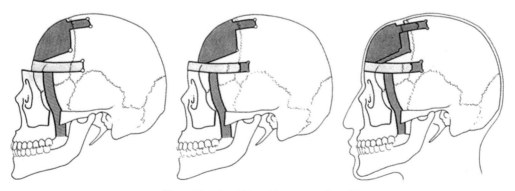

Fig. 44-23　Monobloc procedure.[57]

PHARYNGEAL ARCH SYNDROMES

HEMIFACIAL MICROSOMIA

Hemifacial microsomia is a relatively common birth defect, ranking second behind cleft lip and palate. Although abnormal development of the first and second pharyngeal arches has been identified as the cause of hemifacial microsomia, no chromosomal abnormality has been discovered. Hemifacial microsomia involves underdevelopment of one side of the face (Fig. 44-24). In rare cases it can be bilateral. The condition can vary from extremely mild to severe. Characteristics common to hemifacial microsomia include mandibular hypoplasia, maxillary distortion, orbital dystopia, auricular anomalies, facial nerve weakness, soft tissue deficiency, and skeletal anomalies, especially vertebral (Fig. 44-25). Less common cardiac, neurologic, gastrointestinal, renal, and pulmonary system anomalies have been described.

The manifestations of hemifacial microsomia can be categorized by using the acronym OMENS-Plus, which stands for *orbit*, *mandible*, *ear*, *nerve*, *soft tissue*, *plus* other systemic findings.[58] Orbital distortion can be classified by size and position. Mandibular changes follow the Pruzansky classification[59] (Box 44-2). Auricular changes include microtia and anotia. The facial nerve is separated into upper and lower divisions and should be examined for weakness. Soft tissue deficiency is common in hemifacial microsomia. Patients should also be screened for anomalies such as ventricular septal defects, vertebral anomalies, and renal malformations[58,60,61] (Box 44-3).

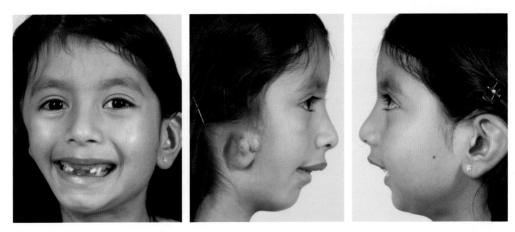

Fig. 44-24   This girl has right hemifacial microsomia with normal orbits, a small, short mandible, right microtia, a normal facial nerve, and severe soft tissue deficiency.

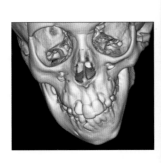
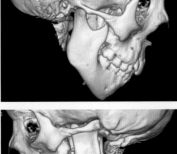
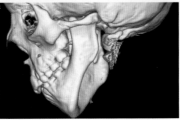
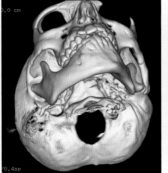
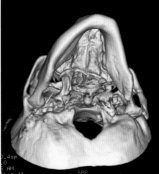

Fig. 44-25   Three-dimensional CT scans of a patient with left hemifacial microsomia.

Box 44-2   Modified Pruzansky Classification of Mandibular Changes

---

I   All mandibular and TMJ components are present and normal in shape, but hypoplastic to a variable degree.

IIA   The mandibular ramus, condyle, and TMJ are present but hypoplastic and abnormal in shape.

IIB   The mandibular ramus is hypoplastic and markedly abnormal in form and location, being medial and anterior. There is no articulation with the temporal bone.

III   The mandibular ramus, condyle, and TMJ are absent. The lateral pterygoid muscle and temporalis, if present, are not attached to the mandibular remnant.

Box 44-3   OMENS-Plus Classification for Hemifacial Microsomia

---

O0: Normal
O1: Abnormal size
O2: Abnormal position
O3: Both abnormal size and position

M0: Normal
M1: Decreased size
M2A: Mandible is small and ramus is short, but TMJ in position
M2B: Mandible is small and ramus is short, and TMJ displaced with hypoplastic condyle
M3: Complete absence of ramus, glenoid fossa, and TMJ

E0: Normal
E1: Minor hypoplasia
E2: Absence of external auditory canal with variable hypoplasia of concha
E3: Malpositioned lobule and absent auricle

N0: Normal
N1: Temporal and zygomatic branch weakness
N2: Buccal, mandibular, and cervical branch weakness
N3: Weakness of all branches of facial nerve

S0: Normal
S1: Minimal soft tissue deficiency
S2: Moderate soft tissue deficiency
S3: Severe soft tissue deficiency

Plus
- Macrostomia
- Skeletal (scoliosis, hemivertebrae/vertebral anomaly, rib anomaly, absent anomalous thumb, anomalous limb, congenital hip deformity)
- Cardiac (murmur, VSD, ASD)
- CNS (hydrocephaly, hemiparesis, microcephaly/partial anencephaly)
- GI (Bilateral inguinal hernia)
- Renal (size discrepancy)
- Pulmonary (tracheoesophageal fistula)

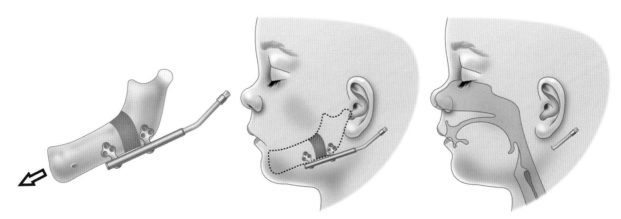

Fig. 44-26   Mandibular distraction osteogenesis. (Courtesy of the Royal Children's Hospital, Victoria, Australia.)

TREATMENT

Hemifacial microsomia patients often need auricular construction. The treatment of choice is repair with an autologous costochondral construct. In suitable cases external auditory canals can be constructed if they are missing. Bone-anchored hearing aids can improve hearing in patients with conductive hearing loss.

Mandibular atrophy or asymmetry can be repaired when the child reaches dental and mandibular maturity. Techniques include bilateral sagittal split osteotomy and distraction osteogenesis (Fig. 44-26). In particular instances, especially if the condyle is minimal or extremely medially displaced, the condyle-ramus unit is constructed with a costochondral graft. With severe mandibular hypoplasia a free vascularized flap may be required, often a fibular flap.

If the facial nerve is weak, the patient can undergo physical therapy. In more severe cases, treatment involves facial reanimation procedures with free gracilis muscular flaps—innervated by cross-facial nerve grafts or grafts from the nerve to the masseter. Botulinum toxin injections contralateral to the affected side can improve symmetry, especially if the mandibular branch is involved.

Soft tissue weakness is difficult to address. Attempts at correction include onlay bone grafts and parascapular free flaps. Techniques in fat grafting have become more established, making it a popular and effective tool for filling facial defects. However, transferred fat still behaves as it would in its original donor site. In children, consideration should be given to hypertrophy of the adipocytes as the child matures or increases in weight.

TREACHER COLLINS SYNDROME

Treacher Collins syndrome affects the middle and lower thirds of the face. The condition is embryologically linked to malformation of the first and second pharyngeal arches but facial nerve function is intact. Common findings include: hypoplasia of the zygomas (89%), micrognathia (78%), microgenia, coloboma of the lower eyelid (69%), absent eyelashes in the medial third of the lower eyelid (53%), downward slanting eyes, microtia (36%), cleft palate (35%), choanal atresia, and hearing loss (40% to 50%).[62]

Three genes are linked to Treacher Collins syndrome. *TCOF1* (5q32) is associated with 70% to 90% of Treacher Collins syndrome and is autosomal dominant. The rest are related to *POLR1D* (13q12.2), which is autosomal dominant, and *POLR1C* (6p21.1), which is autosomal recessive. Sporadic mutations are found in 60% of all Treacher Collins syndrome patients.[62]

Treatment

The chronology of care for Treacher Collins syndrome patients is based on urgency and structural maturation. Airway obstruction is the first priority, and tracheostomy is sometimes necessary. Unlike most nonsyndromic Robin sequence patients, in Treacher Collins syndrome patients the mandible does not exhibit catch-up growth. Early infant mandibular distraction osteogenesis has been used to advance the mandible and expand the posterior pharyngeal space. This can avoid early tracheostomy in some severe cases.

After maturity, bimaxillary orthognathic surgery and advancement genioplasty are usually required to restore a level dental occlusion and facial aesthetics.

Treatment of the eyelid usually begins at an early age with repair of lower eyelid colobomas. In early childhood, tarsoconjunctival flaps can be used to add tissue to the lower eyelid. Lateral canthopexy corrects the downward slanting palpebral fissures (Fig. 44-27).

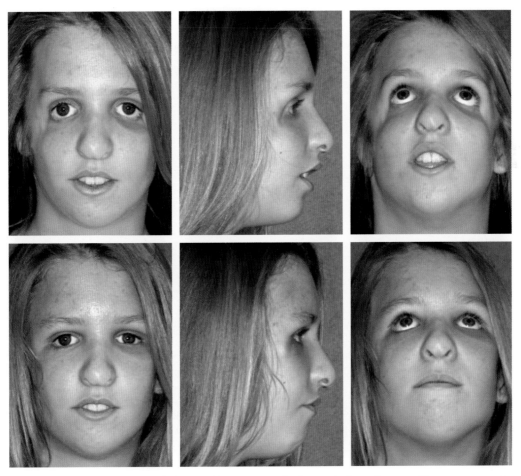

Fig. 44-27   This girl with Treacher Collins sydrome is seen before and after orbitomaxillary augmentation, a subperiosteal midface lift, and canthoplasties.

Hypoplasia of the zygoma (Fig. 44-28) along the Tessier 6, 7, and 8 facial cleft lines can be corrected with autologous bone grafts, often with use of calvarial bone. Later procedures include auricular construction using costochondral constructs and malar implants with porous plastic prostheses or autologous bone (Fig. 44-29).

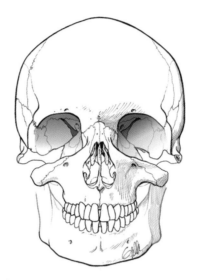

Fig. 44-28 Hypoplastic zygoma in a patient with Treacher Collins syndrome.

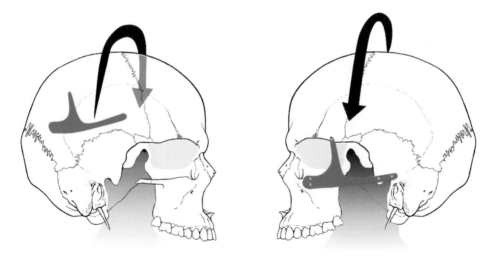

Fig. 44-29 Calvarial bone graft to augment hypoplastic zygoma in a patient with Treacher Collins syndrome.

KEY POINTS

- Nonsyndromic craniosynostosis must be differentiated from the more common deformational plagiocephaly/brachycephaly.
- Craniosynostosis can cause predictable calvarial deformity, increased intracranial pressure, and neurodevelopmental delay.
- Correction of craniosynostosis involves release of the affected suture and restoration of normal anatomy.
- Hemifacial microsomia, a disorder of pharyngeal arches 1 and 2, is classified through the OMENS-Plus classification system.
- There is no genetic cause identified for hemifacial microsomia.
- Treacher Collins syndrome, a disorder of pharyngeal arches 1 and 2, is caused by genetic mutations *TCOF1* (5q32), *POLR1D* (13q12.2), and *POLR1C* (6p21.1).
- Pharyngeal arch syndromes are treated in two ways: With airway procedures such as tracheostomy and/or early mandibular distraction, and using secondary procedures to protect and restore normal anatomy and function.
- Syndromic craniosynostosis mutations are identified as *FGFR1, FGFR2, FGFR3, TWIST,* and *MSX2.* Common findings in these syndromes are complex craniosynostosis, midfacial hypoplasia, airway obstruction, and hearing loss.
- Each craniosynostosis syndrome has unique features:
  - Apert syndrome has symphalangism and syndactyly of digits
  - Crouzon syndrome has no obvious hand findings
  - Crouzon syndrome with acanthosis nigricans has skin changes and jugular foraminal stenosis
  - Pfeiffer syndrome has broad toes and thumbs
  - Muenke syndrome has minimal midfacial hypoplasia and carpal/tarsal fusions
  - Saethre-Chotzen syndrome has upper eyelid ptosis, ear anomalies, low hairline cutaneous syndactyly of the second and third digits, and minimal midfacial hypoplasia
- Treatment of syndromic craniosynostosis includes airway procedures (such as tracheostomy, early LeFort III, later LeFort III, or other maxillary/mandibular osteotomies), calvarial reconstruction, and procedures to repair syndactyly, macrodactyly, dental abnormalities, malocclusion, hearing loss, and strabismus.

REFERENCES

1. Moore KL, Persaud TVN, Torchia MG. The Developing Human: Clinically Oriented Embryology, ed 9. Philadelphia: Elsevier, 2013.
2. Carlson BM. Human Embryology and Developmental Biology, ed 5. Philadelphia: Elsevier, 2013.
3. Lajeunie E, Le Merrer M, Bonaiti-Pellie C, et al. Genetic study of nonsyndromic coronal craniosynostosis. Am J Med Genet 55:500-504, 1995.
4. Renier D, Sainte-Rose C, Marchac D, Hirsch JF. Intracranial pressure in craniostenosis. J Neurosurg 57:370-377, 1982.
5. Shillito J Jr, Matson DD. Craniosynostosis: a review of 519 surgical patients. Pediatrics 41:829-853, 1968.
6. Hunter AG, Rudd NL. Craniosynostosis. I. Sagittal synostosis: its genetics and associated clinical findings in 214 patients who lacked involvement of the coronal suture(s). Teratology 14:185-193, 1976.
7. Rosenberg JB, Tepper OM, Medow NB. Strabismus in craniosynostosis. J Pediatr Ophthalmol Strabismus 50:140-148, 2012.

8. Lee SJ, Dondey J, Greensmith AL, et al. The effect of fronto-orbital advancement on strabismus on children with unicoronal synostosis. Ann Plast Surg 61:178-180, 2008.

9. Kweldam CF, van der Vlugt JJ, van der Meulen JJ. The incidence of craniosynostosis in the Netherlands, 1997-2007. J Plast Reconstr Aesthet Surg 64:583-588, 2011.

10. van der Meulen J. Metopic synostosis. Childs Nerv Syst 28:1359-1367, 2012.

11. Di Rocco F, Arnaud E, Renier D. Evolution in the frequency of nonsyndromic craniosynostosis. J Neurosurg Pediatr 4:21-25, 2009.

12. Ploplys EA, Hopper RA, Muzaffar AR, et al. Comparison of computed tomographic imaging measurements with clinical findings in children with unilateral lambdoid synostosis. Plast Reconstr Surg 123:300-309, 2009.

13. American Academy of Pediatrics AAP Task Force on Infant Positioning and SIDS: Positioning and SIDS. Pediatrics 89:1120-1126, 1992.
    Prone positioning was implicated as a significant risk factor in sudden infant death syndrome; therefore lateral and supine positioning were recommended when putting infants to sleep.

14. Kane AA, Mitchell LE, Craven KP, et al. Observations on a recent increase in plagiocephaly without synostosis. Pediatrics 97:877-885, 1996.

15. Boston Children's Hospital. Craniosynostosis, 2011. Available at *www.childrenshospital.org/az/Site2130/main pageS2130P0.html.*

16. Rogers GF, Oh AK, Mulliken JB. The role of congenital muscular torticollis in the development of deformational plagiocephaly. Plast Reconstr Surg 123:643-652, 2009.

17. Gault DT, Renier D, Marchac D, et al. Intracranial pressure and intracranial volume in children with craniosynostosis. Plast Reconstr Surg 90:377-381, 1992.
    In this study, 20% of children with craniosynostosis were identified with elevated intracranial pressure, which correlates positively with the number of sutures fused.

18. Siddiqi SN, Posnick JC, Buncic R, et al. The detection and management of intracranial hypertension after initial suture release and decompression for craniofacial dysostosis syndromes. Neurosurgery 36:703-708; discussion 708-709, 1995.

19. Thompson DN, Harkness W, Jones B, et al. Subdural intracranial pressure monitoring in craniosynostosis: its role in surgical management. Childs Nerv Syst 11:269-275, 1995.

20. Da Costa AC, Anderson VA, Savarirayan R, et al. Neurodevelopmental functioning of infants with untreated single-suture craniosynostosis during early infancy. Childs Nerv Syst 28:869-877, 2012.
    Extensive neurodevelopmental examinations in 56 patients with unoperated single-suture craniosynostosis demonstrated an association with increased developmental delay in infancy, especially motor function.

21. Jane JA, Edgerton MT, Futrell JW, et al. Immediate correction of sagittal synostosis. J Neurosurg 49:705-710, 1978.

22. Greensmith AL, Holmes AD, Lo P, Maxiner W, Heggie AA, Meara JG. Complete correction of severe scaphocephaly: the Melbourne method of total vault remodeling. Plast Reconstr Surg 121:1300-1310, 2008.

23. Lauritzen CG, Davis C, Ivarsson A, et al. The evolving role of springs in craniofacial surgery: the first 100 clinical cases. Plast Reconstr Surg 121:545-554, 2008.

24. Pyle J, Glazier S, Couture D, et al. Spring-assisted surgery-a surgeon's manual for the manufacture and utilization of springs in craniofacial surgery. J Craniofac Surg 20:1962-1968, 2009.

25. Persing JA, Babler WJ, Nagorsky MJ, et al. Skull expansion in experimental craniosynostosis. Plast Reconstr Surg 78:594-603, 1986.

26. Steinbacher DM, Skirpan J, Puchała J, et al. Expansion of the posterior cranial vault using distraction osteogenesis. Plast Reconstr Surg 127:792-801, 2011.

27. Rozbruch SR, Ilizarov S. Limb Lengthening and Reconstructive Surgery. New York: Informa Healthcare, 2007.

28. Barone CM, Jimenez DF. Endoscopic craniectomy for early correction of craniosynostosis. Plast Reconstr Surg 104:1965-1973; discussion 1974-1975, 1999.
    This landmark paper introduced a minimally invasive technique for removal of craniosynostotic sutures with an endoscope. The authors demonstrated the safety and efficacy of this technique in treating craniosynostosis.

29. Abbott MM, Rogers GF, Proctor MR, et al. Cost of treating sagittal synostosis in the first year of life. J Craniofac Surg 23:88-93, 2012.

30. Jabs EW, Muller U, Li X, et al. A mutation in the homeodomain of the human MSX2 gene in a family affected with autosomal dominant craniosynostosis. Cell 75:443-450, 1993.

31. Bochukova EG, Roscioli T, Hedges DJ, et al. Rare mutations of FGFR2 causing Apert syndrome: identification of the first partial gene deletion, and an Alu element insertion from a new subfamily. Hum Mutat 30:204-211, 2009.

32. Reardon W, Winter RM, Rutland P, et al. Mutations in the fibroblast growth factor receptor 2 gene cause Crouzon syndrome. Nat Genet 8:98-103, 1994.

33. Mulliken JB, Steinberger D, Kunze S, et al. Molecular diagnosis of bilateral coronal synostosis. Plast Reconstr Surg 104:1603-1615, 1999.

34. Muenke M, Schell U, Hehr A, et al. A common mutation in the fibroblast growth factor receptor 1 gene in Pfeiffer syndrome. Nat Genet 8:269-274, 1994.

35. Genetics Home Reference. FGFR1, 2008. Available at *www.ghr.nlm.nih.gov/gene/FGFR1.*

36. Agochukwu NB, Doherty ES, Muenke M. Muenke syndrome. In Pagon RA, Bird TD, Dolan CR, eds. GeneReviews. Seattle: University of Washington, 1993.

37. Paznekas WA, Cunningham ML, Howard TD, et al. Genetic heterogeneity of Saethre-Chotzen syndrome, due to TWIST and FGFR mutations. Am J Hum Genet 62:1370-1380, 1998.

38. Sculerati N, Gottlieb MD, Zimbler MS, et al. Airway management in children with major craniofacial anomalies. Laryngoscope 108:1806-1812, 1998.

   In a large population, this study is one of the first to quantify breathing difficulties in patients with specific craniofacial disorders. Treatment protocols were discussed specific to each diagnosis.

39. Lowe LH, Booth TN, Joglar JM, et al. Midface anomalies in children. Radiographics 20:907-922; quiz 1106-1107, 1112, 2000.

40. Nargozian C. The airway in patients with craniofacial abnormalities. Paediatr Anaesth 14:53-59, 2004.

41. Agochukwu NB, Solomon BD, Muenke M. Impact of genetics on the diagnosis and clinical management of syndromic craniosynostoses. Childs Nerv Syst 28:1447-1463, 2012.

42. Desai U, Rosen H, Mulliken JB, et al. Audiologic findings in Pfeiffer syndrome. J Craniofac Surg 21:1411-1418, 2010.

43. Rosen H, Andrews BT, Meara JG, et al. Audiologic findings in Saethre-Chotzen syndrome. Plast Reconstr Surg 127:2014-2020, 2011.

44. Upton J. Apert syndrome. Classification and pathologic anatomy of limb anomalies. Clin Plast Surg 18:321-355, 1991.

45. Fearon JA, Podner C. Apert syndrome: evaluation of a treatment algorithm. Plast Reconstr Surg 131:132-142, 2013.

46. Renier D, Lajeunie E, Arnaud E, et al. Management of craniosynostoses. Childs Nerv Syst 16:645-658, 2000.

47. Lajeunie E, Bonaventure J, El Ghouzzi V, et al. Monozygotic twins with Crouzon syndrome: concordance for craniosynostosis and discordance for thumb duplication. Am J Med Genet 91:159-160, 2000.

48. Renier D, Arnaud E, Cinalli G, et al. Prognosis for mental function in Apert's syndrome. J Neurosurg 85:66-72, 1996.

49. Cohen MM Jr. Pfeiffer syndrome update, clinical subtypes, and guidelines for differential diagnosis. Am J Med Genet 45:300-307, 1993.

50. Robin NH, Falk MJ, Haldeman-Englert CR. FGFR-related craniosynostosis syndromes. In Pagon RA, Bird TD, Dolan CR, eds. GeneReviews. Seattle: University of Washington, 1993.

51. Stoler JM, Rosen H, Desai U, et al. Cleft palate in Pfeiffer syndrome. J Craniofac Surg 20:1375-1377, 2009.

52. Muenke M, Gripp KW, McDonald-McGinn DM, et al. A unique point mutation in the fibroblast growth factor receptor 3 gene (FGFR3) defines a new craniosynostosis syndrome. Am J Hum Genet 60:555-564, 1997.

53. Gripp KW, McDonald-McGinn DM, Gaudenz K, et al. Identification of a genetic cause for isolated unilateral coronal synostosis: a unique mutation in the fibroblast growth factor receptor 3. J Pediatr 132:714-716, 1998.

54. Whitaker LA, Bartlett SP, Schut L, et al. Craniosynostosis: an analysis of the timing, treatment, and complications in 164 consecutive patients. Plast Reconstr Surg 80:195-212, 1987.

55. Wong GB, Kakulis EG, Mulliken JB. Analysis of fronto-orbital advancement for Apert, Crouzon, Pfeiffer, and Saethre-Chotzen syndromes. Plast Reconstr Surg 105:2314-2323, 2000.

56. Ridgway EB, Wu JK, Sullivan SR, et al. Craniofacial growth in patients with FGFR3Pro250Arg mutation after fronto-orbital advancement in infancy. J Craniofac Surg 22:455-461, 2011.

57. Ortiz-Monasterio F, del Campo AF, Carrillo A. Advancement of the orbits and the midface in one piece, combined with frontal repositioning, for the correction of Crouzon's deformities. Plast Reconstr Surg 61:507-516, 1978.

58. Horgan JE, Padwa BL, LaBrie RA, et al. OMENS-Plus: analysis of craniofacial and extracraniofacial anomalies in hemifacial microsomia. Cleft Palate Craniofac J 32:405-412, 1995.

This landmark paper is the sequel to the original OMENS paper that provided a classification system for hemifacial microsomia. This study revealed an incidence of extracraniofacial anomalies in 55.4% of HFM patients, thus modifying the classification system to OMENS-Plus.

59. Kaban LB, Padwa BL, Mulliken JB. Surgical correction of mandibular hypoplasia in hemifacial microsomia: the case for treatment in early childhood. J Oral Maxillofac Surg 56:628-638, 1998.

60. Vento AR, LaBrie RA, Mulliken JB. The O.M.E.N.S. classification of hemifacial microsomia. Cleft Palate Craniofac J 28:68-76; discussion 77, 1991.

61. Gougoutas AJ, Singh DJ, Low DW, et al. Hemifacial microsomia: clinical features and pictographic representations of the OMENS classification system. Plast Reconstr Surg 120:112e-120e, 2007.

62. Katsanis SH, Jabs EW. Treacher Collins syndrome. In Pagon RA, Bird TD, Dolan CR, et al, eds. GeneReviews. Seattle: University of Washington, 1993.

45

Cleft Lip and Palate Repair

Carolyn R. Rogers ▪ *John G. Meara*

Clefts of the lip and palate have been documented since ancient times, but until modern embryology developed as a field, the nature of clefting was poorly understood. For example, in some ancient cultures a cleft lip was thought to represent the presence of evil spirits. Although surgical correction of cleft lip was performed as early as 390 BC in China, many ancient cultures abandoned children with orofacial clefts. An embryologic, rather than mystical, basis for clefting was first suggested in 1600 AD.[1] The abnormal anatomy in a cleft lip or palate is now better understood, which has facilitated many refinements in surgical treatment of cleft lip and palate over the past six decades. Involvement of orthodontists and speech and language pathologists to create comprehensive cleft teams has improved immediate and long-term care. Afflicted children, who were marginalized in previous times, are now often provided successful surgical correction and better opportunities to live normal, integrated, and productive lives.

EMBRYOLOGY AND ANATOMY

The face begins to form early in embryologic development, arising from paired mandibular and maxillary prominences and a single midline frontonasal prominence emerging around the primitive stomodeum. During the fourth week after conception, nasal pits, or *placodes*, form in the frontonasal prominence. Medial and lateral nasal processes form around these pits. The medial nasal and maxillary processes fuse to form the upper lip and primary palate by the sixth week postconception. Disrupted fusion results in clefting of the lip and alveolus.

Palatal shelves form from the maxillary prominences during the seventh week postconception. These vertically oriented shelves elevate to a horizontal position by the ninth week postconception. They fuse with each other to form the secondary palate and fuse with the primary palate. Failure of elevation and fusion of these shelves results in a cleft palate.[2]

In a normal upper lip, the *orbicularis oris* muscle passes from modiolus to philtrum (see Fig. 1-20). At the philtrum, muscle fibers decussate with fibers from the contralateral side, providing architecture for the philtral ridges and dimple. The major blood supply to the upper lip arises from branches of the paired facial arteries, primarily the superior labial branches. The facial artery continues as the lateral nasal artery to supply to the nasal tip (see Fig. 1-9). The columella is supplied by paired columellar arteries, which represent an anastomosis between the superior labial and dorsal nasal arteries. Upper lip surface anatomy reflects its embryologic formation and underlying muscular anatomy (Fig. 45-1).

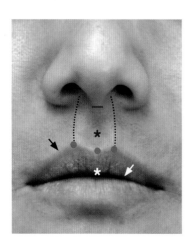

Fig. 45-1   The surface anatomy of the upper lip. The philtral columns *(black dotted lines)*, philtral dimple *(purple star)*, columellar-labial junction *(blue line)*, height of the Cupid's bow *(red dot)*, depth or low point of the Cupid's bow *(green dot)*, median tubercle *(white star)*, white roll *(black arrow)*, and red line or wet-dry junction *(white arrow)*.

Fig. 45-2   Anatomy of a unilateral cleft lip. The orbicularis oris muscle is abnormally oriented toward the alar base laterally and the columella medially. The anterior nasal spine, caudal septum, and columella are displaced toward the noncleft side. The lower lateral cartilage and alar base are displaced inferolaterally on the cleft side.

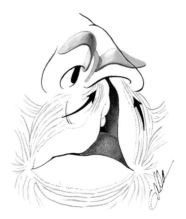

In cases of cleft lip, the tissue is distorted rather than deficient. In a unilateral cleft the nasal tip and ala are displaced inferolaterally, corresponding to deformity of the underlying lower lateral cartilage. The lip is divided where the philtral ridge should be. Orbicularis oris muscle fibers are oriented toward the alar base lateral to the cleft and toward the columella medial to the cleft. The anterior nasal spine and caudal septum deviate away from the cleft and the midseptum bows toward the cleft side. The superior labial artery is discontinuous and oriented along the cleft (Fig. 45-2). In a bilateral cleft lip, orbicularis oris muscle fibers are oriented toward both alar bases laterally and the prolabium has little to no muscle tissue. The superior labial arteries supply lateral lip elements, whereas the columellar and septal arteries supply the prolabium.[3]

PALATE ANATOMY

The hard palate is formed by paired palatine processes of the maxilla and paired palatine bones, articulating with the vomer (see Fig. 1-7). The incisive foramen is located in a midline location just posterior to the alveolus at the junction of the primary and secondary palate (Fig. 45-3).

Structures anterior to the incisive foramen are considered the primary palate, and structures posterior to the incisive foramen are considered the secondary palate. The soft palate is a muscular sling formed by the paired levator veli palatini, palatopharyngeus, palatoglossus, and uvular muscles innervated by the pharyngeal branch of the vagus nerve; it is reinforced by the broad aponeurosis of the tensor veli palatini innervated by the medial pterygoid branch of the mandibular nerve. These muscles work with the superior constrictor to form the velopharyngeal sphincter. Palatal and velopharyngeal blood supply comes from branches of the paired internal maxillary arteries, recurrent pharyngeal arteries, ascending pharyngeal arteries, and ascending palatine arteries. The soft palate and velopharyngeal sphincter muscles have a rich blood supply from branches of these arteries. The greater palatine branches of the internal maxillary artery provide the major blood supply to the hard palate mucoperiosteum.

Cleft palate involves secondary palate structures. The maxillary and palatine bones are separated at the midline, resulting in a large oronasal fistula. The tensor veli palatini aponeuroses, levator veli palatini muscles, and palatopharyngeus muscles are disoriented parallel to the cleft, inserting on the posterior hard palate (Fig. 45-4). In cleft lip and palate, the defect extends along the junction of the primary and secondary palate, resulting in an alveolar gap. If the alveolus is cleft, the lateral incisors are frequently absent and other dental anomalies are common, such as supernumerary teeth.

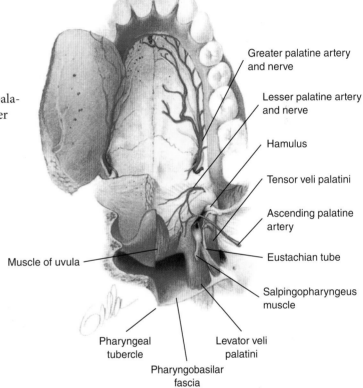

Fig. 45-3   Palatal anatomy, showing the greater palatine neurovascular bundle emerging from the greater palatine foramen.

Greater palatine artery and nerve

Lesser palatine artery and nerve

Hamulus

Tensor veli palatini

Ascending palatine artery

Eustachian tube

Salpingopharyngeus muscle

Levator veli palatini

Pharyngobasilar fascia

Pharyngeal tubercle

Muscle of uvula

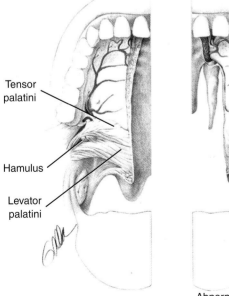
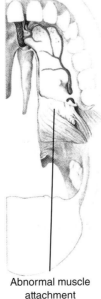

Tensor palatini

Hamulus

Levator palatini

Abnormal muscle attachment

Fig. 45-4   A comparison of normal and abnormal palate anatomy. *Left,* Normal anatomy of the hard and soft palate. The soft palate musculature is oriented toward the midline to complete the velopharyngeal sphincter. The greater palatine artery exits the greater palatine foramen to supply the hard palate. The lesser palatine artery, exiting just posterior to it, contributes to the soft palate. *Right,* Abnormal anatomy of a cleft palate. The vomer is visualized in the cleft. The soft palate musculature inserts on the posterior edge of the hard palate.

CLASSIFICATION

CLEFT LIP

Cleft lip is classified as unilateral or bilateral and further categorized by the extent of the defect. Complete cleft lip involves a separation extending from the nasal floor through the lip and alveolar ridge. In an incomplete cleft lip, there is a connection between the lip elements, ranging from a thin skin bridge (often referred to as *Simonart's band*) to a substantial musculocutaneous connection. Lesser forms of incomplete cleft lip, as defined by Yuzuriha and Mulliken,[4] involve smaller degrees of disruption of the vermilion-cutaneous junction at the peak of the Cupid's bow and the orbicularis oris muscle (Fig. 45-5).

CLEFT PALATE

Cleft palate is often described using the Veau classification,[5] which allows clinicians to communicate the anatomic nature of the defect (Fig. 45-6).

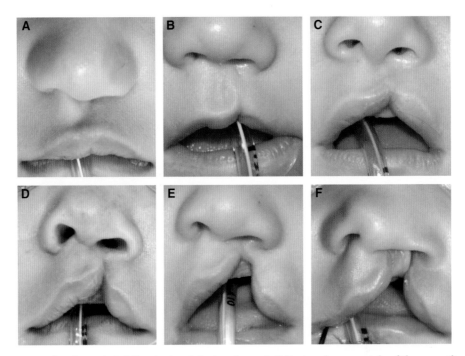

Fig. 45-5 Forms of unilateral cleft lip. **A,** A minimicroform cleft lip involves a notch of the vermilion-cutaneous junction without elevation of the peak of the Cupid's bow. **B,** A microform cleft lip has a disruption of the free margin of the lip with less than 3 mm elevation of the peak of the Cupid's bow. **C,** A minor form cleft lip is a disruption of the free margin of the lip with 3 to 5 mm elevation of the peak of the Cupid's bow. **D,** An incomplete cleft lip involves disruption of the free margin of the lip with greater than 5 mm elevation of the peak of the Cupid's bow. **E,** A wide incomplete cleft lip has a disruption of most of the lip with a small cutaneous band at the nasal floor. **F,** A complete cleft lip is has a disruption of the medial and lateral lip elements resulting in a gap extending from the nasal floor through the free margin of the lip. Note the presence of nasal deformity in all forms of clefting, even microform.

The Kernahan striped-Y system is another frequently used classification for describing cleft palate deformities[6] (Fig. 45-7).

The Kernahan classification addresses the submucous cleft palate, whereas the Veau classification does not. In submucous clefting, which is a lesser form of cleft palate, there is a soft palatal muscular diastasis but the palatal mucosa is intact. The diastasis may be visualized as a bluish zona pellucida or furrow in the soft palate. Other findings may include a bifid uvula and/or a notch in the posterior hard palate. These three findings together constitute Calnan's triad.[7] This type of cleft is often diagnosed during evaluation for abnormal speech.

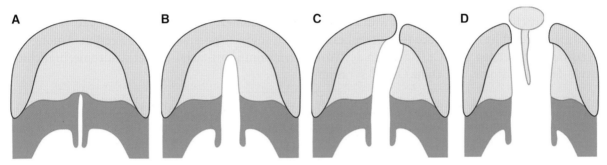

Fig. 45-6   Veau classification of cleft palate. **A,** Veau I is a soft palate cleft only. **B,** Veau II is a soft and hard palate cleft posterior to the incisive foramen. **C,** Veau III is a unilateral cleft lip and palate extending through the alveolus and the hard and soft palates. **D,** Veau IV is a bilateral cleft lip extending through the alveolus bilaterally and the hard and soft palates.

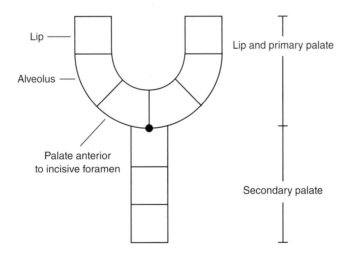

Fig. 45-7   The Kernahan striped-Y classification of the cleft palate. The striped-Y classification allows easy documentation of the involved areas of the lip and palate with stippling of the corresponding location on the Y. (From Kernahan DA. The striped Y—a symbolic classification for cleft lip and palate. Plast Reconstr Surg 47:469-470, 1971.)

EPIDEMIOLOGY

Traditionally, cleft lip (with or without cleft palate) (CL/P) and isolated cleft palate have been considered two separate etiopathogenetic entities,[8] although emerging evidence suggests that the delineation is less distinct.[9,10] In the United States, the estimated prevalence of CL/P is 1 in 940 live births.[11] The condition is twice as common in boys as in girls.[12] The prevalence of CL/P has ethnic heterogeneity, with Asians and Hispanics demonstrating the highest incidence, whites demonstrating intermediate incidence, and blacks manifesting the lowest incidence[13] (Table 45-1).

CL/P is thought to result from a combination of genetic and environmental factors. Environmental factors that are associated with increased risk include maternal smoking, folate deficiency, alcohol consumption, advanced maternal age, and retinoid use. Mutations in multiple candidate genes, such as *IRF6,* Wnt signaling, and *MSX1,* and BMP signaling factors have also been associated with CL/P.[14] The condition is infrequently (10% to 14%) associated with a recognized syndrome,[15,16] but as many as 29% to 45% of patients with a cleft lip have associated anomalies,[15,17] which suggests possible underdetection. Among the syndromes associated with CL/P are Van der Woude syndrome, oro-facial-digital syndrome, branchio-oculo-facial syndrome, and Opitz G/BBB syndrome.[18]

In the United States, the estimated prevalence of isolated cleft palate is 1 in 1570 live births.[11] The condition is twice as common in women and girls[12] and does not have the same ethnic variation that CL/P has (see Table 45-1). Cases of isolated cleft palate are often (12% to 54%) associated with an underlying syndrome,[15,16] and as many as 47% to 72% of isolated cleft palate patients have associated anomalies.[15,17] Among

Table 45-1   Estimated Incidence of Cleft Lip With or Without Cleft Palate and Isolated Cleft Palate in Countries Around the World

Country	Incidence of Cleft Lip ± Palate (Births)	Incidence of Isolated Cleft Palate (Births)
Bolivia	1/440	1/4260
China	1/620	1/4240
Germany	1/720	1/1500
Norway	1/750	1/1800
Argentina	1/810	1/2680
Japan	1/820	1/2200
Brazil	1/840	1/2230
Ecuador	1/1000	1/2370
Finland	1/1000	1/700
England and Wales	1/1620	1/3440
United Arab Emirates	1/2010	1/3150
Australia	1/2480	1/1540
Canada	1/2720	1/1420
South Africa	1/2970	1/5180

Data from World Atlas of Birth Defects, ed 2. Geneva: World Health Organization, 2003.

the 250 or more recognized syndromes associated with cleft palate are 22q deletion spectrum, Stickler syndrome, Cornelia de Lange syndrome, Emanuel syndrome, trisomy 13, Treacher Collins syndrome, and Apert syndrome.[18]

PATIENT EVALUATION AND PREOPERATIVE PLANNING

DIAGNOSIS AND EARLY MANAGEMENT

Cleft lip and palate are increasingly diagnosed prenatally; CLWWCP is well visualized with ultrasound, whereas isolated cleft palate is less frequently diagnosed with ultrasound but may be detected with prenatal MRI. As soon as the diagnosis is made, the expectant mother or newborn infant should be referred to a cleft team for evaluation and counseling.

The concept of team care is one of the most important advances in cleft care in the past several decades. The American Cleft Palate-Craniofacial Association and Cleft Palate Foundation have set standards for designated cleft centers. A cleft team must include a speech and language pathologist, a surgeon trained in cleft lip and palate surgery, and an orthodontist. In addition, to best serve the unique needs of children with cleft lip and palate, the team should have access to practitioners of services in the domains of psychology, social work, psychiatry, audiology, genetics, general and pediatric dentistry, otolaryngology, and pediatrics/primary care.[19]

Many infants with isolated cleft lip are able to breastfeed, but infants with cleft lip and palate or isolated cleft palate often have feeding difficulties early in life. When a cleft palate is present, infants are not able to generate suction because of the large oronasal fistula. These infants are best fed semiupright using cleft feeders such as the SpecialNeeds Feeder (commonly known as the Haberman), Mead Johnson cleft lip/palate nurser, or a Pigeon cleft palate nipple. When possible, feeding instructions for the parents should begin prenatally.

PRESURGICAL ORTHOPEDICS AND LIP ADHESION

Presurgical orthopedic treatment is an essential component of comprehensive care for the patient with a wide complete cleft lip or bilateral cleft lip. Orthopedic devices are designed to bring the displaced alveolar segments or protruding premaxilla into a more normal anatomic position, which means less extensive dissection will be necessary at the time of operation and, when used effectively, the use of such a device often results in the ability to perform a gingivoperiosteoplasty. Presurgical orthopedics measures are initiated in the first month or two of life. Passive appliances, such as removable plates, apply external force on the alveolar segments[20] and are often augmented with lip taping. Nasoalveolar molding is an advanced passive device that employs an intraoral plate with nasal outriggers to shape the lower lateral cartilages and elongate the columella.[21] The Latham device is an active appliance that is fixed intraorally. Screws and elastic chains are used to gradually bring the alveolar segments together[22] (Fig. 45-8).

Lip adhesion is a preliminary surgical procedure that improves alveolar position. This technique can be used if presurgical orthopedics are unavailable or as an adjunct to presurgical orthopedics to improve lip symmetry at the time of formal repair. Lip adhesion is usually performed at 6 to 12 weeks of age and involves closure of skin and oral mucosa. It is important not to manipulate the tissues that will be involved in the future lip repair and to minimize dissection to prevent excessive scarring and distortion, which could compromise the definitive repair.

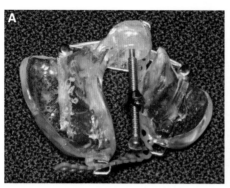
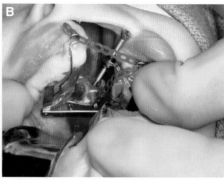

Fig. 45-8   **A,** The Latham appliance is a presurgical orthopedic device consisting of acrylic plates with a screw between the greater and lesser segments in a unilateral cleft (pictured), or between the lateral segments with a chain attached to the premaxilla in a bilateral cleft. **B,** After the device is placed in the operating room, the screw is turned over time, bringing the alveolar segments together. (Courtesy of Stephen Shusterman, DMD, and Veerasathpurush Allareddy, BDS.)

TIMING OF SURGERY

Timing of cleft lip repair varies widely among surgeons. Although cleft lip repair has been attempted in utero, this technique has been abandoned because of the risk of significant morbidity and mortality. Cleft surgeons have historically held to the "rule of 10's" for cleft lip repair: the baby must be at least 10 pounds, 10 weeks of age, and have a hemoglobin of 10 g/dl.[23] A recent survey of bilateral cleft lip practice demonstrated that slightly fewer than 50% of surgeons perform bilateral cleft lip repair on infants who are between 1 and 3 months of age, and approximately 50% perform repair on infants who are between 4 and 6 months of age.[24] Many centers typically perform unilateral cleft lip repair on infants who are between 3 and 5 months of age, or approximately 3 months after a lip adhesion has been performed. For bilateral cleft lip repair, many centers favor later correction on infants who are between 4 and 6 months of age. The benefits of later repair include improved patient safety and the ability to more precisely align anatomic elements.

Timing for cleft palate repair also varies among surgeons. In one study, repair at 6 months of age led to better speech outcomes with fewer compensatory articulations than repair at 12 months.[25] Another study correlated increasing age at repair to velopharyngeal insufficiency requiring corrective surgery, with a major increase when repair was performed on infants who were 13 months or older.[26] One concern with early repair is that manipulation at the younger age more substantially inhibits midfacial growth.[27] The surgeon must balance the potential growth restriction associated with early repair with the potentially poorer speech outcomes associate with late repair. For this reason, most surgeons (85%) perform cleft palate repair on infants who are between 6 and 12 months of age.[28]

ROBIN SEQUENCE

Robin sequence (also called *Pierre Robin sequence* or *syndrome*), defined by the triad of microretrognathia, glossoptosis, and airway obstruction, deserves special mention. Isolated cleft palate is found in 69% to 90% of patients with Robin sequence.[29,30] Robin sequence is often associated with an underlying syndromic diagnosis, most commonly Stickler syndrome, which is present in one third to one half of patients with Robin sequence.[17,31] Other syndromes associated with Robin sequence include 22q deletion spectrum, fetal alcohol syndrome, campomelic dysplasia, Treacher Collins syndrome, and Apert syndrome.

The degree of airway obstruction in Robin sequence is often classified using the Laberge grading system[29]:
- Grade I: Adequate respiration in prone position; able to bottle feed regularly
- Grade II: Adequate respiration in prone position; unable to bottle feed adequately, requiring gavage feeding
- Grade III: Inadequate respiration in prone position requiring intubation; gavage feeding is necessary

Initial management of infants with Robin sequence focuses on lateral and prone positioning to open the airway, and is further assisted if necessary by use of nasopharyngeal airways and gavage feeding. Infants with grade III Robin sequence and some infants with grade II Robin sequence will require a surgical procedure such as mandibular distraction osteogenesis, tongue-lip adhesion, or tracheostomy during infancy to protect the airway. Before either a mandibular distraction or a tongue-lip adhesion, patients require bronchoscopy to rule out a lower airway-based source of obstruction, such as severe laryngomalacia. Airway-based sources of obstruction will not be corrected with distraction osteogenesis or tongue-lip adhesion, therefore tracheostomy should be considered.

For children in whom glossoptosis is determined to be the source of obstruction, first-line treatment involves tongue-lip adhesion. During this procedure, the genioglossus muscle is released, the tongue base is advanced in relation to the mandible, and the ventral surface of the tongue is incised and sutured to the lip; this maneuver maintains the tongue in an anterior position.[32] Some institutions favor mandibular distraction osteogenesis as the first line of treatment, in which an osteotomy is made in the ramus or angle of the mandible, and the mandible is slowly lengthened over a period of 1 to 2 weeks, bringing the mandibular symphysis and body, with the attached tongue musculature, into a more forward position.

Regardless of whether Robin sequence is treated with conservative measures or surgical management, cleft palate repair in this subset of patients should be approached extremely cautiously. Airway problems in the early postoperative period have been reported after cleft palate repair in these patients[33,34]; repair should be delayed if the airway is not clearly secure.

SURGICAL TECHNIQUES

Unilateral Cleft Lip Repair

Early attempts to repair unilateral cleft lip focused on linear closure of labial elements. This approach resulted in a short lip and left the muscle aberrantly oriented. Modern lip repair focuses on lengthening the medial and lateral labial elements and establishing orbicularis oris muscle continuity. Variations of straight-line repair were described by Rose[35] and Thompson,[36] who used angled incisions to lengthen the medial and lateral lip elements. Tennison,[37] Skoog,[38] and Randall[39] lengthened the medial and lateral elements with triangular flaps. In 1957 Millard[40] described *rotation-advancement repair*. With this technique the philtrum and Cupid's bow are rotated into normal position, and a curvilinear scar simulates the philtral ridge. Advancement of the upper lateral lip element maintains favorable rotation and corrects the wide alar base. A C flap elongates the shortened columella (Fig. 45-9). Rotation-advancement repair is adaptable to many anatomical variations in the cleft lip and can be applied to clefts of any severity. The "cut as you go" technique permits incisions to be extended further as needed for tissue mobilization.

Since Millard's original description, variations of the rotation-advancement repair have become the mainstay for unilateral cleft lip repair. Multiple eponymous modifications exist.[41] The differences involve the design of the superior rotation flap and columella, the extent of the incision around the alar base, and handling the vermilion-cutaneous junction. One commonly used modification was described by Mohler[42] and further modified by Cutting and Dayan.[43] The rotation flap incision is carried onto the columella and

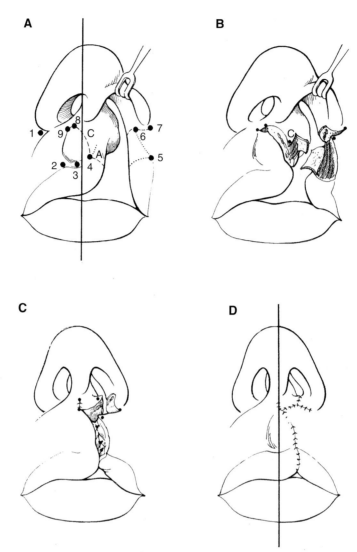

Fig. 45-9   Millard rotation-advancement repair of a unilateral cleft lip. **A,** Markings for the repair. *Point 1:* Alar base of the normal side. *Point 2:* Peak of the Cupid's bow on the normal side. *Point 3:* Low point of the Cupid's bow. *Point 4:* Peak of the Cupid's bow on the medial side of the cleft. The distance from *point 2* to *3* and *point 3* to *4* should be equal. *Point 5:* Peak of the Cupid's bow on the lateral side of the cleft. *Point 6:* Tip of the advancement flap. The distance from point *5* to *6* and from point *4* to *8* to *9* should be equal. *Point 7:* Alar base of the cleft side. The distance from *point 5* to *7* and from *point 1* to *2* should be equal. *Point 8:* Base of the columella. *Point 9:* Backcut point. (The incision often has to be carried from point *4* to *8* and then extended to *point 9* to achieve adequate rotation of the flap.) **B,** Development of the flaps. *C flap:* A triangle of soft tissue from the lip margin that will reconstruct the hemicolumella and nasal floor. **C,** Closure of the cleft. Lip from the normal side is rotated downward to reposition the philtrum, and the lip from the cleft side is advanced medially. Note that a portion of the C flap is closed on itself to lengthen the columella. **D,** Completed repair of the cleft lip.

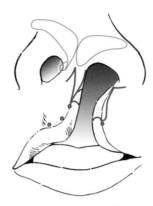

Fig. 45-10   Markings for the modified Mohler variation of rotation-advancement repair. In this variation, the rotation flap extends onto the columella, a long C flap constructs the hemicolumella and nasal floor, and the advancement flap incision does not extend around the alar base.

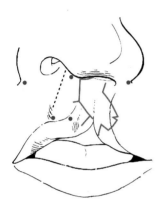

Fig. 45-11   Abbreviated markings for the Fisher anatomic subunit repair. In this unilateral cleft lip repair, releasing incisions near the columellar-labial junction and lower philtral column lengthen the medial lip when lateral triangular flaps are inset.

angulated sharply down leaving a single, vertically oriented incision along the constructed philtral ridge without extension across the superior aspect of the dimple. A long C flap lengthens the hemicolumella and constructs the nasal floor. The incision around the alar base is thus unnecessary because the lateral lip segment does not require significant advancement (Fig. 45-10).

Other current techniques for unilateral cleft lip repair employ elements of the rotation-advancement repair combined with triangular flaps. Mulliken includes small triangular flaps to construct the white roll and augment the vermilion.[44] Fisher described a technique for lip repair that lengthens the medial and lateral segments of the cleft while adhering to an anatomic subunit concept. Anatomic points are marked and small triangular flaps in the vermilion and lower philtral column; this is reminiscent of the Skoog technique to lengthen the lip[45] (Fig. 45-11).

These techniques differ in design of the cutaneous repair. The orbicularis oris muscle is repaired separately, and the technique does not necessarily correspond to a specific named repair. Techniques for muscle repair range from simple linear closure to eversion of the muscle in an attempt to build a philtral ridge.

A hybrid procedure involving elements of techniques described by Millard, Skoog, Fisher, and Mulliken is a favored approach[46] (Box 45-1) (Fig. 45-12).

Box 45-1   Goals of Unilateral Cleft Lip Repair

1. Establish a symmetrical Cupid's bow.
2. Construct a full median tubercle and adequate vermilion height.
3. Construct a philtral ridge mimicking the noncleft lip side.
4. Construct a normal columella and establish a symmetric columellar-labial junction.
5. Reorient and repair the orbicularis oris muscle.
6. Create a labial sulcus.
7. Correct the cleft nasal alar deformity.
8. Perform an atraumatic, nonlinear skin closure.

Data from Meara JG, Andrews BT, Ridgway EB, et al. Unilateral cleft lip and nasal repair: techniques and principles. Iran J Pediatr 21:129-138, 2011.

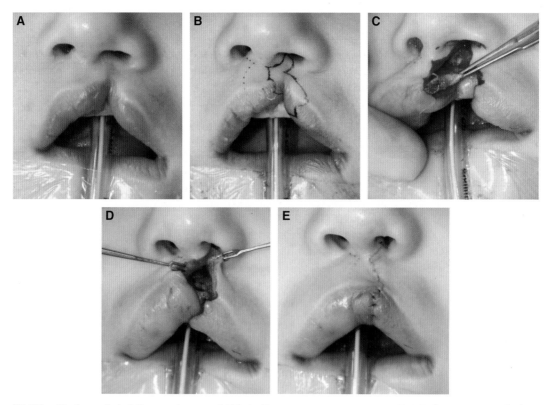

Fig. 45-12   Unilateral cleft lip repair on a child. **A,** Preoperative appearance. **B,** Markings are made for repair. **C,** Cutaneous incisions are made and the orbicularis oris muscle is dissected. **D,** The orbicularis oris muscle is repaired and a hemialar cinch suture is placed. **E,** Immediate postoperative appearance.

Surgical Planning

- Mark (1) the low point of the Cupid's bow, (2) the high point of the Cupid's bow on the noncleft side, (3) the columellar "apron" starting on the noncleft side and mirrored on the cleft side, (4) the red line, and (5) the high point of the Cupid's bow on the lateral lip element (where the vermilion-cutaneous junction begins to curve and dry vermilion begins to diminish).
- Tattoo the markings of the Cupid's bow using a 30-gauge needle and methylene blue or brilliant green dye.
- Inject local anesthetic with epinephrine for hemostasis: bupivacaine 0.25% with 1:200,000 epinephrine (1 ml/kg).
- The medial element mark begins lateral to the "apron" of tissue that curves gently at the columellar-labial junction and extends to the high point of the Cupid's bow. Releasing incisions are designed (1) beneath the apron, (2) just above the white roll, and (3) along the red line.
- The lateral mark starts in the nasal vestibule and extends to the high point of the Cupid's bow. Triangular flaps are designed corresponding to the releasing incisions on the medial segment (1) where the alar skin curves to meet the medial footplate skin, (2) just above the white roll, and (3) in the vermilion.

Surgical Procedure

- Medial skin incisions are made, followed by lateral skin incisions, then an incision in the labial sulcus several millimeters above the attached gingiva.
- The orbicularis oris muscle is sharply dissected medially and laterally, releasing it from the subcutaneous tissue and submucosa and releasing abnormal attachments.
- A small muscular flap is created from the distal aspect of lateral muscle and used to augment the median tubercle.
- Tip rhinoplasty is performed at the time of the initial operation (see discussion under Cleft Rhinoplasty).

Closure

- The lateral lip mucosa is advanced medially and closed with 5-0 chromic sutures intraorally and 6-0 and 7-0 chromic sutures for the vermilion.
- A suture is placed at the inferior aspect of the orbicularis oris muscle and tension is applied to maintain length during closure. Closure continues superiorly with 5-0 PDS interrupted sutures.
- A unilateral alar cinch suture is placed to pull the alar base medially.
- Skin closure begins by approximating the tattooed high points of the Cupid's bow using 6-0 PDS on a taper needle. Precision and accuracy are essential because submillimeter deviations will be noticeable to the casual observer as the child grows. The remaining skin is closed with intradermal sutures followed by 2-octyl cyanoacrylate glue. The nasal floor is closed with 5-0 and 6-0 chromic sutures.

BILATERAL CLEFT LIP REPAIR

Repair of a bilateral cleft lip is more demanding than repair of a unilateral cleft lip. Challenges of a bilateral cleft lip are a wide, flat bilateral nasal deformity, a protruding premaxilla, and a short, wide prolabium devoid of muscle. Historically, the premaxilla was pushed back mechanically with bonnets or other external devices. Operative premaxillary setback involving excision of septal cartilage was later advocated, but concerns arose about midfacial growth disturbance. Many surgeons used the prolabium to reconstruct the columella and united the lateral labial elements in the midline. Others used the prolabium to reconstruct the superior philtrum and united the lateral elements inferiorly.[47,48] Staged repair was also employed and is still used by a small number of surgeons today.[24] Repairing one side of the lip and saving the other for a second stage limits the ability of the surgeon to obtain symmetry.

The middle of the twentieth century brought about major advances in bilateral cleft lip repair with a concentration on widespread use of prolabial tissue only to reconstruct the philtrum. Multiple authors described techniques with similar principles, including reconstructing the philtrum and central tubercle with prolabial skin and vermilion, advancing lateral lip elements to meet the constructed philtrum, and discarding little tissue.[48-53] Marcks et al[52] used releasing incisions to elongate the prolabium. Schultz[51] united the orbicularis oris muscle at the midline, whereas Manchester[48] later advocated uniting it with either side of the constructed philtrum to avoid tension.

Millard turned attention to nasal construction with the use of lateral prolabial skin as "forked flaps" to elongate the columella and was among the early proponents of discarding prolabial vermilion and using lateral lip elements to create the median tubercle.[54-56] His use of forked flaps, however, created a distorted nasal morphology and has since been abandoned by most cleft surgeons. Mulliken further refined bilateral cleft lip repair using direct anthropometry to study and optimize long-term, "fourth-dimension" results.[57-59] He constructed a very narrow philtrum at the time of primary repair with the understanding that it would widen in childhood. In addition he discarded forked flaps in favor of primary rhinoplasty with repositioning of the lower lateral cartilages[57,59-62] (Box 45-2) (Fig. 45-13).

One favored approach is to employ Mulliken's technique with a modification during cutaneous closure (Figs. 45-14 and 45-15).

Box 45-2 Goals of Bilateral Cleft Lip Repair

1. Maintain symmetry.
2. Achieve muscular continuity.
3. Design the philtral flap anticipating that it will bow and elongate with growth.
4. Construct the median tubercle from the lateral labial elements.
5. Position the lower lateral cartilages to construct the nasal tip and columella at the initial operation.

Adapted from Mulliken JB. Bilateral cleft lip. Clin Plast Surg 31:209-220, 2004.

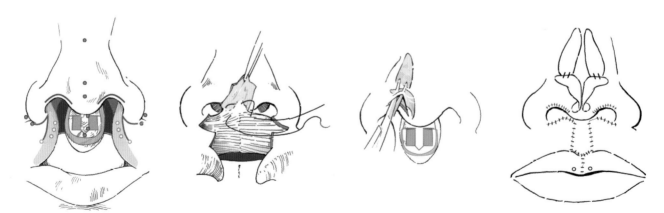

Fig. 45-13   The Mulliken bilateral cleft lip repair.

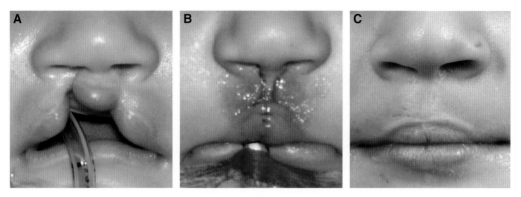

Fig. 45-14   A child with an incomplete bilateral cleft lip. **A,** Preoperative appearance. **B,** Immediate postoperative result. **C,** Result at 5 years of age.

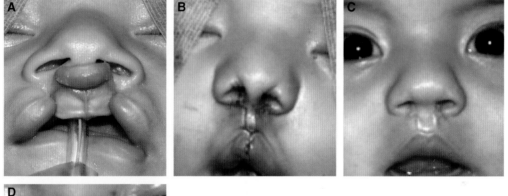

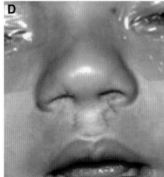

Fig. 45-15   A child with a wide bilateral cleft lip. **A,** Preoperative appearance. **B,** Immediate postoperative result. **C,** Early postoperative result. **D,** Result at 2 years of age.

Surgical Planning

- Identify and mark the anthropometric points: (1) *en* (endocanthion), (2) *n* (nasion), (3) *prn* (pronasale), (4) *c* (highest point of the columella), (5) *al* (alare), (6) *sbal* (subalare), (7) *sn* (subnasale), (8) *cphs* (crista philtri superior), (9) *cphi* (crista philtri inferior), (10) *ls* (labiale superius), and (11) *sto* (stomion). The position of *cphs* and *cphi* are determined such that the distance between *cphs* points is approximately 2 mm and the distance between *cphi* points is approximately 4 mm. The position of *ls* is determined such that the philtral length is approximately 6 to 7 mm.

- The philtral flap is marked out based on *cphs, cphi,* and *ls.* Flanking strips of deepithelialized dermis are left on either side of the flap to build philtral ridges. The high point of the Cupid's bow is determined on the lateral elements and the advancement flaps are marked.

- The following measurements are made and recorded for reference: (1) *en-en* (intercanthal distance), (2) *n-sn* (nasal length), (3) *al-al* (nasal base width), (4) *sn-prn* (nasal protrusion), (5) *sn-c* (columellar length), (6) *c-c* (columellar width), (7) *cphs-cphs* (upper philtral width), (8) *cphi-cphi* (lower philtral width), (9) *sn-ls* (philtral height), (10) *sn-sto* (labial height), and (11) *ls-sto* (vermilion height).
- Tattoo the major landmarks and inject local anesthetic with epinephrine.

Surgical Procedure
- Prolabial incisions are made and the flanking flaps are deepithelialized. The philtral flap is elevated in the subcutaneous plane. Prolabial mucosa is used to deepen the labiogingival sulcus.
- Lateral labial elements are incised and the medial margin of tissue is discarded. The orbicularis oris muscle is sharply dissected.

Closure
- The prolabial mucosa is inset onto the premaxillary periosteum. The lateral labial mucosa is advanced and closed at the midline with 5-0 chromic sutures.
- The midline muscular closure is performed using 5-0 PDS interrupted sutures.
- Tip rhinoplasty is performed (discussed under Cleft Rhinoplasty).
- Alar cinch sutures are placed to pull the alar bases medially until *al-al* is several millimeters less than *en-en* (this widens postoperatively).
- The skin is closed as previously described.
- The vermilion flaps are everted to form a protuberant central tubercle and closed at the midline using 7-0 or 6-0 chromic sutures.
- The previously mentioned distances are measured again; *al-al* narrows, *sn-c* lengthens, and the philtral flap measurements do not change significantly.

Cleft Rhinoplasty

The cleft lip nasal deformity may be considered in terms of the tip deformity caused by distorted lower lateral cartilages present at birth and the deformity of the nasal bones and septum that is present at birth but worsens as the child grows. Treatment of the latter should be delayed until skeletal maturity to prevent growth disturbance and is accomplished with the techniques of adult septorhinoplasty. Treatment of the nasal tip deformity should be performed much earlier. There is debate about the optimal timing for correction. Traditionally, nasal correction was performed after lip repair, but now many surgeons address the lip and nose at the same time. Thus the tip deformity is corrected without another procedure with the patient under general anesthetic, and the nasal stigmata of cleft lips are minimized early in childhood. Nasal growth is unaffected by early tip rhinoplasty.[63,64]

Whether cleft rhinoplasty is performed in a primary or a delayed fashion, the goals are uniform: to reposition the lower lateral cartilages in a way that elevates the lateral crus or crura, elongates the columella, narrows the alar base, and anticipates future growth. The lower lateral cartilages have a predilection to slump after correction, therefore overcorrection is emphasized for long-term symmetry. The lower lateral cartilages can be dissected from a lateral approach through the gingivobuccal sulcus incision made for the lip repair or through separate rim incisions that give direct access to the cartilages. The lower lateral cartilages are elevated with sutures. McComb advocates through-and-through sutures tied over bolsters to medialize the genu and elevate the lateral crus.[63,64] Mulliken prefers internal fixation of the cartilages using an interdomal suture to medialize the genua and intercartilaginous sutures to suspend the lateral crus or crura to the upper lateral cartilage.[44,59,62] Still others employ elements of both techniques. For unilateral cleft lip nasal correction the dissection is performed through the gingivobuccal sulcus incision. There is no need for any additional perialar incisions, because the lower aspect of the nose can be adequately dissected through this approach, combined with a columellar approach. After the lower aspect of the nasal skin has been dissected and separated from the lower lateral cartilages on both sides, multiple through-and-through quilting sutures are used to reposition and resuspend the cartilage. For a bilateral cleft lip the cartilages are approached through a rim incision, internal sutures are used to bring the splayed genua together and suspend the lateral crus, and quilting sutures are used for final elevation and contouring.

Surgical Technique

- The alar base or bases are mobilized along the piriform aperture to allow inferomedial alar rotation.
- The skin over the lower lateral cartilages is degloved through a lateral alar approach combined with a columellar approach from underneath the apron in a unilateral cleft or with rim incisions in a bilateral cleft.
- Quilting sutures (5-0 PDS) are placed along the lower lateral cartilage to reapproximate the degloved nasal skin with the lower lateral cartilage and elevate the lateral crus.
- In a unilateral cleft, quilting sutures are placed between the genua, bringing the domes together, and the knots are tied in the nasal vestibule. In a bilateral cleft, an interdomal suture is used.
- Hemialar cinch sutures bring the cleft alae toward the base of the columella.
- The incisions are closed during lip closure. Additional rim incisions are closed with a 6-0 or 7-0 chromic gut.

CLEFT PALATE REPAIR

Whereas the major goal of cleft lip repair is to restore normal facial appearance, the goals of cleft palate repair are to close the large oronasal fistula and to promote normal speech. Early treatment of the cleft palate included the use of obturators to obstruct the oronasal fistula and simple suture closure of the velum after burning the tissue edges. In 1820, von Graefe described excision of the soft palate cleft edge and closure with sutures.[65] Subsequently, Dieffenbach described mobilizing palatal mucosa and bone to close the hard palate defect. His successor, von Langenbeck, observed that bone regenerates when the periosteum is intact and described subperiosteal mobilization of the mucoperiosteal flaps. In his repair, lateral relaxing incisions allowed bipedicled palatal flaps to medialize, and the levator veli palatini and palatopharyngeus muscles were released to close the soft palate[66] (Fig. 45-16). This technique remains the basis for current cleft palate repair. Palatoplasty technique advanced further when Braithwaite[67] recognized the importance

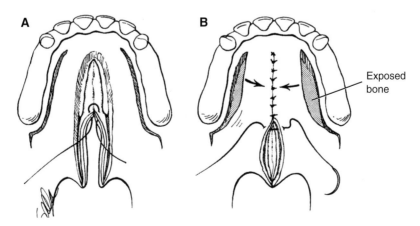

Fig. 45-16   A bipedicled palatoplasty. **A,** Incisions have been made and both the nasal and palatal mucosa have been elevated as bipedicled flaps. Nasal closure is in progress. **B,** The flaps have been mobilized to the midline and palatal closure is nearly complete. The lateral relaxing incisions are left open.

of the abnormally oriented palatal musculature and advocated detaching and retropositioning the muscles to construct the soft palate muscular sling. This procedure was further described by Kriens,[68] who coined the term *intravelar veloplasty* to describe construction of that muscular sling.

The major goals in modern cleft palate repair are the same as those in past centuries: to close the oronasal fistula and to optimize speech through proper palatal musculature positioning. Most surgeons perform soft palate repair at the same time as hard palate repair to better mobilize soft palatal tissue toward the midline. Some centers, however, perform hard and soft palate repair at separate stages. Sommerlad advocated hard palate repair using a single layer vomerine flap in concert with lip repair at age 3 months. Soft palate repair is delayed until 6 months.[69,70] Friede, however, advocated delaying hard palate repair to optimize midfacial growth.[71]

Regardless of timing, soft palate repair is performed in layers: nasal mucosa, velar musculature, and palatal mucosa. The velar musculature is released from its attachments on the posterior hard palate, rotated posteromedially, and sutured at the midline to create a muscular sling, the intravelar veloplasty. An alternative to straight-line repair with intravelar veloplasty is Furlow's double-opposing Z-plasty.[72] In this latter technique, Z-plasties that face opposite directions are designed on the palatal and nasal mucosa. The velar muscles are elevated with the mucosal flaps that rotate posteriorly, creating a muscular sling (Fig. 45-17).

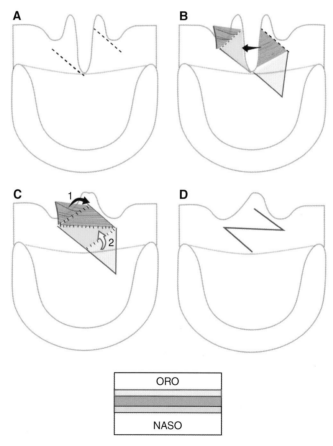

Fig. 45-17   A double-opposing Z-plasty cleft palate repair. In the double-opposing Z-plasty, the abnormally oriented palatal muscles are raised with the mucosal flaps, with the oral mucosal flap on one side and the nasal mucosal flap on the other side. These flaps are rotated posteriorly to overlap the muscles and construct the muscular sling.

To close the hard palate, the nasal lining is elevated from the vomer medially and maxilla and palatine bones laterally and closed to restore nasopharyngeal lining. The palatal mucosa is elevated in a subperiosteal plane and mobilized so that it may be closed as a separate layer in the midline. Von Langenbeck described elevating the palatal mucosa as bipedicled flaps. The two-flap palatoplasty advocated by Bardach[73,74] employs a single pedicle based on the greater palatine arteries (Fig. 45-18). Lateral relaxing incisions with a thin area of exposed palatal bone are left laterally with both the bipedicled and two-flap techniques. In the Veau-Wardill-Kilner or V-Y pushback palatoplasty, the palatal flaps are retropositioned leaving exposed bone anteriorly and lengthening the palate (Fig. 45-19).

One favored approach is to perform two-flap palatoplasty similar to the technique described by Bardach for the oral layer and extended velar muscle repair as described by Sommerlad,[69,70] but using a double-opposing Z-plasty for submucous cleft palate repair and in selected case of velopharyngeal insufficiency.

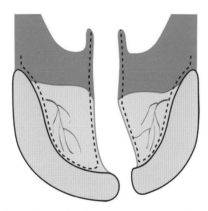

Fig. 45-18   In the two-flap palatoplasty the palatal gingivoperiosteal flaps are marked out on either side based on the greater palatine arteries. The lateral marking is made at the junction of the alveolar gingiva and the palatal mucosa, and the medial marking is made at the junction of the palatal and nasal mucosa, extending from the hard palate to the soft palate.

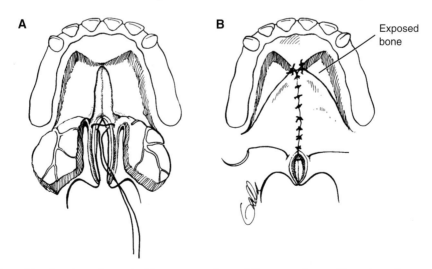

Fig. 45-19   V-Y pushback palatoplasty. **A,** The mucoperiosteal flaps are elevated based on the greater palatine arteries. Closure of the nasal lining is in progress. **B,** As the closure is completed and the palate is lengthened or pushed back, large areas of exposed bone are left on the anterior hard palate.

Surgical Planning

- Position the patient with the neck in slight extension.
- Place a Dingman mouth gag to maintain retraction.
- Mark the two-flap palatoplasty.
- Inject local anesthetic with bupivacaine 0.25% with 1:200,000 epinephrine into the hard and soft palate mucosa (1 ml/kg). Adequate hemostasis is essential, particularly during muscle dissection.

Surgical Procedure

- The soft palate mucosa is incised with a No. 15 blade along the junction of the nasal and oral mucosa extending from the uvula to the hard palate.
- The hard palate is incised laterally and medially.
- The mucoperiosteal flaps are elevated in the subperiosteal plane with care being taken to preserve the greater palatine arteries.
- An incision is made down the midline of the vomer and a periosteal elevator is used to elevate just enough mucoperiosteum to close the nasal lining.
- Afrin nasal spray is sprayed on to the soft palate before the muscle dissection.
- The levator veli palatini and palatopharyngeus muscles are sharply dissected, and their attachments to the posterior hard palate are released. This muscle dissection and repair is performed as described by Sommerlad.

Closure

- The nasal lining is closed using a 5-0 Monocryl suture on a taper needle beginning at the uvula and progressing anteriorly. Care is taken to evert the closure and avoid tearing fragile tissue. A cutting needle should not be used.
- The palatal muscles are approximated with a 4-0 PDS suture.
- The palatal mucoperiosteum and soft palate mucosa are closed using 5-0 Monocryl mattress sutures beginning posteriorly at the uvula and progressing anteriorly.
- A small piece of Surgicel is placed on each side in the recess of the muscle dissection near the eustachian tube before the oral layer closure is completed.
- Several mattress sutures are placed between the oral and nasal layer to hold the oral layer in position. Occasionally a suture can be placed through the soft bone of the hard palate to secure the oral layer anteriorly if needed.

Alveolar Bone Grafting

Closure of the alveolar cleft with bone grafting is performed at approximately 8 to 9 years of age. The timing of this intervention is based on the potential for canine eruption, typically when the tooth root is one half to two thirds formed on radiograph.[75] The benefits of alveolar bone grafting include (1) providing bony support for the erupting canine and the teeth adjacent to the cleft, (2) closing the nasolabial fistula, if it is not primarily closed with gingivoperiosteoplasty, (3) creating a continuous dental arch that permits orthodontic manipulation, (4) providing support for the nasal floor and the alar base, and (5) providing stable bone for future osseointegrated implant placement.

Cancellous bone harvested from the anterior or posterior iliac crest has traditionally been used for the graft material. The latter site is favored because of the large volume of bone available, the ability to simultane-

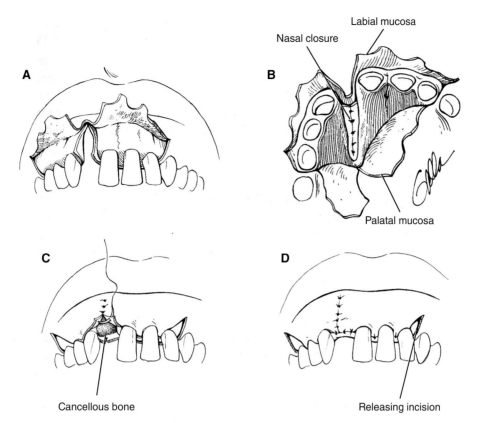

Fig. 45-20   Alveolar bone grafting. **A,** Gingival incisions have been made and labial mucosal flaps have been elevated. **B,** Nasal mucosa has been elevated and sutured to close the nasal floor. The labial and palatal flaps have also been elevated. **C,** Cancellous bone has been packed into the cleft defect. **D,** Advancement of the gingival and mucosal flaps to close the oral side. Releasing incisions may be left, but this is not usually necessary.

ously harvest thick dermal grafts for lip augmentation, and the avoidance of lateral femoral cutaneous nerve injury (Fig. 45-20). Multiple substances for augmenting or replacing traditional cancellous bone graft are currently under study, such as bone morphogenetic protein, platelet rich plasma, and hydroxyapatite paste.

Surgical Planning

- Preoperative orthodontic manipulation to expand the maxillary arch typically begins 6 to 12 months before bone grafting.
- Extraction of remaining deciduous teeth may be necessary.
- When the orthodontic phase is complete, the patient is ready for bone grafting.

Surgical Procedure

- Cancellous and cortical bone is harvested.
- The alveolar gingiva is incised and elevated in the subperiosteal plane on either side of the alveolar cleft.
- Dissection is carried up to the nasal floor.
- The entire area is densely packed with bone, and a small piece of cortical bone used to suspend the nasal floor.

Closure

- The gingiva and mucosa are closed with chromic sutures.
- The hip incision is closed with 4-0 PDS and 6-0 nylon sutures.
- The area is protected using Coe-Pak.

POSTOPERATIVE CARE

A postoperative care protocol that is currently employed is detailed in this section. Arm restraints or elbow immobilizers have been used by many surgeons but their necessity remains in question.

CLEFT LIP AND NASAL REPAIR

- Bottle feeding or breastfeeding is resumed immediately postoperatively.
- Oils and ointments should be avoided (they promote breakdown of the skin glue).
- Careful bathing is allowed after 24 hours; avoid scrubbing or getting soap on the lip.
- If the patient is taking in enough fluids by mouth, discharge him or her home on the first postoperative day.
- The lip and nasal area may be washed with simple soap and water beginning 3 days after surgery.
- Follow up with the patient 1 week after surgery, at which time any remaining chromic suture remnants and/or glue can be removed.
- Antibiotic ointment is applied to the incision for 1 week; sunscreen is applied thereafter.
- At 1 month, begin scar massage for 5 minutes several times daily.

CLEFT PALATE REPAIR

- Clear liquids through a cleft feeder or breastfeeding is allowed immediately after surgery.
- Cardiopulmonary monitoring is used routinely.
- Four doses of antibiotics are given to cover oral flora.
- Formula may be used on the first postoperative day.
- Discharge the patient home on the first postoperative day if he or she is taking in enough fluids by mouth.
- Pureed and soft foods are allowed on discharge. The patient should avoid sharp utensils, straws, crunchy food, and other items that are potentially injurious to the repaired palate.
- Follow up with the patient 3 months after surgery.

ALVEOLAR BONE GRAFT

- The Coe-Pak falls out on its own approximately 2 to 3 days postoperatively.
- The patient should be on a clear liquid diet through the third postoperative day and should be encouraged to drink every 2 to 3 hours to keep the mouth moist.
- A full liquid/blenderized diet begins on postoperative day 4 and continues for 6 weeks.
- The patient should not chew hard or crunchy food or drink from straws for 6 weeks.
- Amoxicillin (Augmentin) is continued for 1 week postoperatively.
- The patient should rinse with chlorhexidine mouthwash twice daily and rinse with water after meals for 10 days.
- The patient should not sneeze or blow his or her nose with the mouth open for 6 weeks after surgery.
- Suture removal from the hip incision should be scheduled for 7 to 10 days postoperatively.
- Ossification of the bone graft should be assessed radiologically 3 months postoperatively.
- Orthodontic manipulation begins 3 to 4 months postoperatively.

COMPLICATIONS

Cleft Lip

Major complications of cleft lip repair, including complete dehiscence, are very rare, but minor complications occur frequently and are mostly related to appearance. Mild asymmetry is common, but when it is significant, it requires revision. Hypertrophic scarring may occur and may be addressed with steroid injections. An overly long lip may require excision of excess tissue, usually vermilion. A short lip ("whistle deformity") is more difficult to correct. The condition may be addressed with a dermal graft or a Z-plasty, but it will often require complete revision of the lip repair. Inadequate repair of the orbicularis oris muscle at the time of the primary repair results in a depression of the philtral column during animation in a unilateral cleft lip and a widening of the constructed philtrum in a bilateral cleft lip. Nostril stenosis may occur at the site of the alar base advancement and nasal floor repair and is very difficult to correct. It is crucial not to overresect the nasal floor in an attempt to reposition the cleft side ala. The ala should be repositioned with a cinch suture, and care must be taken to leave adequate nasal floor skin.

Cleft Palate

Major complications of cleft palate repair are rare, but they include bleeding and airway-threatening edema. Some surgeons leave a stitch in the tongue for retraction in case of an airway emergency. Minor complications are also infrequent but have a substantial functional impact. The two complications most feared by the cleft surgeon are palatal fistulas and velopharyngeal insufficiency. Palatal fistulas occur at areas of tension in the nasal and palatal repairs. The hard palate–soft palate junction is the most common site of unplanned fistula, but they may occur anywhere along the point of repair. Everting the nasal and palatal closures under minimal tension at the time of repair is essential to preventing fistula. Velopharyngeal insufficiency is caused by inadequate closure of the velopharyngeal sphincter during speech, which results in nasal air escape. This may be caused by a short palate or inadequate muscular repair, but often it has no clear cause. With speech therapy many children with velopharyngeal insufficiency will be able to achieve adequate speech, but a small number of children require additional surgical procedures. These procedures may include conversion to a double-opposing Z-plasty, a sphincter pharyngoplasty, a pharyngeal flap, and augmentation of the posterior pharyngeal wall. Other complications of cleft palate repair that are detected late in childhood include injury to tooth buds and maxillary growth deficiency.

Key Points

- Cleft lip and palate result from facial prominences failing to fuse early in embryologic development. Both conditions are associated with genetic and environmental influences. Isolated cleft palate is more likely to be associated with an underlying syndrome.
- Cleft lip repair aims to restore normal lip length, build a symmetrical Cupid's bow, establish orbicularis oris muscle continuity, and construct a symmetric, normal appearing nose.
- Cleft palate repair closes the oronasal fistula and establishes continuity of soft palate musculature to provide the best chance of normal speech development.
- Secondary procedures may be required to address an alveolar cleft, residual nasal deformity, or surgical complication, such as poor speech or palatal fistulas.

REFERENCES

1. Bhattacharya S, Khanna V, Kohli R. Cleft lip: the historical perspective. Indian J Plast Surg 42(Suppl):S4-S8, 2009.

2. Sperber GH, Sperber SM, Guttman GD, eds. Early orofacial development. In Craniofacial Embryogenetics and Development, ed 2. Shelton, CT: People's Medical Publishing House-USA, 2010.

3. Fára M. Anatomy and arteriography of cleft lips in stillborn children. Plast Reconstr Surg 42:29-36, 1968.

4. Yuzuriha S, Mulliken JB. Minor-form, microform, and mini-microform cleft lip: anatomical features, operative techniques, and revisions. Plast Reconstr Surg 122:1485-1493, 2008.

5. Veau V. Division Palatine. Paris: Masson et Cie, 1931.

6. Kernahan DA. The striped Y—a symbolic classification for cleft lip and palate. Plast Reconstr Surg 47:469-470, 1971.

7. Calnan J. Submucous cleft palate. Br J Plast Surg 6:264-282, 1954.

8. Fogh-Andersen P. Inheritance of Hare Lip and Cleft Palate. Copenhagen: Nyt Nordisk Forlag Arnold Busck, 1942.

9. Weinberg SM, Brandon CA, McHenry TH, et al. Rethinking isolated cleft palate: evidence of occult lip defects in a subset of cases. Am J Med Genet 146:1670-1675, 2008.

10. Moreno LM, Mansilla MA, Bullard SA, et al. FOXE1 association with both isolated cleft lip with or without cleft palate, and isolated cleft palate. Hum Mol Genet 18:4879-4896, 2009.

11. National Institute of Dental and Craniofacial Research, National Institutes of Health. Prevalence (Number of Cases) of Cleft Lip and Cleft Palate. Available at *www.nidcr.nih.gov/DataStatistics/FindDataByTopic/CraniofacialBirthDefects/PrevalenceCleft+LipCleftPalate.htm.*

12. Shaw GM, Croen LA, Curry CJ. Isolated oral cleft malformations: associations with maternal and infant characteristics in a California population. Teratology 43:225-228, 1991.

13. International Centre for Birth Defects. World Atlas of Birth Defects, ed 2. Geneva: World Health Organization, 2003.

14. Dixon MJ, Marazita ML, Beaty TH, et al. Cleft lip and palate: understanding genetic and environmental influences. Nat Rev Genet 12:167-178, 2011.

15. Stoll C, Alembik Y, Dott B, et al. Associated malformations in cases with oral clefts. Cleft Palate Craniofac J 37:41-47, 2000.

16. Jones MC. Etiology of facial clefts: prospective evaluation of 428 patients. Cleft Palate J 25:16-20, 1988.

17. Shprintzen RJ, Siegel-Sadewitz VL, Amato J, et al. Anomalies associated with cleft lip, cleft palate, or both. Am J Med Genet 20:585-595, 1985.

18. Genetics Home Reference, National Institutes of Health. Available at *http://ghr.nlm.nih.gov/search?query=cleft+lip&Search=and http://ghr.nlm.nih.gov/search?query=cleft+palate.*

19. American Cleft Palate-Craniofacial Association. Standards for Cleft Palate and Craniofacial Teams, 2010. Available at *www.acpa-cpf.org/team_care/standards/.*

20. Burston WR. The early orthodontic treatment of cleft palate conditions. Dent Pract 9:41-56, 1958.

21. Grayson BH, Cutting C, Wood R. Preoperative columella lengthening in bilateral cleft-lip and palate. Plast Reconstr Surg 92:1422-1423, 1993.

22. Georgiade NG, Latham RA. Maxillary arch alignment in the bilateral cleft lip and palate infant, using pinned coaxial screw appliance. Plast Reconstr Surg 56:52-60, 1975.

23. Wilhelmsen HR, Musgrave RH. Complications of cleft lip surgery. Cleft Palate J 3:223-231, 1966.

24. Tan SP, Greene AK, Mulliken JB. Current surgical management of bilateral cleft lip in North America. Plast Reconstr Surg 129:1347-1355, 2012.

25. Ysunza A, Pamplona MC, Mendoza M, et al. Speech outcome and maxillary growth in patients with unilateral complete cleft lip/palate operated on at 6 versus 12 months of age. Plast Reconstr Surg 102:675-679, 1998.

26. Sullivan SR, Marrinan EM, LaBrie RA, et al. Palatoplasty outcomes in nonsyndromic patients with cleft palate: a 29-year assessment of one surgeon's experience. J Craniofac Surg 20(Suppl 1):S612-S616, 2009.

27. Friede H, Enemark H. Long-term evidence for favorable midfacial growth after delayed hard palate repair in UCLP patients. Cleft Palate Craniofac J 38:323-329, 2001.

28. Katzel EB, Basile P, Koltz PF, et al. Current surgical practices in cleft care: cleft palate repair techniques and postoperative care. Plast Reconstr Surg 124:899-906, 2009.

29. Caouette-Laberge L, Bayet B, Larocque Y. The Pierre Robin sequence: review of 125 cases and evolution of treatment modalities. Plast Reconstr Surg 93:934-942, 1994.

30. Printzlau A, Andersen M. Pierre Robin sequence in Denmark: a retrospective population-based epidemiological study. Cleft Palate Craniofac J 41:47-52, 2004.

31. Herrmann J, France TD, Spranger JW, et al. The Stickler syndrome (hereditary arthroophthalmopathy). Birth Defects Orig Artic Ser 11:76-103, 1975.

32. Rogers GF, Murthy AS, LaBrie RA, et al. The GILLS score: part I. Patient selection for tongue-lip adhesion in Robin sequence. Plast Reconstr Surg 128:243-251, 2011.

33. Antony AK, Sloan GM. Airway obstruction following palatoplasty: analysis of 247 consecutive operations. Cleft Palate Craniofac J 39:145-148, 2002.

34. Dell'Oste C, Savron F, Pelizzo G, et al. Acute airway obstruction in an infant with Pierre Robin syndrome after palatoplasty. Acta Anaesthesiol Scand 48:787-789, 2004.

35. Rose W. On Harelip and Cleft Palate. London: Lewis, 1891.

36. Thompson JE. An artistic and mathematically accurate method of repairing the defects in cases of harelip. Surg Gynecol Obstet 14:498-502, 1912.

37. Tennison CW. The repair of the unilateral cleft lip by the stencil method. Plast Reconstr Surg 9:115-120, 1952.

38. Skoog T. A design for the repair of unilateral cleft lips. Am J Surg 95:223-226, 1958.

39. Randall P. A triangular flap operation for the primary repair of unilateral clefts of the lip. Plast Reconstr Surg Transplant Bull 23:331-347, 1959.

40. Millard DR Jr. The primary camouflage of the unilateral harelip. In Skoog T, Ivy RH, eds. Transactions of the International Society of Plastic Surgeons First Congress Stockholm and Uppsala 1955. Baltimore: Williams & Wilkins, 1957.

41. Stal S, Brown RH, Higuera S, et al. Fifty years of the Millard rotation-advancement: looking back and moving forward. Plast Reconstr Surg 123:1364-1377, 2009.
    The authors discuss the rotation-advancement technique, Millard's monumental contribution to unilateral cleft lip repair. In addition, there is a review of modifications to this technique as described by current authorities in cleft surgery including Byrd, Cutting, Mulliken, and Stal.

42. Mohler LR. Unilateral cleft lip repair. Plast Reconstr Surg 80:511-517, 1987.

43. Cutting CB, Dayan JH. Lip height and lip width after extended Mohler unilateral cleft lip repair. Plast Reconstr Surg 111:17-23, 2003.

44. Mulliken JB, Martínez-Pérez D. The principle of rotation advancement for repair of unilateral complete cleft lip and nasal deformity: technical variations and analysis of results. Plast Reconstr Surg 104:1247-1260, 1999.

45. Fisher DM. Unilateral cleft lip repair: an anatomical subunit approximation technique. Plast Reconstr Surg 116:61-71, 2005.

46. Meara JG, Andrews BT, Ridgway EB, et al. Unilateral cleft lip and nasal repair: techniques and principles. Iran J Pediatr 21:129-138, 2011.

47. Adams WM, Adams LH. The misuse of the prolabium in the repair of bilateral cleft lip. Plast Reconstr Surg 12:225-232, 1953.

48. Manchester WM. The repair of bilateral cleft lip and palate. Br J Surg 52:878-882, 1965.

49. Axhausen G. Technik und Ergebnisse der Lippenplastik. Leipzig: Thieme, 1932.

50. Brown GV. Surgery of Oral and Facial Diseases and Malformations. Philadelphia: Lea & Febiger, 1938.

51. Schultz LW. Bilateral cleft lips. Plast Reconstr Surg 1:338-343, 1946.

52. Marcks KM, Trevaskis AE, Payne MJ. Bilateral cleft lip repair. Plast Reconstr Surg 19:401-408, 1957.

53. Cronin TD. Management of the bilateral cleft lip with protruding premaxilla. Am J Surg 92:810-816, 1956.

54. Millard DR. A primary compromise for bilateral cleft lip. Surg Gynecol Obstet 111:557-563, 1960.

55. Millard DR. Bilateral cleft lip and a primary forked flap: a preliminary report. Plast Reconstr Surg 39:59-65, 1967.

56. Millard DR. Closure of bilateral cleft lip and elongation of columella by two operations in infancy. Plast Reconstr Surg 47:324-331, 1971.

57. Mulliken JB. Bilateral complete cleft lip and nasal deformity: an anthropometric analysis of staged to synchronous repair. Plast Reconstr Surg 96:9-23, 1995.

58. Mulliken JB, Burvin R, Farkas LG. Repair of bilateral complete cleft lip: intraoperative nasolabial anthropometry. Plast Reconstr Surg 107:307-314, 2001.
    The author describes his technique for bilateral cleft lip/nasal repair and provides data detailing how nasolabial features change over time. He emphasizes the concept of the "fourth-dimension" in cleft care and uses the data provided as a rationale for over-lengthening slow-growing nasolabial features (columellar length, nasal tip protrusion, and median tubercle height) and under-lengthening fast-growing features (philtral length and alar base width).

59. Mulliken JB. Primary repair of bilateral cleft lip and nasal deformity. Plast Reconstr Surg 108:181-914, 2001.

60. Mulliken JB. Correction of the bilateral cleft lip nasal deformity: evolution of a surgical concept. Cleft Palate Craniofac J 29:540-545, 1992.

61. Mulliken JB. Repair of bilateral complete cleft lip and nasal deformity--state of the art. Cleft Palate Craniofac J 37:342-347, 2000.

62. Mulliken JB. Bilateral cleft lip. Clin Plast Surg 31:209-220, 2004.

63. McComb H. Primary correction of unilateral cleft lip nasal deformity: a 10-year review. Plast Reconstr Surg 75:791-799, 1985.

64. McComb HK. Primary repair of the bilateral cleft lip nose: a long-term follow-up. Plast Reconstr Surg 124:1610-1615, 2009.

65. May H. The classic reprint. The palate suture. A newly discovered method to correct congenital speech defects. Dr. Carl Ferdinand von Graefe, Berlin. Plast Reconstr Surg 47:488-492, 1971.

66. Goldwyn RM. Bernhard Von Langenbeck. His life and legacy. Plast Reconstr Surg 44:248-254, 1969.

67. Braithwaite F. Cleft palate repair. In Gibson T, ed. Modern Trends in Plastic Surgery. London: Butterworths, 1964.

68. Kriens OB. An anatomical approach to veloplasty. Plast Reconstr Surg 43:29-41, 1969.

69. Sommerlad BC. A technique for cleft palate repair. Plast Reconstr Surg 112:1542-1548, 2003.

70. Sommerlad BC. Cleft palate repair. In Losee JE, Kirschner KE, eds. Comprehensive Cleft Care. New York: McGraw Hill, 2009.

71. Friede HT. Two-stage palate repair. In Losee JE, Kirschner KE, eds. Comprehensive Cleft Care. New York: McGraw Hill, 2009.

72. Furlow LT. Cleft palate repair by double opposing Z-plasty. Plast Reconstr Surg 78:724-738, 1986.

73. Bardach J. Rozszczep wargi: gornej podniebienia. Warsaw: Pánstwowy Zakład Wydawn, 1967.

74. Salyer KE, Sng KW, Sperry EE. Two-flap palatoplasty: 20-year experience and evolution of surgical technique. Plast Reconstr Surg 118:193-204, 2006.

75. Abramowicz S, Katsnelson A, Forbes PW, et al. Anterior versus posterior approach to iliac crest for alveolar cleft bone grafting. J Oral Maxillofac Surg 70:211-215, 2012.

46

Secondary Cleft Palate and Velopharyngeal Function

Derek J. Rogers ▪ *Christopher J. Hartnick*

Secondary cleft palate repair techniques developed in the nineteenth century by pioneers such as von Langenbeck, Wardill, Killner, and Furlow have withstood the test of time. From the time of Schoenborn's innovative pharyngeal flap operation in 1876, modifications have been made to the pharyngeal flap, and sphincter pharyngoplasty and Furlow palatoplasty have emerged as attractive alternatives for the treatment of velopharyngeal dysfunction. Current surgical strategy embraces the concept. The earlier surgical intervention is begun, the better the patient's chances of developing normal speech. However, as with surgical correction of a cleft lip, this advantage must be weighed against the potential detrimental effects that early surgical intervention can have on facial growth in repair of bony clefts of the secondary palate. Regardless of the surgical approach, the production of intelligible speech and prevention of nasal reflux depend on competent velopharyngeal function and remain paramount considerations in the rehabilitation of patients with cleft palate.

ANATOMY

Formation of the secondary palate (the hard palate posterior to the incisive foramen and the soft palate) occurs at week 6 of gestation and continues through week 12. The lateral palatine processes form on the medial aspect of the maxillary processes and grow toward the midline. Fusion first occurs at the incisive foramen by week 8 of gestation and progresses posteriorly toward the uvula, which fuses at approximately week 12. As the palatine processes grow medially, they are deflected in a downward direction because of the presence of the tongue. However, as facial growth continues, the tongue descends and the palatine processes swing upward and migrate toward each other in a more horizontal position to fuse in the palatine raphe. Failure of fusion results in clefting of the secondary palate.[1]

Understanding the anatomic features of clefts of the secondary palate requires a thorough understanding of normal palatal anatomy (Fig. 46-1). The bony portion of the secondary palate is composed of the maxillary bones, the palatine bones, and the pterygoid plates. The tensor veli palatini, levator veli palatini, palatopharyngeus, palatoglossus, musculus uvulae, and superior pharyngeal constrictor are the muscles that attach to the bony palate and form the soft tissue portion of the secondary palate. The anterior third of the soft palate consists of the aponeurosis of the tensor veli palatini muscles with their tendons coursing around the hamulus on their respective sides.

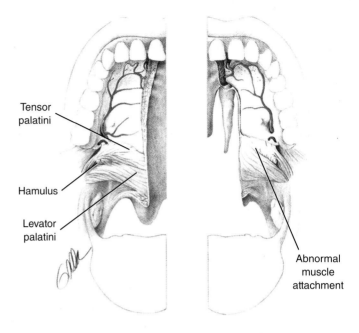

Fig. 46-1 Normal anatomy of the palate. A portion of the levator veli palatini has been removed to show the opening of the eustachian tube *(left)*. Cleft anatomy of the secondary palate. Note the abnormal attachment of the muscles to the edges of the cleft *(right)*.

The tensor veli palatini originates partially from the cartilaginous portion of the eustachian tube. It opens the eustachian tube and provides ventilation of the middle ear during swallowing but is not involved in normal speech function. The paired levator veli palatini muscles originate from the petrous portion of the temporal bone and displace the soft palate superiorly and posteriorly to achieve velopharyngeal closure. They are the primary muscles involved in speech. The musculus uvulae originates and extends posteriorly into the uvula from the posterior nasal spine and the aponeurosis of the tensor veli palatini muscle. The musculus uvulae increases the thickness of the posterior aspect of the soft palate while elevating it against the posterior pharyngeal wall to achieve velopharyngeal closure during speech. The superior pharyngeal constrictor arises from the pterygomandibular raphe and the medial pterygoid plate and inserts into the median raphe in the posterior pharyngeal wall. The superior portion of the superior pharyngeal constrictor contributes to the medial movement of the lateral pharyngeal wall and the forward movement of the posterior pharyngeal wall to facilitate velopharyngeal closure. Contraction of the superior pharyngeal constrictor forms Passavant's ridge, which may play an important role in providing velopharyngeal competence in some cleft patients. Both the palatopharyngeus and the palatoglossus contribute to the downward movement of the palate and medial movement of the pharyngeal wall. However, their contribution in speech is not considered significant when compared with the levator veli palatini.[2]

In patients with a cleft palate, the hard palate is shortened because of the midline defect and the soft palate is shortened because of the faulty anterior attachment of the musculature along the medial margin of the bony defect. The atypical insertion and accompanying hypoplasia of the musculature result in insufficient closure of the velopharynx and poor middle ear ventilation.

EPIDEMIOLOGY AND CLASSIFICATION

Race does not appear to be a factor in clefts of the secondary palate. The incidence is quite constant, at approximately 1 in 2000 live births. When associated with cleft defects of the primary palate, it follows the racial heterogeneity of the primary palate (see Chapter 45). Asian individuals show an increased incidence, at 1 in 500 live births. Clefts of the secondary palate occur 1 in 1000 live births for white individuals and approximately 1 in 2000 live births in black individuals.

The most commonly used classification scheme is the Kernahan "striped Y" system.[3] The incisive foramen is the focal point of the system, and the vertical limb of the Y represents the secondary palate. In general, cleft palate can be classified into two types: overt and submucous. The *overt* cleft can have a variable bony defect with associated hypoplastic musculature and atypical attachments of the muscles along the bony edges of the cleft. The *submucous* cleft may be associated with clinical features such as a bifid uvula, a notched bony defect in the posterior hard palate, and a prominent median raphe (zona pellucida). The submucous cleft may also manifest abnormal muscle attachments to the notched bony defect, similar to the overt cleft. However, some submucous clefts have only mild clefting of the musculature in the soft palate. Known as the *occult submucous cleft,* these clefts may cause velopharyngeal insufficiency after adenoidectomy.

INDICATIONS AND LIMITATIONS

Overt clefts of the secondary palate require surgical correction. Submucous clefts may or may not require surgery, depending on the patient's symptoms. Patients with moderate to severe velopharyngeal insufficiency and a consistently documented anatomical defect usually require surgery.[4] Regardless of the type of procedure chosen, the goal is to recruit or augment adjacent tissue to improve velopharyngeal sphincter closure. Children rarely undergo surgery for velopharyngeal insufficiency before 3 years of age, because they need to have developed conversational speech to be properly diagnosed. A common exception to this rule involves patients with velocardiofacial syndrome and submucous cleft palate, who have severe nasal regurgitation. These patients undergo surgical correction earlier and require preoperative imaging to assess for the presence of medialized carotid arteries.

Overt clefts of the secondary palate are commonly addressed with the von Langenbeck palatoplasty, Wardill-Kilner V-Y pushback palatoplasty, or Furlow palatoplasty. For velopharyngeal insufficiency caused by a submucous cleft or resulting from scarring from previous palatoplasty, surgical options include a superiorly based pharyngeal flap, sphincter pharyngoplasty, Furlow palatoplasty, and posterior pharyngeal wall augmentation. The superiorly based pharyngeal flap pioneered by Schoenborn in 1876 works well for large velopharyngeal gaps with good lateral wall motion. The sphincter pharyngoplasty is indicated for large, central velopharyngeal gaps with poor lateral wall motion. A Furlow palatoplasty is employed for small velopharyngeal gaps and is particularly useful in reorienting the levator veli palatini sling in a submucous cleft palate. Posterior pharyngeal wall augmentation is used for small central velopharyngeal gaps with touch closure, as is commonly seen after adenoidectomy.

Although there are various methods to repair clefts of the secondary palate and to improve velopharyngeal insufficiency, there are still limitations to their success. With a superiorly based pharyngeal flap, the surgeon balances the risk of obstructive sleep apnea against the potential for persistent velopharyngeal insufficiency. In a patient with velocardiofacial syndrome and a large velopharyngeal gap, a sphincter pharyngoplasty or superior based pharyngeal flap may be the best option to improve velopharyngeal function; however, a Furlow palatoplasty may be the safest option due to the fact these patients often manifest medialized carotid arteries. This approach may yield an inadequate result, and a palatal prosthesis may then be required to achieve acceptable function. Patients may also have neuromuscular incoordination or may have learned inappropriate compensatory speech strategies, limiting the success of any surgical procedure. Speech therapy is a high priority in this subgroup of patients.

PATIENT EVALUATION AND PREOPERATIVE PLANNING

Patients with an overt cleft of the secondary palate benefit from palatoplasty. The type of palatoplasty may be surgeon dependent. The most important factor is to ensure good healing after primary surgery to prevent dehiscence, a fistula, and excessive scarring. A Wardill-Kilner V-Y pushback palatoplasty or Furlow palatoplasty may be more appropriate for short palates, because these techniques significantly lengthen the palate.

When patients undergo evaluation for velopharyngeal insufficiency, they require formal perceptual speech evaluation by a speech pathologist with expertise in velopharyngeal insufficiency. The speech pathologist often performs nasometry to grade the amount of nasal air escape during speech and a videofluoroscopic speech evaluation to visualize the velopharynx in motion. Nasoendoscopy is used in cooperative children to directly visualize the velopharynx during speech. A mirror may be placed under the nares to assess for fogging while the patient says oral plosive consonants. Cine MRI has been used in some centers to evaluate patients with velopharyngeal insufficiency.[5]

TECHNIQUE

Surgical management of overt clefts of the secondary palate usually involves closure of both the hard and soft palate in a single stage, and is commonly performed at approximately 10 months of age. However, some surgeons prefer to close the soft palate first to facilitate the development of normal speech, while managing the cleft in the hard palate with an obturator. Closure of the hard palate is postponed until the child is older. This staged procedure is thought to lessen the detrimental effect of surgical manipulation and scarring on facial and maxillary growth.

Clefts of the secondary palate are most commonly repaired using the von Langenbeck palatoplasty (Fig. 46-2), Wardill-Kilner V-Y pushback method (Fig. 46-3), and Furlow palatoplasty (Fig. 46-4) (see Chapter 45 also).

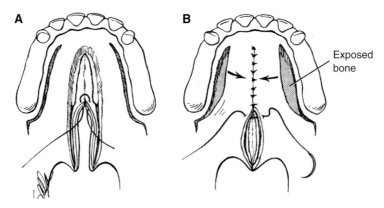

Fig. 46-2   The von Langenbeck repair of a cleft palate. **A,** Incisions have been made, and the palatal and nasal mucosa have been elevated. The levator muscles have been dissected from the abnormal attachment at the edges of the cleft. Closure of the nasal side is nearly completed. **B,** The cleft palate is nearly closed. Note the resulting exposure of the bony palate from advancement of the palatal mucosa medially.

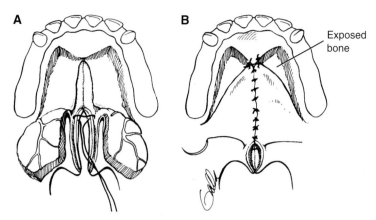

Fig. 46-3   Wardill-Kilner V-Y pushback repair of a cleft palate. **A,** Incisions have been made, the palatal and nasal mucosa have been elevated, and the levator veli palatini muscles have been dissected from the bone edges of the cleft. The greater palatine vessels have been released from the foramen to improve the rotation of the palatal mucosa. The nasal closure has been started. Repair of the soft palate sling involves suturing the levator veli palatini muscles across the midline (intravelar veloplasty). **B,** The cleft palate has been closed. The levator veli palatini muscles have been sutured across the midline. Note the resulting exposure of the bony palate from advancement of the palatal mucosa medially and posteriorly.

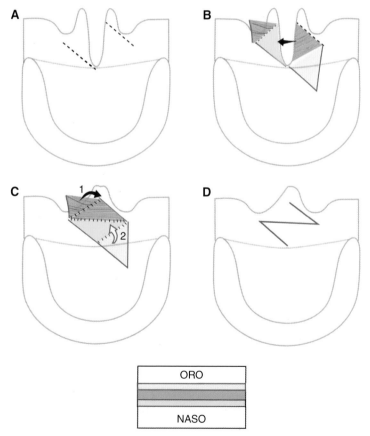

Fig. 46-4   Furlow palatoplasty. **A,** Initially mucosal incisions (for a right-handed surgeon) are made. **B,** A myomucosal flap is elevated on the left and oral mucosal flap on the right and second incisions are shown producing a nasal mucosal flap on the left and a myomucosal flap on the right. **C,** First layer closure reorienting the right levator veli palatini muscle. **D,** Second layer closure reorienting the left levator veli palatini muscle to reproduce a complete sling.

The most important principle is to create a multilayer, tension-free closure that heals well. In general, the Wardill-Kilner pushback method or Furlow palatoplasty is preferred, because either of these achieves closure of the palate while lengthening the soft palate to improve velopharyngeal closure. Patients who have an isolated cleft of the secondary palate do not usually have significant dental problems. However, these patients often have a transverse maxillary deficiency that is thought to be the result of surgical scarring of the palate leading to constriction of maxillary growth. Orthodontic treatment with a palatal prosthesis is sometimes required to widen the maxillary arch.

The superiorly based pharyngeal flap recruits tissue from the posterior pharyngeal wall to bridge a large velopharyngeal gap, leaving two lateral ports for nasal breathing (Fig. 46-5). The width of the pharyngeal flap is based on the extent of lateral pharyngeal wall motion noted on videofluoroscopy or nasoendoscopy. The better the lateral wall motion, the smaller the flap required. Sphincter pharyngoplasty recruits tissue from the lateral pharyngeal walls and places the two flaps along the posterior pharyngeal wall both to tighten the velopharynx circumferentially and to decrease the distance from the posterior edge of the soft palate to the posterior pharyngeal wall (Fig. 46-6). Furlow palatoplasty involves a double-opposing Z-plasty, which reorients the levator veli palatini muscular sling and lengthens the soft palate (see Fig. 46-4). Posterior pharyngeal wall augmentation may be accomplished with a rolled posterior pharyngeal wall flap (Fig. 46-7) or by injection of autologous or nonautologous materials (Fig. 46-8).

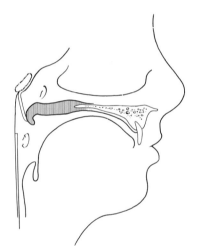

Fig. 46-5 Superiorly based pharyngeal flap. Sagittal view of flap inset muscle-to-muscle into nasal side of soft palate.

Fig. 46-6 Sphincter pharyngoplasty. Flaps are sutured to prevertebral fascia posteriorly and to each other. Flaps may also be sutured end-to-end, depending on the degree of velopharyngeal tightening required.

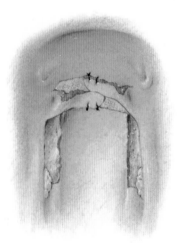

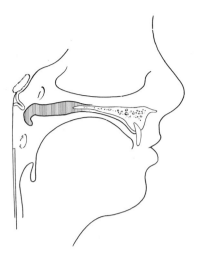

Fig. 46-7   Rolled pharyngeal flap.

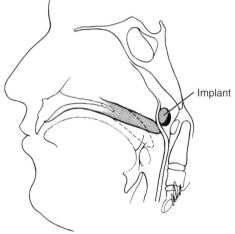

Fig. 46-8   Posterior pharyngeal wall augmentation to facilitate closure of the velopharynx.

ADJUNCTIVE PROCEDURES

Patients who have persistent velopharyngeal insufficiency after surgery may require additional interventions. Revision surgery with the same technique may be indicated in some patients. However, other patients may need a different surgical approach to address residual issues. For instance, a patient who fails a superiorly based pharyngeal flap due to flap dehiscence should undergo a revision superiorly based pharyngeal flap. A patient who originally fails to improve after a Furlow palatoplasty may experience improvement after a superiorly based pharyngeal flap. When velopharyngeal insufficiency fails to improve after multiple surgeries, a daytime palatal lift prosthesis may be indicated.

POSTOPERATIVE CARE

Patients are admitted to the hospital after surgery. For those who have undergone velopharyngeal surgery, continuous pulse oximetry is employed to monitor for obstructive sleep apnea during the first postoperative night. Some children require restraints to ensure they do not place their fingers in their mouths. If a patient is tolerating liquids with adequate pain control, he or she is discharged home on postoperative day 1. Patients remain on a soft diet and the parents and patients are instructed to avoid using straws and sippy cups for at least 2 weeks. Antibiotics are commonly prescribed for 1 week postoperatively.

COMPLICATIONS

Common complications from surgery of the secondary palate include flap dehiscence, fistula, persistent velopharyngeal insufficiency, and excessive scarring. The most feared complication from superiorly based pharyngeal flap surgery is obstructive sleep apnea, which is estimated to occur in 2% to 10% of cases. Patients often have sleep-disordered breathing symptoms for the first few weeks after velopharyngeal surgery, but these symptoms usually resolve.

RESULTS

The von Langenbeck (Fig. 46-9), Wardill-Kilner, and Furlow palatoplasties (Fig. 46-10) represent effective methods of closing clefts of the secondary palate. Becker et al[6] found that there was moderate to severe hypernasality in 7 of 44 patients (16%) after von Langenbeck palatoplasty and in 7 of 22 patients (32%) after Wardill-Kilner palatoplasty; however, the Wardill-Kilner group had fewer fistulas. Williams et al[7] showed that Furlow palatoplasty resulted in better speech results than the von Langenbeck procedure, but fistula occurrence was significantly higher in the Furlow group compared with the von Langenbeck group. Although speech results may be good after Furlow palatoplasty, multiple studies have found that it is not as effective an option in clefts wider than 8 mm.[8,9]

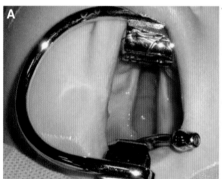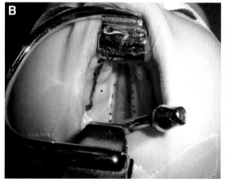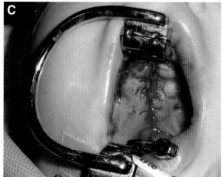

Fig. 46-9   von Langenbeck palatoplasty.

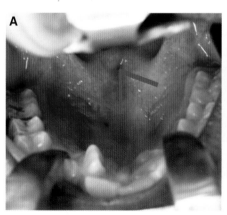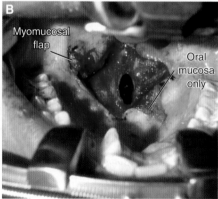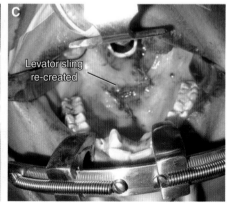

Fig. 46-10   Furlow palatoplasty.

The superiorly based pharyngeal flap has proved to be quite effective in improving velopharyngeal competence through the years. Shprintzen[10] found that regardless of the closure pattern, when a superiorly based pharyngeal flap is used to treat patients with typical velopharyngeal insufficiency, it is up to 80% effective in improving hypernasality. With careful diagnosis and patient selection, this procedure can be up to 97% effective in treating velopharyngeal insufficiency.[10] Armour et al[11] found that although a superiorly based pharyngeal flap may be used to treat a velopharynx with a coronal closure pattern (soft palate closes against posterior pharyngeal wall), it is more effective in patients with noncoronal closure patterns (sagittal closure of lateral pharyngeal walls or circumferential closure of entire velopharyngeal sphincter with or without Passavant's ridge).

Although it is a newer procedure than the superiorly based pharyngeal flap, sphincter pharyngoplasty has proved to be highly effective. Carlisle et al[12] described a success rate of 87% with sphincter pharyngoplasty, which increased to 100% with one revision surgery. Losken et al[13] also achieved an initial success rate of 87%, which increased to 99% after one revision procedure. Riski et al[14] identified a success rate of only 67% in the first 5 years of a 15-year period, but the rate climbed to 86% in the last 5 years, suggesting either a technical learning curve or perhaps more appropriate patient selection. Many centers favor sphincter pharyngoplasty over posterior pharyngeal flaps because of the higher obstructive sleep apnea risk associated with the latter procedure. Sie et al[15] reviewed 24 patients who underwent sphincter pharyngoplasty and found no patients with postoperative obstructive sleep apnea, although the procedure was slightly modified. Witt et al[16] found that only 8 of 58 patients had perioperative or postoperative airway obstruction after sphincter pharyngoplasty, and all but 2 patients resolved these airway symptoms within 3 days postoperatively. Five of these patients also had Pierre Robin sequence.

When used in an ideal patient, the Furlow palatoplasty produces good results. Sie and Gruss[17] reviewed 48 patients who underwent Furlow palatoplasty regardless of velopharyngeal gap size, lateral wall motion, and age, and identified only a 40% incidence of complete resolution of velopharyngeal insufficiency for the entire group. However, Chen et al[18] reviewed 18 patients who underwent Furlow palatoplasty and reported that 89% had complete velopharyngeal closure postoperatively. Fifteen patients in this study had velopharyngeal gaps of less than 5 mm. Lindsey and Davis[19] reviewed 8 patients who underwent Furlow palatoplasty for velopharyngeal dysfunction, and 87% exhibited good palate closure and significant improvement in speech. Half of these patients had undergone previous surgery for cleft palate. In a study of 148 patients, Perkins et al[20] found that 56% of patients had complete resolution of their velopharyngeal insufficiency.

Using posterior pharyngeal wall augmentation in the appropriately selected patient may also be an effective means of achieving velopharyngeal closure. Brigger et al[21] reviewed 12 children who underwent posterior pharyngeal wall augmentation with calcium hydroxyapatite and found that 67% of patients demonstrated successful outcomes 3 months postoperatively. They noted that the ideal patient for this procedure was one with a small central velopharyngeal gap. Additionally, four of the treatment failures occurred early in the senior author's experience with this technique. Sipp et al[22] reviewed 7 patients who underwent injection with calcium hydroxyapatite and achieved a 57% success rate with the procedure 17 months postoperatively. The ideal patients appear to be those with a small velopharyngeal gap and no associated syndrome. Gray et al[23] reviewed 14 patients who underwent rolled posterior pharyngeal wall flap surgery for mild velopharyngeal insufficiency; nasometry scores normalized in 6 of 10 patients who had this variable measured. They found that this procedure was most appropriate in young, nonsyndromic patients with small velopharyngeal gaps. Witt et al[24] reviewed 14 patients who underwent rolled posterior pharyngeal wall flaps for velopharyngeal insufficiency and showed that although this procedure did not result in nasal airway obstruction, it was not effective in improving speech.

KEY POINTS

- Overt clefts of the secondary palate require repair.
- In patients with suspected velopharyngeal insufficiency, a thorough workup is necessary to determine appropriate treatment, including evaluation by a speech pathologist trained in velopharyngeal insufficiency.
- The most essential concept in any cleft surgery is to create a multilayer, tension-free closure that heals optimally after primary surgery.
- A functioning velopharyngeal sphincter is required to prevent nasal air escape and reflux during speech and deglutition, respectively.
- The ideal option in choosing a velopharyngeal surgical approach varies from case to case, depending on the type and size of velopharyngeal gap.

REFERENCES

1. Sadler TW. Langman's Medical Embryology, ed 6. Baltimore: Williams & Wilkins, 1990.
2. Lewin ML, Croft CB, Shiprintzen RJ. Velopharyngeal insufficiency due to hypoplasia of the musculus uvulae and occult submucous cleft palate. Plast Reconstr Surg 65:585-591, 1980.
3. Kernahan DA. The striped Y—a symbolic classification for cleft lip and palate. Plast Reconstr Surg 47:469-470, 1971.
   Kernahan's classification serves as the most commonly used system to describe cleft lip and palate deformities.
4. Costello BJ, Ruiz RL, Turvey TA. Velopharyngeal insufficiency in patients with cleft palate. Oral Maxillofacial Surg Clin N Am 14:539-551, 2002.
   This is an excellent summary of the workup and management of velopharyngeal insufficiency in patients with cleft palate.
5. Silver AL, Nimkin K, Ashland JE, et al. Cine magnetic resonance imaging with simultaneous audio to evaluate pediatric velopharyngeal insufficiency. Arch Otolaryngol Head Neck Surg 137:258-263, 2011.
6. Becker M, Svensson H, Sarnaes KV, et al. Von Langenbeck or Wardill procedures for primary palatal repair in patients with isolated cleft palate—speech results. Scand J Plast Reconstr Surg Hand Surg 34:27-32, 2000.
7. Williams WN, Seagle MB, Pegoraro-Krook MI, et al. Prospective clinical trial comparing outcome measures between Furlow and von Langenbeck palatoplasties for UCLP. Ann Plast Surg 66:154-163, 2011.
   This study suggests that Furlow palatoplasty may result in better speech outcomes compared with von Langenbeck palatoplasty in patients with unilateral cleft lip and palate.
8. Spauwen PH, Goorhuis-Brouwer SM, Schutte HK. Cleft palate repair: Furlow versus von Langenbeck. J Craniomaxillofac Surg 20:18-20, 1992.
9. Losken HW, van Aalst JA, Teotia SS, et al. Achieving low cleft palate fistula rates: surgical results and techniques. Cleft Palate Craniofac J 48:312-320, 2011.
10. Shprintzen RJ. The use of multiview videofluoroscopy and flexible fiberoptic nasopharyngoscopy as a predictor of success with pharyngeal flap surgery. In Ellis F, Flack E, eds. Diagnosis and Treatment of Palatoglossal Malfunction. London: College of Speech Therapists, 1979.
    This chapter discusses the importance of careful preoperative assessment to improve outcomes after pharyngeal flap surgery.
11. Armour A, Fischbach S, Kaiman P, et al. Does velopharyngeal closure pattern affect the success of pharyngeal flap pharyngoplasty? Plast Reconstr Surg 115:45-52, 2005.
12. Carlisle MP, Sykes KJ, Singhal VK. Outcomes of sphincter pharyngoplasty and palatal lengthening for velopharyngeal insufficiency: a 10-year experience. Arch Otolaryngol Head Neck Surg 137:763-766, 2011.
13. Losken A, Williams JK, Burstein FD, et al. An outcome evaluation of sphincter pharyngoplasty for the management of velopharyngeal insufficiency. Plast Reconstr Surg 112:1755-1761, 2003.
14. Riski JE, Ruff GL, Georgiade GS, et al. Evaluation of failed sphincter pharyngoplasties. Ann Plast Surg 28:505-594, 1992.

15. Sie KC, Tampakopoulou DA, De Serres LM, et al. Sphincter pharyngoplasty: speech outcome and complications. Laryngoscope 108:1211-1217, 1998.

16. Witt PD, Marsh JL, Muntz HR, et al. Acute obstructive sleep apnea as a complication of sphincter pharyngoplasty. Cleft Palate Craniofac J 33:183-189, 1996.

17. Sie KC, Gruss JS. Results with Furlow palatoplasty in the management of velopharyngeal insufficiency. Plast Reconstr Surg 109:2588-2589, 2002.

18. Chen PK, Wu JT, Chen YR, et al. Correction of secondary velopharyngeal insufficiency in cleft palate patients with the Furlow palatoplasty. Plast Reconstr Surg 94:933-941, 1994.

19. Lindsey WH, Davis PT. Correction of velopharyngeal insufficiency with Furlow palatoplasty. Arch Otolaryngol Head Neck Surg 122:881-884, 1996.

20. Perkins JA, Lewis CL, Gruss JS, et al. Furlow palatoplasty for management of velopharyngeal insufficiency: a prospective study of 148 consecutive patients. Plast Reconstr Surg 116:72-80, 2005.
    This article reports on a large prospective study of Furlow palatoplasty showing good speech outcomes, especially in patients with small velopharyngeal gaps.

21. Brigger MT, Ashland JE, Hartnick CJ. Injection pharyngoplasty with calcium hydroxylapatite for velopharyngeal insufficiency: patient selection and technique. Arch Otolaryngol Head Neck Surg 136:666-670, 2010.

22. Sipp JA, Ashland J, Hartnick CJ. Injection pharyngoplasty with calcium hydroxyapatite for treatment of velopalatal insufficiency. Arch Otolaryngol Head Neck Surg 134:268-271, 2008.

23. Gray SD, Pinborough-Zimmerman J, Catten M. Posterior wall augmentation for treatment of velopharyngeal insufficiency. Otolaryngol Head Neck Surg 121:107-112, 1999.

24. Witt PD, O'Daniel TG, Marsh JL, et al. Surgical management of velopharyngeal dysfunction: outcome analysis of autogenous posterior pharyngeal wall augmentation. Plast Reconstr Surg 99:1287-1296, 1997.

SUGGESTED READINGS

Dorf SO, Curtin JW. Early cleft palate repair and speech outcome. Plast Reconstr Surg 70:74-79, 1982.
    The authors found that children whose palates were repaired before the onset of speech production demonstrated significantly better speech than those who underwent palatoplasty between 12 and 27 months of age.

Golding-Kushner KJ, Argamaso RV, Cotton RT, et al. Standardization for the reporting of nasopharyngoscopy and multiview videofluoroscopy: a report from an International Working Group. Cleft Palate J 27:337; discussion 347-348, 1990.
    The authors devised criteria to describe the velopharyngeal gap and closure pattern as a movement ratio of one structure relative to the resting position of the structure at the opposite side of the valve, with the movement of each structure rated separately.

47

Congenital Vascular Anomalies of the Head and Neck

Milton Waner ▪ *Teresa M. O*

CLASSIFICATION OF CONGENITAL VASCULAR LESIONS

The importance of accurately identifying and naming a vascular lesion cannot be overstated. A correct initial diagnosis will provide an understanding of the natural history of the lesion and guide overall management. An incorrect diagnosis on the other hand, may lead to incorrect treatment. Mulliken and Glowacki initially proposed a biologic and functional classification.[1] They recognized two groups, *hemangiomas* and *vascular malformations*. Hemangiomas were considered distinct from vascular malformations because of their ability to proliferate. Vascular malformations do not proliferate. These lesions were further subclassified according to the primary vessel involved: arterial, venous, capillary, and lymphatic. Before this, all vascular lesions were diagnosed as hemangiomas. This led to incorrect diagnoses and treatments.

Mulliken and Glowacki's biologic classification led to a renaissance in the study of congenital vascular anomalies. The fundamental difference between hemangiomas and vascular malformations was recognized. This classification, which became the official schema accepted by the International Society for the Study of Vascular Anomalies (ISSVA), was further modified and updated in 1996 and 2014 to include other vascular tumors (Box 47-1).

Vascular Tumors

Infantile Hemangiomas

Natural History

Infantile hemangiomas (IH) are the most common type of hemangiomas and are benign stem cell tumors.[2-4] They occur in 1 of 10 births and are more common in girls, fair-skinned individuals, and multiple, premature, and low-birth-weight infants.[5] At birth, there is often nothing visible, or perhaps a hypopigmented macule. This is followed by a period of rapid postnatal growth of the lesion beginning 1 to 2 weeks after birth. The growth or proliferation phase will depend on the type of hemangioma.

Lesions may be focal (localized) or segmental (dermatomal) in distribution[6] (Fig. 47-1). Focal lesions are made up of tumors whose parenchyma consists of a mass of proliferating endothelial cells. These lesions proliferate for up 10 months. This is followed by a quiescent phase, and then a decade-long process of involution or shrinkage.

Box 47-1   ISSVA Classification of Vascular Anomalies

Vascular Tumors

Infantile hemangiomas (IH)

Congenital hemangiomas

Rapidly involuting congenital hemangioma (RICH)

Partially involuting congenital hemangioma (PICH)

Noninvoluting congenital hemangioma (NICH)

Tufted angioma (± Kasabach-Merritt syndrome)

Kaposiform hemangioendothelioma
(± Kasabach-Merritt syndrome)

Spindle cell hemangioendothelioma

Other rare hemangioendotheliomas
(such as epithelioid, composite, retiform,
polymorphous, Dabska tumor, and
lymphangioendotheliomatosis)

Acquired vascular tumors (such as pyogenic
granuloma, targetoid hemangioma, glomeruloid
hemangioma, and microvenular hemangioma)

Vascular Malformations

Capillary malformation (CM)

Port-wine stain

Telangiectasia

Angiokeratoma

Venous malformation (VM)

Common sporadic VM

Familial cutaneous and mucosal venous malformation
(VMCM)

Glomuvenous malformation (GVM) (glomangioma)

Blue rubber bleb nevus syndrome

Maffucci syndrome

Lymphatic malformation (LM)

Fast-flow vascular malformation:

    Arterial malformation (AM)

    Arteriovenous fistula (AVF)

    Arteriovenous malformation (AVM)

Complex-combined vascular malformation:
    CMV, CLM, LVM, CLVM, AVM-LM, CM-AVM

A, Arterial; *C,* capillary; *ISSVA,* International Society for the Study of Vascular Anomalies; *L,* lymphatic; *M,* malformation; *V,* venous.

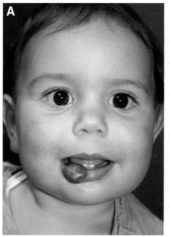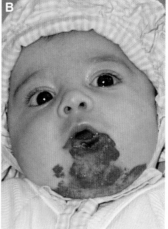

Fig. 47-1 **A,** A child with a focal lip infantile hemangioma. **B,** A baby with a segmental lip infantile hemangioma.

Segmental lesions are more aggressive and grow within dermatomal segments for as long as 18 to 36 months. During this phase, they may ulcerate (up to 35%), which can lead to extensive necrosis and tissue loss, especially of fibrocartilage (Fig. 47-2). When this heals, these children are often severely disfigured. IH may also be superficial (epidermis only), deep (subcutaneous), or compound.

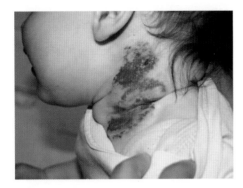

Fig. 47-2   A child with an ulcerated cervical infantile hemangioma.

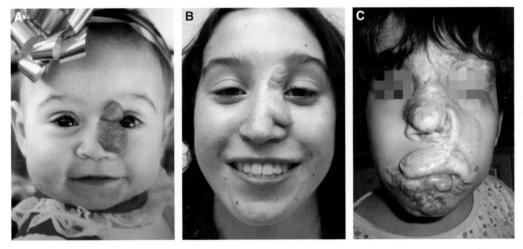

Fig. 47-3   A child with a left paranasal infantile hemangioma. **A,** During the proliferative phase, age 6 months. **B,** A 16-year-old girl with the same lesion after involution. Note the residual fibrofatty mass, with overlying atrophic scarring. **C,** A child with an extensive left segmental facial infantile hemangioma. Note the areas of previous ulceration and scarring. No previous treatment had been administered.

After a period of quiescence, the hemangioma will begin to involute. Vascular channels diminish in size and number and are eventually replaced with fibrofatty, vascular stroma. Histologically, proliferating vascular endothelial cells undergo apoptosis and are replaced by hypervascular fibrofatty tissue. Concomitant clinical changes include a diminution in the size of the mass. The mass will "disappear" in about 50% of cases and in the remainder, a fibrofatty mass will remain.[7] If the overlying skin was involved, then reduced vascularity brought about by involution will translate into a reduction in erythema. At times, all of the erythema will disappear, but in approximately 50% of cases erythema will persist, often in the form of telangiectasias.

During the proliferation phase, the papillary dermis is often replaced with hemangioma. This layer contains the adnexal structures (sweat glands, sebaceous glands, and hair follicles) that are essential to normal healing. In addition, the dermal layer is rich in collagen and elastin. During involution, the papillary dermis does not regenerate. The skin becomes atrophic because of an absence of normal dermal collagen.[8] Therefore, in 50% of cases, an atrophic scar overlying a fibrofatty mass will persist, even though this lesion has "involuted." *Involuted* therefore does not necessarily mean the lesion will disappear; it means it will shrink (Fig. 47-3).

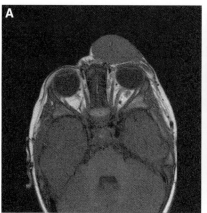 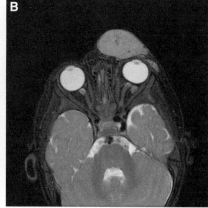

Fig. 47-4 An axial MRI of left upper eyelid and brow infantile hemangioma. **A,** The lesion is isointense on a T1-weighted image. **B,** Infantile hemangioma has an intermediate signal on a T2-weighted image.

Diagnosis

A diagnosis of IH is made largely from the history and physical examination. Unlike vascular malformations, IHs are usually not present at birth. Their typical growth pattern is postnatal proliferation followed by involution. Focal hemangiomas grow as well-defined lobulated masses that occur in sites of predilection.[6] Superficial lesions have characteristic bright erythematous staining, whereas deep lesions may be flesh colored or a bluish hue. Compound lesions will exhibit variable signs with both superficial and deep lesion characteristics.

Segmental hemangiomas are more diffuse and involve one or more dermatomal segments. Within these segments, involvement is almost always superficial, in which case the lesion is diffuse, macular or papular, and erythematous. The dermatome may be filled with disease, or it may only be partially involved.

Radiologic features are consistent. On MRI these are parenchymatous, lobulated, well-defined masses with intermediate signal intensity on T1-weighted images and increased signal intensity on T2-weighted images[8a,8b] (Fig. 47-4). Vascular flow voids are evident on spin echo sequences. The signal intensity enhances with the administration of gadolinium. Ultrasound will show a hypervascular soft tissue mass within skin or subcutaneous fat.

Biopsy is rarely necessary, because in the vast majority of cases the diagnosis is straightforward. However, histologically, cellular markers are evident during proliferation and involution. The primary cellular components include vascular endothelial cells, mast cells, macrophages, plasma cells, and pericytes.[9,10] During proliferation, there are masses of endothelial cells and pericytes with erythrocytes within their lumen. High mitotic figures are evident.

During involution, the endothelial cells become flattened, mitotic activity decreases, basement membranes are thickened, and there is an abundance of loose fibroadipose tissue surrounding the few remaining capillaries. Cellular mediators are involved, including vascular endothelial growth factor, fibroblast growth factor, tissue inhibitor of metalloproteinase type I, type IV collagenase, urokinase, and insulinlike growth factor.[9,11-14] Another marker is the SKI oncogene protein, which is differentially expressed according to growth phase and is consistent with IH as a tumor. It is not expressed in pyogenic granuloma or other vascular tumors or malformations.[15]

Glucose transporter 1 (GLUT1) is the currently used marker for hemangiomas in all phases of growth.[11] It is only expressed by hemangiomas, not other vascular tumors or malformations. GLUT1 is a surface protein that is highly expressed in most embryonic and fetal endothelial cells, but is lost in most tissues except at the blood-tissue barrier (CNS and placenta).[11,16] This finding spawned a hypothesis that hemangiomas are derived from placental tissue.[17,18] Current research points to hemangiomas as stem cell tumors.[2-4,19]

ASSOCIATED SYNDROMES

PHACES SYNDROME

In about 30% of segmental hemangiomas, a constellation of developmental abnormalities may be associated. These are collectively known as PHACES syndrome: *p*osterior fossa structural malformations, *h*emangiomas (segmental), *a*rterial anomalies (such as agenesis, hypoplasia, and stenosis of vessels), *c*ardiac defects, *e*ye abnormalities, and *s*ternal and other midline abnormalities.

A diagnosis of PHACES syndrome can be made when one or more of these conditions is present with a segmental hemangioma.[20,21] Hemangiomas of the posterior midline or paramedian areas may be associated with neural tube defects. These should be excluded by ultrasound within the first 6 months.

RAPIDLY INVOLUTING CONGENITAL HEMANGIOMA

Rapidly involuting congenital hemangiomas (RICH) are congenital vascular tumors that are fully formed at birth. They are high-flow lesions and may precipitate high output cardiac failure either in utero or after birth. Once the child is born, these lesions begin to involute. This process is typically complete by the time the child is 18 months of age, and is usually associated with extensive atrophy of the surrounding tissues. In contrast to IHs, both RICHs are GLUT1 negative[22] (Fig. 47-5).

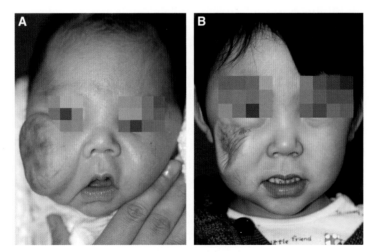

Fig. 47-5   A child with a rapidly involuting congenital hemangioma. **A,** Early stages. **B,** Later stages. Note the extensive soft tissue atrophy. (Courtesy of Ho Yun Chung, MD.)

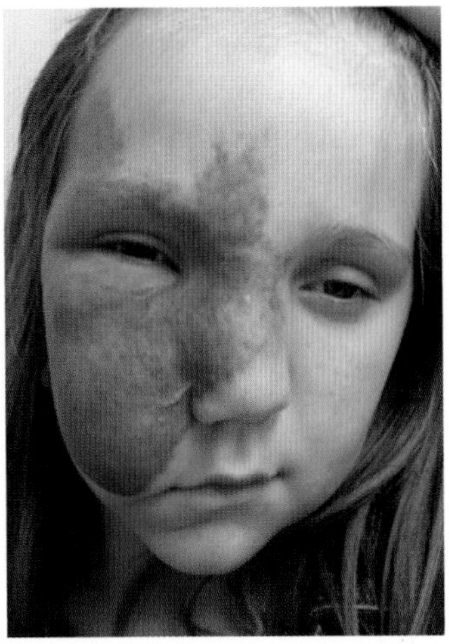

Fig. 47-6   A 10-year-old girl with a right-sided facial noninvoluting congenital hemangioma. The lesion has grown proportionally with the patient.

NONINVOLUTING CONGENITAL HEMANGIOMA

Noninvoluting congenital hemangiomas (NICH) are also fully formed at birth, but unlike hemangiomas and RICH lesions, these never involute. Instead, they are stable over the lifetime of the patient. Observation over the first few months of life will often help to distinguish a RICH from a NICH. These lesions are high flow and often exhibit shunting. NICHs are also GLUT1 negative[22] (Fig. 47-6).

TUFTED ANGIOMA (± KASABACH-MERRITT SYNDROME)

Tufted angioma (± Kasabach-Merritt syndrome) is a rare vascular tumor that may present as a solitary tumor or erythematous violaceous plaque.[23] Spontaneous involution may occur, however, when associated with Kasabach-Merritt syndrome, and may be present at birth or over the first year of life.[24] Histologic examination reveals a proliferation of endothelial cells forming lobules with typical "shotgun" distribution.[24] Clinical findings include thrombocytopenia, hypofibrinogenemia, and coagulopathy with vascular tumor, and at times with lymphatic malformation.[25]

KAPOSIFORM HEMANGIOENDOTHELIOMA (KHE ± KASABACH-MERRITT SYNDROME)

Kaposiform hemangioendothelioma is a rare childhood tumor often associated with Kasabach-Merritt phenomenon (KMP) and occasionally lymphangiomatosis. Lesions are slightly raised and blue-red in color.[26] Clinical findings include thrombocytopenia, hypofibrinogenemia, and coagulopathy with vascular tumor and at times with lymphatic malformation.[25]

Spindle cell hemangioendothelioma is a superficially located mass, some with Maffucci syndrome.[27] Histologic findings include cavernous blood-filled spaces and spindle cells.[28]

VASCULAR MALFORMATIONS

In contrast with vascular tumors, vascular malformations are true congenital malformations of the vascular system; they are present at birth. They do not proliferate, nor do they involute. Instead, they expand with advancing age and are influenced by factors such as hormonal changes. Expansion is not associated with

Box 47-2   Vascular Malformations by Vessel Type

Slow-Flow Vascular Malformations
Capillary Malformations
Port-wine stains
Telangiectasia

Venous Malformations
Common sporadic
Familial cutaneous and mucosal venous
    malformations

Glomuvenous Malformations
Blue rubber bleb nevus syndrome
Maffucci syndrome

Lymphatic Malformations
Fast-Flow Vascular Malformations
Arteriovenous malformations
Arteriovenous fistulas

Complex-Combined Vascular Malformations
    (mixed malformations)

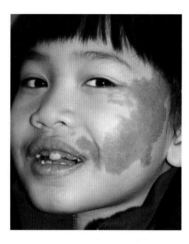

Fig. 47-7   A child with a left facial V2
maxillary port-wine stain.

cellular proliferation but rather hypertrophy of existing vascular channels. Vascular malformations are sub-divided by their vessel type in accordance with the previously mentioned ISSVA classification (Box 47-2).

Recent work has highlighted the role of genetic mutations in causing these lesions. This is an area that was uncharted until recently, and in which major advances are expected.[29,30]

CAPILLARY MALFORMATIONS

Port-wine stains are by far the most common examples in this group of lesions. They occur in 0.3% of the population.[31] They present as macular cutaneous vascular stains that vary in intensity from a light pink to a dark purple (Fig. 47-7).

They are dermatomal/segmental lesions caused by the dilation of the vessels in the dermal plexus of post-capillary venules.[32,33] This results from an absence of autonomic innervation, which causes a loss of ve-nomotor tone.[34] The net effect of this loss is vasodilation that progresses over the patient's lifetime. The port-wine stain will therefore darken as the patient gets older. Within the dermatome, the distribution of the vascular stain can vary from a confluent lesion involving the entire dermatome to a geographic distri-bution of scattered islands of staining within an otherwise normal dermatome.[35] In addition to darkening, as the patient ages, about 30% will form nodules or cobblestones with or without thickening.[36] Although the causes of these are unknown, they are focal collections of ectatic vessels.

A small percentage of port-wine stains are associated with soft tissue overgrowth, the cause of which is unknown. In these cases, there is overgrowth of all of the components of the dermatome, including bone.

Port-wine stains may also involve ocular structures and in some cases, if left untreated, can lead to blindness. Patients with lesions involving one or both eyelids (V1 alone or V1 and V2) should be seen by an ophthalmologist for evaluation and follow-up.[32] These patients may develop glaucoma, but blindness can be prevented if it is detected early and treated aggressively. Children with port-wine stains may also have Sturge-Weber syndrome.[37] This syndrome refers to a triad of port-wine stain in the V1 distribution, ipsilateral leptomeningeal vascular malformation, and a choroidal vascular lesion of the eye. Between 3% and 10% of patients with V1 port-wine stains will have Sturge-Weber syndrome,[37] which is characterized by contralateral seizures, hemiplegia or hemiparesis, cerebral atrophy, and mental impairment.[38,39] Developmental delays occur in about half of these patients. Ocular manifestations include glaucoma, choroidal vascular lesions of the eye, coloboma, cataract formation, iris heterochromia, and myopia.[40,41]

Capillary malformation–arteriovenous malformation (CM-AVM) is a rare autosomal dominant lesion caused by a mutation in the *RASA1* gene.[30] These patients present with small multifocal capillary malformation overlying arteriovenous malformation.

LYMPHATIC MALFORMATIONS

Lymphatic malformations (also called *lymphangiomas* and *cystic hygromas*) result from an abnormality of lymph flow across an area.[42] This may be caused by an overdevelopment or an underdevelopment of lymph tissue in an area. The net result of this is focal or diffuse edema of the involved area. If the disease process extends to the skin or mucosa, this manifests as small lymph-filled and/or blood-filled vesicles. There can be devastating consequences for these patients, including craniofacial distortion and severe functional abnormalities such as airway obstruction and dysphagia. Tongue and/or floor of mouth disease can lead to glossoptosis, and multiple vesicles will leak lymph or a mixture of blood and lymph. Lymphatic malformations can also lead to craniofacial bony distortion. This is a result of a mass effect or bony overgrowth. These patients often have dental hygiene issues and an open bite, which will lead to drooling, feeding difficulties, and poor speech intelligibility.[43,44]

Lymphatic malformations are frequently diagnosed in utero. A large craniofacial lesion will alert the treating physician that an airway obstruction is likely and that an exit tracheostomy may be necessary[45] (Fig. 47-8).

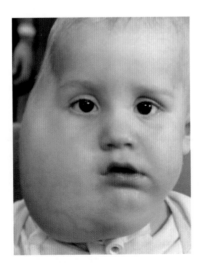

Fig. 47-8   A child with a right hemifacial lymphatic malformation. Note the tracheotomy.

VENOUS MALFORMATIONS

Venous malformations (VM) are a result of an inborn error in the development of the venous system. The veins in a VM are thin walled and dilated.[46] The flow rate of blood through this system is significantly slowed, and whether this or some other factor is responsible, intravascular clotting takes place (Fig. 47-9). Phleboliths thus form, which are often tender. If the amount of intravascular clotting is extensive, a consumptive coagulopathy may result; this is known as *localized intravascular coagulation*.[47-49]

VMs may be focal or diffuse, and in 90% of cases they are solitary. These are sporadic in nature. In 10% of cases there is a familial factor; 80% of these are glomuvenous malformations and the remaining 20% are cases of cutaneomucosal venous malformations (CMVMs).[50]

Glomuvenous malformation is an autosomal dominant lesion with glomuslike cells along the vessel wall. These lesions are typically superficial and involve cutaneous and subcutaneous structures, and can be painful on palpation. CMVMs are multifocal autosomal dominant small lesions (less than 5 cm) involving the head and neck in 50% of cases (Fig. 47-10).

VMs are typically bluish, soft, compressible lesions that expand when in a dependent position. Phleboliths are commonly palpated within these lesions and their presence is a diagnostic feature of a venous malformation. A venous malformation involving the face or scalp, with a transcalvarial dural communication with an intracranial sinus, is known as *sinus pericranium*.

Blue rubber bleb nevus syndrome is a rare condition in which multiple small (less than 2 cm) cutaneous lesions and gastrointestinal lesions are present.[51,52] Severe gastrointestinal bleeding is the major complication associated with this syndrome.[53]

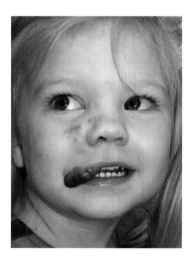

Fig. 47-9   A child with right premaxillary and upper lip venous malformation.

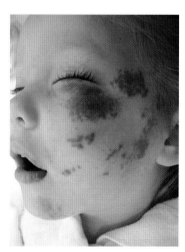

Fig. 47-10   A child with a left facial glomuvenous malformation.

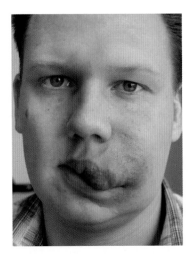

Fig. 47-11   A patient with a left upper lip and premaxillary small vessel arteriovenous malformation.

ARTERIOVENOUS MALFORMATIONS

Arteriovenous malformations (AVMs) are vascular anomalies in which there is abnormal shunting from the arterial side to the venous side. This takes place across an abnormal capillary bed in which we believe the normal regulatory mechanisms have been lost. In the normal circulation, the flow of blood into a capillary bed is regulated according to the local needs of the tissue. Loss of this regulation results in continuous shunting of blood across the capillary bed. This constant perfusion brings about the clinical changes. Constant perfusion results in slow expansion of the capillary bed, also known as the *nidus*. This causes venous dilation and arterial hypertrophy, which are secondary changes.[54]

AVMs may be focal or diffuse. Focal lesions commonly occur in "choke zones," which are areas between angiosomes (Fig. 47-11). An angiosome is the three-dimensional block of tissue supplied by branches of a single source artery.[55] As an expansion of this theory, we believe that the capillary beds within these choke zones are the primary sites of the nidus. Autoregulation of the flow through these capillary beds is most likely to be deficient, and this becomes the nidus of an AVM.

Clinically, AVMs present as firm vascular masses. Although they may not be apparent at birth, they are always present and increase in size during the patient's lifetime. Tissue ischemia occurs despite the high perfusion rate. This may cause ulceration of the overlying tissue, thus placing the patient at risk for infection and bleeding. The vascular mass may or may not pulsate, and often a fluid thrill can be found within the nidus.

THE TREATMENT OF INFANTILE HEMANGIOMAS

Infantile hemangiomas (IH) should only be treated if active treatment offers a distinct advantage over conservative management. A number of factors must be considered when deciding how and when to treat a hemangioma. First and foremost, the natural history must be taken into account. All hemangiomas involute, but the degree and speed with which the lesion will involute is unpredictable. It is generally accepted that involution can take up to 12 years to complete. Furthermore, there is no way of predicting how far the lesion will regress spontaneously. In approximately half of cases, the degree of spontaneous involution is satisfactory; in the other half, some form of treatment is necessary (Fig. 47-12). It is believed that a patient showing early involution will fall into the former group, whereas late involuters (involution that takes longer than 5 years) will generally fall into the latter group.[7]

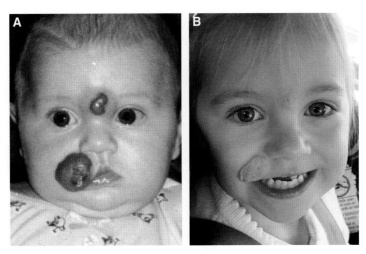

Fig. 47-12   **A,** A child with a midglabellar and right upper lip focal infantile hemangioma. **B,** Same child at age 3 with involution of the IH. There is atrophic scarring with fibrofatty residuum.

A second factor concerns the degree of disfigurement. Today's standards far exceed what was once considered acceptable. We are therefore more likely to treat a disfiguring lesion now than we were 20 years ago.

Third, our understanding of differential wound-healing environments in children and adults has changed. Infants and very young children produce more type III collagen in a fine reticular pattern. It is also laid down more rapidly, and mesenchymal stem cells are more readily mobilized during the healing process than in an older child.[56-59] All of this translates into less scarring and underscores the value of treatment at a younger age. An incised wound in an infant will heal with little or no scar tissue.

Further, medical and surgical options have advanced over the past decades for the treatment of vascular lesions. Today, fine electrocautery devices, novel hemostatic agents, improved anesthesia, and refined surgical techniques have offered a safe approach to obtain a cosmetically acceptable result.

Finally, the anatomic location of the lesion is of paramount importance. A 2 cm lesion on the tip of a child's nose has much more visual impact than the same size lesion on the neck or back.

In general, the following lesions need to be considered for treatment:
1. Facial or clearly exposed hemangiomas; 60% of hemangiomas occur in the central face[6]
2. Any hemangioma that is unlikely to involute to a satisfactory degree and in whom intervention will result in a more favorable outcome
3. Any complication (such as ulceration, functional impairment, cardiac failure, and disfigurement) will warrant treatment
4. Airway lesions
5. Periocular lesions warrant special attention because of their propensity to cause amblyopia and even blindness

Factors that will determine the modality for treatment include:
- The child's age (this will determine if the lesion is proliferating or involuting)
- The anatomic location of the lesion
- The type of the lesion (focal versus segmental)
- The depth of the lesion (superficial, deep, or compound)

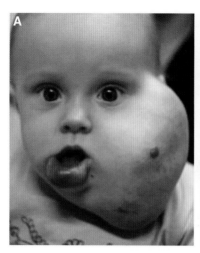
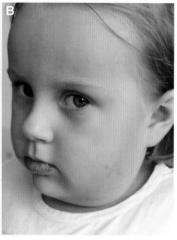

Fig. 47-13 **A,** A child with a left parotid compound hemangioma. **B,** After 12 months of treatment with propranolol only. There is residual asymmetry, which will be treated surgically.

MEDICAL TREATMENT
Propranolol

Since 2008, propranolol has become an extremely useful drug, rapidly surpassing all other medical modalities in the treatment of infantile hemangiomas.[60] In most centers propranolol has become the first-line therapy (Fig. 47-13).

Propranolol is a nonselective beta-1, beta-2 antagonist. Its exact mechanism of action is still unknown. As with many new therapies, the basic scientific explanation is still nascent and evolving with clinical experience. Current theories address effects on vascular endothelial cells and hemangioma stem cells.[61-64] The medication is taken two or three times a day and is well tolerated. Side effects of particular concern include bronchospasm and hypoglycemia.[65-67] At present, there is no consensus on the initiation of the drug. After cardiology evaluation, some centers routinely admit children and others do not.

Topical beta-blockers have also been reported to be an effective alternative treatment for very superficial hemangiomas. Several case reports have been published, all of which show encouraging results, but there are valid concerns regarding the bioavailability of the drug in neonates and infants. Timolol gel-forming solution (Timolol GFS), the more popular form, appears to be up to 10 times more potent than propranolol. Although precise correlates are unknown, each drop of topical timolol may represent between 2 and 8 mg of oral propranolol. Significant amounts may be systemically absorbed when applied near a mucous membrane or to an ulcerated surface. For this reason, Timolol gel is used for very small (1 to 2 cm) cutaneous, superficial lesions only (Fig. 47-14). Current studies are exploring the use and efficacy of selective beta-1 antagonists.

Corticosteroids

Although some physicians still advocate the use of oral corticosteroids,[68] their role has been significantly reduced by the advent of propranolol. Steroids are now rarely prescribed unless propranolol is contraindicated, or as an adjuvant in airway disease.

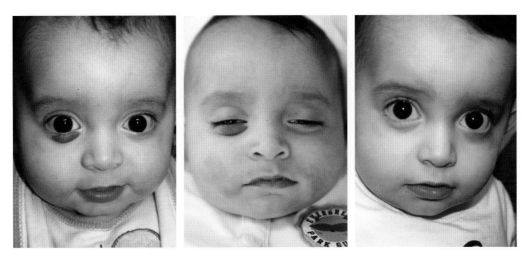

Fig. 47-14   A child with a superficial infantile hemangioma of the right lower eyelid treated with five pulsed-dye laser treatments.

Vincristine

Systemic vincristine is a microtubule-disrupting agent that inhibits angiogenesis. This drug became popular in cases of steroid failure, or as an adjuvant to steroids in cases in which their long-term use was becoming problematic.[69,70] Vincristine was also useful in treating kaposiform hemangioendotheliomas.[71] Vincristine is rarely used today. Propranolol contraindication or failure warrants the consideration of systemic vincristine use.

Interferon Alfa

Interferon alfa is mentioned as a historical footnote. Because of the high risk of complications (including hepatic and renal dysfunction and central nervous system disorders such as spastic diplegia) and the availability of other safer medical treatments, this drug should no longer be used.

LASER TREATMENT

Laser treatment emerged as the treatment of choice for port-wine stains in the early 1980s.[35,72] The theory of selective photothermolysis and subsequent clinical experience made pulsed-dye lasers (PDLs) the treatment of choice for port-wine stains. Within a few years, physicians began treating hemangiomas with PDLs.[73,74] The parameters used in these studies were similar to those used to treat port-wine stains. Since hemangiomas are tumors and are vastly different from port-wine stains, the same concepts do not apply. Despite this, several authors have reported successful treatment for early superficial hemangiomas and the superficial component of a deep hemangioma.[75] Complications have also been reported. These include atrophic scarring, a direct consequence of laser destruction of dermis, and severe and extensive ulceration, the cause of which we still do not understand. From this, we know the following:

- Pulsed-dye laser treatment of superficial hemangiomas is effective.
- Treatment complications appear to be uncommon.
- The mechanism of action of laser treatment is not well understood.

PDLs emit light at 585 nm. The effective depth of penetration of light at this wavelength (2 mm at best) will be sufficient to treat only the most superficial lesions or the superficial component of a deeper lesion.[75] This means that only the erythematous (red) component of the hemangioma can be treated with a PDL. Several treatments may be necessary to eliminate the red component of a hemangioma. Neodymium-doped

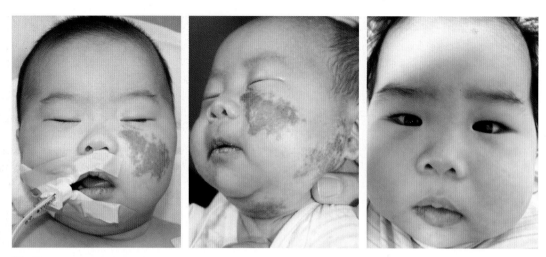

Fig. 47-15 A child with V2 and V3 segmental infantile hemangioma treated with propranolol and serial PDL treatment.

yttrium aluminum garnet (Nd:YAG) lasers emit light in the near infrared spectrum (1064 nm), which penetrates far deeper and thus is more effective for the deeper component. The higher risk of scarring with these lasers has precluded them from widespread use.

The role for laser treatment has become largely secondary, since both topical and systemic beta-blockers have become the first line of treatment for hemangiomas and are able to eliminate the erythematous component. PDL can be used as an adjuvant to beta-blockers to eliminate superficial hemangiomas and has been shown to have a synergistic effect[76] (Fig. 47-15). PDL is also used in cases in which parents object to the long-term use of an oral medication, or for small lesions that would respond to one or two treatments with a PDL.

In some cases, a telangiectatic pattern of larger vessels persists after propranolol and/or PDL treatment. These vessels can be seen as discrete ectatic vessels and generally are greater than 200 μm in diameter. Thus they require a greater thermal load to obliterate them. This can be done with either a diode laser with a smaller spot size (1 mm) or an Nd:YAG laser (in conjunction with dynamic skin cooling). Intense pulsed light emitting devices can also be used.

Involuted IH skin is atrophic and hypopigmented. CO_2 Fraxel dermabrasion is used to generate subepidermal fibrosis, which leads to new collagen deposition and improved skin texture.

THE SURGICAL TREATMENT

The indications for surgery are not uniform and vary from center to center. In general, indications for surgery include the following:

1. *Failed conservative therapy.* This category includes lesions that have been allowed to proliferate and then involute without any form of treatment. At some point it becomes obvious that the lesion is unlikely to involute adequately. Another reason may be that the child has reached a level of maturity at which he or she is aware of the lesion and is psychologically affected by it.
2. *Failed medical therapy.* In our experience, propranolol is more efficacious with segmental IHs than with focal lesions. In many instances, propranolol will fail to shrink an IH completely. Surgery is therefore indicated.

3. *Complications.* Ulcerated lesions cause severe pain, may become secondarily infected, and bleed. Immediate surgical excision may obviate weeks of medical therapy and discomfort for the child. Areas of ulceration lead to atrophic scarring, which will ultimately require scar revision. Congestive heart failure is a complication of very large IHs and may require urgent removal. Airway hemangiomas require close monitoring and possible intervention to prevent airway obstruction. Eyelid hemangiomas also tend to cause astigmatism or visual obstruction and need early intervention.

4. *Surgery is likely to provide the best outcome.* In some instances, especially in focal hemangiomas, treatment with propranolol will, at best, merely shrink the hemangioma. In these instances surgery may provide a better outcome.[77] The timing of surgery takes into consideration the location of the lesion, the type and extent of the lesion (focal/segmental), and the age of the patient.

For simplicity, the surgical management of IH will be discussed by anatomic sites:

- Eyelid and orbit
- Nasal
- Cheek
- Lip
- Forehead and scalp
- Parotid gland
- Airway

In all cases, attention should be directed to the normal anatomic subunits of the face. Often, the hemangioma has expanded the tissues, and thus primary closure may be achieved even in very large lesions. When this is not the case, staged surgical excision is possible to prevent overresection. With the combined use of preoperative and postoperative laser therapy, treated hemangioma-infiltrated skin may be left in place.

Periocular Hemangiomas

Periocular hemangiomas occur in 24% of cases[6]; specifically 8.5% involve the upper eyelid. Like airway hemangiomas, orbit, eyelid, and conjunctival hemangiomas constitute a special category because of their anatomic location. These hemangiomas threaten visual development, significantly affect facial expression, and have an impact on psychological development. The threat of permanent visual loss *(amblyopia),* spectacle dependence *(astigmatism),* strabismus, eyelid deformity, and orbit distortion must be considered when treating periocular IH. The most serious cause of amblyopia is direct visual axis obstruction. Cases of partial obstruction should be managed according to the amount and frequency of visual axis obstruction.

Astigmatism, which occurs from pathologic warping of the cornea, may be caused by either upper or lower eyelid hemangiomas. It can be reversed with early intervention before 9 months of age, but not beyond 13 months (unpublished data).

Strabismus may result from mechanical obstruction of extraocular motility or direct invasion of extraocular muscles. Medial rectus involvement is most common, producing esotropia. Superior oblique involvement is seen in typical superonasal orbit cases, but this is more subtle and may require special testing to diagnose.

Permanent eyelid deformity results from direct invasion, vascular steal, or prolonged pressure of adjacent structures. Most sensitive are the levator palpebrae superioris, tarsus, eyelash follicles, and lamina papyracea. The levator muscle can be salvaged with early treatment, but prolonged invasion produces a fatty, atrophic muscle. The tarsus, lash follicles, and bones of the orbit also respond well to early excision, allowing them to resume unimpeded growth and development. Preservation of the tarsus ensures eyelid margin stability, whereas maintenance of the bony socket prevents globe displacement.

Like all facial hemangiomas, periocular IH should be categorized according to subtype. The most common location of focal periocular hemangiomas is the superomedial orbit. These lesions always involve the eyelid and frequently invade the dermis. They compress the globe and produce medial upper eyelid ptosis. MRI frequently reveals an unexpectedly large lesion that envelops the superior oblique muscle. Surgical extirpation is best accomplished through a lid crease approach (Fig. 47-16).

Hemangiomas involving the central upper lid tend to expand the pretarsal space and distort lash follicles; in many cases they wrap around the tarsus to involve the conjunctiva. Even a small IH in this location can produce astigmatism. Surgical dissection requires careful attention to lash follicles and proper placement of a lid crease incision.

A consistent challenge in the removal of lower eyelid IH is prevention of postoperative ectropion or retraction. Early surgery takes advantage of natural tissue expansion to reduce this risk. Occasionally tissue rotation, such as a Tenzel rotation flap, is required, especially if surgery has been delayed.

The upper lid is commonly involved in V1 segmental hemangiomas. The full thickness of the eyelid is involved in addition to orbital soft tissues and bone. Propranolol is typically effective if given early. Nevertheless, surgical correction of upper lid ptosis is often necessary (Fig. 47-17).

Early surgery is the most effective way to eliminate or decrease the risk of amblyopia, and dramatically improves the chances for preservation of the extraocular muscle, eyelid, and orbit. Nevertheless, diffuse orbital hemangiomatosis is not amenable to surgery but may respond well to oral propranolol treatment.

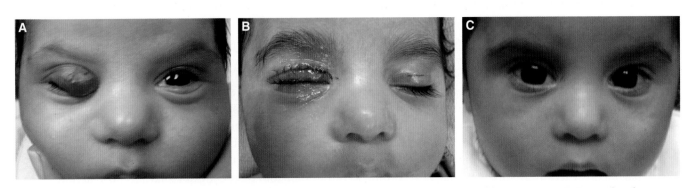

Fig. 47-16   A child with a focal upper eyelid infantile hemangioma. **A,** Upper eyelid hemangioma. **B,** Immediately after resection. **C,** Result 6 months postoperatively.

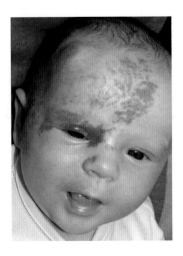

Fig. 47-17   A child with a segmental upper eyelid infantile hemangioma with ptosis and severe astigmatism.

Nasal Hemangiomas

About 16% of facial IHs occur on the nose. Most are focal and involve the nasal tip.[6] The nose may also be involved as part of a segmental lesion. Both frontonasal and V2 segmental hemangiomas may involve the nose. In these cases, more than one nasal subunit is usually affected. Left untreated, most of these children experience social ridicule from both society at large and the medical profession. Terms such as *harlequin nose* and *Cyrano nose* are frequently used to describe these lesions. Early intervention is thus clearly indicated. Prevention of these deformities with timely medical therapy is preferable, but if this has not happened or the lesion has failed to respond, surgical treatment is necessary.

Timing of surgical intervention is important. One should not intervene until proliferation has clearly ceased. This would mean not earlier than the tenth month and up to at least 18 months of life for a segmental lesion. Although it is tempting to wait until the child is much older, this should be discouraged for two reasons. The psychosocial trauma inflicted on these children can be avoided with early intervention. The likelihood of scarring is diminished if surgery is performed when the child is about 1 year old as opposed to 5 or 6 years of age.

Nasal tip hemangiomas occur in 5% of cases and have many features in common. They almost all distort the nasal tip by separating and displacing the lower lateral cartilages laterally and rotating them outward. In most cases the overlying skin is not involved. Most of these lesions are midline but a minority may involve one side more than the other. Many surgical approaches have been described. Of these, we prefer the modified subunit approach as described by Waner et al, which is an incision extending across the columella and then up just past the soft triangle to the space between the ala and the nasal tip. This approach allows access to the lower lateral cartilages and the ability to trim excess skin that has been expanded by the hemangioma. Two or three dome-binding sutures and a columella transfixion suture will be needed to correct the deformity of the nasal tip. An extension of this incision may be necessary in cases that involve more than one subunit. Laser treatment of the overlying skin may precede or follow the surgical resection. If the skin is extensively infiltrated, raising a flap will be difficult, if not impossible. In these cases laser treatment that is aimed at eradicating the cutaneous component should precede surgery (Fig. 47-18).

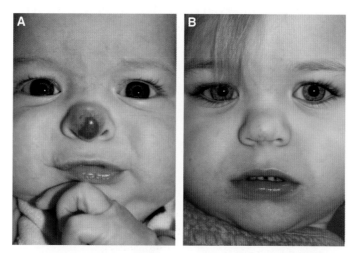

Fig. 47-18   A child with nasal tip infantile hemangioma. **A,** Preoperative view. **B,** After excision through a modified subunit approach. Residual erythematous staining is treated with PDL.

Hemangiomas of the Lip

The lip is involved in 20% of facial hemangiomas.[6] Hemangiomas of the lip may often impede function (such as speech and feeding) and lead to disfigurement. Additionally, there is a high incidence of ulceration. When this occurs, treatment should be administered as soon as possible, because ulceration can present with pain, bleeding, and infection.

As with all anatomic sites, lip hemangiomas can be classified into focal and segmental patterns of tissue involvement with distinct sites of occurrence. Segmental IHs may involve the maxillary, frontonasal, or mandibular segments. The lower lip is the most common site of both focal and segmental lip IHs.[78]

Because of these sites of predilection, the anatomic extent and distortion of the lip can be predicted. With this in mind, surgical guidelines have been developed for their management.[78] Regarding the upper and lower lips, apart from skin staining, the lip may be elongated in its vertical or its horizontal dimension. There may be inversion or eversion of the lip with oral incompetence. These dimensions can be corrected, and the surgical approach will depend on the site of the IH. Oftentimes, the lip has been expanded (especially in focal lesions), and thus more than 30% of the lip can be excised without causing microstomia. Incisions are placed along the boundaries of facial subunits (such as the alar groove, philtrum, vermiliocutaneous junction, and wet-dry mucosal margin), because there is easy access to the lesion, and any redundant tissue can then be removed with an acceptable cosmetic result (Fig. 47-19).

Lower lip focal hemangiomas are the most common focal lip hemangiomas and tend to involve the lateral aspect of the lower lip. These lesions will frequently lengthen and evert the lower lip. The lip can be lengthened by as much as 50%, depending on the size of the hemangioma. These lesions can normally be resected by using a through-and-through wedge excision.

Propranolol has made the most impact on the treatment of segmental hemangiomas. With early treatment, most of the deformities can be prevented. However, all too often treatment is not initiated at an early stage, which results in devastating functional and aesthetic abnormalities.

Frontonasal segmental lesions are the most difficult, because they distort the philtrum. The vertical height of the upper lip is usually lengthened. These can be approached through the vermiliocutaneous junction (VCJ) and/or the inferior border of the columella and the nasal sill.

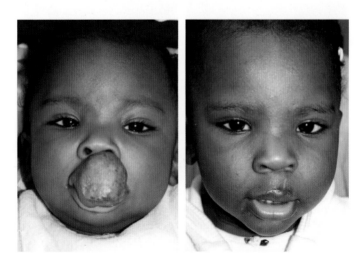

Fig. 47-19   A child with local lip infantile hemangioma before and after surgical excision.

Maxillary or V2 segmental lesions elongate the hemilip and invert the VCJ. They are usually approached along the VCJ, extending up the philtrum and across the nasal sill and ala.

The most common segmental lip hemangioma involves the entire lower lip (mandibular segment). Since ulceration is frequent, the VCJ is usually distorted, and the concavity between the VCJ and the labiomental crease is obliterated. These lesions also lengthen the lower lip. A wedge resection of the lower lip will correct the horizontal lengthening. An incision along the VCJ will correct the inversion and the convexity below the VCJ. A specially modified suture technique will help to recreate the natural sulcus of the lower lip (OTM).

Each of these procedures may require a staged approach to prevent overresection. Postoperative PDL therapy is used for superficial areas, and CO_2 fractional dermabrasion is used to treat atrophic scarring from an involuted hemangioma.

Hemangiomas of the Cheek

The midcheek is one of the most common locations for focal hemangiomas, and these occur in 11% of cases.[6] The majority of cheek IHs that are surgically removed are focal lesions that have not improved with conservative treatment or have never been treated. Midcheek lesions are the most common, and are usually lateral to the nasolabial fold. Most of these lesions are cutaneous/subcutaneous. They frequently extend down to the fascial layer overlying the buccal fat space. Facial nerve involvement is not uncommon, thus facial nerve monitoring is highly recommended. These lesions can be removed through an elliptical incision, encompassing involved skin and parallel with relaxed tension lines of the face. If the degree of skin involvement is too extensive to remove without facial disfigurement, some involved skin can be left in one of the flaps. This can be treated with laser at a later stage. Extensive mobilization of the flaps is essential before closing, and unless one is removing a proliferating lesion, truncation of the lesion may be necessary to avoid a contour deformity. The remaining lesion will, over time, become fibrofatty tissue (Fig. 47-20).

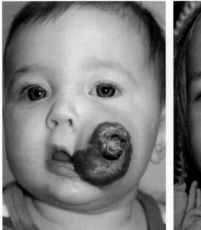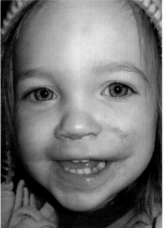

Fig. 47-20   A child with an ulcerated cheek infantile hemangioma treated with surgical excision through direct elliptical incision with intraoperative facial nerve monitoring.

Hemangiomas of the Forehead and Scalp

Both focal and segmental IHs can involve the forehead. Segmental involvement is caused by either fronto-nasal or frontal (V1) segmental involvement. Early treatment with propranolol is indicated, with or without concomitant laser treatment. Focal lesions are usually paramedian or involve the midforehead on one side or the other. Since the relaxed tension lines of the forehead are horizontal, the axis of surgical resection should ideally be parallel to them. This may result in displacement of the brow if the lesion is compound and the vertical dimension of the superficial component is larger than 2 cm. By virtue of the bulk of the hemangioma, tissue expansion will often avoid brow and/or hairline displacement. In cases in which there is a large hemangioma and brow displacement is likely, the placement of a tissue expander should be considered. At times, a vertical incision may be necessary. Even this will heal well in young children and be of minimal aesthetic significance.

In addition to this, these lesions almost always extend to the fascial layer of the frontalis or the procerus muscle. Resection of these muscles should obviously be avoided. However, if necessary, acellular dermis may be placed to avoid a soft tissue defect. Alternatively, autologous tissue is preferred; fat injections may be performed at a later date.

Scalp hemangiomas can grow to very large dimensions, and when they involute they almost always leave an area of alopecia overlying a soft doughy mass. This clearly calls for intervention. In addition to this, in infants younger than 4 months, the absence of a thick fibrous galeal layer will leave the skin of the scalp extremely lax. The galeal layer develops around 4 to 5 months of age and the skin loses its laxity. Because of this, it is much easier to remove very large scalp lesions before 4 months of age. This should clearly be weighed against the added anesthetic risks seen in this age group.

Parotid Hemangiomas

Hemangiomas of the parotid gland are the most common benign salivary gland tumors in children. The parotid gland appears to be the only major salivary gland that may be affected by hemangiomas. This is because the parotid gland is ectodermal in origin, whereas the submandibular and sublingual glands are endodermal in origin. Minor salivary glands are also frequently involved, especially in mandibular V3 segmental hemangiomas. These minor salivary glands are also ectodermal in origin.

Involvement of the parotid gland may be a result of a focal or segmental V3 hemangioma.[79] With focal hemangiomas, the entire parotid gland (deep and superficial lobes) is involved, and there may or may not be overlying skin involvement. Segmental V3 hemangiomas are frequently bilateral, and there is always preauricular skin involvement and involvement of the lower lip. In these cases, the entire parotid gland is involved. All segmental V3 patients should be evaluated by laryngoscopy since almost a third of these patients will have airway involvement. In addition to this, there is a high association with PHACES syndrome.

Treatment of Parotid Hemangiomas

Parotid hemangiomas may be extremely disfiguring. In addition to this, in segmental involvement the incidence of ulceration and airway issues are significant.[79] Furthermore, congestive high-output heart failure from excessive shunting through a massive parotid hemangioma is not unusual. For these reasons, parotid hemangiomas should be treated. Parotid IHs involve the entire salivary gland and deep and superficial lobes. There is also often associated skin staining.

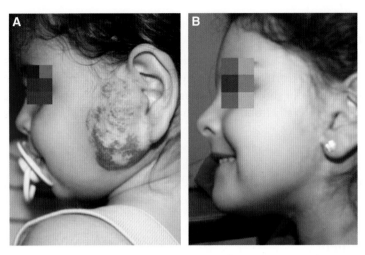

Fig. 47-21   A child with a parotid infantile hemangioma. **A,** After treatment with propranolol. **B,** After surgical excision.

Propranolol is the first line of therapy, and the likelihood of response with segmental hemangiomas is high (Fig. 47-21).

Unfortunately, not all focal lesions respond to propranolol. Treatment failures or residual disease after the cessation of propranolol should be treated surgically. The surgery should be undertaken by a surgeon with experience in the treatment of vascular anomalies in children for several reasons, including that the position of the branches of the facial nerve are frequently displaced, the inherent vascularity of the mass, and the perineurium is frequently infiltrated by hemangioma, which makes neural dissection more challenging. Preoperative embolization may reduce the vascularity of the hemangioma and facilitate surgical excision.

Intralesional corticosteroid injection using a combination of triamcinolone (40 mg/ml) and betamethasone (6 mg/ml) has been used successfully to treat parotid hemangiomas.[80] This may be an option if propranolol is contraindicated or has failed. Although corticosteroid is injected locally, there is still significant systemic absorption, and thus the side effects commonly seen with systemic corticosteroids may occur. PDL is used to treat the superficial component of a compound hemangioma as an adjuvant to propranolol and surgery.

Airway Hemangiomas

The airway may be involved as either an isolated focal lesion (most frequently in the subglottis) or as part of a segmental manifestation. In these cases, airway involvement may include all areas of the upper aerodigestive tract. At least one third of patients with a V3 segmental cutaneous pattern also have airway findings. Thus it is essential that all patients with this distribution of disease undergo endoscopy.

For all of these reasons, we avoid the term *subglottic* hemangiomas, because this is an oversimplification and only describes focal airway hemangiomas. We believe that a more precise term is *airway infantile hemangiomas,* which are further described as either focal or segmental.[82]

Focal Airway Hemangiomas

Oral propranolol is the first-line therapy. Response is usually rapid, and in most cases intubation and/or tracheotomy may be avoided.[81] Corticosteroids may be used as adjuvant therapy in cases of airway obstruction. Typically, this is used in short pulses, whereas propranolol is used in sustained treatment until 9 to 10 months of age. It is especially important to monitor the child for hypoglycemia when steroids are used in tandem.

If propranolol is contraindicated or fails to produce an adequate effect, other treatment options should be considered. These include intralesional corticosteroid injection, CO_2 laser ablation, and surgical resection. The treatment bias will be determined by the experience of the surgeon.

Segmental Involvement

Segmental airway involvement will vary from diffuse mucosal staining to extensive bulky disease and airway obstruction. Tracheal staining is also not uncommon[82] (Fig. 47-22). There is no way to predict which patients will progress. They should all be closely monitored. Propranolol is the drug of choice for those who warrant treatment. The vast majority of patients will respond to medication alone. Because of this, tracheostomy is performed less frequently.

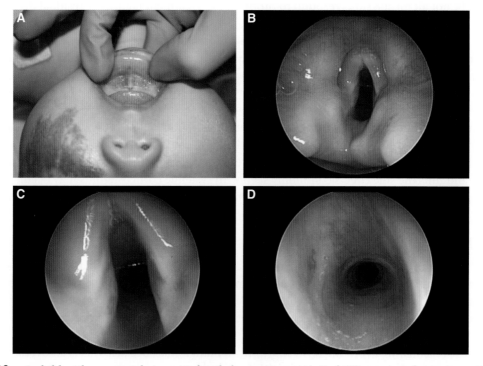

Fig. 47-22   A child with segmental airway infantile hemangioma. **A,** Left V2 segmental cutaneous IH and lip/gingival staining. **B,** Direct rigid laryngoscopy. **C,** Diffuse staining of the false vocal folds and true vocal folds. **D,** The tracheal wall.

TREATMENT OF VASCULAR MALFORMATIONS

No single modality should ever be considered as the benchmark for the treatment of vascular malformations. On the contrary, the treatment of vascular malformations is a multidisciplinary endeavor. The goal of treatment is to improve facial symmetry and a patient's quality of life. Very small lesions may be cured, but more diffuse lesions are inactivated and may require maintenance therapy throughout a patient's lifetime.

PORT-WINE STAINS (VENULAR OR CAPILLARY MALFORMATION)

Port-wine stains or venular or capillary malformations are vascular malformations characterized by ectatic vessels in the papillary and reticular dermis. They may cause soft tissue hypertrophy in all tissue layers, including skin, subcutaneous fat, and muscle.

Laser Treatment

Serial laser treatment is the mainstay for the treatment of port-wine stains because of its proven efficacy and safety. Specifically PDL with dynamic cooling using the principle of selective photothermolysis has become the standard device, and its use is widespread.[72,83] PDL will lighten the port-wine stain (Fig. 47-23). A small percentage of patients will have complete clearance of their birthmark. The vast majority of patients will lighten considerably. About 20% to 30% of patients will have resistant lesions that will only marginally improve.[84]

The best age to begin treatment is debatable. Some groups advocate for early treatment, and others have found no advantage. It is widely accepted that all port-wine stains will eventually recur.[35]

Alexandrite laser (755 nm ms pulsed Alexandrite laser, MSPAL) has been used for resistant lesions, but the therapeutic index is narrower with a higher risk of scarring. The laser preferentially targets deoxyhemoglobin that is found in venous vessels, which may explain its efficacy for darker lesions.[85]

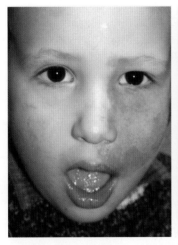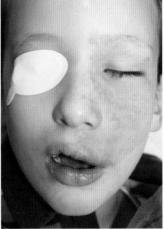

Fig. 47-23   A child with a left V2 maxillary confluent port-wine stain before and after eight PDL treatments. Although the lesion has not completely disappeared, it is considerably lighter. Involvement of the skin of the upper lip and midcheek is not as responsive because the skin is thicker.

Photodynamic Therapy

Photodynamic therapy has been studied extensively in China. A two-step drug delivery system is used involving an intravenous hematoporphyrin-based photosensitizer, followed by irradiation with coherent or noncoherent light. This combination generates oxygen-derived free radicals, which damage endothelial cells in port-wine stain vessels of all sizes. Patients are advised to avoid direct sun exposure for 2 weeks after treatment to prevent photosensitivity. Studies have shown that photodynamic therapy is as effective as PDL for treating light port-wine stains, and more effective for darker port-wine stains.[86-88] The main reported side effects include hyperpigmentation and scarring. In one series, 5-year follow-up showed no recurrence.[87]

Surgical Management

A proportion of patients with port-wine stains have soft tissue hypertrophy in the same dermatomal distribution as their port-wine stains.[36] This hypertrophy appears to involve the entire dermatome. As a result, mesodermal and ectodermal elements are involved. The upper lip and maxilla are commonly involved with skeletal hypertrophy in addition to muscle and subcutaneous fat hypertrophy (Fig. 47-24). A frequent finding is cobblestone or soft tissue nodule formation, which appears to be composed of hypertrophic vascular tissue (Fig. 47-25). In early cobblestones, the lesion is clearly vascular and empties on compression. This may be treated with PDL or Nd:YAG laser. An established cobblestone, however, is more fibrous and less compressible.

Soft tissue hypertrophy and established cobblestones are treated surgically. The surgical approach should be zonal and problem oriented. Incisions are placed in the boundaries of facial subunits or in the direction of the relaxed skin tension lines.

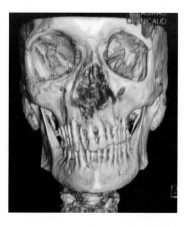

Fig. 47-24   A three-dimensional CT reconstruction showing skeletal hypertrophy of the right maxilla and nasal bones.

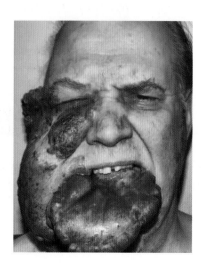

Fig. 47-25   A man with a right V2 maxillary and bilateral lower lip port-wine stain with nodules and soft tissue hypertrophy.

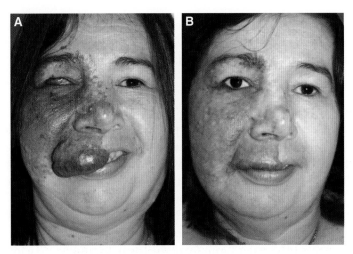

Fig. 47-26 **A,** A patient with a right V2 maxillary port-wine stain and upper lip hypertrophy. **B,** A wedge of vermilion, submucosa, and muscle was removed to correct the hypertrophy.

The most commonly affected areas are the upper and lower lip. The affected lip is usually elongated horizontally and thickened in the anteroposterior dimension. The length is usually addressed through a full thickness wedge resection, and the thickness through a wet/dry margin or a VCJ debulking procedure. It is often necessary to remove a wedge of muscle together with submucosal or subcutaneous tissues (Fig. 47-26).

The cheek is accessed through a nasolabial incision and the forehead can be approached through a coronal flap or a suprabrow incision. In these instances, subcutaneous fat is usually reduced, leaving intact muscle and nerves. The nasal tip is often deviated to the opposite side with enlargement of the nasal vestibule and thickening of the ala. A traditional rhinoplasty may be performed in addition to repositioning of the nasal ala. Maxillary or zygomatic bone may be burred down to improve symmetry.

Staged procedures spaced 4 to 6 weeks apart are common, because correction in more than one vector is needed. If the patient is still growing, a repeat procedure should be anticipated. The procedure is aimed at improving the patient's quality of life. Although there is a possibility of a repeat procedure, this should not discourage the surgeon from intervening early. Removal of disfiguring tissue will improve the patient's self-esteem and therefore his or her quality of life.

VENOUS MALFORMATIONS

The decision as to when and how to treat venous malformations should take into account the natural history of the disease. Venous malformations will naturally increase in size over the life of the patient. The rate of expansion varies. "High grade" or "active" lesions expand more rapidly, whereas other lesions expand in a more benign fashion. Trauma, hemorrhage, sepsis, hormonal fluctuations (puberty and pregnancy), and thrombosis will result in a more rapid expansion. Advancing age results in a thinning of the supporting connective tissue, leading to more rapid expansion.

Three modalities have a role in the management of venous malformations: laser treatment (Nd:YAG laser), sclerotherapy (transcutaneous or transmucosal), and surgical resection. The choice of modality will depend on the depth of the lesion and its anatomic location. In general, superficial lesions and the superficial component of a compound lesion are treated with an Nd:YAG laser.[89,90] Deep lesions will either be treated with sclerotherapy as a primary modality, or sclerosed preoperatively and then surgically removed 24 hours later.[91-93] Sclerotherapy is advocated in anatomic locations where surgery will add significant morbidity. It is important to realize that although sclerotherapy may seem innocuous, it carries significant risk of morbidity and mortality and may require several treatments.[94,95] The risks and benefits should be carefully weighed before a treatment plan is selected.

LASER TREATMENT

Our laser of choice is a 1064 nm Nd:YAG laser. It is possible to use a similar wavelength from a different laser source.[89,96] At this wavelength, light will penetrate to a depth of approximately 1 cm. It is therefore only effective for superficial lesions. When used transcutaneously, a larger spot size with dynamic surface cooling is preferable (Fig. 47-27). The cryogen coolant cools the skin surface and thereby prevents thermal necrosis. The laser pulse follows the coolant by about 40 ms. The endpoint should be vasoconstriction, darkening, or intravascular coagulation of the lesion. No blanching of the overlying skin should be allowed, because this will lead to necrosis and the risk of scarring. A bare fiber is preferred for disease in the posterior oropharynx. The fiber is held about 1 mm from the treated surface, and a grid or "snowstorm" pattern of treatment spaced 5 to 8 mm apart is delivered [96] (Fig. 47-28).

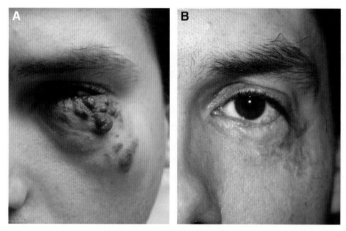

Fig. 47-27 A patient with a left lower eyelid venous malformation. **A,** View before treatment. **B,** View after multiple Nd:YAG laser treatments and surgical excision with preoperative sclerotherapy.

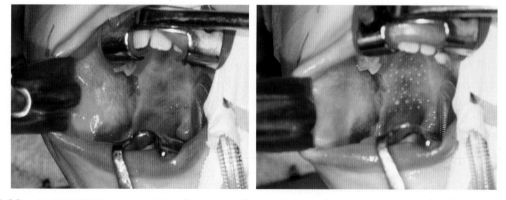

Fig. 47-28 An Nd:YAG laser is used in a "snowstorm" pattern on oral mucosa. NOTE: Each white spot represents a site of impaction.

This treatment can be a primary treatment for superficial lesions or an adjunct for compound lesions. In these cases, laser treatment is used to treat the superficial component of a compound lesion. With treatment skin or mucosa, a layer of intentional subcutaneous or submucosal scarring is achieved. This will enable the surgeon to raise a mucosal or skin flap during surgery. Laser treatment should precede surgery by about 6 weeks.

A 600 μm quartz fiber taped to a zero-degree telescope can be used to treat laryngeal disease. We usually place the airway in suspension and deliver the laser pulses with the fiber/telescope apparatus. It is important not to deliver too many pulses during one treatment session, because treatment invariably produces edema, which will reach a maximum over 18 to 24 hours. The patient should be admitted postoperatively for observation, and steroids should be administered intraoperatively and postoperatively for 4 days.

Sclerotherapy

Sclerotherapy may be used as primary or adjuvant therapy.[94,95] Intramuscular VM with no overlying contour deformity may be treated with primary sclerotherapy to inactivate disease. Once the lesion is expanded, however, sclerotherapy alone will not be adequate. Combined surgical excision removes disease and provides facial symmetry.

The overall treatment will depend on the bias of the multidisciplinary group. Eyelid and orbital lesions may be treated with a combination of laser, sclerotherapy, and surgery. Recently, bleomycin has been used to treat orbital lesions with minimal swelling and good effect.[97]

Surgical Resection

Lesions of the head and neck should be considered by anatomic site. We have divided these lesions into facial and cervical. Facial lesions can be focal or diffuse. Focal lesions should be approached according to their anatomic location and depth. Diffuse lesions are generally treated in stages; during each stage the area being treated is approached in accordance with its depth and anatomic location. Superficial lesions and the superficial component of a complex lesion are treated with an Nd:YAG laser as described earlier.

Facial lesions may involve one or more of the following: parotid space, masseteric/temporal space, buccal fat space, and premaxillary/premandibular space.

The approach to each of these spaces should be considered separately, because each space has distinct anatomic considerations.

The Parotid Space

Small focal lesions of the parotid may be sclerosed or surgically removed. We have no firm guidelines for this decision and feel that the preference of the multidisciplinary team is the overriding factor. Focal lesions may be completely removed or even cured. Diffuse lesions within the parotid can be extremely difficult to resect without intraoperative hemorrhage and facial nerve damage. We may treat these primarily with sclerotherapy, or if a decision is made to proceed with surgery, the lesion should be sclerosed 24 to 48 hours preoperatively. The surgical approach should be through a parotidectomy incision. The facial nerve main trunk can be found at the stylomastoid foramen. Oftentimes, the individual branches can be

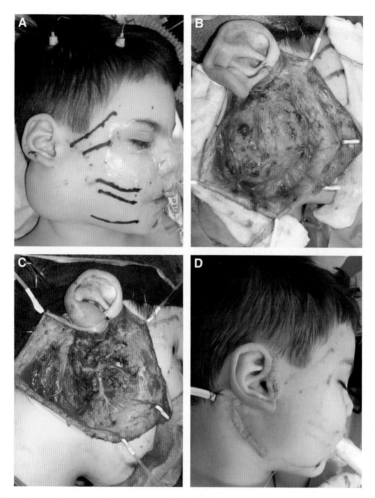

Fig. 47-29   A child with a right parotid venous malformation. **A,** Preoperative view. Note the facial nerve mapping on the skin, which denotes facial nerve branches. **B,** The skin flap is elevated in the parotideomasseteric plane. **C,** The facial nerve branches are dissected and preserved. The venous malformation is removed. **D,** Result immediately after surgery.

found distally, anterior to the parotid gland, over the fascia on the masseter, and then traced retrograde to the foramen. We prefer this approach, because it may avoid a bloody dissection. The parotid gland is then removed in the same fashion as it is in tumor dissection (Fig. 47-29).

THE MASSETER

Focal lesions of the masseter are not uncommon. These lesions have been referred to erroneously as *intramuscular hemangiomas.* In general, sclerotherapy will not reduce the size of the lesion. Therefore if the lesion protrudes and is disfiguring, it should be surgically resected. An extended parotidectomy incision is made. The flap is raised over the parotideomasseteric fascia over the parotid and the masseter. The facial nerve branches will be found in the fascial layer on the surface of the masseter. These branches can be dissected and carefully elevated, exposing the masseter. The muscle is removed from its inferior attachments on the mandible and the superior attachment to the zygomatic arch. The remaining soft tissue defect is corrected with an autologous fat graft.

THE BUCCAL FAT SPACE

The buccal fat space is a common site for venous malformations. The buccal fat space is enclosed in an investing layer of fascia. The facial nerve branches are within this fascial layer. Venous malformation may involve a portion of the space or the whole space. More commonly, the lesion extends to the masseter or the premaxilla. The surgical approach to the buccal fat space is similar to that of the masseter. An extended parotidectomy incision with elevation of a flap will expose the masseter and the buccal fat space. The facial nerve branches can be found on the surface of the masseter or in the fascia of the fat space. The fascia between the facial nerve branches should be incised, and the buccal fat can be teased out and removed. In most cases, we prefer not to sclerose the malformation preoperatively, because the edema makes the dissection more difficult. This space may also be accessed through an intraoral approach.

THE PREMAXILLA/PREMANDIBULAR SPACE

It is common for lesions of the premaxilla and premandibular spaces to also involve the adjacent lip. They can be treated through an intraoral approach. Our usual approach is preoperative sclerotherapy followed by surgical resection within 24 to 48 hours. Resection of the sclerosed mass is undertaken during surgery. If the sclerotherapy was complete, this will include the entire lesion. Since venous malformation is commonly intramuscular, it may also be necessary to remove muscle during surgery. The extent of muscle removal should not be sufficient to affect function (Fig. 47-30).

Cervical lesions can also be removed surgically. These dissections are more familiar to head and neck surgeons and therefore should pose very little difficulty. Preoperative sclerotherapy can also be advantageous.

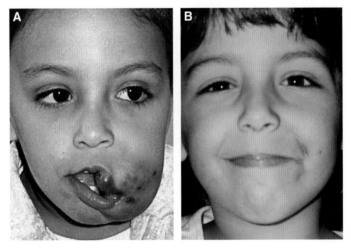

Fig. 47-30   **A,** A child with a facial venous malformation who will be treated with an Nd:YAG laser. **B,** Same patient after sclerotherapy and surgical excision through an intraoral approach, which was performed 6 weeks after laser therapy.

COAGULATION ABNORMALITIES

Localized intravascular coagulation is a coagulation disorder associated with vascular lesions, especially venous malformations.[47] The presence of a venous malformation may cause microthrombosis within the venous malformation, which in turn results in a chronic consumptive coagulopathy. This is a chronic condition that is usually well compensated for by the patient. Any increase in consumption could potentially distress the system and the patient will decompensate. This may happen after surgery, sclerotherapy, trauma, or prolonged immobilization. If the consumption is severe, this could lead to disseminated intravascular coagulation. These patients typically have an elevated D-dimer level caused by the chronic consumption. The degree of D-dimer elevation appears to correlate with the size of the venous malformation.

Localized intravascular coagulation decompensation can usually be prevented and/or treated with low-molecular-weight heparin.[47,49] This should be started 2 days before any form of treatment that may produce coagulation, and should be continued for several days after the procedure. The timing of treatment is empirical, and currently there are no data to confirm this.

GLOMUVENOUS MALFORMATION

Glomuvenous malformations are low-flow vascular malformations that affect the epidermal, dermal, and subcutaneous fat layers. They are often dermatomal. They can be treated with a combination of laser (Nd:YAG) and surgical excision. Depending on the cutaneous extent of the lesion, the incisions will be direct, or more ideally, placed along facial subunits or relaxed skin tension lines.

LYMPHATIC MALFORMATIONS

Lymphatic malformations (LMs) are congenital abnormalities of the lymphatic system in which the flow of lymph is retarded across the affected area. The degree of retardation varies from case to case. A high-grade lesion is one in which there is a marked abnormality. Since the flow of lymph in these cases is significantly slowed, these patients will manifest with clinical features of an LM at birth. In low-grade lesions, there may be no clinical manifestation of an LM until some event later in life causes an increase in the production of lymph. This may not occur until the second decade of life. An intermediate lesion usually manifests within the first 18 to 24 months of life.

An LM presents clinically as a firm, flesh-colored or bluish mass. The most notable features are that these lesions do not fill in a dependent position and are not compressible. They are prone to exacerbations and remissions, and these are usually associated with upper respiratory infections. During exacerbations, the lesion can become swollen, inflamed, and tender. LMs expand over time and frequently cause severe disfigurement.

Mucosal and/or skin involvement results in the presence of vesicles. These are commonly seen on the tongue and mucosa. The vesicles are filled with lymph, which is transparent. Whether they are mucosal or deep, LMs have a variable concentration of veins in the walls of their cysts. During an exacerbation, bleeding into one or more of these cysts may occur, resulting in a reddish or purple discoloration of some of the vesicles. Hemorrhage may cause an expansion of the lesion, and this in turn will cause a variable degree of pain.[98] Tongue and/or floor of mouth involvement frequently causes glossoptosis. In evaluating a patient with glossoptosis, it is important to differentiate between frank macroglossia and glossoptosis caused by floor of mouth disease. Oral cavity, floor of mouth, and parapharyngeal disease cause deformation of the mandible and or the maxilla. An increase in the angle of the mandible and an open bite will result from the mass effect. An open bite deformity is seen in severe cases. These children have difficulty with chewing, and their alimentation often needs to be supplemented. They commonly drool, and their

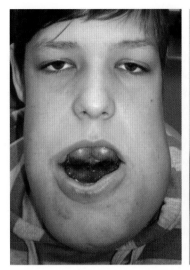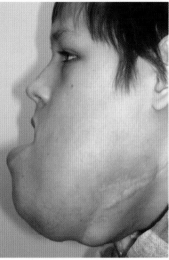

Fig. 47-31   A patient with bilateral cervicofacial lymphatic malformation. Note the vertical lengthening of the lower third of the face with glossoptosis, class III malocclusion, and tracheotomy.

speech intelligibility is severely compromised. LMs are therefore among the most challenging of lesions. Almost half of patients with head and neck LM will have airway involvement. A significant percentage of these patients also have airway obstruction, which is always supraglottic.[43] No cases manifest with glottic, subglottic, or tracheal disease. Presumably this is because of the paucity of lymph tissue in these areas. Many of these patients will have a tracheotomy[44] (Fig. 47-31).

Radiologic features of a lymphatic malformation are unique. They are multiseptated cystic masses that are "soft" lesions, and therefore invaginate between structures. Cyst sizes range from small to large. This appears to be largely dependent on the consistency of the surrounding tissue. Furthermore, a cyst may vary in size depending on whether the MRI was taken during an exacerbation or quiescent period. Much has been made of whether the lesion is *macrocystic* (greater than 2 cm) or *microcystic*.[99] This merely refers to the likely response of a lesion to sclerotherapy with Picibanil (OK-432). Smith et al[99] found that macrocystic lesions responded best; hence the distinction. Lymphatic malformations are prone to internal hemorrhage, and it is common to find fluid-fluid levels caused by separation of the blood and lymph within a cyst. This is a diagnostic feature of LMs. Gadolinium staining is limited to the capsule or the septae, and therefore is not as intense as other vascular malformations.

The management of lymphatic malformations is multidisciplinary. Sclerotherapy, surgery, and mechanical ablation (laser ablation, coblation, and radiofrequency ablation) are all useful, and are often all used in a single patient. Sclerotherapy has become the first line of treatment for LMs.[99,100] A number of agents are popular, including OK-432, doxycycline, 98% ethanol, sodium morrhuate/Ethiodol (3:1), and sodium tetradecyl/ethiodol (3:1). Of these, OK-432, doxycycline, and bleomycin are the most widely used. It has become clear that macrocystic lesions (cysts greater than 2 cm) respond best to sclerotherapy. In our institution doxycycline is the preferred agent, with or without bleomycin. The advantage of bleomycin is that it causes minimal postinjection swelling, and therefore can be used in the retroorbital space or around the airway. In addition to this, bleomycin appears to be effective in treating microcystic lesions.

Extensive experience in treating macrocystic lesions with OK-432 has also been encouraging. In one series it was found to be much more likely to be successful than surgery, with considerably less morbidity. In addition to this, long-term control of macrocystic lesions treated with OK-432 was excellent. A metaanalysis of data on sclerotherapy shows that inconsistent presentation of data and inconsistency between case series hinders the development of uniform guidelines for the management of these difficult lesions. In more than 60% of papers, the reduction in size of the LMs is not clearly defined.[101]

SURGICAL RESECTION

For most extensive lesions, surgery is used in conjunction with sclerotherapy. Surgical resection is useful in reducing the size of the lesion, and in some cases surgical resection can completely eradicate the lesion. However, in the majority of cases, surgical removal is incomplete, especially in cervicofacial lesions. Control should be undertaken with sclerotherapy wherever disease is left behind. If both surgery and sclerotherapy will be needed, it is preferable to perform surgery first, since operating in a field that has been previously sclerosed is extremely difficult. The fibrosis caused by sclerosing agents distorts surgical planes and makes it challenging to define and preserve important structures. This is especially true in the parotid gland. Sclerotherapy will distort the perineural anatomic plane and embed the facial nerve in a block of fibrosis, making it extremely difficult to dissect out the nerve.

The surgical approach to disease involving the various zones of the face should be the same as those mentioned in the approach to VMs.

In cases of glossoptosis the surgeon must determine whether this is caused by frank macroglossia or disease involving the floor of the mouth, which may also cause tongue protrusion. If the latter is the dominant cause, sclerotherapy treatment is indicated for the floor of the mouth. If this is unsuccessful, surgery may be necessary. If there is true macroglossia, however, a tongue reduction is indicated. Two procedures have been described, a wedge resection and a keyhole procedure. We prefer the former.

Mucosal involvement of the tongue is commonly symptomatic. Symptoms include pain, especially when acidic food or carbonated drinks are ingested. These patients also have frequent lymph seepage and bleeding from the vesicles. The presence of these vesicles is therefore an indication for intervention. Several modalities are available. CO_2 laser ablation is preferred in our institution, but good results have also been reported with coblation.[96,102] No direct comparison of these two modalities has ever been undertaken. Both treatments will improve the quality of life in these patients, but it must be understood that they are temporary and only address the superficial vesicles. Patients can be symptom free for 1 to 5 years. However, the vesicles will invariably recur because the deep component still persists. Recent work with intralingual injections of bleomycin appears to provide more lasting relief. Further work is necessary to verify this.

SCLEROTHERAPY

The use of sclerosing agents is essential in the treatment of lymphatic malformations. This form of therapy is evolving. In earlier times, absolute alcohol was used as a sclerosant. More recently, agents such as doxycycline, OK-432, and bleomycin are being used with good results and fewer side effects. Bleomycin is the most recent entry into this field and appears to have significant advantages. Unlike the other sclerosants, treatment with bleomycin is followed with little or no posttreatment edema. This is especially useful for areas such as the orbit and airway. Its main disadvantage is that it has a maximum lifetime dosage and risk of pulmonary fibrosis.

Sclerotherapy is predicated on the percutaneous/transmucosal penetration of the cyst, followed by drainage and the injection of a sclerosant into the cyst to destroy the cyst wall. Since larger cysts are more easily targeted, larger or macrocysts (greater than 2 cm) respond best. Microcysts are naturally more difficult to target and respond poorly. As a consequence of this, lymphatic malformations are commonly referred to as either macrocystic or microcystic. This classification is based purely on their differential response to sclerotherapy. In reality, the size of the cysts can vary from month to month, depending on whether the lesion is active or quiescent. In addition to this, we believe that the size of the cysts is likely to be related

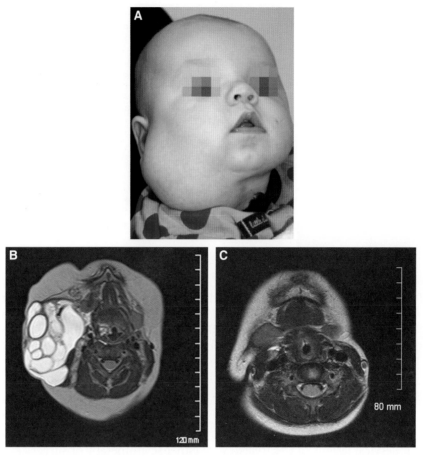

Fig. 47-32   **A,** An infant with a right cervical lymphatic malformation with parapharyngeal and retropharyngeal involvement. **B,** T2-weighted axial MRI before doxycycline sclerotherapy to the cervical portion and bleomycin injection to the airway compartment. **C,** MRI after sclerotherapy.

to the anatomic location of the lesion and hence the surrounding tissue. Cervical lesions are more likely to be macrocystic, whereas facial lesions are more likely to be microcystic. Nevertheless, most head and neck lesions are made up of both macrocysts and microcysts.

Because sclerotherapy appears to be noninvasive when compared with surgery, it has become more popular and is often the first line of treatment for lymphatic malformations. However, a meta-analysis of published data showed significant inconsistencies in reporting outcomes of treatment. Multiple treatments are the norm, and the outcomes are variable. Although sclerotherapy can reduce the bulk of a lesion, surgery is frequently necessary as an adjuvant to sclerotherapy. However, when surgery is performed after sclerotherapy, the normal tissue planes are adherent and anatomic landmarks are usually very difficult to find. This makes facial nerve preservation during parotid surgery a real challenge. For this reason, we advocate surgery as the first line of therapy. Residual disease can then be sclerosed, and since surgical resection has reduced the volume of disease, this will in turn reduce the number of sclerotherapy events.

Lesions of the orbit and retropharyngeal or parapharyngeal lesions are, however, best treated with sclerotherapy as a primary treatment, and bleomycin should be used in these cases because it produces the least amount of postoperative edema[103,104,105] (Fig. 47-32).

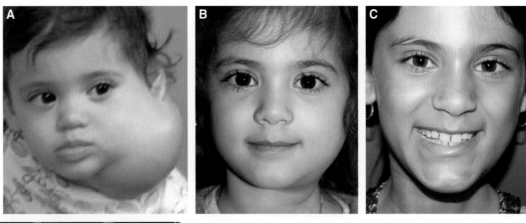

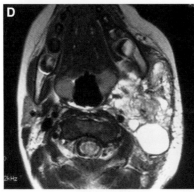

Fig. 47-33   **A** and **B,** A child with a left neck mixed microcystic/ macrocystic lymphatic malformation treated with surgical excision only. **C,** The child 10 years after surgery, with no recurrence. **D,** Axial MRI showing mixed macrocystic and microcystic disease involving left parotid, masseteric, and parapharyngeal disease.

Large macrocystic cervical lesions can be treated with either sclerotherapy or surgery as a primary treatment, but mixed cervicofacial lesions are best treated with surgical debulking followed with sclerotherapy to sclerose the residual disease (Fig. 47-33).

After surgery, the healing response in LMs is exaggerated. An excess of scar tissue forms. Surgical excision is followed by corticosteroid injection (a combination of betamethasone [Celestone] 6 mg/kg and triamcinolone [Kenalog] 40 mg/kg, 1:1) 4 to 6 weeks later to quell the response.

ARTERIOVENOUS MALFORMATIONS

Arteriovenous malformations (AVMs) are among the most challenging lesions to treat. They may be focal or diffuse, and high grade or low grade. Low-grade lesions present during the second, third, or fourth decades of life, whereas high-grade lesions are obvious at birth. The underlying abnormality appears to be an absence of control of blood flow across a capillary network. This results in continuous shunting of blood across the capillary bed, which in turn leads to dilation of the vessels. A number of "secondary" changes also occur, such as venous dilation and arterial hypertrophy, which accommodate this increased blood flow across the AVM. Over time, the volume of blood shunting across this area will increase as the capillary bed dilates. This will lead in turn to "secondary" dilation of the surrounding vessels, and in time, this could lead to flow reversal upstream and a steal syndrome.[106]

The underlying pathology—that is, the abnormal capillary bed—is known as the *nidus.* Treatment should be directed at the nidus. The dilated vessels surrounding the nidus are secondary changes and need not necessarily be treated. In reality, when faced with a large lesion, the surgeon may often find it difficult to determine where the nidus is centered. Combining the findings of an angiogram with an MRI is helpful in this regard. The area of shunting is the nidus.

Treatment of AVMs is best approached in a multidisciplinary setting; the participation of both an interventional radiologist and a surgeon is essential. Both embolization and surgical resection are necessary treatment modalities.[107,108] In general, preoperative sclerotherapy followed by surgical resection of the nidus is advocated. In treatment of localized or focal lesions, this may be curative. In more diffuse lesions, a "cure" is unrealistic. In these cases, an attempt should be made to improve the patient's quality of life. This is usually accomplished by surgery or a combination of embolization and surgical resection. An attempt is usually made to address problem areas, such as areas that have ulcerated and are bleeding, and to improve the appearance of the patient.

Surgical resection can be extremely challenging and should be accompanied by preoperative embolization. The choice of embolic agents depends on the experience of the interventional radiologist and whether embolization is being performed as a primary or preoperative treatment (Figs. 47-34 and 47-35).

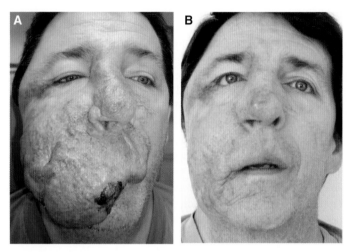

Fig. 47-34   **A,** An adult with a diffuse right facial arteriovenous malformation. Preoperative view with no prior treatment. **B,** After two serial debulking surgeries, each preceded by embolization and direct puncture sclerotherapy 24 hours before surgery. Incisions were placed along the boundaries of facial subunits and along relaxed skin tension lines.

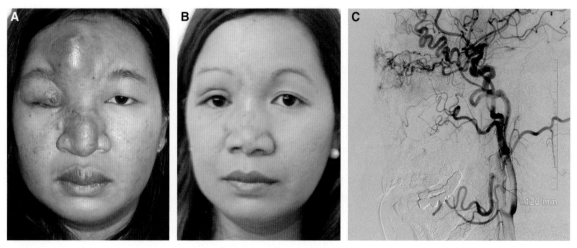

Fig. 47-35   **A,** A woman with a focal frontonasal and right upper eyelid arteriovenous malformation. **B,** Results after staged resection. **C,** Lateral angiogram imaging shows multifocal nidus with several choke areas with shunting in brow, forehead, and nasal dorsum.

REFERENCES

1. Mulliken JB, Glowacki J. Hemangiomas and vascular malformations in infants and children: a classification based on endothelial characteristics. Plast Reconstr Surg 69:412-422, 1982.
2. Khan ZA, Melero-Martin JM, Wu X, et al. Endothelial progenitor cells from infantile hemangioma and umbilical cord blood display unique cellular responses to endostatin. Blood 108:915-921, 2006.
3. Bischoff J. Progenitor cells in infantile hemangioma. J Craniofac Surg 20 Suppl 1:695-697, 2009.
4. Xu D, O TM, Shartava A, et al. Isolation, characterization, and in vitro propagation of infantile hemangioma stem cells and an in vivo mouse model. J Hematol Oncol 4:54, 2011.
5. Amir J, Metzker A, Krikler R, et al. Strawberry hemangioma in preterm infants. Pediatr Dermatol 3:331-332, 1986.
6. Waner M, North PE, Scherer KA, et al. The nonrandom distribution of facial hemangiomas. Arch Dermatol 139:869-875, 2003.
7. Finn MC, Glowacki J, Mulliken JB. Congenital vascular lesions: clinical application of a new classification. J Pediatr Surg 18:894-900, 1983.
8. Waner M, Suen JY. The natural history of hemangiomas. In Waner M, Suen JY, eds. Hemangiomas and Vascular Malformations of the Head and Neck. New York: Wiley-Liss, 1999.
8a. Meyer JS, Hoffer FA, Barnes PD, Mulliken JB. Biological classification of soft-tissue vascular anomalies: MR correlation. AJR Am J Roentgenol 157:559-564, 1991.
8b. Barnes PD, Burrows PE, Hoffer FA, Mulliken JB, Hemangiomas and vascular malformations of the head and neck: MR characterization. AJNR Am J Neuroradiol 15:193-195, 1994.
9. Takahashi K, Mulliken JB, Kozakewich HP, et al. Cellular markers that distinguish the phases of hemangioma during infancy and childhood. J Clin Invest 93:2357-2364, 1994.
10. Glowacki J, Mulliken JB. Mast cells in hemangiomas and vascular malformations. Pediatrics 70:48-51, 1982.
11. North PE, Waner M, Mizeracki A, et al. GLUT1: a newly discovered immunohistochemical marker for juvenile hemangiomas. Hum Pathol 31:11-22, 2000.
12. Bielenberg DR, Bucana CD, Sanchez R, et al. Progressive growth of infantile cutaneous hemangiomas is directly correlated with hyperplasia and angiogenesis of adjacent epidermis and inversely correlated with expression of the endogenous angiogenesis inhibitor, IFN-beta. Int J Onco 14:401-408, 1999.
13. Ritter MR, Dorrell MI, Edmonds J, et al. Insulin-like growth factor 2 and potential regulators of hemangioma growth and involution identified by large-scale expression analysis. Proc Natl Acad Sci U S A 99:7455-7460, 2002.
14. Yu Y, Wylie-Sears J, Boscolo E, et al. Genomic imprinting of IGF2 is maintained in infantile hemangioma despite its high level of expression. Mol Med 10:117-123, 2004.
15. O TM, Tan M, Tarango M, et al. Differential expression of SKI oncogene protein in hemangiomas. Otolaryngol Head Neck Surg 141:213-218, 2009.
16. Farrell CL, Yang J, Pardridge WM. GLUT-1 glucose transporter is present within apical and basolateral membranes of brain epithelial interfaces and in microvascular endothelia with and without tight junctions. J Histochem Cytochem 40:193-199, 1992.
17. Barnes CM, Huang S, Kaipainen A, et al. Evidence by molecular profiling for a placental origin of infantile hemangioma. Proc Natl Acad Sci U S A 102:19097-19102, 2005.
18. North PE, Waner M, Brodsky MC. Are infantile hemangioma of placental origin? Ophthalmology 109:223-224, 2002.
19. Yu Y, Flint AF, Mulliken JB, et al. Endothelial progenitor cells in infantile hemangioma. Blood 103:1373-1375, 2004.
20. Mizuno Y, Kurokawa T, Numaguchi Y, et al. Facial hemangioma with cerebrovascular anomalies and cerebellar hypoplasia. Brain Dev 4:375-378, 1982.
21. Frieden IJ, Reese V, Cohen D. PHACE syndrome. The association of posterior fossa brain malformations, hemangiomas, arterial anomalies, coarctation of the aorta and cardiac defects, and eye abnormalities. Arch Dermatol 132:307-311, 1996.
22. North PE, Waner M, James CA, et al. Congenital nonprogressive hemangioma: a distinct clinicopathologic entity unlike infantile hemangioma. Arch Dermatol 137:1607-1620, 2001.
23. Ferrandiz-Pulido C, Mollet J, Sabado C, et al. Tufted angioma associated with Kasabach-Merritt phenomenon: a therapeutic challenge. Acta Derm Venereol 90:535-537, 2010.

24. Alberola FT, Betlloch I, Montero LC, et al. Congenital tufted angioma: case report and review of the literature. Dermatol Online J 16:2, 2010.
25. Alvarez-Mendoza A, Lourdes TS, Ridaura-Sanz C, et al. Histopathology of vascular lesions found in Kasabach-Merritt syndrome: review based on 13 cases. Pediatr Dev Pathol 3:556-560, 2000.
26. Lyons LL, North PE, Mac-Moune Lai F, et al. Kaposiform hemangioendothelioma: a study of 33 cases emphasizing its pathologic, immunophenotypic, and biologic uniqueness from juvenile hemangioma. Am J Surg Pathol 28:559-568, 2004.
27. Perkins P, Weiss SW. Spindle cell hemangioendothelioma. An analysis of 78 cases with reassessment of its pathogenesis and biologic behavior. Am J Surg Pathol 20:1196-1204, 1996.
28. Terashi H, Itami S, Kurata S, et al. Spindle cell hemangioendothelioma: report of three cases. J Dermatol 18:104-111, 1991.
29. Boon LM, Ballieux F, Vikkula M. Pathogenesis of vascular anomalies. Clin Plast Surg 38:7-19, 2011.
30. Boon LM, Mulliken JB, Vikkula M. RASA1: variable phenotype with capillary and arteriovenous malformations. Curr Opin Genet Dev 15:265-269, 2005.
31. Esterly NB. Cutaneous hemangiomas, vascular stains and associated syndromes. Curr Probl Pediatr 17:1-69, 1987.
32. Barsky SH, Rosen S, Geer DE, et al. The nature and evolution of port wine stains: a computer-assisted study. J Invest Dermatol 74:154-157, 1980.
33. Motley RJ, Lanigan SW, Katugampola GA. Videomicroscopy predicts outcome in treatment of port-wine stains. Arch Dermatol 133:921-922, 1997.
34. Smoller BR, Rosen S. Port-wine stains. A disease of altered neural modulation of blood vessels? Arch Dermatol 122:177-179, 1986.
35. Orten SS, Waner M, Flock S, et al. Port-wine stains. An assessment of 5 years of treatment. Arch Otolaryngol Head Neck Surg 122:1174-1179, 1996.
36. Klapman MH, Yao JF. Thickening and nodules in port-wine stains. J Am Acad Dermatol 44:300-302, 2001.
37. Hennedige AA, Quaba AA, Al-Nakib K. Sturge-Weber syndrome and dermatomal facial port-wine stains: incidence, association with glaucoma, and pulsed tunable dye laser treatment effectiveness. Plast Reconstr Surg 121:1173-1180, 2008.
38. Sturge WA. A case of partial epilepsy, apparently due to a lesion of one of the vaso-motor centres of the brain. Trans Clin Soc Lond 12:162-167, 1879.
39. Comi AM. Sturge-Weber syndrome and epilepsy: an argument for aggressive seizure management in these patients. Expert Rev Neurother 7:951-956, 2007.
40. Baselga E. Sturge-Weber syndrome. Semin Cutan Med Surg 23:87-98, 2004.
41. Celebi S, Alagoz G, Aykan U. Ocular findings in Sturge-Weber syndrome. Eur J Ophthalmol 10:239-243, 2000.
42. Levine C. Primary disorders of the lymphatic vessels—a unified concept. J Pediatr Surg 24:233-240, 1989.
43. O TM, Diallo AM, Scheuermann-Poley C, et al. Lymphatic malformations of the airway. Otolaryngol Head Neck Surg 149:156-160, 2013.
44. Padwa BL, Hayward PG, Ferraro NF, et al. Cervicofacial lymphatic malformation: clinical course, surgical intervention, and pathogenesis of skeletal hypertrophy. Plast Reconstr Surg 95:951-960, 1995.
45. Otteson TD, Hackam DJ, Mandell DL. The Ex Utero Intrapartum Treatment (EXIT) procedure: new challenges. Arch Otolaryngol Head Neck Surg 132:686-689, 2006.
46. Mihm M Jr, North PE. The surgical pathology approach to pediatric vascular tumors and anomalies. In Waner M, Suen JY, eds. Hemangiomas and Vascular Malformations of the Head and Neck. New York: Wiley-Liss, 1999.
47. Dompmartin A, Acher A, Thibon P, et al. Association of localized intravascular coagulopathy with venous malformations. Arch Dermatol 144:873-877, 2008.
48. Dompmartin A, Ballieux F, Thibon P, et al. Elevated D-dimer level in the differential diagnosis of venous malformations. Arch Dermatol 145:1239-1244, 2009.
49. Mazoyer E, Enjolras O, Laurian C, et al. Coagulation abnormalities associated with extensive venous malformations of the limbs: differentiation from Kasabach-Merritt syndrome. Clin Lab Haematol 24:243-251, 2002.
50. Vikkula M, Boon LM, Carraway KL III, et al. Vascular dysmorphogenesis caused by an activating mutation in the receptor tyrosine kinase TIE2. Cell 87:1181-1190, 1996.
51. Oranje AP. Blue rubber bleb nevus syndrome. Pediatr Dermatol 3:304-310, 1986.
52. Bean WB. Vascular Spiders and Related Lesions of the Skin. Springfield, IL: Charles C Thomas, 1958.
53. Fishman SJ, Smithers CJ, Folkman J, et al. Blue rubber bleb nevus syndrome: surgical eradication of gastrointestinal bleeding. Ann Surg 241:523-528, 2005.

54. Waner M, Suen JY. The natural history of hemangiomas. In Waner M, Suen JY, eds. Hemangiomas and Vascular Malformations of the Head and Neck. New York: Wiley-Liss, 1999.

55. Mitchell EL, Taylor GI, Houseman ND, et al. The angiosome concept applied to arteriovenous malformations of the head and neck. Plast Reconstr Surg 107:633-646, 2001.

56. Lo DD, Zimmermann AS, Nauta A, et al. Scarless fetal skin wound healing update. Birth Defects Res C Embryo Today 96:237-247, 2012.

57. Adzick NS, Harrison MR, Glick PL, et al. Comparison of fetal, newborn, and adult wound healing by histologic, enzyme-histochemical, and hydroxyproline determinations. J Pediatr Surg 20:315-319, 1985.

58. Viljanto J, Penttinen R, Raekallio J. Fibronectin in early phases of wound healing in children. Acta Chir Scand 147:7-13, 1981.

59. Gay S, Vijanto J, Raekallio J, et al. Collagen types in early phases of wound healing in children. Acta Chir Scand 144:205-211, 1978.

60. Leaute-Labreze C, Dumas de la Roque E, Hubiche T, et al. Propranolol for severe hemangiomas of infancy. N Engl J Med 358:2649-2651, 2008.

61. Lamy S, Lachambre MP, Lord-Dufour S, et al. Propranolol suppresses angiogenesis in vitro: inhibition of proliferation, migration, and differentiation of endothelial cells. Vascul Pharmacol 53:200-208, 2010.

62. Itinteang T, Withers AH, Leadbitter P, et al. Pharmacologic therapies for infantile hemangioma: is there a rational basis? Plast Reconstr Surg 128:499-507, 2011.

63. Wong A, Hardy KL, Kitajewski AM, et al. Propranolol accelerates adipogenesis in hemangioma stem cells and causes apoptosis of hemangioma endothelial cells. Plast Reconstr Surg 130:1012-1021, 2012.

64. Zou HX, Jia J, Zhang WF, et al. Propranolol inhibits endothelial progenitor cell homing: a possible treatment mechanism of infantile hemangioma. Cardiovasc Pathol 22:203-210, 2012.

65. Breur JM, de Graaf M, Breugem CC, et al. Hypoglycemia as a result of propranolol during treatment of infantile hemangioma: a case report. Pediatr Dermatol 28:169-171, 2011.

66. Holland KE, Frieden IJ, Frommelt PC, et al. Hypoglycemia in children taking propranolol for the treatment of infantile hemangioma. Arch Dermatol 146:775-778, 2010.

67. Fusilli G, Merico G, Gurrado R, et al. Propranolol for infantile haemangiomas and neuroglycopenic seizures. Acta Paediatr 99:1756, 2010.

68. Greene AK, Couto RA. Oral prednisolone for infantile hemangioma: efficacy and safety using a standardized treatment protocol. Plast Reconstr Surg 128:743-752, 2011.

69. Moore J, Lee M, Garzon M, et al. Effective therapy of a vascular tumor of infancy with vincristine. J Pediatr Surg 36:1273-1276, 2001.

70. Fawcett SL, Grant I, Hall PN, et al. Vincristine as a treatment for a large haemangioma threatening vital functions. Br J Plast Surg 57:168-171, 2004.

71. Haisley-Royster C, Enjolras O, Frieden IJ, et al. Kasabach-Merritt phenomenon: a retrospective study of treatment with vincristine. J Pediatr Hematol Oncol 24:459-462, 2002.

72. Garden JM, Polla LL, Tan OT. The treatment of port-wine stains by the pulsed-dye laser. Analysis of pulse duration and long-term therapy. Arch Dermatol 124:889-896, 1988.

73. Ashinoff R, Geronemus RG. Capillary hemangiomas and treatment with the flash lamp-pumped pulsed-dye laser. Arch Dermatol 127:202-205, 1991.

74. Sherwood KA, Tan OT. Treatment of a capillary hemangioma with the flashlamp pumped-dye laser. J Am Acad Dermatol 22:136-137, 1990.

75. Waner M. Laser photocoagulation of hemangiomas. In Waner M, Suen JY, eds. Hemangiomas and Vascular Malformations of the Head and Neck. New York: Wiley-Liss, 1999.

76. Reddy KK, Blei F, Brauer JA, et al. Retrospective study of the treatment of infantile hemangiomas using a combination of propranolol and pulsed-dye laser. Dermatol Surg 39:923-933, 2013.

77. Buckmiller LM, Munson PD, Dyamenahalli U, et al. Propranolol for infantile hemangiomas: early experience at a tertiary vascular anomalies center. Laryngoscope 120:676-681, 2010.

78. O TM, Tan M, Waner M. The distribution, clinical characteristics, and surgical treatment of lip infantile hemangiomas. JAMA Facial Plast Surg 15:292-304, 2013.

79. Weiss I, O TM, Lipari BA, et al. Current treatment of parotid hemangiomas. Laryngoscope 121:1642-1650, 2011.

80. Waner M, Suen JY. Treatment for the management of hemangiomas. In Waner M, Suen JY, eds. Hemangiomas and Vascular Malformations of the Head and Neck. New York: Wiley-Liss, 1999.

81. Buckmiller L, Dyamenahalli U, Richter GT. Propranolol for airway hemangiomas: case report of novel treatment. Laryngoscope 119:2051-2054, 2009.

82. O TM, Alexander RE, Lando T, et al. Segmental hemangiomas of the upper airway. Laryngoscope 119:2242-2247, 2009.

83. Tan OT, Sherwood K, Gilchrest BA. Treatment of children with port-wine stains using the flashlamp-pulsed tunable dye laser. N Engl J Med 320:416-421, 1989.

84. Jasim ZF, Handley JM. Treatment of pulsed-dye laser-resistant port wine stain birthmarks. J Am Acad Dermatol 57:677-682, 2007.

85. Tierney EP, Hanke CW. Alexandrite laser for the treatment of port wine stains refractory to pulsed-dye laser. Dermatol Surg 37:1268-1278, 2011.

86. Gao K, Huang Z, Yuan KH, et al. Side-by-side comparison of photodynamic therapy and pulsed-dye laser treatment of port-wine stain birthmarks. Br J Dermatol 168:1040-1046, 2013.

87. Xiao Q, Li Q, Yuan KH, et al. Photodynamic therapy of port-wine stains: long-term efficacy and complication in Chinese patients. J Dermatol 38:1146-1152, 2011.

88. Huang Z. Photodynamic therapy in China: over 25 years of unique clinical experience. Part 2: Clinical experience. Photodiagnosis Photodyn Ther 3:71-84, 2006.

89. Scherer K, Waner M. Nd:YAG lasers (1,064 nm) in the treatment of venous malformations of the face and neck: challenges and benefits. Lasers Med Sci 22:119-126, 2007.

90. Enjolras O, Ciabrini D, Mazoyer E, et al. Extensive pure venous malformations in the upper or lower limb: a review of 27 cases. J Am Acad Dermatol 36(2 Pt 1):219-225, 1997.

91. Glade RS, Richter GT, James CA, et al. Diagnosis and management of pediatric cervicofacial venous malformations: retrospective review from a vascular anomalies center. Laryngoscope 120:229-235, 2010.

92. Dubois J, Garel L. Imaging and therapeutic approach of hemangiomas and vascular malformations in the pediatric age group. Pediatr Radiol 29:879-893, 1999.

93. Buckmiller LM, Richter GT, Suen JY. Diagnosis and management of hemangiomas and vascular malformations of the head and neck. Oral Dis 16:405-418, 2010.

94. Berenguer B, Burrows PE, Zurakowski D, et al. Sclerotherapy of craniofacial venous malformations: complications and results. Plast Reconstr Surg 104:1-11; discussion 12-15, 1999.

95. Siniluoto TM, Svendsen PA, Wikholm GM, et al. Percutaneous sclerotherapy of venous malformations of the head and neck using sodium tetradecyl sulphate (Sotradecol). Scand J Plast Reconstr Surg Hand Surg 31:145-150, 1997.

96. Waner M, Suen JY. Treatment options for the management of vascular malformations. In Waner M, Suen JY, eds. Hemangiomas and Vascular Malformations of the Head and Neck. New York: Wiley-Liss, 1999.

97. Yue H, Qian J, Elner VM, et al. Treatment of orbital vascular malformations with intralesional injection of pingyangmycin. Br J Ophthalmol 97:739-745, 2013.

98. Edwards PD, Rahbar R, Ferraro NF, et al. Lymphatic malformation of the lingual base and oral floor. Plast Reconstr Surg 115:1906-1915, 2005.

99. Smith MC, Zimmerman MB, Burke DK, et al. Efficacy and safety of OK-432 immunotherapy of lymphatic malformations. Laryngoscope 119:107-115, 2009.

100. Burrows PE, Mitri RK, Alomari A, et al. Percutaneous sclerotherapy of lymphatic malformations with doxycycline. Lymphat Res Biol 6:209-216, 2008.

101. Adams MT, Saltzman B, Perkins JA. Head and neck lymphatic malformation treatment: a systematic review. Otolaryngol Head Neck Surg 147:627-639, 2012.

102. Grimmer JF, Mulliken JB, Burrows PE, et al. Radiofrequency ablation of microcystic lymphatic malformation in the oral cavity. Arch Otolaryngol Head Neck Surg 132:1251-1256, 2006.

103. Kamijo A, Hatsushika K, Kanemaru S, et al. Five adult laryngeal venous malformation cases treated effectively with sclerotherapy. Laryngoscope 123:2766-2769, 2013.

104. Shen CY, Wu MC, Tyan YS, et al. Preliminary experience of percutaneous intralesional bleomycin injection for the treatment of orbital lymphatic-venous malformation refractory to surgery. Clin Radiol 67:182-184, 2012.

105. Endoscopic transmucosal direct puncture sclerotherapy for management of airway vascular malformations (in press).

106. Waner M, Suen JY. The treatment of vascular malformations. In Waner M, Suen JY, eds. Hemangiomas and Vascular Malformations of the Head and Neck. New York: Wiley-Liss, 1999.

107. Eivazi B, Werner JA. Management of vascular malformations and hemangiomas of the head and neck—an update. Curr Opin Otolaryngol Head Neck Surg 21:157-163, 2013.

108. Richter GT, Suen JY. Pediatric extracranial arteriovenous malformations. Curr Opin Otolaryngol Head Neck Surg 19:455-461, 2011.

PART IV

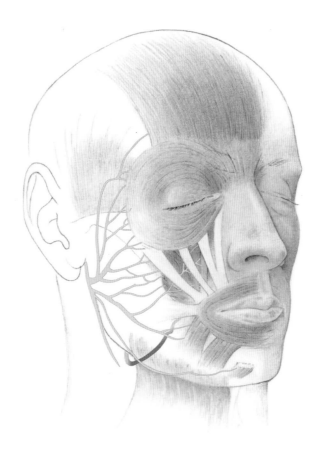

Progress lies not in enhancing what is,
but in advancing toward what will be.
–Khalil Gibran
(1883-1931)

Emerging Trends and New Directions in Facial Plastic Surgery

48

Facial Transplantation

Daniel S. Alam ▪ *John J. Chi*

Remarkable strides have been made in the field of facial reconstruction over the past century. Injuries and defects that were once considered impossible to reconstruct have become amenable to modern techniques. The evolution of these techniques began with the early development of local soft tissue flaps and rigid fixation, and progressed substantially with the advent of microsurgical free tissue transfer. Complex three-dimensional facial defects can now be repaired using free flaps. This technology has allowed us to effectively replace significant amounts of missing tissue. From early reports of free flaps in the 1970s through the complex reconstructions of present day, flap design has evolved significantly. Flaps may be molded, prelaminated, and modified extensively to provide accurate reconstructions. Despite all of these advances, certain defects and injuries encountered in clinical practice remain difficult challenges.

The first human face allograft was performed in France in 2005 on a patient who had been mauled by a dog, resulting in amputation of her distal nose, lips, chin, and portions of the midface. The patient developed mild signs of rejection postoperatively but recovered well after additional treatment with corticosteriods.[1] The first full-face transplant was performed in 2010 in Barcelona, Spain, on a 30-year-old man with facial deformity as a result of ballistic trauma.[2] The success of these cases, coupled with decades of scientific research, has resulted in international interest in facial transplantation.

LIMITATIONS OF CONVENTIONAL RECONSTRUCTION

The difficulty in subtotal facial reconstruction arises from the complexity of the face both in form and function. The face is composed of unique three-dimensional structures consisting of multiple tissue types. Because of its unique color, texture, and consistency, facial skin is often best reconstructed from adjacent areas within the face. Skin from distal extremities, although effectively transferred through microvascular techniques, is not usually appropriately color-matched to the face and results in noticeable disfigurement. The face has unique structures that lack homologs in other parts of the body, such as eyelashes and eyelids. The complex spatial relationships and varied tissue types of facial components, such as the nasal base to the upper lip and the junction of the red and white lip at the vermilion, create reconstructive challenges that are not easily overcome. Microvascular reconstruction of the face is usually most optimal in cases of subcutaneous or bony reconstruction in which the skin and superficial musculoaponeurotic system (SMAS) envelope of the face are unaffected by the injury or surgical resection. When the neuromotor components of the face or facial skin are missing, the reconstruction of these areas becomes more difficult. Flap modification and revision may achieve a progressive molding of the tissue to better approximate the desired endpoints, although there are significant limitations to this approach. In addition to difficulties in achieving the exact structural form of the face, the most significant limitation to conventional reconstruction

Adapted from Alam DS, Chi JJ. Facial transplantation for massive traumatic injuries. Otolaryngol Clin North Am. 2013 Oct;46(5):883-901. Epub 2013 Sep 4.

involves restoration of function, which is a much larger obstacle. In general, free flaps are static structural tissue transfers. Any motor function is related to residual muscle function in the face. An example would be a mandibular reconstruction with a fibula flap that relies on native function of the muscle of mastication to work. The face moves under the control of an intricate neuromuscular roadmap that directs its activity. We smile, laugh, eat, speak, and blink according to impulses traveling from the brain, through the motor branches of the facial nerve, to the facial musculature. The ability to communicate emotions with our facial functions has no substitute. Any successful reconstruction of the face from a functional standpoint cannot simply be limited to a replication of form, but must make this essential connection to the brain.

Movement of the central face is the critical component of all of its functional roles. Almost every facet of human communication and socialization relies on proper function of this zone. The central face presents the window to human emotions. We express anger, joy, grief, and love through the subtle and delicate movements of this part of the face. Injuries to this area not only affect the afflicted individual, but also observers who interact with them.

Although surgeons have mastered moving bone, skin, and soft tissue from one region of the body to another, we are still limited in our ability to execute effective neuromuscular reconstruction. The only widely used clinical application of a neuromuscular flap in the face is the gracilis muscle for smile reconstruction (see Chapter 43). Although the results are excellent for this indication, the limitations of this procedure are obvious. The gracilis muscle is used primarily to reconstruct only the smiling action in the face, and the remaining soft tissues and other structures must be intact and uninjured to achieve optimal results. The procedure is in principle solely the replacement of the zygomaticus major and minor complex. We are not yet capable of reconstructing muscular facial defects involving orbicularis oculi and oris, and have limited options when facial skin and soft tissue are missing in addition to muscle.

Restoration of bony landmarks and closure of soft tissue wounds is often not possible after ballistic trauma because of the loss of viable soft tissue and bone. Additionally, the inherently poor vascularity of the severely traumatized tissues that remain and the associated evolving tissue necrosis and infection make a challenging situation worse. The paradigm must shift, from the classical conceptions of injury repair, to rebuilding. Successful restoration of form and function can only be achieved by recruiting tissues to rebuild the deficient structures of the face.

The treatment approach for extensive traumatic head and neck injuries has shifted away from delayed repair to early repair with local tissue and free tissue transfer reconstructions. Staged early definitive reconstruction allows for fewer surgeries and shorter hospitalizations. The initial repair may involve some elements of healing by secondary intention or primary closure, but usually requires early recruitment of healthy tissue into the face through local tissue rearrangement, pedicled regional flap, or free tissue transfer. Local tissue advancement with a cervicofacial flap can be used to reduce the soft tissue deficit and provide skin coverage. Although this flap brings healthy adjacent tissue into the defect, it is a randomly based flap and susceptible to vascular compromise and distal flap necrosis. Pedicled regional flaps (for example, paramedian forehead flap, deltopectoral flap, and latissimus dorsi flap) are supplied by a vascular pedicle allowing for greater tissue viability and versatility. The paramedian forehead flap can be used for nasal reconstruction. The deltopectoral flap and latissimus dorsi flap can be used to reconstruct large skin defects of the neck, lateral face, and scalp.

The evolving success and reliability of microvascular surgery has led to the early use of healthy vascularized free tissue transfer for trauma reconstruction. The advantages of recruiting nontraumatized native tissue for the reconstruction include a more physiologic restoration of function and a reduction in scar contracture. Free tissue transfer also allows for the reconstruction of varying tissue defects (such as mucosa, bone, skin, and soft tissue) with comparable vascularized tissue. The anterolateral thigh flap can be used to reconstruct large skin and soft tissue defects. The osteocutaneous fibula flap can be used to reconstruct orbitomaxillary and mandibular defects. (Many of these cases are illustrated in Chapter 32.)

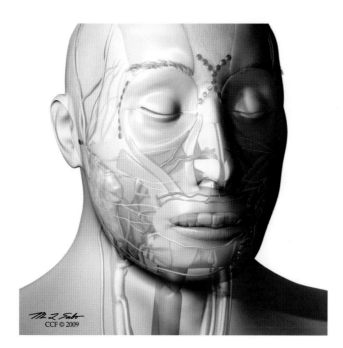

Fig. 48-1   Facial anatomy of the neuromuscular region of the face. The colored segment shows the portion of the craniofacial soft tissues that are integrally connected to the brain motor cortex for complex functional purposes. The black and white regions that include the lateral face and scalp are relatively static structures. (From Alam DS, Chi JJ. Facial transplantation for massive traumatic injuries. Otolaryngol Clin North Am 46:883-901, 2013.)

Conventional microsurgical reconstruction cannot effectively provide a neuromuscular reconstruction of significant central facial defects, since this zone has significant neuromuscular functions and uniquely complex structures that are quite distinct (Fig. 48-1). In this zone, traditional techniques are grossly inadequate.

HISTORY OF ALLOTRANSPLANTATION

Although the specific limitations of conventional reconstructive approaches have been a strong driving force toward the development of facial transplantation, the history of allotransplantation extends a few decades before its consideration for use in the face. The concept of transferring tissues to match complex difficult-to-reconstruct structures (such as the hands, larynx, and tongue) had been studied extensively before this approach was considered for use in the face. The primary concerns with allografts rested with the increased antigenicity of skin and the rejection risks. A groundbreaking study in 1985 showing long-term survival of a hind limb transplant in rats first brought forth the feasibility of skin transplantation.[3] The development of protocols in higher animals led to a series of successful human composite allograft transplants.[4] This critical step in the proof of concept of allograft transplantation was the precursor to the development of animal models and the consideration of human face transplants. The Semionow lab at the Cleveland Clinic developed a rat model of transplantation and conducted basic science immunology trials as a precursor to the Institutional Review Board (IRB) submission for the human trial in 2005. The ultimate justification for this procedure, despite its significant risk to the recipient, was based on the remarkable importance of the face to human identity and quality of life.

THE IMPORTANCE OF THE CENTRAL FACE

The consequence of our limitations in facial reconstruction of the central face is magnified by the incredible importance this area has for maintaining quality of life. The functional significance of the area is obvious. Speech communication is dependent on the function of our lips and mouth. Labial sounds such as "B" and "P," common in almost all languages, cannot be articulated without lip function. The function of the orbicularis oris is critical for eating and drinking. Nasal form and function are important to establish

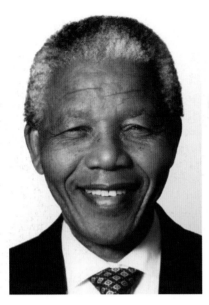
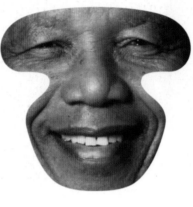

Fig. 48-2   The central face is essential for recognizing an individual's identity. Nelson Mandela is shown. The left panel shows his entire face and the right isolates the neuromuscular zone. Despite representing only 5% of the body surface area, this region conveys the entire identity of the individual.

a safe and appropriate airway. Eyelid function is critical for maintaining vision and corneal protection. These represent just a few of the many vital functions of our faces in our daily existence.

The central face is important to our physical identity. We are recognized by the interplay of the structural relationship between our eyes, nose, and lips—more so than any other part of the body. Within this small region, which comprises less than 5% of our body surface area, lies the foundation of our personal identity (Fig. 48-2).

The precision of human facial recognition is noteworthy. We are able to distinguish more than 200,000 faces from each other. Within 50 hours of birth, newborn infants are able to distinguish their own mothers from other individuals.[5] The secondary consequences of this recognition ability are profound. A mother shown images of her children experiences activation of reward and socialization centers of the brain, associated with feelings of positive emotions. These responses are unique and distinct from those seen when these mothers are shown images of other people's children or strangers. The face offers a key to our human connection; the bonds we develop among our friends and families are based on recognition of this critical region. There are data to suggest that neurochemical relationships of human emotions are based initially on facial recognition, and serve as the foundation for subsequent synaptic relationships to other centers of the brain.

Patients with significant midfacial injuries and severe disfigurement often feel disconnected from society.[6] The neurophysiologic data suggest that this problem arises from behavior with the observers rather than the patient. If an individual does not have a somewhat normal-appearing face, it is almost impossible for observers to develop a normal human relationship with him or her. Most patients with significant midfacial loss who seek complex facial reconstruction are not seeking a surgical procedure to return them to their preinjury state; they simply would like to have the ability to return to human society.

THE RATIONALE FOR FACIAL TRANSPLANTATION

The complex movement of the midface and its critical importance to human interaction requires that effective central facial reconstruction involve neuromuscular reconstruction. Simply replacing like tissue with like, without reestablishing the connections to the brain, results in a suboptimal masklike outcome. This effect can be more disturbing than the defect itself in certain cases.

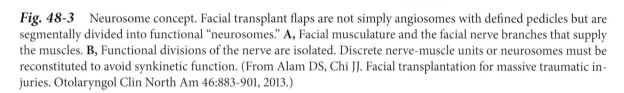

Fig. 48-3   Neurosome concept. Facial transplant flaps are not simply angiosomes with defined pedicles but are segmentally divided into functional "neurosomes." **A,** Facial musculature and the facial nerve branches that supply the muscles. **B,** Functional divisions of the nerve are isolated. Discrete nerve-muscle units or neurosomes must be reconstituted to avoid synkinetic function. (From Alam DS, Chi JJ. Facial transplantation for massive traumatic injuries. Otolaryngol Clin North Am 46:883-901, 2013.)

The solution to this complex reconstructive challenge has been to employ allograft flaps. Facial transplantation has been used to reconstruct severe facial trauma injuries when massive loss of facial structures occurs. Although technically more challenging than the typical free tissue transfer and requiring lifelong immunosuppression for the recipient, face transplantation allows composite transfer of skin, soft tissue, and bone that replaces the lost tissue with precise anatomic and functional match.

Traditionally, free flaps are considered to comprise the tissue that is recruitable within the angiosome of its pedicle vessel. To understand the rationale for facial transplantation, we must expand this idea to involve the concept of the *angioneurosome* (Fig. 48-3).

The design of the flap is based not only on the tissue nourished by its blood supply, but also on the concept of transferring a neuromuscular unit and its muscular origin and insertion, including rigid facial structures and cutaneous ligaments. If this angioneurosome can be transferred in its entirety, it may be used to functionally replace deficient tissue. Vascularization leads to tissue viability and selective coaptation to the corresponding peripheral nerve restoring movement and sensation. In both vascular and neural coaptations, the possibility exists of not simply reconstructing a masklike facial form, but also restoring the face from a functional perspective. Isolating each of the divisions of the facial nerve within an allograft specimen, for example, allows the surgeon to sequentially and segmentally rehabilitate the face.

MEDICAL RISKS

Facial transplantation procedures require lifelong immunosuppression, yielding significant morbidity. Some of the adverse effects and risks associated with this therapy are listed in Fig. 48-4, and must be weighed heavily when considering this approach to facial reconstruction.[7-9]

Immunosuppression is associated with an increased risk of cancer recurrence and the development of new cancers; a history of active cancer or a potential risk for recurrent tumor is an absolute contraindication

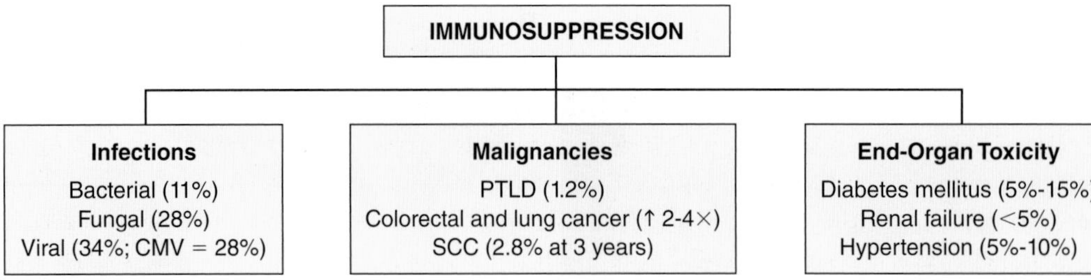

```
                    ┌─────────────────────────┐
                    │   IMMUNOSUPPRESSION      │
                    └─────────────────────────┘
```

Infections	Malignancies	End-Organ Toxicity
Bacterial (11%)	PTLD (1.2%)	Diabetes mellitus (5%-15%)
Fungal (28%)	Colorectal and lung cancer (↑ 2-4×)	Renal failure (<5%)
Viral (34%; CMV = 28%)	SCC (2.8% at 3 years)	Hypertension (5%-10%)

Fig. 48-4 The medical risks of long-term immunosuppression. (*CMV,* Cytomegalovirus; *PTLD,* posttransplant lymphoproliferative disease; *SCC,* squamous cell carcinoma.) (Data from Morris et al,[7] Wiggins et al,[8] and Vasilic et al.[9]) (From Alam DS, Chi JJ. Facial transplantation for massive traumatic injuries. Otolaryngol Clin North Am 46:883-901, 2013.)

for allograft procedures. Facial transplantation is currently reserved within the context and protection of experimental protocols.

Tissue rejection, both acute and chronic, is a serious potential complication of any transplant procedure and may result in organ loss. Appropriate salvage plans and backup protocols are essential steps in planning facial transplantation. To date there have been no transplanted faces lost because of chronic rejection in compliant patients. However, acute rejection is a common phenomenon, reported with multiple events in every case in the literature. Fortunately, these episodes are manageable with relative ease using short-term immunomodulation.

ETHICAL CONSIDERATIONS

The medical risks associated with transplantation highlight the contemporary dilemma clinicians encounter when weighing the appropriateness of the procedure.[3] At this time, face transplant surgery remains experimental, and ethical considerations are paramount in the development of surgical protocols.[10] The ethical implications of this procedure warrant considering the general principles of autonomy, beneficence, and nonmalfeasance, which form the foundations of the ethics of medicine. The possible life-threatening complications of face transplantation are a current reality. The potential gain must outweigh this risk. The surgery should only be considered in individuals who report a loss in their quality of life that warrants acceptance of these risks. Proper evaluation of the capacity of recipients to make this decision, their understanding of the risks and benefits, and their potential compliance with lifelong therapy are critical.

Beyond the difficult assessment of risk/benefit, facial transplantation presents other considerations. The concept of personal facial identity is inextricably connected to facial transplantation. Do recipients lose their identity in the procedure? Do the donors transfer their identity? Or is it a hybrid of these two phenomena? The preclinical data and clinical experience both indicate that identity confusion is less problematic than initially predicted. Although the recipients of full-face transplants share similarities to the donor, variations in skeletal structure and facial shape result in a composite appearance, neither firmly donor nor recipient in origin.

The recipient's identification with and connection to his or her new face is a transformation in and of itself. Fortunately, this has not been a difficult adjustment for patients to make.

SURGICAL INDICATIONS FOR FACIAL TRANSPLANTATION

Facial transplantation should be reserved for individuals with significant midfacial neuromuscular injuries. Complete absence or loss of the function of the orbicularis oris muscles with a concurrent complete nasal defect is currently the minimal indication for considering allograft-based reconstructions. Defects may extend beyond these limits to include eyelids and the full face, but the minimum deficit requiring allograft is the central neuromuscular segment of the midface. At present, the inclusion criteria comprise only ballistic and physical trauma (such as burns). The potential risk of the loss of cancer surveillance under immunosuppression precludes postsurgical ablation of malignancy as a potential indication.

ALLOGRAFT DESIGN AND CLASSIFICATION SCHEME

Numerous allograft procurement protocols have been described in the literature.[11-13] At this relative stage of infancy of this procedure, most allografts have been tailored to the defects of the individual patients. To date, only 25 facial transplantation procedures have been performed worldwide. Despite the variability of cases, some common themes are present across all procedures. The facial artery alone provides the arterial inflow in most (18 of 25) cases, though in a few cases the external carotid artery has been used. Angiographic studies and clinical experience have shown that the facial artery is sufficient to supply a full-face transplant, including the maxilla. The palate, although primarily supplied by palatine vessels from the internal maxillary system, can easily be perfused through oral mucosal vascular networks from the facial artery. The venous outflow has been based on the common facial veins, as well as the external jugular venous system. Some surgeons have chosen to use the internal jugular vein, but it is clear that the common facial vein is adequate for venous drainage of the inferior facial structures. The cross circulation in the face is so well established that vascular reconstitution of one side of the face alone will provide sufficient perfusion of both sides across the midline.

The depth of the allograft harvest must be below the plane of the facial musculature and the facial nerve. The facial nerve must be carefully dissected and preserved to achieve a neuromuscular reconstruction. Individual facial nerve branches are isolated and a sequential and segmental series of neurorrhaphies are performed.

The various facial procurement protocols are combinations of traditional surgical approaches. For example, the combination of a bicoronal flap, a LeFort III level osteotomy, and bilateral superficial parotidectomy plan elevation is a full-face procurement (see Fig. 48-3). The bicoronal flap, which is a component of all facial procurement protocols, and the other surgical approaches that are used preserve allograft vascularity and nerve function. With the use of a combination of surgical approaches, a blueprint can be created for the allograft procurement appropriate for the patient's facial defects. The procurement procedures are not novel surgical techniques, but merely a combination of accepted surgical approaches.

CLINICAL EXPERIENCE

Currently, the worldwide clinical experience in facial transplantation is too limited to provide significant data to support its long-term efficacy.[1,6,14-19] The largest reported clinical series includes only three patients. The reports are essentially proof-of-concept papers and anecdotal experience. The evolution of the surgical procedure during the time between two illustrative cases, performed only months apart, demonstrates the rapidly advancing nature of this field.

This 46-year-old woman underwent 23 reconstructive procedures after a gunshot wound, including four failed free flaps, resulting in the clinical presentation seen in Fig. 48-5, *A* through *C*. She continued to have significant disfigurement and functional limitation after these procedures and therefore was seen for evaluation by the multidisciplinary Cleveland Clinic Face Transplant Team.

Her entire midface was functionally absent or surgically altered. The extent of the defect included a complete absence of any nasal or septal structure. She had undergone a paramedian forehead flap. She had no maxilla, zygomatic arches, or inferior orbital rims. Additionally, scar contracture in the midface and the prior flap coverage eliminated a nasal passageway, rendering the patient anosmic and an obligate mouth breather. The absence of any mimetic musculature in the midface left her with a functional bilateral facial paralysis and significant oral incompetence. She had extensive scarring and fibrosis in the soft tissue of the neck, and depletion of native vessels.

Preoperative evaluations were undertaken by the departments of transplant surgery, transplant psychiatry, and bioethics. The complex skeletal loss presented the unique challenge of having to incorporate vascularized maxilla into the transplanted face. The design of the donor facial skin and soft tissue envelope incorporated the entire cheek subunit, the entire nose, and the entire upper lip (Fig. 48-5, *D*). The flap was planned as a full-thickness flap, including the buccal mucosa of the midface. In the lower third, where the patient had existing viable tissue, the allograft flap was procured in the subplatysmal plane, with incorporation of both the parotid and portions of the submandibular glands for safe preservation of the neurovascular pedicles (Fig. 48-5, *E*). This design intentionally incorporated redundant glandular tissue, which will require future excision. The donor's hypoglossal nerves were also included as motor nerve cable grafts to bridge the gap between the recipient's midface division branch of the facial nerve and the donor facial nerve trunk created by the redundant parotid gland tissue. Since the inflow axons are only midface in origin, this neurorrhaphy would reduce potential synkinesis and inappropriate facial movement. The surgical steps of the transplant procedure are illustrated in Fig. 48-5, *F* through *I*.

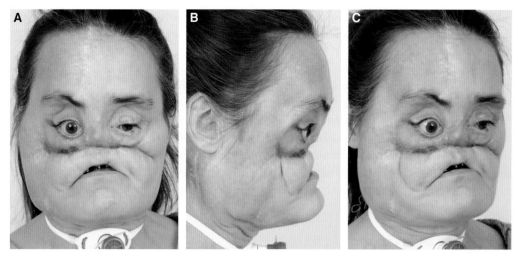

Fig. 48-5   Preoperative views of a 46-year-old face transplant patient whose midface injuries resulted from a gunshot wound. **A,** Frontal view. **B,** Lateral view. **C,** Oblique view. (From Alam DS, Chi JJ. Facial transplantation for massive traumatic injuries. Otolaryngol Clin North Am 46:883-901, 2013.)

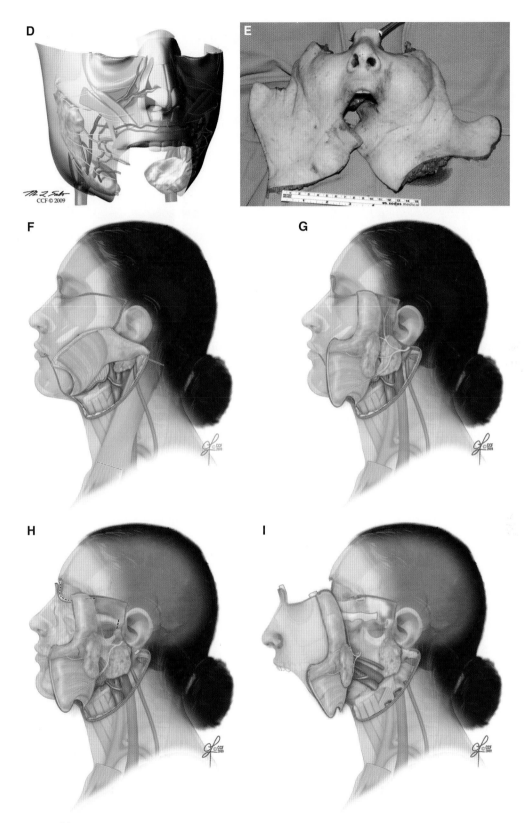

Fig. 48-5, cont'd   **D,** Design for the harvested donor tissue. **E,** Allograft specimen intraoperatively, before inset. **F-I,** Transplant procedure. The dissection was done in a superior to inferior fashion. **F,** Skin incisions and the initial dissection. **G,** Parotid and facial nerve dissection. **H,** Isolation of the bony skeletal framework of the midface for osteotomy. **I,** Facial mobilization after osteotomy at the LeFort III level. (From Alam DS, Chi JJ. Facial transplantation for massive traumatic injuries. Otolaryngol Clin North Am 46:883-901, 2013.)

Continued

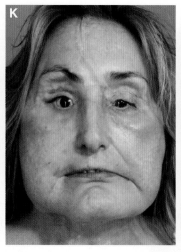
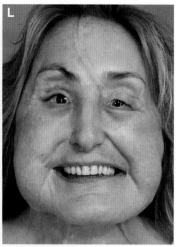

Fig. 48-5, cont'd   **J,** Preoperative view. **K** and **L,** The patient is seen 4 years postoperatively. (From Alam DS, Chi JJ. Facial transplantation for massive traumatic injuries. Otolaryngol Clin North Am 46:883-901, 2013.)

The incorporation of the allograft was complete 4 years postoperatively, with no graft loss (Fig. 48-5, *K*). The patient has recovered facial nerve function and facial sensation. She has experienced restoration of all of her midfacial functions lost after her injury, including smiling and laughing (Fig. 48-5, *L*). The aesthetic outcome is limited by her preexisting eyelid trauma that was not addressed by the transplant. She also has redundant parotid tissue requiring excision, and her facial nerve recovery has been asymmetrical, with greater functional recovery on her left side. Despite these limitations, she is able to function well in social environments.

This 56-year-old woman was the victim of a chimpanzee attack that resulted in a near-total facial avulsion (Fig. 48-6, *A*). She was initially managed with debridement and wound care to stabilize her infected wounds. She retained normal cognitive function 1 month after her injury. Subsequently she underwent interval reconstruction with local advancement flaps and an anterolateral thigh free flap with costal cartilage grafting to temporize her condition.

The extent of injury in this case required a full-face transplant. Although the procedure for the patient in Fig. 48-5 was planned by defining a novel surgical approach to the exact defect, the design of the transplant for this woman was based on traditional surgical approaches. The extent of her injury justified full-face replacement. The allograft was a composite of a bicoronal flap, bilateral parotid dissections, LeFort III level osteotomies, and oral mucosal release (Fig. 48-6, *B* through *H*). The neck plane was executed in the subplatysmal plane, with dissection of the facial arterial and venous vascular system. The superficial parotid glands were removed in this case, eliminating the need for revision parotid surgery.

With full-face transplantation, isolation of individual facial nerve branches is a critical step. Neural coaptation was performed at distal locations to prevent synkinesis and to improve selective motor function. (Patients with injury to the facial nerve proximal to the pes anserinus are poor candidates for full-face transplantations for this reason.)

The immediate postoperative outcome of this patient is seen in Fig. 48-6, *J*. At nearly 2 years after transplantation, she has full graft take and excellent functional recovery. She has restored facial movement bilaterally, although her facial nerve function remains paretic. She has been able to effectively reintegrate into society, although her blindness and loss of hands remain significant residual disabilities.

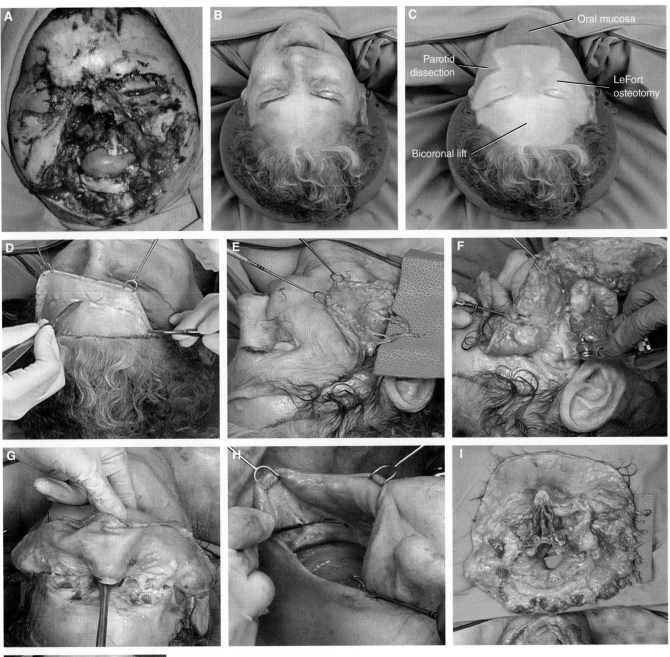

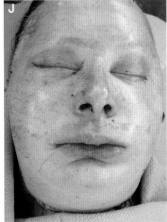

Fig. 48-6   **A,** This face transplant patient is seen preoperatively. **B** and **C,** General planning components of the surgery, including a bicoronal flap, bilateral parotid dissections, LeFort III osteotomy, and an oral mucosal release. **D,** Bicoronal flap. **E,** Parotid dissection. **F** and **G,** Osteotomy approaches. **H,** Oral mucosal release. **I,** The entire specimen from its inner surface. **J,** The patient is seen immediately after face transplant surgery. The graft take was successful, and her facial movement function was restored bilaterally. (From Alam DS, Chi JJ. Facial transplantation for massive traumatic injuries. Otolaryngol Clin North Am 46:883-901, 2013.)

CONCLUSION

Despite the relative infancy of the field of facial transplantation, the optimism for its role in facial reconstruction continues. This optimism is a response both to successful early outcomes and the complex nature of the problem that the surgery is designed to address. We currently have no means to repair complex neuromuscular injuries of the face. Although free flaps have offered us an effective tool to transfer tissue, we remain unable to functionally connect the transferred tissues to the brain to make it perform properly. The gracilis free flap reconstruction begins to scratch the surface of this issue, but has a limited indication for a single function. In massive injuries, there are still no ideal options. This futility provides the strongest impetus for facial transplantation.

The technique has improved over the first 25 cases of facial transplantation; and this trend should continue as more cases are performed and long-term follow-up of early cases becomes possible. The true success of this operation remains an unanswered question at this stage, although the early outlook remains promising.

KEY POINTS

- The clinical limitation of conventional microvascular reconstruction of the face is our inability to effectively reconstruct the neuromotor complex of the midface.
- Midface structure and function is critical for human social and communicative functions, and breathing, eating, and emotional expression.
- The central midface is essential to facial identity, which provides in turn the basis of human relationships.
- Facial transplantation permits restoration of a neuromotor function of the midface, with outcomes that allow patients to reintegrate into society.
- Facial transplantation remains experimental surgery, and long-term follow up will determine its ultimate role in facial reconstruction.

REFERENCES

1. Devauchelle B, Badet L, Lengele B, et al. First human face allograft: early report. Lancet 368:203-209, 2006.
   This is the first report of human facial transplantation in the medical literature.
2. Barret JP, Gavalda J, Bueno J, et al. Full face transplant: the first case report. Ann Surg 254:252-256, 2011.
3. Black KS, Hewitt CW, Fraser LA, et al. Composite tissue (limb) allografts in rats. II. Indefinite survival using low-dose cyclosporine. Transplantation 38:365-368, 1985.
4. Strome M, Stein J, Esclamado R, et al. Laryngeal transplantation and 40-month follow-up. N Engl J Med 344:1676-1679, 2001.
5. Bushneil IW, Sai F, Mullin JT. Neonatal recognition of the mother's face. Br J Dev Psychol 7:3-15, 1989.
6. Soni CV, Barker JH, Pushpakumar SB, et al. Psychosocial considerations in facial transplantation. Burns 36:959-964, 2010.
7. Morris P, Bradley A, Doyal L, et al. Face transplantation: a review of the technical, immunological, psychological and clinical issues with recommendations for good practice. Transplantation 83:109-128, 2007.
8. Wiggins OP, Barker JH, Martinez S, et al. On the ethics of facial transplantation research. Am J Bioeth 4:1-12, 2004.
9. Vasilic D, Alloway RR, Barker JH, et al. Risk assessment of immunosuppressive therapy in facial transplantation. Plast Reconstr Surg 120:657-668, 2007.
10. Alexander AJ, Alam DS, Gullane PJ, et al. Arguing the ethics of facial transplantation. Arch Facial Plast Surg 12:60-63, 2010.

11. Alam DS, Papay F, Djohan R, et al. The technical and anatomical aspects of the world's first near-total human face and maxilla transplant. Arch Facial Plast Surg 11:369-377, 2009.

    This study highlights the specifics behind the first successful transfer of a complete bony framework and soft tissue envelope of the face.

12. Meningaud JP, Paraskevas A, Ingallina F, et al. Face transplant graft procurement: a preclinical and clinical study. Plast Reconstr Surg 122:1383-1389, 2008.

13. Pomahac B, Lengele B, Ridgway EB, et al. Vascular considerations in composite midfacial allotransplantation. Plast Reconstr Surg 125:517-522, 2010.

14. Dubernard JM, Lengele B, Morelon E, et al. Outcomes 18 months after the first human partial face transplantation. N Engl J Med 357:2451-2460, 2007.

15. Siemionow M, Papay F, Alam D, et al. Near-total human face transplantation for a severely disfigured patient in the USA. Lancet 374:203-209, 2009.

16. Guo S, Han Y, Zhang X, et al. Human facial allotransplantation: a 2-year follow-up study. Lancet 372:631-638, 2008.

17. Lantieri L, Meningaud JP, Grimbert P, et al. Repair of the lower and middle parts of the face by composite tissue allotransplantation in a patient with massive plexiform neurofibroma: a 1-year follow-up study. Lancet 372:639-645, 2008.

18. Pomahac B, Pribaz J, Eriksson E, et al. Restoration of facial form and function after severe disfigurement from burn injury by a composite facial allograft. Am J Transplant 11:386-393, 2011.

19. Lantieri L, Hivelin M, Audard V, et al. Feasibility, reproducibility, risks and benefits of face transplantation: a prospective study of outcomes. Am J Transplant 11:367-378, 2011.

49

Evaluating Patient Outcomes in Facial Plastic Surgery

Richard Gliklich ▪ *Regan Bergmark* ▪ *Prabhat K. Bhama*

Although the goal of facial plastic and reconstructive surgical interventions is to improve patient outcomes, to date the evaluation of these outcomes has not been systematic, but rather has been anecdotal, subjective, selective, or simply ignored by most surgeons and institutions. However, given the visibility of form and criticality of the functions of facial structures, facial plastic surgery may lend itself more readily to systematic evaluation of patient outcomes than many other medical disciplines. "Quality of care" was defined by the Institute of Medicine as "the degree to which health services for individuals and populations increase the likelihood of desired health outcomes and are consistent with current professional knowledge," a definition that has remained widely quoted over the past several decades.[1]

EVOLUTION OF OUTCOMES ASSESSMENT

Outcomes refer to the "crucial link between the care that is provided and its effects on health."[1] Systematic assessment refers to the use of a valid set of methodologies, applied in a consistent manner across one or more practices to collect uniform information on either all or a representative sample of patients and procedures. By contrast, the common practice of collecting and displaying before and after photographic documentation may be illustrative of what could be achieved in a surgical procedure, but the use of photographs from selected patients presented for visual assessment is neither representative nor objective in the outcomes that might be implied.

ROLE OF OUTCOMES ASSESSMENT IN FACIAL PLASTIC AND RECONSTRUCTIVE SURGERY

A system to evaluate patient outcomes would document before and after states for all patients in a standardized, uniform, valid, and reproducible manner and allow those measures to be tracked over time, benchmarked with other surgeons or institutions. Such a system would provide information on the safety and clinical, comparative, and cost effectiveness of those procedures compared with alternative treatments or expenditures of health care funds. At the aggregate level, it would also provide key information on learning curves, volume-outcome relationships, patient or disease characteristics that predict better or worse outcomes, and opportunities for improvement in processes and procedures. From a public health perspective, such systems enhance our safety net by identifying earlier issues with implants or new treatments. From a patient perspective, outcome measurements may be reported in a manner that facilitates patient choice of procedures as well as facilities and surgeons (as is the case with the Society of Thoracic Surgeons Database).[2]

Historically, outcomes measurement has been performed in an ad hoc and incomplete manner in facial plastic surgery. Humans have attempted to assess beauty for millennia; Greek writings describe definitions of beauty (see Chapter 2). Modern facial plastic surgeons have evaluated results through a multitude of outcomes measures, including anthropomorphic measures, clinician-reported outcomes, complication rates, and more recently patient-reported outcomes.[3] This chapter outlines examples of currently available facial plastics outcomes measures and outlines a new comprehensive model for national outcomes measurement.

TYPES OF OUTCOMES MEASURES

Outcomes evaluation in facial plastic surgery is a nascent field. Holistic outcomes measurement models may include both the response of the patient and the disease to treatment and are measured by variables such as mortality, disease response (for example, change in tumor volume on CT scans), and adverse events. Traditionally, many treatments have been measured by clinician-reported measures. During the past 20 years, patient-reported outcomes (PROs) measures have become more prevalent, enabling more quantitative assessment of treatment outcomes when PROs are applicable (as is the case in most of facial plastic and reconstructive surgery). In addition, societal impact factors such as health care utilization are becoming increasingly important. Both clinician- and patient-reported measures exist in facial plastic surgery, and their roles merit thorough understanding.

CLINICIAN-REPORTED OUTCOMES

Clinician-reported measures have historically been used for assessment of outcomes in plastic surgery. Unlike a CT scan measurement or laboratory result, clinician reports are subjective. Although many historical studies reported results by clinicians and thus lack rigorous validity, today there are several validated clinician-reported measures that can and should be used where applicable. Similar to PROs, there is a scientific process for developing an observer-based metric, with clear standards for reasonable agreement among different observers, which renders such measurements useful. The key is that the measurement be appropriately validated and have reasonable performance characteristics for test-retest reliability and inter-rater reliability, among other parameters. There are some measurements that have been validated both for reliability and responsiveness to change; for certain outcomes, such as subtle improvements in facial rhytids, such scales may be preferable to other alternatives.

PATIENT-REPORTED OUTCOMES

Patient-centered care is becoming a cardinal principle of health care. Furthermore, significant differences exist between patient and clinician assessments of disease symptoms and response to treatment.[4-7] A PRO is a measurement that is based on information that comes directly from the patient without interpretation. As PRO measures have become more user friendly, they are rapidly being incorporated into routine measurement of outcomes during clinical care.

The use of PRO instruments typically involves a general health assessment combined with a disease- or condition-specific assessment. The former assessment allows a level setting of the degree of disability versus other conditions and focuses on issues that are common across many diseases (for example, pain, ability to perform daily functions). The latter assessment aims to evaluate more specific issues associated with a particular condition. Typically, the specialized measure will also be more responsive to changes in clinical status. Together, they provide a more holistic impression of the patient's overall functioning and well-being. Some instruments will combine both dimensions into one form, such as the University of Washington Quality of Life (UWQOL) instrument for head and neck cancer. More often, commonly used general measures, such as the EuroQol Group's EQ5D or Medical Outcomes Study Short Form 36 or 12 instruments, will be combined with the specific measure to achieve the same result and also allow comparisons with other diseases. In some cases, a specific measure is sufficient to evaluate the question of interest. The resources and expertise required to create these instruments are substantial; a brief guide to some of the existing measures is identified next.

DEVELOPMENT OF APPROPRIATE OUTCOMES MEASURES

A multitude of ad-hoc questionnaires have been used, but thoroughly validated instruments are sparse in facial plastic surgery. Several PRO measures have been tested and found reliable, valid, and able to detect real clinical change. The following concepts are crucial when developing a PRO measure and are highlighted with an example from *Laryngoscope,* "Validation of a Patient-Graded Instrument for Facial Nerve Paralysis: the FaCE Scale"[8]:

1. Item generation: As with any questionnaire, the source of the questions or items is critical to understanding how comprehensive the questions are likely to be. For many instruments it is not disclosed how items were chosen for measurement. Expert opinion is often used for item generation but may fail to capture critical aspects of patient outcomes.

2. Reliability: Reliability describes the degree to which the results would be reproducible. Reliability is a measure of precision of the instrument. Measures should be tested for interobserver and/or intraobserver agreement and test-retest reliability. Instruments should be internally consistent.

3. Validity: Validity is the degree to which the assessment measures what it intends to measure. Measures require formal validation. Validity has multiple components, including content, criterion, construct, and internal and external validity. Validation is a process of using logical constructs to evaluate these components. Examples include whether the questions make sense to someone with skill in the art; whether the measurement is internally consistent from question to question; and whether it yields similar results to either objective measurements or other validated questionnaires that address similar patient issues.

4. Ability to detect clinical change: Instruments should be able to detect change when real clinical change has occurred. This is typically measured and reported with standard metrics such as the standardized response mean (SRM).

EXAMPLE OF PROM (PATIENT-REPORTED OUTCOMES MEASURES) DEVELOPMENT WITH THE FACIAL CLINIMETRIC EVALUATION (FACE) SCALE

Facial nerve injury has a multidimensional impact on patients, and other than protection from eye injury, patient functioning and well-being make up the most relevant clinical outcomes. Although the House-Brackmann (HB) scale and more recently others such as the American Academy of Otolaryngology–Head and Neck Surgery Facial Nerve Disorders committee's Facial Nerve Grading System 2.0 (FNGS2) have gained acceptance among clinicians for the evaluation of recovery, these clinician-reported scales do not incorporate the patient's perspective and are less useful for providing insight into disability or for conducting long-term evaluations when patients may not return to the clinic.

FaCE was developed to measure facial disability rather than facial impairment. This validated outcomes instrument contains 15 items from which the patient must select a number on an ordinal scale and one item to assess the side of dysfunction. (The FaCE Scale is available for use with permission from the Massachusetts Eye and Ear Infirmary.) The description below of the validation of the FaCE scale outlines and illustrates the general steps used in developing and validating most PRO measures today:

1. Item generation: A literature search and interviews with physicians, nurses, and physical rehabilitation specialists were used to obtain background information for item generation. Six patients with facial nerve injury were then interviewed with questions developed by the authors of the cited study. Initially, 51 individual items were included in the FaCE scale.

2. Reliability: The scale was completed by 86 patients with facial nerve paralysis, most of whom repeated the questionnaire 2 weeks later. Reliability of the total score and domain scores was calculated with a Spearman's rank-order correlation.

3. Validity: Content validity was achieved as described in the "item generation" section above. The 86 patients also completed the Facial Disability Index (FDI) and the Medical Outcomes Study Short Form 36-Item Questionnaire (SF-36), which helped assess construct validity. A small subset also presented for evaluation with the HB scale to help establish criterion validity. In addition, the test was given to control subjects. The instrument was then scaled to contain only 15 primarily Likert scale items to assess their level of dysfunction with exploratory factor analysis. Internal consistency was assessed with Cronbach's alpha coefficient. Overall the development of this scale included construct, criterion, content, convergence, and internal and external validity measures.

4. Ability to detect clinical change. Potential uses for the scale include assessment of the natural history of facial paralysis, success of surgical or nonoperative interventions, and understanding outcomes of surgeries in which facial nerve function may be compromised. Examination of sensitivity to clinical change was beyond the scope of the initial validation study of this scale, although subsequent studies have examined sensitivity to clinical change. For example, one study compared morbidity of patients with Bell's palsy to those with vestibular schwannoma.

EXISTING PROMS FOR FACIAL PLASTIC SURGERY

Currently several condition- or procedure-specific instruments are available in the facial plastic surgery literature; undoubtedly over time more instruments will be developed and their use standardized, which will permit more robust comparisons within and between practices. A recent review by Rhee and McMullin[3] identified 23 patient-reported, 35 observer-reported, and 10 objective measure instruments in the plastics literature. The authors concluded that the quality of validation was significantly varied among the instruments and that validity was the most powerful in the PRO measures. Kosowski et al[9] identified only nine PRO measures designed for facial cosmetic surgery and nonsurgical facial rejuvenation from a broad literature search. Forty-seven PRO measures were identified, although 38 of these assessed general or psychological health and were not tailored toward aesthetic outcomes. All nine of the questionnaires that passed the authors' inclusion criteria were limited by development, validation, or content.

Although experts agree that numerous useful instruments are available in facial plastic surgery, a full complement of reliable measures across the breadth of facial plastic surgery remains lacking. Some PROs useful in facial plastic surgery are included in Table 49-1.

Table 49-1 Selected Patient-Reported Outcomes Measures

Study	Authors, Year	Brief Description
Derriford Appearance Scale (DAS59/DAS24)	Harris and Carr, 2001[10]	Assess psychological and physical distress and disability before or after intervention in patients with disfigurement, aesthetic concerns, history of trauma and repair, or aesthetic surgery. General scales; some questions are not relevant to patients undergoing facial plastic surgery.
Glasgow Benefit Inventory (GBI)	Robinson et al, 1996[11]	Eighteen-item questionnaire assesses general psychological, physical, and emotional well-being after intervention. Developed originally in a population of patients having tonsillectomy, otoloplasty, and facial nerve paralysis, this measure was validated only in patients undergoing rhinoplasty.
Rhinoplasty Outcome Evaluation (ROE)	Alsarraf et al, 2001[12]	Six-item assessment of patient-reported satisfaction with appearance, functional outcome, patient's perception of family satisfaction with outcome, and breathing difficulty.
Nasal Obstruction Septoplasty Effectiveness (NOSE)	Stewart et al, 2004[13]	Five-item quality of life questionnaire used for septoplasty.
Blepharoplasty Outcomes Evaluation (BOE)	Alsarraf et al, 2001[12]	Six-item assessment of patient-reported satisfaction with appearance, functional outcome, and patient's perception of family satisfaction with outcome.
Facelift Outcomes Evaluation (FOE)	Alsarraf et al, 2001[12]	Six-item assessment of patient-reported satisfaction with appearance, functional outcome, and acceptance after surgery.
Facial Lines Treatment Satisfaction	Cox et al, 2003[14]	Fourteen item assessment of patient satisfaction with treatment outcomes and side effects of treatment.
Skindex-61, Skindex-29, and Skindex-16	Chren et al, 1996, 1997[15-17]	61-, 29-, and 16-item questionnaires regarding quality of life for general dermatology, cutaneous malignancy, and botulinum toxin treatment.
Skin Rejuvenation Outcomes Evaluation	Alsarraf et al, 2001[12]	Six-item assessment of patient-reported satisfaction with appearance, functional outcome, and acceptance after surgery.
Dermatology Life Quality Index (DLQI)	Finlay and Khan, 1994[18]	Ten-item assessment of quality of life for general dermatologic disease, cutaneous malignancy, acne, and laser treatment of rosacea.
Facial Clinimetric Evaluation Scale (FaCE)	Kahn et al, 2001[8]	Fifteen-item assessment of disability and quality of life in patients with facial paralysis.
Facial Disability Index (FDI)	VanSwearingen and Brach, 1996[19]	Ten-item assessment of disability and quality of life in patients with facial paralysis.

Continued

Table 49-1 Selected Patient-Reported Outcomes Measures—cont'd

Study	Authors, Year	Brief Description
Synkinesis Assessment Questionnaire (SAQ)	Mehta et al, 2007[21]	Nine items evaluating functional status in patients with facial synkinesis.
Bock Quality of Life Questionnaire for patients with keloid and hypertrophic scarring	Bock et al, 2006[22]	Fifteen-item qualify of life assessment for patients with hypertrophic scarring.
Patient and Observer Scar Assessment Scale (POSAS)	Draaijers et al, 2004[23]	Eleven-item assessment of body image for patients with hypertrophic scarring and keloids.
Melasma Quality of Life scale (MelasQOL)	Balkrishnan 2003[24]	Ten-item assessment of quality of life related to skin resurfacing and laser treatment.
Skin Cancer Index (SCI)	Rhee et al, 2007[25]	Fifteen-item assessment of quality of life related to cutaneous malignancy and associated dermatologic treatment.

GLOBAL ASSESSMENT MEASURES
Derriford Appearance Scale 59 (DAS59)

The DAS59 is a global psychometric scale of 59 items in Likert format that was developed to evaluate the psychological distress and loss of function caused by disfigurement, deformities, and problems with appearance. The main limitation of this instrument with regard to applicability to facial plastic surgery is that many of the items are not directed at facial assessment. For instance, one entire subscale of nine items is directed at assessment of body appearance. Thus this instrument may be less responsive to interventions performed by the facial plastic and reconstructive surgeon.[10]

SEPTORHINOPLASTY
Nasal Obstruction Septoplasty Effectiveness (NOSE)

The NOSE scale is a five-item questionnaire on a Likert scale, validated for the assessment of patients with nasal obstruction. The scale was developed because the use of objective measurements of nasal airflow has been controversial and because no validated instrument was designed for subjective measurement of nasal obstruction. The instrument has been demonstrated to be valid, reliable, and responsive to intervention.[26] It has been used in the clinical setting since its implementation in the mid-2000s and has been found to be effective after septoplasty in a prospective study.[13] This instrument is excellent for the assessment of nasal obstruction, but does not address the aesthetic issues coinciding with rhinoplasty.

AGING FACE
Skindex

The Skindex was first published in the dermatology literature as a 61-item instrument to assess quality of life as impacted by skin disease and has been modified over time; several versions exist.[15,26] The instrument underwent validation and was found to be both reliable and responsive to clinical change. The study was initially performed on 201 patients with various skin disorders such as cutaneous carcinoma, benign neoplasms, acne, and alopecia. One obvious disadvantage with this scale is that the items are not specific to facial skin—rather, they refer to the skin envelope of the entire body.

FACIAL NERVE DISORDERS

Synkinesis Assessment Questionnaire (SAQ)

The SAQ is another instrument used to assess patients with facial movement disorders. Although other instruments exist that incorporate synkinesis into the assessment, they have been found to have low reliability. The SAQ is a 10-item questionnaire that was designed specifically to assess those patients who have developed synkinesis of the facial muscles as a result of facial nerve insult and recovery. It has been validated and has demonstrated reliability.[21]

SCARRING

Patient and Observer Scar Assessment (POSAS)

The POSAS is a two-part numeric scale—one for the observer and one for the patient. It consists of 11 total items graded on a scale from 1 to 10, assessing pain, pruritus, color, thickness, irregularity, and pliability of the scar. The instrument was initially developed to evaluate all scars but was only found to be reliable for rating burn scars.[23]

COMPREHENSIVE OUTCOMES MEASUREMENT FRAMEWORK

The evaluation of outcomes in facial plastic surgery requires two key components: A systematic approach to collect and analyze data and standards-based measures of relevant patient outcomes.

COLLECTION OF DATA

The collection of useful data to evaluate patient outcomes is best accomplished prospectively with the use of a patient registry. A patient registry is "an organized system that uses observational study methods to collect uniform data (clinical and other) on a population defined by an exposure to meet a specific scientific, clinical or policy purpose."[26] The ideal registry for collecting outcomes in clinical practice would enroll all or a representative sample of patients with similar conditions undergoing the same procedure. The registry would collect clinically rich data including risk factors, treatments, and outcomes at key points depending on the procedure or condition. It should collect such data from multiple sources, including patients, physicians, and hospitals, and use standardized methods to ensure a representative sample, data quality, and comparability (Fig. 49-1). Because facial plastic surgery interventions are delivered largely in an outpatient setting and not all patients return to the same providers over the long term, well-considered methods must be in place both to obtain longer-term follow-up from all sampled patients and to clearly understand losses to follow-up and how they are similar to or different from those patients who continue to be measured.

Outcome Measures Framework

An extremely difficult task that requires national consensus efforts is to define outcome measures for facial plastic surgery procedures. Recent work from the Agency for Healthcare Research and Quality (AHRQ) has led to the development of a proposed model for outcomes measures across all health fields.[28] A pictorial representation of such a framework, adapted to facial plastic surgery, is shown in Fig. 49-2. To populate the model for a specific procedure, one must complete the relevant framework elements.

The ideal model would incorporate PROs within a comprehensive framework. Such a model would allow assessment of patient and provider characteristics, disease characteristics, treatment options, and selection. PROs would be one outcome measure; other outcomes measures could include mortality, disease response, adverse events, and health system use.

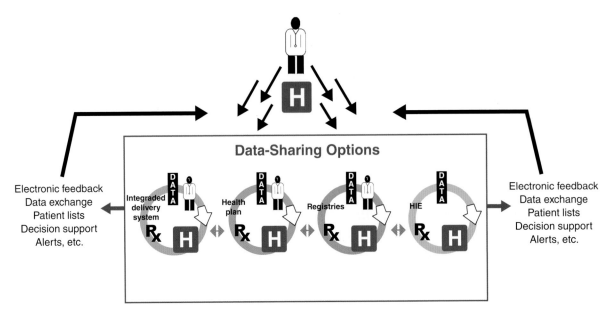

Fig. 49-1 Model of registry for the collection of outcomes in clinical practice.

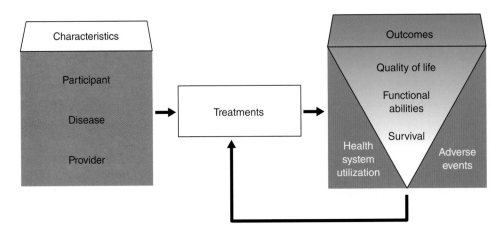

Fig. 49-2 A framework applied to facial plastic and reconstructive surgery.

Example: Facial Nerve Paralysis

Participant Characteristics The model would include demographic data and may expand to include genetic data. Patient comorbidities, especially those that might predispose to the disease (for example, neurofibromatosis) or would affect surgical success, would be included.

Disease Characteristics The model would record clinical cause and disease characteristics affecting facial function, such as tumor involvement, surgical sacrifice of the nerve, Ramsay-Hunt syndrome, viral disease, or other causes. The model would also record onset characteristics and duration of paralysis and prior treatments, including surgical intervention, botulinum toxin therapy, or physical therapy. The degree of paralysis as determined by standardized PROs such as the FaCE scale and clinical measures of degree of recovery such as the House-Brackmann score would be noted.

Provider Characteristics Surgeon experience, including training, the number of facial nerve–related operations completed, average annual volume, and so on, would likely affect the treatment offered and patient outcomes. Geographic location and academic versus private practice setting would also be recorded.

Treatment   Treatment rendered would include conservative treatment such as physical therapy, botulinum toxin chemodenervation therapy, and operative management (for example, static slings, alternative source nerve grafting, cross-face nerve grafting, and free and regional muscle transfer).

Outcomes   Mortality, both disease related and unrelated, would be included. Disease response as measured by PROs such as the FaCE scale and clinician-reported measures such as the House-Brackmann Scale are major endpoints. Adverse event recording and measurements of health system use, including inpatient hospitalizations, office and emergency visits, additional procedures, absenteeism from work and direct costs, would be recorded.

Example: Rhinoplasty

Participant Characteristics   Demographics, ethnicity, health behaviors (including smoking and recreational drug use), family history, occupation, and so on, would be included. Systemic disease would include those that affect any surgery (for example, comorbidities such as diabetes) and nasal surgery (for example, sarcoidosis, Wegener's granulomatosis, and skin diseases); relevant environmental exposures would also be included. For patients undergoing aesthetic procedure, a history of prior aesthetic surgeries for the face and body may be relevant.

Disease Characteristics   A detailed, diagnostic evaluation is important, including functional issues (for example, nasal valve stenosis and septal deviation) and nasal form distortions or asymmetries (for example, saddle nose deformity, dorsal hump, bifid tip, skin deficit, etc.). Skin thickness and history of prior nasal surgery would be particularly relevant. Radiologic assessment of fractures could be included to demonstrate the degree of deformity in trauma patients.

Provider Characteristics   Again, we would include training, rhinoplasty case volume (primary and revision) over the provider's career and per year, geography, and practice setting.

Treatment   Surgical treatment such as components of rhinoplasty such as tip rhinoplasty, dorsal hump reduction, the use of grafts (type/donor site and location used), and use of alloplasts would be included. Surgical goals should be identified because some patients' goals will vary from the norm.

Outcomes   Response to treatment as measured by PROs such as the Rhinoplasty Outcomes Evaluation and clinician-reported outcomes if validated would be included. Procedure-related adverse events (for example, skin loss, graft extrusion, or worsened breathing) and need for any subsequent revisions should be recorded.

How Might the Data Be Used?

Ideally, surgeons performing facial plastic and reconstructive procedures will soon have the tools to systematically evaluate their outcomes in practice, much as they currently obtain photographs or videographs of their patients. Such data at an aggregate level will provide tremendous information on the types of patients who seek care, patterns and approaches to treatment, outcomes achieved, which patients are most likely to benefit from certain procedures or treatments, and which are most likely to suffer complications (see Fig. 49-1). At a specialty level, we will better understand the duration to become competent in a particular procedure, how many procedures a surgeon should perform per year to maintain reasonable outcomes, and which procedures or implants should be phased out because of effectiveness or safety concerns. Recording and scrutinized outcomes data have repeatedly been shown to facilitate quality improvement.

Public Reporting

In the modern health care climate, patients and payers will increasingly request information regarding outcomes of the procedures they are seeking. This phenomenon has already become commonplace in some surgical fields, including thoracic surgery, and is likely to become the norm over time. One must accept the reality of this trend, and practitioners of facial plastic and reconstructive surgery should be educated about rigorous participation in the outcomes movement as it relates to facial plastic surgery.

CONCLUSION

The field of facial plastic surgery is poised to move beyond the ad-hoc, unstructured assessment of patient outcomes, which until now has been commonplace. Models are emerging for regular outcomes assessment across all health care fields and should be used in facial plastic surgery. Already validated instruments exist to begin to assess PROs in a rapid and accurate way and more are being created. The routine use of standardized and comprehensive outcomes measurements in our field will create tremendous opportunities to analyze and ultimately improve our treatments and procedures.

KEY POINTS

- Although our goal as facial plastic surgeons is to have excellent outcomes, we have not been systematic in measuring or defining outcomes.
- PROMs, when used systematically, are often more useful than clinician-reported outcomes.
- PROMs must be developed and validated in a systematic manner, testing reliability, validity, and sensitivity to clinical change.
- There are many PROMs of varying quality. Some of the more validated or widely used instruments are outlined here.
- A national database should be used to measure outcomes in facial plastics and throughout medicine.
- A national database would include significant background and demographic information. Outcomes would include PROMs and information on mortality, complications, rehospitalization rates, and other critical outcomes.

REFERENCES

1. Lohr K. Medicare: A Strategy for Quality Assurance, vols 1 and 2. Washington, DC: National Academy Press, 1990.
2. Society of Thoracic Surgeons Database. Available at *http://www.sts.org/national-database.*
3. Rhee JS, McMullin BT. Measuring outcomes in facial plastic surgery: a decade of progress. Curr Opin Otolaryngol Head Neck Surg 16:387-393, 2008.
   This is a large review of available outcomes measures in facial plastic surgery.
4. Basch E, Iasonos A, McDonough T, et al. Patient versus clinician symptom reporting using the National Cancer Institute Common Terminology Criteria for Adverse Events: results of a questionnaire-based study. Lancet Oncol 7:903-909, 2006.
5. Bushmakin AG, Cappelleri JC, Taylor-Stokes G, et al. Relationship between patient-reported disease severity and other clinical outcomes in osteoarthritis: a European perspective. J Med Econ 14:381-389, 2011.
6. Cleeland CS, Sloan JA; ASCPRO Organizing Group. Assessing the Symptoms of Cancer Using Patient-Reported Outcomes (ASCPRO): searching for standards. J Pain Symptom Manage 39:1077-1085, 2010.

7. Pakhomov SV, Jacobsen SJ, Chute CG, et al. Agreement between patient-reported symptoms and their documentation in the medical record. Am J Manag Care 14:530-539, 2008.

8. Kahn JB, Gliklich RE, Boyev KP, Stewart MG, Metson RB, McKenna MJ. Validation of a patient-graded instrument for facial nerve paralysis: the FaCE scale. Laryngoscope 111:387-398, 2001.
    This article demonstrates how validity and reliability can be established for a new PROM.

9. Kosowski TR, McCarthy C, Reavey PL, et al. A systematic review of patient-reported outcome measures after facial cosmetic surgery and/or nonsurgical facial rejuvenation. Plast Reconstr Surg 123:1819-1827, 2009.
    Another review of facial plastic surgery outcomes, this article concludes that few validated instruments are available.

10. Harris DL, Carr AT. The Derriford Appearance Scale (DAS59): a new psychometric scale for the evaluation of patients with disfigurements and aesthetic problems of appearance. Br J Plast Surg 54:216-222, 2001.

11. Robinson K, Gatehouse S, Browning GG. Measuring patient benefit from otorhinolaryngological surgery and therapy. Ann Otol Rhinol Laryngol 105:415-422, 1996.

12. Alsarraf R, Larrabee WF Jr, Anderson S, et al. Measuring cosmetic facial plastic surgery outcomes: a pilot study. Arch Facial Plast Surg 3:198-201, 2001.

13. Stewart MG, Smith TL, Weaver EM, et al. Outcomes after nasal septoplasty: results from the Nasal Obstruction Septoplasty Effectiveness (NOSE) study. Otolaryngol Head Neck Surg 30:283-290, 2004.

14. Cox SE, Finn JC, Stetler L, et al. Development of the Facial Lines Treatment Satisfaction Questionnaire and initial results for botulinum toxin type A-treated patients. Dermatol Surg 29:444-449; discussion 449, 2003.

15. Chren MM, Lasek RJ, Quinn L, et al. Skindex, a quality-of-life measure for patients with skin disease: reliability, validity, and responsiveness. J Invest Dermatol 107:707-713, 1996.

16. Chren MM, Lasek RJ, Flocke SA, et al. Improved discriminative and evaluative capability of a refined version of Skindex, a quality-of-life instrument for patients with skin diseases. Arch Dermatol 133:1433-1440, 1997.

17. Chren MM, Lasek RJ, Quinn LM, et al. Convergent and discriminant validity of a generic and a disease-specific instrument to measure quality of life in patients with skin disease. J Invest Dermatol 108:103-107, 1997.

18. Finlay AY, Khan GK. Dermatology Life Quality Index (DLQI)—a simple practical measure for routine clinical use. Clin Exp Dermatol 19:210-216, 1994.

19. VanSwearingen JM, Brach JS. The Facial Disability Index: reliability and validity of a disability assessment instrument for disorders of the facial neuromuscular system. Phys Ther 76:1288-1298; discussion 1298-1300, 1996.

20. Chren MM. The Skindex instruments to measure the effects of skin disease on quality of life. Dermatol Clin 30:231, 2012.

21. Mehta RP, WernickRobinson M, Hadlock TA. Validation of the Synkinesis Assessment Questionnaire. Laryngoscope 117:923-926, 2007.

22. Bock O, Schmid-Ott G, Malewski P, et al. Quality of life of patients with keloid and hypertrophic scarring. Arch Dermatol Res 297:433-438, 2006.

23. Draaijers LJ, Tempelman FR, Botman YA, et al. The patient and observer scar assessment scale: a reliable and feasible tool for scar evaluation. Plast Reconstr Surg 113:1960-1965; discussion 1966-1967, 2004.

24. Balkrishnan R, McMichael AJ, Camacho FT, et al. Development and validation of a health-related quality of life instrument for women with melasma. Br J Dermatol 149:572-577, 2003.

25. Rhee JS, Matthews BA, Neuburg M, et al. The skin cancer index: clinical responsiveness and predictors of quality of life. Laryngoscope 117:399-405, 2007.

26. Coulson SE, Croxson GR, Adams RD, O'Dwyer NJ. Reliability of the "Sydney," "Sunnybrook," and "House-Brackmann" facial grading systems to assess voluntary movement and synkinesis after facial nerve paralysis. Otolaryngol Head Neck Surg 132:543-549, 2005.

27. Gliklich R, Dreyer NE. Registries for Evaluating Patient Outcomes: A User's Guide. Rockville, MD: Agency for Healthcare Research and Quality, Sept 2007.

28. Outcome Measures Framework (OMF) Design Document. Agency for Healthcare Research and Quality. Available at *http://effectivehealthcare.ahrq.gov/ehc/products/311/1223/OMF-Design-Document_DraftReport_20120814.pdf.*

50

Tissue Engineering for Facial Plastic Surgery

Cathryn A. Sundback ▪ *Joseph P. Vacanti*

The craniomaxillofacial (CMF) region has a complex structure, consisting of bone, cartilage, skeletal muscle, fat, and a rich neurovascular network. Numerous conditions, including trauma, tumor resections, and congenital malformations lead to loss of function and deformity. Despite state-of-the-art medical and surgical therapies, clinical outcomes following reconstructive procedures may be suboptimal, in part because of the lack of biologic replacement parts.

The use of bioengineered tissues holds promise for the repair of craniomaxillofacial defects. Over the past several decades, significant advances have been realized toward replacing damaged organs by guiding and exploiting the body's innate capacity for regeneration.[1] The concept of tissue engineering was introduced more than two decades ago, when it was defined as "an interdisciplinary field that applies the principles of engineering and the life sciences toward the development of biologic tissues that restore, maintain, or improve tissue function."[2] These basic tissue engineering principles initially proposed by Langer and Vacanti in 1993 continue to be relevant.[2] In CMF surgery, clinical success has been demonstrated with engineered bone, cartilage, and soft tissues.[3]

SIGNIFICANCE

Engineering of tissues and organs is governed by complex interactions within the "tissue engineering triad," which includes three components: isolated cells, biochemical signals, and biomimetic scaffold materials[3] (Fig. 50-1). Increasing overlap exists between the roles of cells, signals, and scaffolds. For example, new generation matrices provide structural support as well as induce cell behavior. The cells contribute to tissue formation and secrete factors that promote blood vessel ingrowth.

ISOLATED CELLS

Cells used for tissue engineering are capable of enhancing the reparative and regenerative processes of tissues. Cells are isolated from tissues, typically autologous, and are often expanded ex vivo and differentiated. Today, cells span the gamut from embryonic stem cells (hES cells) to fully differentiated mature cells, like chondrocytes (Fig. 50-2). Although hES cells are pluripotent and capable of differentiating into any cell type, their use in the United States has been severely limited by ethical and regulatory guidelines.

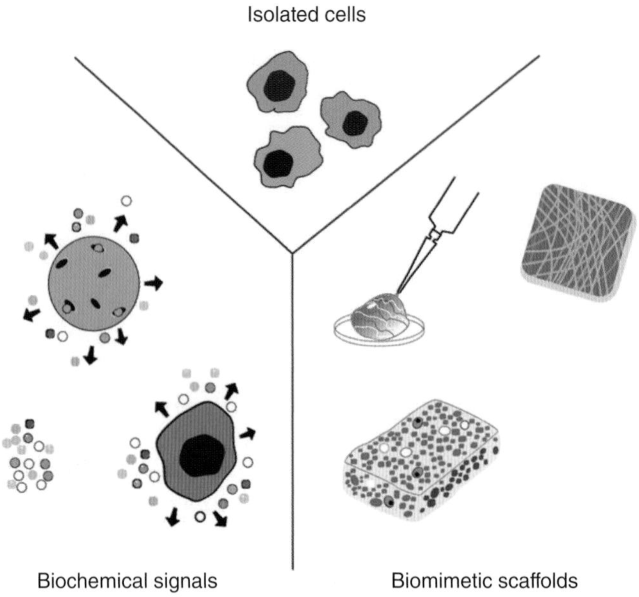

Isolated cells

Fig. 50-1 The core principles of tissue engineering. Tissue engineering is based on complex interactions between isolated cells, biochemical factors, and biomimetic scaffolds.

Biochemical signals   Biomimetic scaffolds

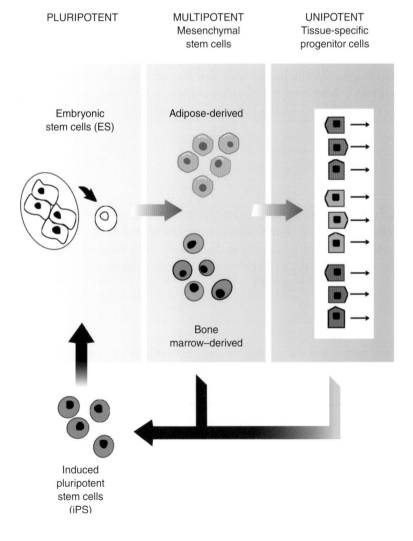

PLURIPOTENT

MULTIPOTENT
Mesenchymal
stem cells

UNIPOTENT
Tissue-specific
progenitor cells

Embryonic
stem cells (ES)

Adipose-derived

Bone
marrow–derived

Induced
pluripotent
stem cells
(iPS)

Fig. 50-2 Types of stem cells available for tissue engineering. Embryonic stem (ES) cells are pluripotent and can be differentiated into multipotent mesenchymal stem cells (MSCs). MSCs, which are harvested from adipose tissue or bone marrow, can be differentiated to adult tissue-specific progenitor cells. MSCs and tissue-specific progenitor cells can be reprogrammed to induced pluripotent stem (iPS) cells. iPS cells, like ES cells, can be differentiated to cells of the endoderm, ectoderm, or mesoderm germ layers.

Consequently, adult stem cells are most often used as the source of progenitor cells. Mesenchymal stem cells (MSCs), commonly harvested from bone marrow or adipose tissue, are multipotent progenitor cells capable of differentiating into tissues of mesodermal origin, such as bone, cartilage, fat, muscle, and blood vessels.[4] Interest is developing in the potential use of induced pluripotent stem (iPS) cells, which are produced through genetic reprogramming of adult cells into an embryonic-like state.[5] The use of these pluripotent *dedifferentiated* cells does not cause the ethical concerns associated with embryonic stem cells. However, significant characterization of the genetic alterations incurred during cellular reprogramming is required before this emerging technology may be applied clinically.

Biochemical Signals

Soluble factors, including growth factors, cytokines, and synthetic small molecules, provide highly regulated biochemical and environmental cues that control cell behavior and fate. The precise delivery of these factors modulates tissue regeneration, so must be tightly regulated. The release pattern of biochemical signals is designed to imitate normal development and to direct proper cell lineage differentiation. These agents may be delivered through nanoparticulates or controlled release microspheres, or through overexpression by genetically modified cells.

Biomimetic Scaffold Materials

Engineered scaffolds re-create the extracellular environment required for organogenesis.[6] A biomimetic scaffold serves as a three-dimensional template for cell attachment and proliferation and provides inductive cues to enhance progenitor cell differentiation. Scaffolds should be biocompatible, nonimmunogenic, provide mechanical support, enable blood vessel ingrowth from the host (angiogenesis), and eventually undergo resorption.[6] Scaffolds have an extensive macroarchitecture and microarchitecture that supports cellular migration and blood vessel ingrowth and should provide channels for delivery of biofactors. However, the benefit of this porosity must be balanced against the need to protect the regenerating tissue until it develops sufficient mechanical integrity.

Natural and synthetic materials have been used as scaffold materials. Natural scaffold materials from autologous, allogenic, and xenogenic sources have frequently been combined with isolated cells and/or soluble factors.[7] However, the supply of natural substitutes is limited, and the mechanical properties of these materials are insufficient in many applications. Consequently, synthetic biomaterials are frequently employed either as porous structural polymers or as hydrogels.[8] Often these engineered scaffolds are produced with advanced fabrication technologies such as microfabrication, three-dimensional printing, and nanotechnology. The resulting extracellular biosystems provide structural support and deliver soluble and tethered factors which actively guide, respond to, and modulate the cell-scaffold interactions necessary for tissue formation.[9]

The ability to cultivate a regenerative environment in engineered tissue constructs depends on inducing the cells and surrounding cues to re-create the programming present during tissue and organ morphogenesis. Because of the biologic and regulatory complexities, tissue engineering approaches have been slow to transition toward clinical applications. However, several craniofacial reconstruction challenges have benefited from tissue engineering methodologies, including skeletal and auricle reconstruction and dermal augmentation (Fig. 50-3).

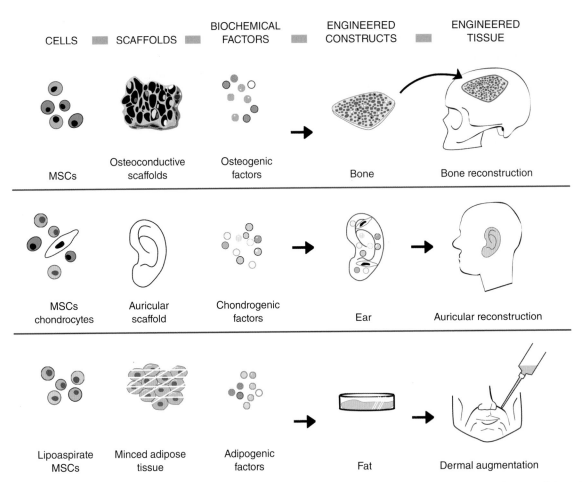

Fig. 50-3   Strategies for engineering specific craniomaxillofacial tissues: bone, auricular cartilage, and fat. Although each is unique, all strategies combine progenitor cells or fully differentiated cells with biomimetic scaffolds and appropriate biochemical factors to engineer tissue-specific cellularized constructs. These constructs are implanted into the appropriate locations in the body, where the scaffolds are resorbed or remodeled and the cells mature into replacement tissue.

CRANIOFACIAL SKELETON RECONSTRUCTION

Whether from congenital malformations, trauma, or cancer extirpation, loss of bone in the craniofacial skeleton has significant structural and functional consequences. The current clinical standard for repair is reconstruction with autologous bone harvested from the iliac crest, fibula, scapula, and other sites. Bone is highly vascularized and contains osteocytes, osteoblasts, and osteoclasts, which are surrounded by a matrix composed of hydroxyapatite (HAP), collagens, glycoproteins, proteoglycans, and sialoproteins.[10] Thus bone grafts are osteoconductive, osteoinductive, and osteogenic. The osteoconductive bone graft serves as a scaffold for new bone replacement by the host. Osteoblasts at the margin of the graft invade the bone graft framework and generate new bone. During osteoinduction, biochemical signals, including bone morphogenetic proteins (BMPs), stimulate osteoprogenitor cells to differentiate into osteoblasts that form new bone. In osteogenesis, surviving osteogenic cells form new bone.

The autologous bone graft is ostensibly the ideal option for facial bone reconstruction. However, bone graft use is constrained by significant donor site morbidity, operative risk, resorption, and the limited volume of available donor bone, particularly in pediatric patients. Allografts have been used in craniofacial reconstruction to overcome the limitations of autologous bone grafts. Bone allografts have similar properties to that of autografts but carry a risk of disease transmission and immunologic rejection, which results in unpredictable outcomes. Consequently, small to midsized craniofacial defects are often repaired using inert, nonosteoconductive, synthetic materials, such as polymethylmethacrylate and porous polyethylene.[11] Initial outcomes can be excellent, but these materials do not induce new bone formation. Consequently, these implants carry lifetime risks of mechanical failure, mobility, and infection.

The optimal bone replacement should replicate lost structure and restore function, be easily remodeled by the host, be biocompatible, and be reliable in repair sites compromised by infection, irradiation, scarring, or extensive trauma. Many bone studies have been conducted based on the principles of tissue engineering, using scaffolds alone, scaffolds combined with soluble factors or cells, and constructs that are a combination of all three components: scaffolds, cells, and soluble factors. Bone tissue engineering studies are reviewed next, highlighting outcomes of pilot scale through clinical human studies.

BIOMIMETIC SCAFFOLDS

A variety of biomaterials have been tested for bone engineering applications,[12-18] as described in Table 50-1. Although engineered human bone studies have been conducted with many of these scaffolds, only a single clinical study used a scaffold without isolated cells or soluble factors; clinical studies based on combinations of scaffolds, cells, and/or soluble factors are described in later sections.

Chao et al[18] reported that composite scaffolds were effective for augmenting cranial defects in craniosynostosis patients. PLA/PGA mesh layers were placed on either side of cranial defects, which were filled with osteoconductive demineralized bone void filler. Promising results were obtained in 82% of their patients (9 of 11); 2 patients had small residual defects at 18-month follow-up. Cranial vault reconstruction cases are typically well managed with autologous bone grafts.[19]

Traditional scaffold fabrication techniques are uncontrolled processes that produce scaffolds that can restrain tissue regeneration. Technologies are under development to produce customized three-dimensional engineered scaffolds with precise external shapes and tightly controllable porous architectures. Patient-specific digital information, either from CT scans or MRI, is converted to virtual implants using computer-aided technologies. From these data, customized scaffolds are fabricated for each patient with solid free-form technologies. The scaffolds are either seeded with exogenous cells and biologic factors before implantation into tissue defects, or the macroarchitecture and microarchitecture of the scaffold support endogenous cell migration.[20] In a case study, a calvarial defect was reconstructed with a customized biodegradable scaffold. The implant was well integrated after 6 months, and bony consolidation was observed.[21]

BIOCHEMICAL SIGNALS

Osteogenic growth factors, such as bone morphogenetic proteins (BMPs), enhance the osteoinductive properties of scaffolds. The original BMPs were derived from demineralized bone matrix but today are synthesized as recombinant human proteins.

Recombinant human BMP-2 (rhBMP-2) has been approved for clinical use in the United States for oral implantology, specifically sinus augmentation and alveolar ridge augmentation.[22] In multiple case studies and clinical trials, patients were treated with rhBMP-2/acellular collagen sponge (ACS) for alveolar ridge augmentation or maxillary sinus floor augmentation or to repair mandibular defects. Denser bone formed in rhBMP-2/ACS–treated patients in comparison with patients treated either with ACS alone or with autologous bone grafts. In most cases, sufficient bone formation had occurred for placement and functional loading of endosseous dental implants.[23,24]

Table 50-1   Classes of Biomaterials Used for Engineering Bone Tissue

Material Types	Examples	Advantages	Disadvantages	Comments
Natural polymers	Collagen Hyaluronic acid Calcium alginate Chitosan	Osteoconductive Natural affinity for BMPs and other growth factors[12]	Lack mechanical strength Degrade rapidly Can be immunogenic[13]	
Inorganic materials	Demineralized bone matrix Tricalcium phosphates (beta-TCP) Bioactive glasses Hydroxyapatite (HAP)	Osteoconductive Biocompatible Not immunogenic Sufficient mechanical strength	Porous scaffolds are brittle and not for load-bearing applications[14]	
Synthetic polymers	Polyglycolide (PGA) Poly(D,L-lactide-co-glycolide) (PLGA) Polylactide (PLA) Polycaprolactone (PCL) Polyethylene glycol (PEG) Polyurethanes[15]	Biocompatible Predictable biodegradation Excellent chemical properties	Lack biologic function Degradation byproducts can induce significant inflammatory responses	Often combined or coated with ceramic material such as HAP to increase composite mechanical strength and osteoconductivity[16]
Composite materials	One of many: HAP/collagen/PLA	Build on desirable properties of each material		HAP mimics natural extracellular matrix (ECM) of bone Collagen provides template for apatite formation; PLA mechanically supports regenerating tissue[17]

In addition to these approved indications, promising results have been obtained using rhBMP-2/ACS in adult alveolar cleft repairs, which are more challenging than in children.[25] At 1 year after repair, improved healing and enhanced mineralization and bone volume were observed in adult patients treated with rhBMP-2/ACS compared with patients receiving bone grafts.

Autologous growth factors have been clinically applied as platelet-rich plasma (PRP). This concentrated source of platelets and their growth factors has biologic effects which impact differentiation of osteoprogenitor cells, osteogenesis, and osseous healing; these growth factors include platelet-derived growth factor BB (PDGF-BB), transforming growth factor beta (TGF-beta), vascular endothelial growth factor (VEGF), basic fibroblast growth factor (bFGF), epidermal growth factor (EGF), and insulinlike growth factor 1 (IGF-1).[22]

PRP has been clinically used in a large number of oral and maxillofacial applications because of its potential to promote effective bone repair. Nearly 30 controlled randomized clinical trials have been conducted to determine the efficacy of PRP for treatment of periodontal intraosseous defects and gingival recession as well as in sinus augmentation and other oral-maxillofacial reconstruction procedures.[26] The outcomes are controversial: 9 studies found a positive effect of PRP, whereas in 20 studies little effect was observed.

These inconsistencies are likely related to variable PRP preparation and delivery methods. Standardized and characterized PRP preparations and delivery methods are essential to improve outcome predictability and to decipher the role each component plays in bone regeneration.[22]

Other growth factors have shown promise in preclinical investigations in craniofacial bone repair. The most widely tested factor is recombinant human osteogenic protein 1 (rhOP-1), also known as BMP-7. Calvarial bone formation in nonhuman primates was effectively promoted after repair with either an HA or a collagen scaffold combined with rhOP-1.[27,28] However, variable results were observed when ovine mandibular osteoperiosteal continuity defects were repaired with a collagen scaffold combined with rhOP-1.[29] In a small clinical study, the maxillary sinus floor of three patients was elevated using a collagen scaffold combined with rhOP-1, but bone formed in only one patient.[30] Sufficiently powered clinical trials are necessary to accurately assess the clinical utility of rhOP-1 in craniofacial applications. Several additional growth factors have undergone preclinical testing for repair of craniofacial defects, including parathyroid hormone covalently bonded to polyethylene glycol (PEG) hydrogel and IGF-1 in combination with PDGF-BB in a methylcellulose hydrogel.[31-33] Some local bone formation was observed, but randomized clinical trials are required to adequately assess efficacy.

Biologic and regulatory challenges exist for widespread application of recombinant growth factors in craniofacial reconstruction, as these factors must be delivered at appropriate doses and at rates which enable a beneficial biologic response and effective repair. Growth factor usage raises safety concerns because they have significant roles in normal growth and development, the healing response, and in certain diseases. Although BMP-2 is known as an osteoinductive growth factor, it is also biologically active in human malignancies.[34] Consequently, the delivered dose must be neither excessively high nor low, since either will negatively affect short-term and long-term outcomes. Preclinical safety testing is essential to assess the reproductive and developmental toxicities, immunogenicity, and carcinogenicity of relevant recombinant human growth factors.[35,36]

CELL SOURCES

To date, osteogenic differentiation potential has been best characterized in multipotent mesenchymal stem cells (MSCs). MSCs have been derived from bone marrow (BMSCs) and adipose tissue (AdMSCs) as well as from skeletal muscle and human umbilical cord cells. Following induction with osteogenic cytokines including BMP-2 and bFGF, BMSCs differentiated toward osteoblasts.[37] BMP-induced BMSCs delivered on a variety of biologically active scaffolds have been used to repair critical-sized craniofacial bone defects in small animal models.[38]

In a small case study, a customized vascularized bone flap was engineered on the back of a patient to reconstruct a large critical-sized frontal bone defect. A three-dimensional polyamide mold was fabricated to match the geometry of the frontal bone defect. A portion of the latissimus dorsi muscle was placed into the mold and the muscle was impregnated with rhBMP-2 in a hyaluronic acid–fibrin–collagen gel. Ground autologous bone was placed on the periphery of the mold. Although the expectation was that the MSCs in the skeletal muscle would contribute to ossification, insufficient bone volume had formed after 4 months. Consequently, the flap was augmented with a porous polyethylene (PE) implant. At 6 months the vascularized engineered bone/PE flap with vascular pedicle was transferred to the frontal bone defect, and revascularized using standard microvascular techniques.[39] Although the repair was successful, bone formation could be enhanced through optimization of the osteoinductive and osteogenic components of the flap.

In later clinical craniofacial applications, expanded BMSCs in an autogenous fibrin-rich and PRP clot with a mineral base of beta-TCP and HAP were used to treat three patients with (1) maxillary and mandibular radionecrosis; (2) a nonhealed fracture, bone loss, and bilateral paresthesia; and (3) maxillary bone deficiency. In all cases, bone formation was observed along with nerve, skin, and blood vessel regeneration.[40]

AdMSCs are rapidly gaining popularity among plastic surgeons, because large quantities can be harvested by minimally invasive liposuction and can be differentiated into osteoblasts with proper signaling. Cowan et al[41] reported that MSCs from bone marrow and adipose tissues on apatite-coated PLGA scaffolds supported similar levels of healing of critical-sized calvarial bone defects in small animals.

A few case reports describe the use of AdMSCs to treat craniomaxillofacial defects. Widespread calvarial defects in a pediatric patient were successfully repaired using autogenous AdMSCs seeded in bone grafts.[42] In another case study, bilateral orbitozygomatic defects in adult patients were successfully treated with a combination of human bone allograft, AdMSCs, rhBMP-2, and periosteal grafts which formed healthy bone.[43] This approach may provide an alternative to osteocutaneous free flaps and large structural allografts, with less morbidity and improved long-term results.

Multipotent stem cells and osteogenic growth factors have also been combined with bone grafts and microvascular free flaps. AdMSCs combined with rhBMP-2–containing beta-TCP granules were placed in a titanium cage, which was implanted in the rectus abdominis muscle. After 8 months in vivo, the flap had developed mature bone and vasculature, and was transplanted to the maxillary defect. Postoperative healing was uneventful.[44] (Fig. 50-4) A similar approach was used for mandibular repair. HAP blocks infiltrated with BMSCs and rhBMP-2 were loaded into a titanium mesh cage shaped to match the mandibular defect. The construct was implanted into the latissimus dorsi muscle for seven weeks and then transplanted as a free bone-muscle flap to reconstruct a critical-sized mandibular defect. Satisfactory aesthetic outcome with improved mastication was achieved[45] (Fig. 50-5). These studies demonstrate the promise of progenitor cells and osteogenic biochemical factors when used in combination with proven surgical procedures to enhance osseous healing.

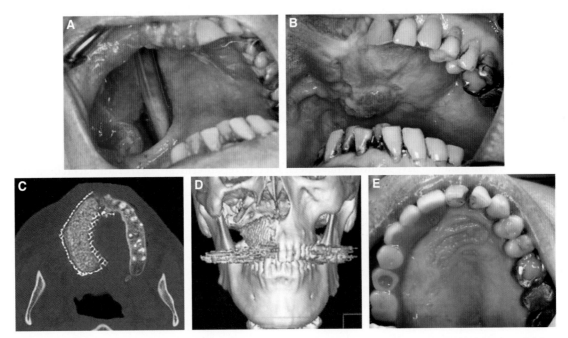

Fig. 50-4   Maxillary reconstruction with ectopic bone formation using AdMSCs. A microvascular custom-made bone flap was engineered in the rectus abdominis muscle using autologous AdMSCs on beta-TCP scaffolds with rhBMP-2. **A,** After 8 months of ectopic implantation, the vascularized bone flap was transplanted to the maxillary defect area. **B,** Axial and **C,** three-dimensional CT scans depict the shape and normal bone density of the regenerated maxilla. **D,** One year after reconstruction, the mechanical integrity of the repaired maxilla was sufficient to support temporary dental implants. **E,** Two months after the defect repair, epithelialization was nearly complete; only a small area in the molar region remained unepithelialized. (From Mesimaki K, Lindroos B, Törnwall J, et al. Novel maxillary reconstruction with ectopic bone formation by GMP adipose stem cells. Int J Oral Maxillofac Surg 38:201-209, 2009.)

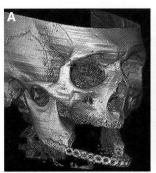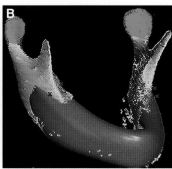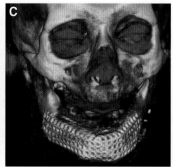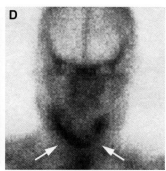

Fig. 50-5   Mandibular reconstruction with ectopic bone formation. **A,** A three-dimensional CT scan was used to produce **B,** a virtual replacement for the mandibular defect. From these data, a titanium mesh cage was manufactured that was filled with bone mineral blocks, infiltrated with rhBMP-7 and autologous bone marrow, and transplanted into the patient's latissimus dorsi muscle. After 7 weeks' implantation, the free bone-muscle flap was transplanted to repair the mandibular defect. **C,** A three-dimensional CT scan after transplantation revealed enhanced soft tissue formation, and **D,** skeletal scintigraphy with tracer enhancement showed bone remodeling and mineralization *(arrows).* (From Warnke PH, Springer IN, Wiltfang J, et al. Growth and transplantation of a custom vascularised bone graft in a man. Lancet 364[9436]:766-770, 2004.)

Bone tissue has been successfully engineered from pluripotent cell sources in small animal studies. hES cells and iPS cells represent potential sources of osteogenic cells. However, major obstacles remain to their clinical implementation, particularly isolation of the desired cell types, the lack of markers for osteogenic progenitors, immunocompatibility, and significant tumorigenicity risks.[46]

To date, the application of MSCs to promote bone regeneration has been restricted to case studies. The FDA has approved the use of hES cells for clinical trials in only three applications: amyotrophic lateral sclerosis, acute spinal cord injury, and Stargardt macular dystrophy. However, the use of adult stem cells has not been approved for any clinical trials: stem cell therapy has not reached the standard of care for treatment of human disease.[47]

The field of bone tissue engineering has improved craniofacial reconstruction with the development of biomimetic scaffolds, the incorporation of biologic factors, and the implementation of adult stem cell therapies. In future work, biomaterials and cellular techniques must be refined based on an enhanced mechanistic understanding of bone tissue regeneration while taking into consideration ethical and safety concerns. Once translated to clinical therapies, these novel approaches will augment craniofacial bone reconstruction.

AURICULAR RECONSTRUCTION

One of the greatest challenges in plastic and reconstructive surgery is total external ear reconstruction, which is required to treat congenital conditions such as microtia-atresia as well as acquired conditions related to trauma, infection, or tumor resections. The standard clinical treatment is a two-stage procedure in which autologous costal cartilage is harvested and carved to shape by a highly trained surgeon. On implantation, the carved framework is resurfaced with flaps and skin grafts.[48] This technique, although generally successful in experienced hands, yields unpredictable cosmetic results and donor site morbidity.

To reduce the necessity of advanced surgical skill, reconstructive procedures have been developed that use a prosthetic auricle anchored by an osteointegrated titanium implant.[49] In another approach, an ear-shaped framework manufactured from alloplastic materials, typically porous polyethylene (PE), has been employed for external ear reconstruction. Although PE is a stable material and can be easily shaped, a PE ear-shaped framework is predisposed to extrusion and infection when implanted subcutaneously. Cover-

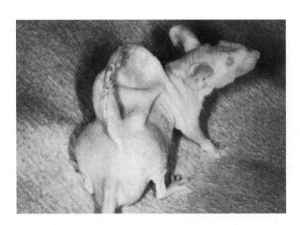

Fig. 50-6   Pioneering image of an "ear on the back of a mouse," taken 12 weeks after implantation in a nude mouse. Bovine articular chondroyctes were seeded onto PGA/PLLA scaffolds of the size and shape of a human child's auricle. The seeded constructs were subcutaneously implanted on the back of nude mice for 12 weeks, with external stenting for the first 4 weeks of implantation. On harvest, the overall geometry of the cartilaginous specimens closely resembled the complex structure of a child's auricle. (From Cao Y, Vacanti JP, Paige KT, et al. Transplantation of chondrocytes using a polymer-cell construct to produce tissue-engineered cartilage in the shape of a human ear. Plast Reconstr Surg 100:297-302; discussion 303-304, 1997.)

ing this implant with temporoparietal fascial flap has been shown to reduce the rate of complications, but not eliminate them altogether.[50] Additionally, both carved cartilage and alloplastic frameworks are rigid, and the resulting aesthetic appearance and mechanical properties do not match those of the native ear. The ideal auricle reconstruction would be aesthetically pleasing and structurally stable over the lifetime of the patient. This framework would eliminate the morbidity associated with donor cartilage harvest and closely match the characteristics of human cartilage.

A tissue engineering approach has the potential to generate structurally stable ear replacements with an improved match to the qualities and appearance of native ears. In principle, adult auricular cartilage has a simple morphology: it is an avascular, single cell type of tissue with a matrix reinforced by collagen and elastin fiber networks. Highly differentiated nonproliferating chondrocytes are sparsely distributed within this stable matrix, with a limited number of progenitor cells. Although the "ear on the back of a nude mouse" was first reported in the 1990s[51,52] (Fig. 50-6), few clinical case studies have been reported which used engineered cartilage for auricular reconstruction. Research has focused on optimizing selection of the scaffold material, cell source, and soluble factors.

Engineering auricular cartilage has been exceedingly challenging because of the response raised to the transplanted cartilaginous construct in immunocompetent animals. The subcutaneous environment of these animals is characterized by active inflammatory and immunologic responses. Inflammatory cytokines like interleukin-1 (IL-1) have been shown to play significant roles in chondrogenesis inhibition in vitro and in autologous-engineered cartilage resorption.[53]

Maturation of neocartilage in vitro may enhance engineered graft survival because of the resistance of cartilage extracellular matrix (ECM) to IL-1 exposure.[54] The impact of in vitro precultivation on engineered cartilage properties has been investigated with articular cartilage in nude mice and in immunocompetent species as well as tracheal cartilage in rabbits and auricular cartilage in sheep.[55-58] Construct precultivation improved neocartilage properties and alleviated postimplantation inflammation. Many of the engineered auricular cartilage studies described next used in vitro culture to mature neocartilage before implantation.

BIOMIMETIC SCAFFOLDS

Natural and synthetic biomaterials have been used to support chondrogenesis in vivo in immunodeficient and immunocompetent animals. However, chondrogenesis is negatively impacted by in vivo inflammatory responses to the material and its degradation products. Thus in vitro and in vivo results obtained in immunodeficient animal models have not been predictive of in vivo outcomes obtained in immunocompetent animal models.

Many scaffold materials are natural polymers that mimic cartilage ECM. Their three-dimensional fibrous structures can be highly hydrated and their surface characteristics promote increased cell adhesion and proliferation.[59] The use of these materials is limited by the same issues that are problematic for engineering bone: their low mechanical strength, fast degradation rate, and possible antigenicity. Natural materials used for auricular cartilage engineering include hydrogels and fibrous collagen derivatives.

Biocompatible hydrogel polymers such as fibrin gel, calcium alginate, Pluronic F-127, hyaluronic acid, and chitosan have been tested as chondrocyte carriers.[50] Cell suspensions encapsulated in these hydrogels can be injected and molded, permitting noninvasive delivery and facile creation of complex three-dimensional shapes.[60] Chondrocyte suspensions in fibrin gel, calcium alginate, or chitosan demonstrated robust cartilage formation in immunodeficient animals over 24 to 38 weeks' implantation.[61-63] Shape maintenance was poor, with significant shrinkage in both fibrin gel and calcium alginate constructs. However, shape retention improved with extended in vitro culture and with external stenting in vivo.[61,64] Improved shape maintenance was observed in chitosan constructs but the construct size slowly decreased with implantation time.[63]

Hydrogel scaffolds have been used in immunocompetent animals, but the cartilaginous constructs were sequestered in vivo to minimize inflammatory degradation. In an initial study, autologous auricular chondrocytes suspended in Pluronic F-127 formed only fibrovascular tissue when injected subcutaneously in swine.[65] In a later study, autologous auricular chondrocytes were suspended in Pluronic F-127 or calcium alginate. Each construct type was placed into human ear–shaped molds to maintain three-dimensional structure and was implanted into subcutaneous pockets in porcine or ovine animal models. Neocartilage formed in the alginate constructs, which best maintained their ear shapes and sizes. The Pluronic F-127 constructs also produced neocartilage, but their shapes were not well maintained.[66]

Synthetic poly(alphahydroxy ester) polymers, in the form of highly porous sponges and fibrous scaffolds, have commonly been used for auricular cartilage engineering. Ear-shaped scaffolds were fabricated from PGA/PLA, PCL, P4HB (poly-4-hydroxybutyrate) and PLA/PCL polymers; chondrocyte-seeded ear-shaped scaffolds were extensively cultured in vitro and implanted in nude mice.[67] Neocartilage was observed in all materials 40 weeks after implantation, but all constructs were moderately to severely distorted; PCL and PLA/PCL scaffolds were not fully degraded and best maintained their initial ear shape. However, in autologous cartilaginous constructs of these materials severe shape deformation occurred without cartilage formation in a rabbit model.[67]

Degradable and nondegradable biomaterials have been combined to overcome deficiencies of current auricular engineering approaches. Using chondrocytes suspended in fibrin gel or in alginate gel, cartilage bioshells have been engineered around rigid alloplastic implants in nude mice to decrease the extrusion risk of the implants.[68] To increase construct flexibility and to potentially maintain complex ear geometry, cartilage was engineered in the pores of nondegradable, flexible polyvinyl alcohol (PVA) scaffolds in nude mice; the compressive modulus of the PVA was significantly increased by the cartilage, potentially promoting improved shape maintenance.[69]

To date, only a single scaffold has demonstrated precise maintenance of complex auricular geometry: a composite ear-shaped fibrous collagen scaffold with a stabilizing embedded titanium wire framework.[58,70] Autologous auricular chondrocyte constructs were cultured in vitro for 2 weeks and implanted into nude mice or immunocompetent large animals. In nude mice at 6 weeks after implantation, robust homogenous cartilage was observed in chondrocyte-seeded scaffolds with and without embedded frameworks. However, in cartilaginous constructs with embedded frameworks, minimal dimensional change occurred (4%

or less in any dimension), whereas those without embedded frameworks shrank approximately 15% in all dimensions[70] (Fig. 50-7). In immunocompetent sheep at 20 weeks after implantation, stable elastic neocartilage had formed and less than 5% shrinkage was observed in any dimension[58] (Fig. 50-8). The thin wire framework did not impede twisting and bending of the cartilaginous construct, and the neocartilage was elastically deformable.

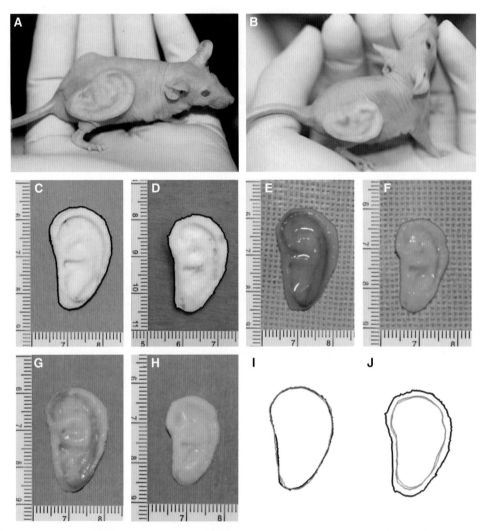

Fig. 50-7   Composite scaffolds maintain ear size and shape in immunocompromised animals. Human ear–shaped constructs, **A,** with and **B,** without embedded framework supports, on the backs of nude mice, retained characteristic ear shape after 6 weeks' implantation. Gross images of ear-shaped constructs: **C** and **D,** before seeding, **E** and **F,** after 2 weeks' in vitro preculture, and **G** and **H,** after 6 weeks' in vivo. **I** and **J,** Comparison of sizes at different stages. **C, E, G,** and **I** constructs had embedded wire frameworks, and **D, F, H,** and **J** had no wire frameworks. The construct size was maintained in scaffolds with wire frameworks (**I**) but was not maintained in scaffolds without wire frameworks (**J**) after 2 weeks' in vitro culture. (From Zhou L, Pomerantseva I, Bassett EK, et al. Engineering ear constructs with a composite scaffold to maintain dimensions. Tissue Eng Part A 17:1573-1581, 2011.)

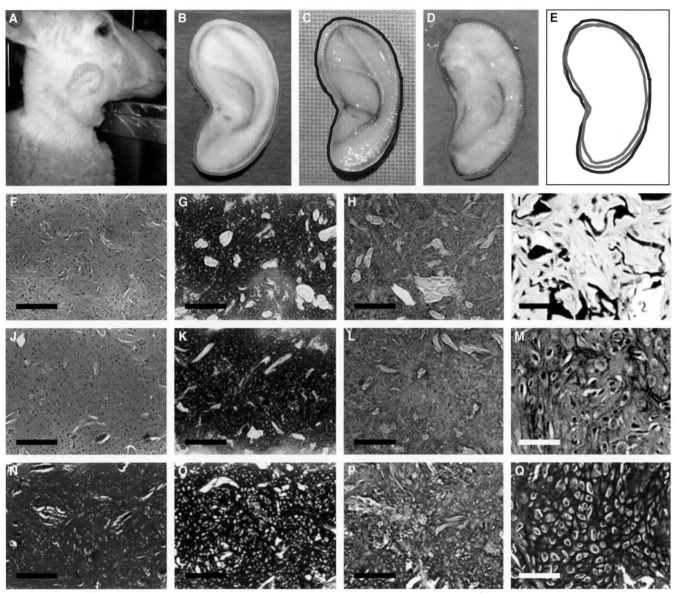

Fig. 50-8 Composite scaffolds maintain ear size and shape in a large animal ovine model and support formation of stable elastic neocartilage. **A,** Human ear–shaped constructs with embedded framework supports, implanted subcutaneously in a sheep's neck, retained characteristic ear shape after 20 weeks of implantation. Gross images of ear-shaped constructs demonstrate little change in the two-dimensional shape when comparing **B,** before seeding, **C,** after 2 weeks of in vitro preculture, and **D,** after 20 weeks in vivo. **E,** Less than 5% shrinkage was observed, based on a comparison of sizes at different stages. In addition, robust stable elastic neocartilage formed and the quality improved with implantation time as demonstrated in samples explanted **F-I,** at 6 weeks, **J-M,** 12 weeks, and **N-Q,** 20 weeks. Sample sections were stained with safranin O (**F, J,** and **N**) and toluidine blue (**G, K,** and **O**) or immunohistochemically stained with collagen II (**H, L,** and **P**) and elastin (**I, M,** and **Q**). Scale bars were 200 μm in **F-H, J-L,** and **N-P,** and 100 μm in **I, M,** and **Q.** (From Bichara DA, Pomerantseva I, Zhao X, et al. Successful creation of tissue-engineered autologous auricular cartilage in an immunocompetent large animal model. Tissue Eng Part A 20:303-312, 2014.)

ISOLATED CELLS

Chondrocytes

Auricular chondrocytes have been used primarily in engineered ear cartilage studies. Alternative cartilage sources have also been explored, since auricular cartilage may not be available in certain patient populations. Porcine and bovine articular, auricular, costal, and nasoseptal chondrocytes were tested in fibrin gel and PLA/PCL scaffolds in nude mice over 20 to 40 weeks' implantation. Auricular, costal, and nasoseptal chondrocytes were superior to articular chondrocytes: greater expressions of cartilage-specific genes (type II collagen and aggrecan) were observed, and the construct sizes and shapes were better maintained.[71] Notably, at 40 weeks' implantation, rigid nodules of mineralized cartilage protruded from the costal chondrocyte constructs, which expressed high levels of bone sialoprotein; these data suggested that cartilage engineered from costal chondrocytes could result in heterotopic ossification. From these studies, nasoseptal and auricular chondrocytes appeared to be suitable chondrocyte cell sources for engineering auricular replacements.

Engineering of human auricular cartilage has been explored. Neocartilage engineered from adult human auricular chondrocytes in PGA/PLA scaffolds shrank a small but significant amount after 8 weeks' implantation.[72] In a separate study, the biologic potentials of pediatric microtic and normal auricular chondrocytes were compared. Similar-quality neocartilage was observed in Pluronic F-127 constructs engineered with both chondrocyte sources.[73]

Large numbers of cells (approximately 200 million chondrocytes) are required to engineer an adult human auricle-shaped replacement. Yet only 2 to 3 million human chondrocytes can be harvested from a small biopsy (a 200 to 300 mg sample), so extensive cell expansion (approximately 100-fold) is required. However, chondrocytes dedifferentiate when expanded beyond four passages in monolayer culture, losing their ability to form cartilage.[74]

A significant number of soluble factors have been used to control chondrocyte differentiation and promote cartilage formation in vivo in nude mice. These factors were either added to the culture medium or encapsulated into scaffolds so the factors were released as the scaffold degraded. TGF-beta improved chondrocyte dedifferentiation and matrix formation in conjunction with IGF-1.[67,75] Connective tissue growth factor (CCN2/CTGF) promoted proliferation and differentiation of auricular chondrocytes while preventing mineralization and apoptosis.[76] bFGF prevented chondrocyte dedifferentiation and promoted elastic cartilage formation.[77]

Microspheres encapsulating bFGF were included in ear-shaped chondrocyte-seeded PLA/PCL scaffolds. Enhanced chondrogenesis as well as neovascularization in the surrounding tissue was observed in constructs containing encapsulated bFGF, relative to their bFGF-free controls.[78] Subsequently, ear-shaped constructs cultured with bFGF and implanted into nude mice demonstrated more homogenous neocartilage than constructs cultured without bFGF.[79]

Although these findings are promising, results in nude mice cannot be confidently extrapolated to predict results in immunocompetent animals or humans. None of these soluble factors have been used or approved for clinical use in the United States, although bFGF was clinically employed to engineer auricular cartilage in Japan (reviewed later).

Stem Cells

Adult stem cells have been examined as possible sources of chondrogenic cells because of the dedifferentiation that chondrocytes can undergo on extensive proliferation. Regenerating auricular cartilage with MSCs has been challenging, because the subcutaneous environment lacks a proper chondrogenic niche, in contrast to injured articular cartilage.[80] Consequently, MSCs targeted for auricular repair must be cultured with chondrogenic induction factors, such as TGF-beta, bFGF, PDFG-b, or BMP-2[75,81-83]; prolonged exposure to these differentiation and growth factors is both costly and tumorigenic.[84] Furthermore, chondrogenic induced BMSCs developed a hypertrophic chondrocyte phenotype in vivo, with extensive calcification of the neocartilage extracellular matrix.[4,80]

Co-transplantation of MSCs and chondrocytes has been examined for regeneration of cartilaginous tissues, as chondrocytes produce chondrogenic induction factors.[85] In a co-transplantation study in nude mice, enhanced cartilage formation was observed in PLA/PLCL constructs containing AdMSCs primed in a chondrocyte-conditioned medium in comparison with a TGF-beta–containing medium. However, co-transplantation of chondrocytes with chondrocyte-conditioned MSCs had a profound effect on neocartilage formation; the resulting cartilage approached the biochemical contents and cellular morphology of cartilage engineered with primary chondrocytes. No engineered cartilage hypertrophy was observed, suggesting that co-transplantation with fully differentiated chondrocytes inhibited the hypertrophic and ossification processes.[84] With further development, an MSC/chondrocyte co-transplantation strategy will likely produce engineered cartilage of similar quality and stability to that engineered with chondrocytes alone.

Clinical Engineered Auricular Cartilage

In comparison with orthopedic applications, the clinical application of engineered auricular cartilage has not been well established. During articular repair, engineered cartilage constructs are implanted into immunoprivileged regions of joints, so they are not subjected to aggressive host immune attack. Engineered auricular cartilage constructs are subcutaneously implanted in the head and neck region, with its well-recognized potential for strong inflammatory responses. Consequently, clinically implemented engineered replacement auricles have met with limited success. Nasoseptal chondrocytes suspended in fibrinogen were seeded into PLGA/PLA ear-shaped scaffolds and gelled with thrombin. These ear-shaped cartilaginous constructs successfully formed stable cartilage in mice.[86] However, Rotter et al[87] described failure of a similar autologous construct in a human study; the construct was completely resorbed 3 weeks after implantation. In Peiseler's case study,[88] a partial ear defect was similarly treated with cartilage engineered from autologous costal chondrocytes. Again, the constructs completely resorbed after several months of implantation. Clearly, successful cartilage engineering in a nude mouse is not predictive of clinical outcome.

A radically different approach was recently demonstrated that circumvented the immune response of the head and neck region. Auricular chondrocytes were isolated from four pediatric microtia patients. After 1 month in vitro culture in an FGF-containing medium, the cells without scaffolds were injected into a subcutaneous abdominal pocket in each patient.[89] After 6 months, the neocartilage mass was harvested, sculpted into an auricle shape, and reimplanted in the temporal region. No resorption of the implanted cartilage was observed in any patient during the five-year monitoring period. Engineering the cartilaginous matrix in minimally manipulated abdominal pockets produced mature, stable neocartilage, capable of surviving transplantation to the head and neck environment. The reconstructed ears were elevated in two patients and grafted with split-thickness skin grafts; skin grafting was successful because neoperichondrium-like tissue with a vascular supply had formed around the neocartilage.[77] Although the engineered cartilage was stable, the aesthetic appearance of these reconstructed ears did not mimic native ear architectures[89] (Fig. 50-9).

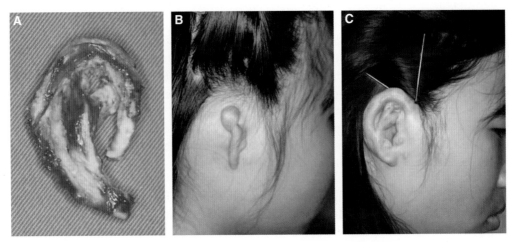

Fig. 50-9   Ear repair with ectopic auricular formation. Robust neocartilage was formed when autologous microtic chondrocytes were cultured in vivo in the patient's lower abdomen. **A,** After 6 months' implantation, the cartilage was surgically harvested, sculpted into an ear framework, and implanted subcutaneously into the auricular defect area. **B,** The aesthetic appearance of a microtic patient is improved 4½ years after implantation, and **C,** 3 years after ear elevation. No adsorption of the cartilage was reported. (From Yanaga H, Koga M, Imai K, et al. Generating ears from cultured autologous auricular chondrocytes by using two-stage implantation in treatment of microtia. Plast Reconstr Surg 124:817-825, 2009.)

Future clinical studies for auricular reconstruction must focus both on stable quality elastic cartilage formation from a clinically relevant cell source, and on the maintenance of complex geometry. Fibrous collagen scaffolds with embedded titanium wire frameworks could be used; as discussed earlier, stable elastic ovine neocartilage, excellent shape retention, and nativelike mechanical properties have been demonstrated from autologous sheep auricular chondrocytes in these composite scaffolds.[58,70] Additional work is required to identify the optimal cell source for human use. Possible cell sources include: autologous auricular or naso-septal chondrocytes expanded in the presence of soluble factors like bFGF to minimize dedifferentiation, or a mixture of chondrocytes and chondrocyte-conditioned MSCs.

FACIAL DERMAL AUGMENTATION

Facial dermal augmentation is achieved through injections of fillers of naturally derived tissue or synthetic materials to correct contour deformities and rhytids due to loss of soft tissue and aging. Current fillers include microspheres of calcium HAP, PLA, or polymethylmethacrylate (PMMA) as well as collagen derived from xenografts and allografts, and freeze-dried acellular dermal tissue.[90] Injectables must be biocompatible and must not induce immunogenic or inflammatory responses. Calcium HAP, PMMA, and PLA degrade slowly, and reinjection is required only every 6 to 12 months. However, injection of HAP, PMMA, and PLA is limited to the subdermal space and subcutaneous tissue; intradermal implantation is not possible, based on the needle size required to avoid clogging and the flow behavior of the injectate. As with all particulate injectable fillers, the risk exists of clumping and localized foreign body reactions.

Extracellular matrix components, particularly collagen-based materials, decellularized dermal allografts, and particulate fascia lata allograft and xenogenic materials were tested as dermal fillers. Collagen-based fillers degraded rapidly so required repeated frequent injection; significant foreign body responses occurred in some patients.[91] Consequently, slowly degrading, naturally occurring, biocompatible materials such as hyaluronic acid (HA) have been clinically used, but periodic injections were still required.[92]

To avoid the need for repeat injections, autologous adipose tissue was transplanted to fill soft tissue defects, including facial defects. However, the clinical longevity of adipose grafts was highly variable. Histologically, progressive loss of transplanted adipocytes was observed as the grafts were converted to fibrous tissue. Free adipose tissue transfer rarely achieved sufficient tissue augmentation. Adipocytes poorly tolerated the ischemia that developed during the slow revascularization of adipose tissue transplants; adipocytes ultimately underwent apoptosis or necrosis, which led to graft volume shrinkage.[93] Postoperative volume reduction after adipose tissue transfer was as high as 70%.[94]

Tissue engineering has been used to address these limitations and to provide new therapeutic paradigms in which engineered adipose tissue can be tailored for specific tissue repair types.[95] Initial studies focused on the use of scaffolds seeded with preadipocytes (adipocyte precursor cells), harvested from autologous adipose tissue biopsies or liposuction aspirates.[96] Long-term persistence of generated adipose tissue remained elusive. In rat studies, the volume of engineered adipose tissue was stable up to 2 months in preadipocyte-PLGA foam scaffolds, but complete resorption occurred by 5 months, which correlated with complete scaffold degradation.[97] Stable engineered adipose tissue in a rat was observed in a very small preadipocyte–fibrin glue construct.[98] Although the degradation rate of the scaffold material affected engineered tissue stability, adipose growth was inhibited by the pressure of overlying tissues, by implantation in a heterotopic site devoid of fat, and by foreign body response.

Adipose tissue was engineered with preadipocytes in scaffolds of natural materials. Preadipocytes were seeded onto collagen scaffolds with directionally aligned pores as well as in HA sponges and nonwoven fiber scaffolds.[99,100] After 8 months' implantation in mice, more adipocytes were found in the HA sponge scaffold than in the collagen scaffold or the HA nonwoven scaffold as the larger, more connected pores better supported adipogenesis. Alginate and collagen hydrogels have also been used for adipose tissue engineering.[101,102] Preadipocytes suspended in alginate gel were injected into the necks of sheep. Well-defined adipose tissue was observed at 1 and 3 months after implantation, although the cellular source of the adipose tissue could not be determined.[101]

Most adipogenesis studies have used AdMSCs, because these cells can be harvested in large quantities from adipose tissue, eliminating the need for cell expansion. AdMSCs are easily differentiated to adipocytes as well as direct angiogenesis and vasculogenesis.[103] Many studies have examined in vivo engineering of adipose tissue using AdMSCs. In immunocompetent rats, engineered adipose tissue was observed at 2 months after implantation in AdMSCs-PLGA constructs but was fully resorbed by 5 to 12 months after implantation.[97] Using another approach, AdMSCs were mixed with minced fat tissue scaffolds and implanted into immunocompetent mice; the AdMSCs were either freshly isolated or cultured in vitro before seeding. Six months after implantation, freshly isolated AdMSCs-fat constructs had significantly greater mass than cultured AdMSCs-fat or fat-only constructs. Histologically, the freshly isolated AdMSCs-fat constructs maintained their adipocyte-rich appearance and were vascularized; these data suggested that freshly isolated AdMSCs support rapid formation of a functional vasculature within the fat implants.[104] In Japan, freshly isolated AdMSCs-fat constructs were successfully used for breast augmentation in 23 patients; only one patient showed evidence of fibrosis after 26 months.[105]

In a promising recent study, the impact of multiple cells and biochemical signals on adipose tissue transplantation was examined. Harvested from adipose tissue, the stromal vascular fraction (SVF) was used, which contains a heterogeneous cell population, including endothelial cells, stromal cells, and AdMSCs.[106] Platelet-rich fibrin (PRF) was incorporated, which contains multiple growth factors, including angiogenic and adipogenic factors such as PDGF-BB, VEGF, bFGF, EGF, IGF-1, and TGF-beta; these growth factors are slowly released from the PRF fibrin matrix in comparison with release rates from PRP.[107] Mixtures of freshly harvested SVF, PRF, and autologous adipose granules were injected subcutaneously into rabbit auricles. The volume of adipose tissue transplants was maintained after 24 weeks, with good adipose structures and vasculature[108] (Fig. 50-10).

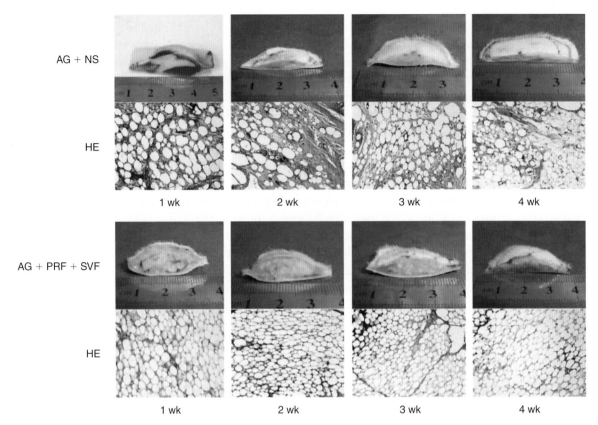

Fig. 50-10 The impact of a stromal vascular fraction (SVF) and platelet-rich fibrin (PRF) on autologous adipose tissue transplantation. Autologous adipose granules (AG) were mixed with SVF and PRF or with normal saline (NS) (negative control) and injected subcutaneoulsy into auriculae of rabbit ears. Gross samples and H&E-stained sections were examined at 1, 2, 3, and 4 weeks after implantation. In the AG + NS group, the transplanted adipose tissue was encapsulated by fibrous tissue, and significant inflammatory infiltrate was observed 1 week after implantation. By 3 weeks after implantation, significant neovascularization and adipose tissue fibrosis were found. Substantial adipose tissue resorption occurred by 4 weeks after implantation, along with reduced inflammation. In the AG + PRF + SVF group, less inflammatory infiltrate and adipose tissue fibrosis were found 1 week after implantation in comparison with the control. Neovascularization occurred earlier than in the control, developing 1 to 2 weeks after implantation. Little adipose tissue fibrosis was observed at 3 weeks after implantation. Substantial vacularized adipose tissue structure formed by 4 weeks after implantation. By 24 weeks, significantly less resorption was found in the AG + PRF + SVF group (17% ± 6%) relative to the control group (49% ± 9%) (data not shown). (From Liu B, Tan XY, Liu YP, et al. The adjuvant use of stromal vascular fraction and platelet-rich fibrin for autologous adipose tissue transplantation. Tissue Eng Part C Methods 19:1-14, 2013.)

This SVF-PRF-adipose tissue system is a cell-based therapy that could be readily translated to clinical application to restore facial defects.[108] Uncultured SVF is an inexpensive, minimally manipulated cell source that overcomes the key commercialization and regulatory hurdles associated with cultured cells. PRF provides a pool of endogenous growth factors and serves as a space-filling matrix for adipose implantation and localization.[109]

In a recent Korean study, the impact of uncultured SVF–assisted autologous fat grafting on cosmetic outcome and fat graft survival was examined in nine patients, who were monitored over 12 weeks after treatment.[110] Improved cosmetic outcomes were observed in facial areas augmented with SVF-fat grafts in comparison with fat grafts alone, particularly in deep facial wrinkles. Although these results are promising, a randomized clinical study with larger numbers of patients monitored for longer periods is required to accurately assess the impact of SVF on the long-term survival of fat grafts for augmentation of facial soft tissue.

THE MAJOR CHALLENGE FOR THE FIELD OF TISSUE ENGINEERING: VASCULARIZATION

Historically, engineered cellularized constructs have relied on extrinsic vascularization to meet the metabolic needs of seeded cells.[111] Ischemia can develop in constructs thicker than 2 to 3 mm, thus compromising cell viability. Cellular and surgical approaches are being developed to enhance the vascularization potential of engineered cellularized constructs before implantation. Although these techniques are generally applicable to engineered tissues, much of the development has focused on rapidly vascularizing bone constructs.

Multiple approaches have been examined in preclinical studies to enhance the vascularization potential of engineered cellularized constructs before implantation (Fig. 50-11). These approaches, some of which have directly targeted engineered bone, include the following:

1. Seeding endothelial progenitor cells into scaffolds with surface-immobilized vascular endothelial growth factor (VEGF) to enhance angiogenesis,[112]
2. Co-implanting MSCs on deproteinized bone scaffold along with a vascular bundle,[113]
3. Co-seeding endothelial and smooth muscle cells in PLA scaffolds to produce vascular networks through vasculogenesis,[114]
4. Co-seeding endothelial cells and MSCs in PLGA scaffolds with a separate MSC population differentiated toward an osteogenic lineage to form bone. The MSCs act as vascular stromal cells as well as secrete trophic factors which direct angiogenesis and vasculogenesis[115] (Fig. 50-12).

In all cases, vascularization of the engineered constructs was significantly accelerated. Enhanced bone formation was observed in studies that implanted MSCs to form bone and used an approach to promote rapid construct vascularization.

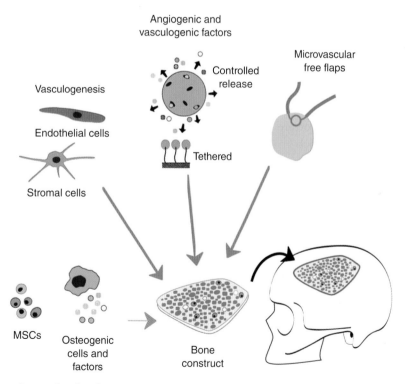

Fig. 50-11   Approaches under development to promote rapid perfusion in engineered constructs using bone constructs as an example. Vasculogenesis can be fostered by the addition of endothelial cells and supporting stromal cells. Angiogenesis and vasculogenesis have been promoted by appropriate biochemical factors, either released in a controlled fashion or tethered to scaffold surfaces. Early perfusion was enhanced by implanting the engineered construct within a host microvascular free flap, which was subsequently reconnected to the host systemic circulation.

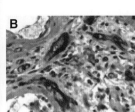
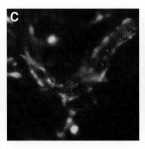
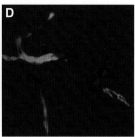

Fig. 50-12   Perfused vascular network engineered using vasculogenesis. **A,** Physical interaction of human mesenchymal stem cells (hMSCs) *(green)* with endothelial cell (EC) network *(red)* in bone scaffold at 28 days after seeding. **B,** Human-specific CD31 immunohistochemical staining of scaffolds explanted 11 days after implantation; lumens were filled with red blood cells. **C,** DiD-labeled blood cells *(blue)* easily flowed through engineered vessels *(yellow).* **D,** The engineered vessels *(red)* were clearly anastomosed with host mouse vessels (*blue* from dye-labeled serum). (From Tsigkou O, Pomerantseva I, Spencer JA, et al. Engineered vascularized bone grafts. Proc Natl Acad Sci U S A 107:3311-3316, 2011.)

The use of autologous microvascular free flaps has been explored to circumvent the need to create de novo vasculature in engineered constructs. The native capillary structure served as the basis for the engineered construct as the surrounding perivascular tissue was dissected from the soft tissue bed, leaving the vasculature intact. These explanted microcirculatory beds (EMBs) consisted of an afferent artery, capillary beds, an efferent vein, and some surrounding parenchymal tissue. The EMBs were maintained ex vivo in a perfusion bioreactor to preserve viability and function, and were seeded with adult stem cells before reimplantation at an injury site. This technique offers the potential to manipulate autologous tissue ex vivo with tissue-specific cells and soluble factors and to engineer tissue at heterotopic locations on reimplantation.[116,117] This methodology will ultimately be scaled to provide vascular support to soft tissue constructs in complex reconstructive applications.

Noncellular approaches can also be used to promote rapid vascularization of implanted engineered constructs. Vasculogenic growth factors and stimulatory ligands have been incorporated into scaffolds to encourage angiogenesis into the implanted engineered construct.[118] Stimulatory cues for endogenous cell recruitment and differentiation toward endothelial and smooth muscle cells have been used to produce a proangiogenic environment, which facilitates graft vascularization.[119]

EMERGING APPLICATIONS OF TISSUE ENGINEERING TECHNOLOGY IN FACIAL RECONSTRUCTION

Many individual craniofacial tissues are being engineered in preclinical animal models that will ultimately be used in the fields of plastic and reconstructive surgery; the status of the efforts to engineer skeletal muscle is described below as an example. In addition, tissue engineering is being conceptualized to reconstruct composite tissues and tissues with extensive defects.

SKELETAL MUSCLE ENGINEERING

Skeletal muscle is highly complex tissue, with a trilevel architecture of aligned myofibers intermixed with a rich microvascular network that supports the metabolic requirements of the tissue. Each muscle fiber is innervated by a host nerve through a neuromuscular junction that allows the muscle to generate contractile force on neural stimulation. Engineering skeletal muscle must address the challenge of recreating this complex architecture as well as recapitulating vascular, microelectrical and contractile networks.[120]

Most current experimental strategies to engineer muscle use myoblasts, progenitor cells of skeletal muscle, along with supporting cells on biocompatible scaffolds. In response to mechanical strain or injury, quiescent satellite cells in native muscle are activated to myoblasts which effect muscle repair; satellite cells sparsely populate muscle at approximately 2×10^5 cells/g muscle.[121] In addition to myoblasts, skeletal muscle tissue contains fibroblasts and muscle derived stem cells (the predecessor of satellite cells).[122,123] Fibroblasts secrete trophic factors that support myogenic processes and myotube viability; many skeletal muscle engineering studies have used a combination of fibroblasts and myoblasts. However, myoblasts undergo dedifferentiation in vitro after several cell cycles, so that sufficient numbers of myoblasts cannot be obtained from autologous muscle donor sites to regenerate a complete muscle.[124] Consequently, MSCs and iPS cells are being examined for engineering skeletal muscle.[125]

Myofibers that form on myoblast fusion must be aligned and parallel to generate maximum contractile force. Myofiber alignment has been achieved in three-dimensional porous scaffolds with aligned microarchitecture and macroarchitectures or through application of mechanical strain or magnetic strain to muscle constructs.[120,126-128] In these systems, muscle fibers reorganized along the lines of force or through static magnetic fields.[123,127,129-130] Cell sheet technology was developed toward solid organ engineering but has been used to generate muscles with geometries similar to those of facial muscles. Cell sheets, cultured on temperature-responsive two-dimensional scaffolds, lifted on exposure to minor temperature changes and were stacked to create three-dimensional constructs.[131]

To enhance vascularization of engineered muscle, endothelial networks have been produced within muscle constructs in vitro by the addition of endothelial cells and supporting stromal cells.[132] On implantation, these prevascularized muscle constructs exhibited improved integration, were perfused at earlier time points, and had enhanced survival. Engineered muscle cell sheets have also been prevascularized by intermixing layers of muscle with vascular layers.[133]

The greatest challenge faced by the field of skeletal muscle engineering is the development of functional, controllable contractile forces. Effective innervation requires formation of neuromuscular junctions which transmit neural signals from the host to the myofiber, inducing contraction. The development of fully functional neuromuscular junctions is impacted by electrical and mechanical stimulation.[126,134-135] Although progress has been made, innervated three-dimensional muscle with predictable and controllable innervation remains the major hurdle for transitioning engineered skeletal muscle into clinical therapies.

HYBRIDIZATION OF COMPOSITE TISSUE ALLOTRANSPLANTATION AND TISSUE ENGINEERING

Recent advances in craniofacial surgery and immunotherapy have spurred the development of composite tissue allotransplantation (CTA) for face transplants, which permits reconstruction of massive composite craniomaxillofacial defects. However, it requires lifelong immunosuppression, with its associated severe health risks. Even if immunotolerance could be developed to the transplanted tissue, the donor skeletal framework and the host tissues may be mismatched, resulting in suboptimal occlusion and soft tissue anthropometrics. Through tissue engineering approaches, irregular defects could be tailored to be conforming and the size of large defects could be decreased and more easily reconstructed. For example, engineered bone could be used to facilitate maxillofacial CTA planning and establish appropriate nasoorbital projection, maxillary sagittal position, and vertical midface position. In patients with extensive neurologic injury, engineered peripheral nerve constructs could be used to span the gap between donor and recipient nerves and the addition of Schwann cells and nerve growth factors could improve functional recovery. Thus application of hybrid CTA-tissue engineering techniques could reestablish occlusion, facial function, and aesthetic form.[136]

Whole Tissue Decellularized Extracellular Matrix for Engineering Composite Facial Tissue

A topic of great interest in the field of tissue engineering is the use of decellularized extracellular matrices (ECM) for regeneration of large tissue defects or for engineering whole organs. Native ECM plays a central role during development in mediating biophysical stimuli, delivering molecular signals, and defining spatial organization. Derived from xenogenic or cadaveric tissue sources following immersion in detergents, native ECM has been used to support regeneration of a number of human tissues. However, this immersion decellularization process can inflict significant damage on ECM three-dimensional geometry. Consequently, whole organs are gently decellularized by perfusing detergents through the vasculature of the organ; vascular pathways remain intact and native ECM structure and cues are maintained. To establish organ function after ECM decellularization, vascular networks and tissue are seeded with autologous vascular cells and parenchymal cells. To date, these experimental procedures have been applied to engineering liver, heart, lung, and pancreas; some return of function, albeit short lived, has been demonstrated in small animal models.[137,138] To be applicable to composite tissues, perfusion decellularization protocols must be refined and tailored to composite tissue size, type, and species. To recapitulate development, the decellularized composite tissue would be seeded with clinically relevant progenitor cell types and the construct exposed to appropriate growth, mechanical and electrical stimuli in vitro. Generating sufficient progenitor cell numbers for regeneration of human-sized composite tissues exceeds current progenitor cell technology and would require significant advances in induced pluripotency cellular technology.

Composite tissue regeneration based on decellularized native ECM scaffolds holds great promise for reconstructing facial features but requires significant breakthroughs in cellular and developmental biology technologies. However, if successful, these autologous engineered composite tissues could revolutionize facial reconstruction. Since these engineered autologous composite tissues would eliminate the need for immunosuppression, their use would complement or eliminate the need for CTA.

Key Points

- The field of tissue engineering has made significant progress for craniofacial reconstruction with successful human demonstrations in the areas of bone regeneration, auricular cartilage replacement, and dermal augmentation.
- All studies were based on the principles of tissue engineering: isolated cells, biochemical signals, and biomimetic scaffolds.
- Major obstacles remain that impede widespread clinical translation of engineered tissues.
- Adult MSCs as well as iPS cells are being considered as cellular platforms to overcome the limitations of fully differentiated cells or tissue-specific progenitor cells.
- Stem cell fate must be better characterized and controlled following ex vivo manipulation and subsequent implantation before stem cells can be safely used in clinical trials.
- Large-scale tissue constructs are limited by insufficient blood supply on implantation. Vascularization strategies are under development but must be scaled and efficacy demonstrated in preclinical studies.
- Sophisticated biomaterials/biochemical signal systems must be optimized to precisely present structural and biochemical cues to support recapitulation of normal development.
- These challenges are further constrained by increasing regulatory restrictions, ethical concerns, and health care costs.
- Engineering of individual and composite tissues remains an exciting and dynamic field that will continue to advance based on collaborative multidisciplinary approaches between cell biologists, biomaterialists, and surgeons.

REFERENCES

1. Gurtner GC, Callaghan MJ, Longaker MT. Progress and potential for regenerative medicine. Ann Rev Med 58:299-312, 2007.

2. Langer R, Vacanti JP. Tissue engineering. Science 260(5110):920-926, 1993.
   Revolutionary article that defined the field of tissue engineering, based on the triad of isolated cells, tissue-inducing substances, and matrices.

3. Wong VW, Rustad KC, Longaker MT, et al. Tissue engineering in plastic surgery: a review. Plast Reconstr Surg 126:858-868, 2010.

4. Pittenger MF, Mackay AM, Beck SC, et al. Multilineage potential of adult human mesenchymal stem cells. Science 284(5411):143-147, 1999.

5. Takahashi K, Tanabe K, Ohnuki M, et al. Induction of pluripotent stem cells from adult human fibroblasts by defined factors. Cell 131:861-872, 2007.

6. Seeherman H, Wozney JM. Delivery of bone morphogenetic proteins for orthopedic tissue regeneration. Cytokine Growth Factor Rev 16:329-345, 2005.

7. Chan BP, Leong KW. Scaffolding in tissue engineering: general approaches and tissue-specific considerations. Eur Spine J 17(Suppl 4):467-479, 2008.

8. Drury JL, Mooney DJ. Hydrogels for tissue engineering: scaffold design variables and applications. Biomaterials 24:4337-4351, 2003.

9. Furth ME, Atala A, Van Dyke ME. Smart biomaterials design for tissue engineering and regenerative medicine. Biomaterials 28:5068-5073, 2007.

10. Kneser U, Schaefer DJ, Polykandriotis E, et al. Tissue engineering of bone: the reconstructive surgeon's point of view. J Cell Mol Med 10:7-19, 2006.

11. Moreira-Gonzalez A, Jackson IT, Miyawaki T, et al. Clinical outcome in cranioplasty: critical review in long-term follow-up. J Craniofac Surg 14:144-153, 2003.

12. Lee SH, Shin H. Matrices and scaffolds for delivery of bioactive molecules in bone and cartilage tissue engineering. Adv Drug Deliv Rev 59:339-359, 2007.

13. Li X, Feng Q, Liu X, et al. Collagen-based implants reinforced by chitin fibres in a goat shank bone defect model. Biomaterials 27:1917-1923, 2006.

14. Porter JR, Ruckh TT, Popat KC. Bone tissue engineering: a review in bone biomimetics and drug delivery strategies. Biotechnol Prog 25:1539-1560, 2009.

15. Lichte P, Pape HC, Pufe T, et al. Scaffolds for bone healing: concepts, materials and evidence. Injury 42:569-573, 2011.

16. Cancedda R, Giannoni P, Mastrogiacomo M. A tissue engineering approach to bone repair in large animal models and in clinical practice. Biomaterials 28:4240-4250, 2007.

17. Hu YY, Zhang C, Lu R, et al. Repair of radius defect with bone-morphogenetic-protein loaded hydroxyapatite/collagen-poly(L-lactic acid) composite. Chin J Traumatol 6:67-74, 2003.

18. Chao MT, Jiang S, Smith D, et al. Demineralized bone matrix and resorbable mesh bilaminate cranioplasty: a novel method for reconstruction of large-scale defects in the pediatric calvaria. Plast Reconstr Surg 123:976-982, 2009.

19. Bartlett SP, Foo R. Demineralized bone matrix and resorbable mesh bilaminate cranioplasty. Plast Reconstr Surg 125:416-417, 2010.

20. Schantz JT, Machens HG, Schilling AF, et al. Regenerative medicine: implications for craniofacial surgery. J Craniofac Surg 23:530-536, 2012.

21. Probst FA, Hutmacher DW, Müller DF, et al. [Calvarial reconstruction by customized bioactive implant] Handchir Mikrochir Plast Chir 42:369-373, 2010.

22. Alvarez P, Hee CK, Solchaga L, et al. Growth factors and craniofacial surgery. J Craniofac Surg 23:20-29, 2012.

23. Herford AS, Boyne PJ. Reconstruction of mandibular continuity defects with bone morphogenetic protein-2 (rhBMP-2). J Oral Maxillofac Surg 66:616-624, 2008.

24. Triplett RG, Nevins M, Marx RE, et al. Pivotal, randomized, parallel evaluation of recombinant human bone morphogenetic protein-2/absorbable collagen sponge and autogenous bone graft for maxillary sinus floor augmentation. J Oral Maxillofac Surg 67:1947-1960, 2009.

25. Davies SD, Ochs MW. Bone morphogenetic proteins in craniomaxillofacial surgery. Oral Maxillofac Surg Clin North Am 22:17-31, 2010.

26. Kotsovilis S, Markou N, Pepelassi E, et al. The adjunctive use of platelet-rich plasma in the therapy of periodontal intraosseous defects: a systematic review. J Periodontal Res 45:428-443, 2010.

27. Ripamonti U, Van Den Heever B, Crooks J, et al. Long-term evaluation of bone formation by osteogenic protein 1 in the baboon and relative efficacy of bone-derived bone morphogenetic proteins delivered by irradiated xenogenic collagenous matrices. J Bone Miner Res 15:1798-1809, 2000.

28. Ripamonti U, Crooks J, Rueger DC. Induction of bone formation by recombinant human osteogenic protein-1 and sintered porous hydroxyapatite in adult primates. Plast Reconstr Surg 107:977-988, 2001.

29. Abu-Serriah M, Ayoub A, Wray D, et al. Contour and volume assessment of repairing mandibular osteoperiosteal continuity defects in sheep using recombinant human osteogenic protein 1. J Craniomaxillofac Surg 34:162-167, 2006.

30. van den Bergh JP, ten Bruggenkate CM, Groeneveld HH, et al. Recombinant human bone morphogenetic protein-7 in maxillary sinus floor elevation surgery in 3 patients compared to autogenous bone grafts. A clinical pilot study. J Clin Periodontol 27:627-636, 2000.

31. Valderrama P, Jung RE, Thoma DS, et al. Evaluation of parathyroid hormone bound to a synthetic matrix for guided bone regeneration around dental implants: a histomorphometric study in dogs. J Periodontol 81:737-747, 2010.

32. Giannobile WV, Hernandez RA, Finkelman RD, et al. Comparative effects of platelet-derived growth factor-BB and insulin-like growth factor-I, individually and in combination, on periodontal regeneration in Macaca fascicularis. J Periodontal Res 31:301-312, 1996.

33. Howell TH, Fiorellini JP, Paquette DW, et al. A phase I/II clinical trial to evaluate a combination of recombinant human platelet-derived growth factor-BB and recombinant human insulin-like growth factor-I in patients with periodontal disease. J Periodontol 68:1186-1193, 1997.

34. Jin Y, Tipoe GL, Liong EC, et al. Overexpression of BMP-2/4,-5 and BMPR-IA associated with malignancy of oral epithelium. Oral Oncol 37:225-233, 2001.

35. Schellekens H. How to predict and prevent the immunogenicity of therapeutic proteins. Biotechnol Annu Rev 14:191-202, 2008.

36. Singh A, Morris RJ. The yin and yang of bone morphogenetic proteins in cancer. Cytokine Growth Factor Rev 21:299-313, 2010.

37. Minamide A, Yoshida M, Kawakami M, et al. The effects of bone morphogenetic protein and basic fibroblast growth factor on cultured mesenchymal stem cells for spine fusion. Spine 32:1067-1071, 2007.

38. Hou LT, Liu CM, Liu BY, et al. Tissue engineering bone formation in novel recombinant human bone morphogenic protein 2-atelocollagen composite scaffolds. J Periodontol 78:335-343, 2007.

39. Arnander C, Westermark A, Veltheim R, et al. Three-dimensional technology and bone morphogenetic protein in frontal bone reconstruction. J Craniofac Surg 17:275-279, 2006.

40. Mendonça JJ, Juiz-Lopez P. Regenerative facial reconstruction of terminal stage osteoradionecrosis and other advanced craniofacial diseases with adult cultured stem and progenitor cells. Plast Reconstr Surg 126:1699-1709, 2010.

41. Cowan CM, Shi YY, Aalami OO, et al. Adipose-derived adult stromal cells heal critical-size mouse calvarial defects. Nat Biotechnol 22:560-567, 2004.

42. Lendeckel S, Jödicke A, Christophis P, et al. Autologous stem cells (adipose) and fibrin glue used to treat widespread traumatic calvarial defects: case report. J Craniomaxillofac Surg 32:370-373, 2004.

43. Taylor JA. Bilateral orbitozygomatic reconstruction with tissue-engineered bone. J Craniofac Surg 21:1612-1614, 2010.

44. Mesimäki K, Lindroos B, Törnwall J, et al. Novel maxillary reconstruction with ectopic bone formation by GMP adipose stem cells. Int J Oral Maxillofac Surg 38:201-209, 2003.

45. Warnke PH, Springer IN, Wiltfang J, et al. Growth and transplantation of a custom vascularised bone graft in a man. Lancet 364(9436):766-770, 2004.

46. Kuznetsov SA, Cherman N, Robey PG. In vivo bone formation by progeny of human embryonic stem cells. Stem Cells Dev 20:269-287, 2011.

47. Oppenheimer AJ, Mesa J, Buchman SR. Current and emerging basic science concepts in bone biology: implications in craniofacial surgery. J Craniofac Surg 23:30-36, 2012.

48. Brent B. Technical advances in ear reconstruction with autogenous rib cartilage grafts: personal experience with 1200 cases. Plast Reconstr Surg 104:319-334; discussion 335-338, 1999.

49. Albrektsson T, Brånemark PI, Jacobsson M, et al. Present clinical applications of osseointegrated percutaneous implants. Plast Reconstr Surg 79:721-731, 1987.

50. Nayyer L, Patel KH, Esmaeili A, et al. Tissue engineering: revolution and challenge in auricular cartilage reconstruction. Plast Reconstr Surg 129:1123-1137, 2012.

51. Vacanti CA, Cima LG, Ratkowski D, Upton J, Vacanti JP. Tissue engineered growth of new cartilage in the shape of a human ear using synthetic polymers seeded with chondrocytes. In Cima LG, Ron ES, eds. Tissue-Inducing Biomaterials. Proceedings of the Materials Research Society Symposium. Pittsburgh: The Society, 1992.
    Initial attempt to tissue engineer cartilage in the shape of a human ear.

52. Cao Y, Vacanti JP, Paige KT, et al. Transplantation of chondrocytes using a polymer-cell construct to produce tissue-engineered cartilage in the shape of a human ear. Plast Reconstr Surg 100:297-302; discussion 303-304, 1997.
    First successful demonstration of functional engineered tissue. Human ear shaped cartilage was demonstrated which retained the appearance of the original ear geometry throughout implantation.

53. Lima EG, Tan AR, Tai T, et al. Differences in interleukin-1 response between engineered and native cartilage. Tissue Eng Part A 14:1721-1730, 2008.

54. Francioli S, Cavallo C, Grigolo B, et al. Engineered cartilage maturation regulates cytokine production and interleukin-1β response. Clin Orthop Relat Res 469:2773-2784, 2011.

55. Deponti D, Di Giancamillo A, Mangiavini L, et al. Fibrin-based model for cartilage regeneration: tissue maturation from in vitro to in vivo. Tissue Eng Part A 18:1109-1122, 2012.

56. Miot S, Brehm W, Dickinson S, et al. Influence of in vitro maturation of engineered cartilage on the outcome of osteochondral repair in a goat model. Eur Cell Mater 23:222-236, 2012.

57. Luo X, Zhou G, Liu W, et al. In vitro precultivation alleviates post-implantation inflammation and enhances development of tissue-engineered tubular cartilage. Biomed Mater 4:025006, 2009.

58. Bichara DA, Pomerantseva I, Zhao X, Zhou L, Kulig KM, Tseng A, Kimura AM, Johnson MA, Vacanti JP, Randolph MA, Sundback CA. Autologous auricular cartilage engineered in an ovine model using a fibrous collagen scaffold. Unpublished manuscript, 2012.

59. Ahmed TA, Dare EV, Hincke M. Fibrin: a versatile scaffold for tissue engineering applications. Tissue Eng Part B Rev 14:199-215, 2008.

60. Peretti GM, Xu JW, Bonassar LJ, et al. Review of injectable cartilage engineering using fibrin gel in mice and swine models. Tissue Eng 12:1151-1168, 2006.

61. Ting V, Sims CD, Brecht LE, et al. In vitro prefabrication of human cartilage shapes using fibrin glue and human chondrocytes. Ann Plast Surg 40:413-420; discussion 420-421, 1998.

62. Chang SC, Rowley JA, Tobias G, et al. Injection molding of chondrocyte/alginate constructs in the shape of facial implants. J Biomed Mater Res 55:503-511, 2001.

63. Jeon YH, Choi JH, Sung JK, et al. Different effects of PLGA and chitosan scaffolds on human cartilage tissue engineering. J Craniofac Surg 18:1249-1258, 2007.

64. Xu JW, Johnson TS, Motarjem PM, et al. Tissue-engineered flexible ear-shaped cartilage. Plast Reconstr Surg 115:1633-1641, 2005.

65. Saim AB, Cao Y, Weng Y, et al. Engineering autogenous cartilage in the shape of a helix using an injectable hydrogel scaffold. Laryngoscope 110(10 Pt 1):1694-1697, 2000.

66. Kamil SH, Vacanti MP, Aminuddin BS, et al. Tissue engineering of a human sized and shaped auricle using a mold. Laryngoscope 114:867-870, 2004.

67. Shieh S, Terada S, Vacanti JP. Tissue engineering auricular reconstruction: in vitro and in vivo studies. Biomaterials 25:1545-1557, 2004.

68. Lee SJ, Broda C, Atala A, et al. Engineered cartilage covered ear implants for auricular cartilage reconstruction. Biomacromolecules 12:306-313, 2011.

69. Bichara DA, Zhao X, Hwang NS, et al. Porous poly(vinyl alcohol)-alginate gel hybrid construct for neocartilage formation using human nasoseptal cells. J Surg Res 163:331-336, 2010.

70. Zhou L, Pomerantseva I, Bassett EK, Bowley CM, Zhao X, Bichara DA, Kulig KM, Vacanti JP, Randolph MA, Sundback CA Engineering ear constructs with a composite scaffold to maintain dimensions. Tissue Eng Part A 17:1573-1581, 2011.

71. Kusuhara H, Isogai N, Enjo M, et al. Tissue engineering a model for the human ear: assessment of size, shape, morphology, and gene expression following seeding of different chondrocytes. Wound Repair Regen 17:136-146, 2009.

72. Park SS, Jin HR, Chi DH, et al. Characteristics of tissue-engineered cartilage from human auricular chondrocytes. Biomaterials 25:2363-2369, 2004.

73. Kamil SH, Vacanti MP, Vacanti CA, et al. Microtia chondrocytes as a donor source for tissue-engineered cartilage. Laryngoscope 114:2187-2190, 2004.

74. Schulze-Tanzil G. Activation and dedifferentiation of chondrocytes: implications in cartilage injury and repair. Ann Anat 191:325-338, 2009.

75. Li WJ, Tuli R, Huang X, et al. Multilineage differentiation of human mesenchymal stem cells in a three-dimensional nanofibrous scaffold. Biomaterials 26:5158-5166, 2005.

76. Fujisawa T, Hattori T, Ono M, et al. CCN family 2/connective tissue growth factor (CCN2/CTGF) stimulates proliferation and differentiation of auricular chondrocytes. Osteoarthritis Cartilage 16:787-795, 2008.

77. Yanaga H, Imai K, Fujimoto T, et al. Generating ears from cultured autologous auricular chondrocytes by using two-stage implantation in treatment of microtia. Plast Reconstr Surg 124:817-825, 2009.

78. Isogai N, Morotomi T, Hayakawa S, et al. Combined chondrocyte-copolymer implantation with slow release of basic fibroblast growth factor for tissue engineering an auricular cartilage construct. J Biomed Mater Res A 74:408-418, 2005.

79. Isogai NY, Nakagawa K, Suzuki R, et al. Cytokine-rich autologous serum system for cartilaginous tissue engineering. Ann Plast Surg 60:703-709, 2008.

80. Pelttari K, Winter A, Steck E, et al. Premature induction of hypertrophy during in vitro chondrogenesis of human mesenchymal stem cells correlates with calcification and vascular invasion after ectopic transplantation in SCID mice. Arthritis Rheum 54:3254-3266, 2006.

81. Ma HL, Hung SC, Lin SY, et al. Chondrogenesis of human mesenchymal stem cells encapsulated in alginate beads. J Biomed Mater Res A 64:273-281, 2003.

82. Dragoo JL, Samimi B, Zhu M, et al. Tissue-engineered cartilage and bone using stem cells from human infrapatellar fat pads. J Bone Joint Surg Br 85:740-747, 2003.

83. Ho ST, Cool SM, Hui JH, et al. The influence of fibrin based hydrogels on the chondrogenic differentiation of human bone marrow stromal cells. Biomaterials 31:38-47, 2010.

84. Hwang NS, Im SG, Wu PB, et al. Chondrogenic priming adipose-mesenchymal stem cells for cartilage tissue regeneration. Pharm Res 28:1395-1405, 2011.

85. Liu X, Sun H, Yan D, et al. In vivo ectopic chondrogenesis of BMSCs directed by mature chondrocytes. Biomaterials 31:9406-9414, 2010.

86. Haisch A, Kläring S, Gröger A, et al. A tissue-engineering model for the manufacture of auricular-shaped cartilage implants. Eur Arch Otorhinolaryngol 259:316-321, 2002.

87. Rotter N, Haisch A, Bücheler M. Cartilage and bone tissue engineering for reconstructive head and neck surgery. Eur Arch Otorhinolaryngol 262:539-545, 2005.

88. Peiseler B. Ohrmuscheln und Gelenke aus Zellkultur. Baseler Zeitung 16:55-57, 2001.

89. Yanaga H, Koga M, Imai K, et al. Clinical application of biotechnically cultured autologous chondrocytes as novel graft material for nasal augmentation. Aesthetic Plast Surg 28:212-221, 2004.

90. Cheng JT, Perkins SW, Hamilton MM. Collagen and injectable fillers. Otolaryngol Clin North Am 35:73-85, vi, 2002.

91. Kawaguchi N, Toriyama K, Nicodemou-Lena E et al. De novo adipogenesis in mice at the site of injection of basement membrane and basic fibroblast growth factor. Proc Natl Acad Sci U S A 95:1062-1066, 1998.

92. Monheit GD, Coleman KM. Hyaluronic acid fillers. Dermatol Ther 19:141-150, 2006.

93. Ersek RA. Transplantation of purified autologous fat: a 3-year follow-up is disappointing. Plast Reconstr Surg 87:219-227; discussion 228, 1991.

94. Billings E Jr, May JW Jr. Historical review and present status of free fat graft autotransplantation in plastic and reconstructive surgery. Plast Reconstr Surg 83:368-381, 1989.

95. Choi JH, Gimble JM, Lee K, et al. Adipose tissue engineering for soft tissue regeneration. Tissue Eng Part B Rev 16:413-426, 2010.

96. Patel PN, Patrick CW. Materials employed for breast augmentation and reconstruction. In Ma PX, Elisseeff J, eds. Scaffolding in Tissue Engineering. New York: Marcel Dekker, 2005.

97. Patrick CW Jr, Zheng B, Johnston C, et al. Long-term implantation of preadipocyte-seeded PLGA scaffolds. Tissue Eng 8:283-293, 2002.

98. Wechselberger G, Russell RC, Neumeister MW, et al. Successful transplantation of three tissue-engineered cell types using capsule induction technique and fibrin glue as a delivery vehicle. Plast Reconstr Surg 110:123-129, 2002.

99. von Heimburg D, Zachariah S, Heschel I, et al. Human preadipocytes seeded on freeze-dried collagen scaffolds investigated in vitro and in vivo. Biomaterials 22:429-438, 2001.

100. von Heimburg D, Zachariah S, Low A, et al. Influence of different biodegradable carriers on the in vivo behavior of human adipose precursor cells. Plast Reconstr Surg 108:411-420; discussion 421-422, 2001.

101. Halberstadt C, Austin C, Rowley J, et al. A hydrogel material for plastic and reconstructive applications injected into the subcutaneous space of a sheep. Tissue Eng 8:309-319, 2002.

102. Huss FR, Kratz G. Mammary epithelial cell and adipocyte co-culture in a 3-D matrix: the first step towards tissue-engineered human breast tissue. Cells Tissues Organs 169:361-367, 2001.

103. Lin RZ, Moreno-Luna R, Zhou B, et al. Equal modulation of endothelial cell function by four distinct tissue-specific mesenchymal stem cells. Angiogenesis 15:443-455, 2012.

104. Zhu M, Zhou Z, Chen Y, et al. Supplementation of fat grafts with adipose-derived regenerative cells improves long-term graft retention. Ann Plast Surg 64:222-228, 2010.

105. Moseley TA, Zhu M, Hedrick MH. Adipose-derived stem and progenitor cells as fillers in plastic and reconstructive surgery. Plast Reconstr Surg 118(3 Suppl):121-128, 2006.

106. Yoshimura K, Sato K, Aoi N, et al. Cell-assisted lipotransfer for facial lipoatrophy: efficacy of clinical use of adipose-derived stem cells. Dermatol Surg 34:1178-1185, 2008.

107. Dohan Ehrenfest DM, Bielecki T, Jimbo R, et al. Do the fibrin architecture and leukocyte content influence the growth factor release of platelet concentrates? An evidence-based answer comparing a pure platelet-rich plasma (P-PRP) gel and a leukocyte- and platelet-rich fibrin (L-PRF). Curr Pharm Biotechnol 13:1145-1152, 2012.

108. Liu B, Tan XY, Liu YP, et al. The adjuvant use of stromal vascular fraction and platelet-rich fibrin for autologous adipose tissue transplantation. Tissue Eng Part C Methods 19:1-14, 2013.

109. Chen FM, Zhang M, Wu ZF. Toward delivery of multiple growth factors in tissue engineering. Biomaterials 31:6279-6308, 2010.

110. Lee SK, Kim DW, Dhong ES, et al. Facial soft tissue augmentation using autologous fat mixed with stromal vascular fraction. Arch Plast Surg 39:534-539, 2012.

111. Cassell OC, Hofer SO, Morrison WA, et al. Vascularisation of tissue-engineered grafts: the regulation of angiogenesis in reconstructive surgery and in disease states. Br J Plast Surg 55:603-610, 2002.

112. Singh S, Wu BM, Dunn JC. Accelerating vascularization in polycaprolactone scaffolds by endothelial progenitor cells. Tissue Eng Part A 17:1819-1830, 2011.

113. Zhao M, Zhou J, Li X, et al. Repair of bone defect with vascularized tissue engineered bone graft seeded with mesenchymal stem cells in rabbits. Microsurgery 31:130-137, 2011.

114. Hegen A, Blois A, Tiron CE, et al. Efficient in vivo vascularization of tissue-engineering scaffolds. J Tissue Eng Regen Med 5:e52-e62, 2011.

115. Tsigkou O, Pomerantseva I, Spencer JA, Redondo PA, Hart AR, O'Doherty E, Lin Y, Friedrich CC, Daheron L, Lin CP, Sundback CA, Vacanti JP, Neville C. Engineered vascularized bone grafts. Proc Natl Acad Sci U S A 107:3311-3316, 2010.

116. Rustad KC, Sorkin M, Levi B, et al. Strategies for organ level tissue engineering. Organogenesis 6:151-157, 2010.

117. Levi B, Glotzbach JP, Wong VW, et al. Stem cells: update and impact on craniofacial surgery. J Craniofac Surg 23:319-322, 2012.

118. Xu Y, Shi Y, Ding S. A chemical approach to stem-cell biology and regenerative medicine. Nature 453:338-344, 2008.

119. Kawamoto A, Asahara T. Role of progenitor endothelial cells in cardiovascular disease and upcoming therapies. Catheter Cardiovasc Interv 70:477-484, 2007.

120. Bach AD, Beier JP, Stern-Staeter J, et al. Skeletal muscle tissue engineering. J Cell Mol Med 8:413-422, 2004.

121. Morgan JE, Partridge TA. Muscle satellite cells. Int J Biochem Cell Biol 35:1151-1156, 2003.

122. Brady MA, Lewis MP, Mudera V. Synergy between myogenic and non-myogenic cells in a 3D tissue-engineered craniofacial skeletal muscle construct. J Tissue Eng Regen Med 2:408-417, 2008.

123. Li M, Dickinson CE, Finkelstein EB, Neville CM, Sundback CA. The role of fibroblasts in self-assembled skeletal muscle. Tissue Eng Part A 17:2641-2650, 2011.

124. Yaffe D. Retention of differentiation potentialities during prolonged cultivation of myogenic cells. Proc Natl Acad Sci U S A 61:477-483, 1968.

125. Koning M, Harmsen MC, van Luyn MJ, et al. Current opportunities and challenges in skeletal muscle tissue engineering. J Tissue Eng Regen Med 3:407-415, 2009.

126. Powell CA, Smiley BL, Mills J, et al. Mechanical stimulation improves tissue-engineered human skeletal muscle. Am J Physiol Cell Physiol 283:C1557-C1665, 2002.

127. Huang YC, Dennis RG, Larkin L, et al. Rapid formation of functional muscle in vitro using fibrin gels. J Appl Physiol 98:706-713, 2005.

128. Moon du G, Christ G, Stitzel JD, et al. Cyclic mechanical preconditioning improves engineered muscle contraction. Tissue Eng Part A 14:473-482, 2008.

129. Matsumoto T, Sasaki J, Alsberg E, et al. Three-dimensional cell and tissue patterning in a strained fibrin gel system. PLoS One 2:e1211, 2007.

130. Coletti D, Teodori L, Albertini MC, et al. Static magnetic fields enhance skeletal muscle differentiation in vitro by improving myoblast alignment. Cytometry A 71:846-856, 2007.

131. Masuda S, Shimizu T, Yamato M, et al. Cell sheet engineering for heart tissue repair. Adv Drug Deliv Rev 60:277-285, 2008.

132. Levenberg S, Rouwkema J, Macdonald M, et al. Engineering vascularized skeletal muscle tissue. Nat Biotechnol 23:879-884, 2005.

133. Asakawa N, Shimizu T, Tsuda Y, et al. Pre-vascularization of in vitro three-dimensional tissues created by cell sheet engineering. Biomaterials 31:3903-3909, 2010.

134. Pedrotty DM, Koh J, Davis BH, et al. Engineering skeletal myoblasts: roles of three-dimensional culture and electrical stimulation. Am J Physiol Heart Circ Physiol 288:1620-1626, 2005.

135. Huang YC, Dennis RG, Baar K. Cultured slow vs. fast skeletal muscle cells differ in physiology and responsiveness to stimulation. Am J Physiol Cell Physiol 291:C11-C17, 2006.

136. Susarla SM, Swanson E, Gordon CR. Craniomaxillofacial reconstruction using allotransplantation and tissue engineering: challenges, opportunities, and potential synergy. Ann Plast Surg 67:655-661, 2011.

137. Ott HC, Matthiesen TS, Goh SK, et al. Perfusion-decellularized matrix: using nature's platform to engineer a bioartificial heart. Nat Med 14:213-221, 2008.

138. Petersen TH, Calle EA, Zhao L, et al. Tissue-engineered lungs for in vivo implantation. Science 329:538-541, 2010.

The Role of Facial Plastic Surgery in Global Health and Surgical Education

Roy Ahn ▪ *Nadia Shaikh*
Wendy Williams ▪ *Thomas F. Burke*

Of all the forms of inequality, injustice in health care is the most shocking and inhumane.
–Dr. Martin Luther King
Second National Convention
of the Medical Committee for Human Rights
Chicago, March 25, 1966

GLOBAL FACIAL SURGERY: PRAXIS, PROCESS, AND POLICY

Paul E. Farmer and Mack L. Cheney

Plastic and reconstructive surgery of the head and neck has enormous potential transformative power. The importance of this surgical subspecialty in the overall continuum of global health should be without dispute. Burns and congenital deformities account for more than one third of the "global burden of disease" and are second only to traumatic injuries—the leading cause of death among children and young adults in much of the world.[1,2] Many acquired and congenital deformities are rarely seen among adults here in Boston but are common in many regions of the globe. By some estimates, more than 1 in 1000 children in the world are born with congenital deformities such as cleft lip or cleft palate.[3] So why do we see more people reach adulthood with these untreated afflictions in one part of the world but not the other? The variance in facial reconstructive treatment between Haiti or rural Ecuador and Boston is largely one of *access* to modern subspecialty surgery (Lancet Commission on Global Surgery, 2014).

Living with a facial deformity can lead to lifelong disability, psychological trauma, social isolation—and, too often, early death. Thus those who survive suffer what some medical anthropologists and sociologists would call a "social death." Modern surgical care—by which we mean not only surgeons, but also the multidisciplinary teams they lead—can readily treat facial deformities, but surgical treatment rarely reaches those in greatest need: the poorest one third of the world's population benefits from only 3.5% of all surgical procedures performed.[4]

As William Foege, an early champion of global health equity, has observed, "improvement does not just happen by chance, it happens because of a plan."[5] Child mortality from all causes (and not simply from polio, measles, and other vaccine-preventable illness) has plummeted in recent decades. Since the early 2000s, fatality rates for chronic infectious diseases such as AIDS and tuberculosis have fallen precipitously as well. The creation of delivery platforms able to integrate prevention, diagnosis, and effective treatment for these and other conditions spurred rapid and dramatic improvements in life expectancy across many low-income settings. Yet these achievements have not been immediately followed by similar investments in addressing the burden of untreated surgical disease, which is increasingly concentrated among the world's poorest.[6]

So what is the equity plan for surgical care? What might transform problems as straightforward as an abscess—or as complicated as cleft palate—from untreatable in Haiti or rural Ecuador to treatable anywhere in the world? The approach endorsed in this chapter is to strive for the highest standard of care, especially for the most vulnerable, and to execute a coordinated strategy to bring improvement to surgical training and care delivery everywhere in the world.

Thus praxis, process, and policy packaged in a comprehensive and strategic manner offer hope for meaningful impact in surgical skills training, evaluation of quality and outcomes, and enhanced funding in the developing world guided by a clear articulation of vision, need, and policy.

REFERENCES

1. Institute for Health Matrics and Evaluation. Global vision of disease 2010 interactive visualizations: arrow diagram. Available at *http://vishubhealthdata.org/rank/arrow.php*.
2. Debas HT. Disease Control Priorities in Developing Countries, ed 2. Washington, DC, The World Bank Group, 2006.
3. Khajanchi MU, Shah H, Thakkar P, Gerdin M, Roy N. Unmet burden of cleft lip and palate in rural Gujarat, India: a population-based study. World J Surg. 2014 May 8. [Epub ahead of print]
4. Weiser TG, Regenbogen SE, Thompson KD, et al. An estimation of the global volume of surgery: a modeling strategy based on available data. Lancet 372:139-144, 2008.
5. Foege W. Keynote Speech for the Fiftieth Anniversary Program for the Thomas Francis Medal in Global Public Health, University of Michigan, Ann Arbor, April 12, 2005.
6. Farmer P. Chronic infectious disease and the future of health care delivery. N Engl J Med 369:2435-2447, 2013.

The concept of global health represents efforts at collaboration among nations for health care delivery, regardless of income or development status.[1] The origins of global health trace back to nineteenth century imperial powers' efforts to control the spread of infectious diseases.[2] The kaleidoscope of diseases has shifted over the years, from smallpox and polio to HIV, tuberculosis, and malaria, to today's "neglected diseases." Yet disease control has remained the dominant focus of global public health and has greatly influenced the direction of public policy, governmental priorities, and funding. The HIV/AIDS epidemic is a modern-day example of the relevance of global health efforts to prevent the spread of deadly disease. The emergence of HIV/AIDS galvanized global health efforts, bridging the gap between clinical medicine and public health, and triggering the commitment of a wide variety of academic and financial resources.[3] Characterized as a threat to global security, the spread of HIV/AIDS prompted unprecedented investment in health care funding for developing countries by the World Bank, the support of individual governmental resources such as the U.S. president's Emergency Plan for AIDS Relief (PEPFAR), and private philanthropy from organizations led by the Bill and Melinda Gates Foundation. Sources of financial support and a groundswell of public interest in turn facilitated the involvement of academic medical centers, schools of public health, and universities, institutionalizing global health as an academic field.

Surgery had long been considered a First World luxury and therefore not a critical component of primary health care. In the past decade, the importance of surgical interventions in advancing population health has received renewed attention in the global health community. Increased representation of the subject in the medical literature has been accompanied by high-profile surgical interventions in recent disaster relief efforts, with reports providing data on the unmet surgical disease burden, and cost-effectiveness studies demonstrating the pragmatism of improving access to surgical care. The nongovernmental organization Médecins Sans Frontières reported performing 4000 surgical procedures in the aftermath of the 2010 Haiti earthquake alone.[4] The Global Burden of Disease Studies conducted in 1990 and 2010 show a continued rise in the prevalence of noncommunicable diseases and injuries, which will soon overtake infectious diseases and malnutrition as the major sources of global death and disability. Although surgical procedures are in high demand everywhere, most of the world's global surgical interventions take place in wealthier countries, not in the lowest-income countries, where need is greatest.[5] With emerging data, the importance of surgery in global health has been made incontrovertible.

Until recently, facial plastic and reconstructive surgery sat on the periphery of global health efforts. Although plastic surgery has a long track record within the international community, its contributions over the past 40 years have been largely restricted to individual nongovernmental organizations (NGOs) dedicated to short-term, disease-specific insertions by volunteer surgeons, characterized by the activities of organizations such as Operation Smile, Smile Train, and ReSurge International.[6] The past decade has seen a shift in global health policy and public opinion, ushering in large-scale commitments to changing health care infrastructure and laying the foundation for long-term sustainability of developing nations' health systems. This has been reflected in the course corrections of these same NGOs, as they expand beyond the short-term medical mission model to incorporate local training, improve integration with local health care systems, and prioritize monitoring and assessment plans to track outcomes and demonstrate the cost-effectiveness of surgical interventions.[7-9]

To fully gauge the cost effectiveness of surgical interventions compared with other health reforms, we must better understand the nature of the surgical disease burden and how to measure its impact on a country's nationwide health and economy. Recognizing the critical lack of methodology for assessing the impact of surgical care, the Global Burden of Surgical Disease Working Group (GBSDWG) proposed using cumulative disability-adjusted life-years (DALYs) as the measurement of the burden of surgical conditions and unmet need for surgical care.[10] Assigning a DALY value to each condition deemed surgical and a DALY averted value to each surgical intervention provides a common language for comparing the value and cost-effectiveness of surgical interventions of more widely supported public health initiatives. One DALY represents 1 lost year of "healthy" life with the disease burden as the gap between the current health status of a population and the ideal. Under this metric, surgery has become recognized as a reasonable extension of health care reform in the developing world, comparing favorably with other public health interventions, such as vaccinations and antiretroviral therapy for HIV.[11] These metrics also reveal the impact and cost-effectiveness of facial plastic and reconstructive surgical interventions in alleviating disability years, increasing productivity, and improving quality of life.[9,12-14]

Barriers exist to the delivery of surgical care in the developing world. The poor condition of health facilities serves as an additional barrier to surgical care.[15] Shortages of surgical supplies, drugs, anesthesia capability, and other critical items are common in resource-poor areas.[16] Moreover, many hospitals in developing countries set their fee structure for surgery at rates that many people simply cannot afford.[17,18] There is a severe shortage of skilled surgeons relative to the demand for surgical services[19-21] (Fig. 51-1). The mi-

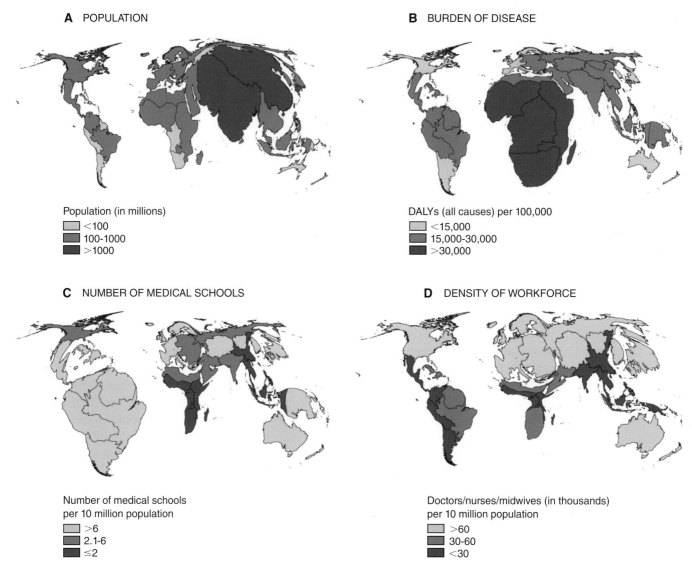

Fig. 51-1 World maps resized by population. **A,** Population. **B,** Burden of disease. **C,** Number of medical schools. **D,** Density of workforce. (*DALYs,* Disability-adjusted life-years.) (From Frenk J, Chen L, Bhutta, ZA, et al. Health professionals for a new century: transforming education to strengthen health systems in an interdependent world. Lancet 376:1923-1958, 2010.)

gration of physicians from developing countries to the United States, the United Kingdom, Canada, and Australia, resulting in a so-called brain drain, has been well documented as a threat to the health and human resource capacity of developing countries.[22-24] Additionally, most physicians in developing countries are located in urban areas, whereas most of the population in developing countries lives in rural regions.

ROLE OF FACIAL PLASTIC SURGICAL INTERVENTIONS

There is a substantial role for facial plastic surgical interventions in alleviating human suffering in developing countries. The developing world sees high rates of burns, traumatic injuries, and congenital anomalies, conditions that have great potential for recovery if overseen by skilled specialty surgeons.[6,11,18] Much attention has focused on addressing the plight of patients afflicted with cleft lip and palate, but there are numerous other conditions that require surgical correction (Box 51-1).

> **Box 51-1** Common Facial Plastic Surgical Conditions in the Developing World
>
> - Cleft lip and palate
> - Facial, nasal, orbital, and mandibular fractures
> - Face, scalp, lip, and neck lacerations and burns
> - Auricular deformities
> - Skin cancers in the head and neck region
> - Congenital vascular birthmarks and nevi

Burns are a leading cause of DALYs in sub-Saharan Africa and South Asia, often eclipsing those resulting from tuberculosis, malaria, and HIV/AIDS, especially among women and children. Although initial care may fall under general surgery, lifelong disability may persist without more specialized knowledge of early burn excision, skin grafting, and other methods of managing burn scar contractures.[11,25] Facial burns are on the rise in regions where incidents of acid violence directed toward women are increasing, such as in Bangladesh.[26] With trauma set to become the third leading contribution to the global disease burden, road traffic injuries in particular have taken on a more highlighted role.[27] As first response treatment improves in developing countries, there should be an even greater increase in reported facial injuries as a result of increased survival rates. In 2008 alone, there were approximately 35,000 new cases of cleft lip and cleft palate in sub-Saharan Africa. Health economists estimate that treating these new cleft cases would economically benefit the region by between $252 million and $441 million.[28]

GLOBAL FACIAL PLASTIC SURGERY INITIATIVES

NONGOVERNMENTAL ORGANIZATION-LED INITIATIVES

The World Health Organization created the Global Initiative for Emergency and Essential Surgical Care (GIEESC),[29] which aims to build surgical capacity at district hospitals in developing countries through public/private partnerships. More than 30 low-income and middle-income countries (in addition to high-income countries) currently participate in this initiative, which targets 34 surgical procedures to which every person in the world should have access[30] (Box 51-2). The GIEESC has also developed guidelines for care delivery in resource-poor health care settings.[29,31]

Many facial plastic surgery initiatives for global health focus on the treatment of specific conditions, including cleft lip, cleft palate, and burns. Specialized NGOs such as Smile Train, Operation Smile, and ReSurge International (formerly known as Interplast) have a long history of providing surgical care in developing countries and their reach is significant. Smile Train performed more than 800,000 cleft repair procedures over 14 years,[32] Operation Smile reported 18,000 procedures in a single year, and provided adjunct services beyond cleft surgery (such as speech pathology, otolaryngology specialty care, and psychological counseling).[33] ReSurge International performed more than 2000 surgical interventions for burn-related issues. Large NGOs such as these are increasingly placing a strong emphasis on training local medical providers to perform these procedures as part of their organizational strategies to build local capacity and provide the necessary multidisciplinary treatment required for long-term positive outcomes.

The number of smaller independent medical mission organizations in the market is striking; more than 500 organizations advertise short-term medical mission opportunities, and the American College of Surgeons posts a web directory of international volunteer opportunities for its members, including many relevant

Box 51-2 World Health Organization's Clinical Procedures in "Tool for Situational Analysis to Assess Emergency and Essential Surgical Care"

Resuscitation (airway, hemorrhage, peripheral percutaneous intravenous access, peripheral venous cut down)

Cricothyroidotomy/tracheostomy

Chest tube insertion

Removal of foreign body (throat/eye/ear/nose)

Acute burn management

Incision and drainage of abscess

Suturing (for wounds, episiotomy, cervical and vaginal lacerations)

Wound debridement

Cesarean section

Dilation and curettage/vacuum extraction (obstetrics/gynecology)

Obstetric fistula repair

Tubal ligation/vasectomy

Biopsy (lymph node, mass, other)

Appendectomy

Hernia repair (strangulated, elective, congenital)

Hydrocelectomy

Cystostomy

Urethral stricture dilation

Laparotomy (uterine rupture, ectopic pregnancy, acute abdomen, intestinal obstruction, perforation, injuries)

Male circumcision

Neonatal surgery (abdominal wall defect, colostomy, imperforate anus, intussusceptions)

Cleft lip repair

Clubfoot repair

Contracture release/skin grafting

Closed treatment of fracture

Open treatment of fracture

Joint dislocation treatment

Drainage of osteomyelitis/septic arthritis

Amputation

Cataract surgery

Regional anesthesia blocks

Spinal anesthesia

Ketamine intravenous anesthesia

General anesthesia inhalational

Adapted from World Health Organization. WHO Global Health Expenditure Atlas, 2012. Available at *http://www.who.int/nha/atlas.pdf.*

to facial plastic surgery. The American Academy of Facial Plastic and Reconstructive Surgery's "FACE TO FACE" program includes an international component that facilitates volunteer trips involving facial plastic surgeons. FACE TO FACE provided direct surgical care to 1000 patients, and its U.S.-based medical providers work closely with local providers in the regions where they work to build long-term capacity.[34]

Drawbacks of narrowly focused, disease-specific programs are that they usually operate outside existing national and local health care infrastructures. By building their own facilities and providing independent delivery mechanisms in developing countries, they may adversely affect a country's ability to determine its own health care priorities.[35,36] Although vertical interventions provide rapid implementation, efficient delivery of services, and are attractive to donors, they may compete with each other and do not necessarily aid in the long-term development of the nation's infrastructure and workforce needed. Bias and varying degrees of follow-up data also invite criticism.[36a]

For these reasons, a number of cleft palate–focused NGOs are gradually subscribing to a diagonal model of care delivery, whereby cleft-focused missions are integrated into sustainable, locally based programs.[37] Websites and short-term continuing medical education trips have been used to instruct local physicians on specific procedures or topics,[7] and the model has shifted from one in which 100% of patients are treated by international teams to one in which increasing numbers of patients receive treatment from local providers.[38]

ACADEMIC INITIATIVES

Buoyed by many surgeons' growing interest in global health, numerous global educational and training initiatives for surgery have emerged in the Unites States, Canada, Europe, and Australia. Many of these programs, which involve a university partner in a high-income country and a developing country university/hospital partner, provide opportunities for mutual benefit and introduce American surgical faculty and surgical trainees to clinical and research experiences in developing countries (Table 51-1).

Table 51-1   Selected Surgical Training Collaborations

Collaborative Partners	Description of Method
University of Makerere/Mulago Hospital (Kampala, Uganda)–Global Partners in Anesthesia and Surgery and University of California at San Francisco	Increased recruitment number of general surgery and anesthesia trainees All sponsored trainees successfully graduated and remained in the region Postgraduate academic positions were created and filled to promote workforce retention Developed local research agenda
National University of Rwanda–McGill University Health Centre	Developed system-based curriculum divided into 2-week modules (lectures, resident case presentations, journal club, morbidity and mortality rounds, and module evaluation by residents) Rotations of McGill University surgeons (matched with subspecialty module) participate in academic and clinical activities as educators, moderators, and facilitators of the program—not replacing local faculty, who supervise all activity

Data from Lipnick et al, 2013; Deckelbaum et al, 2012; Quershi JS et al, 2011; Mutabdzic D et al, 2013; Cameron BH et al, 2010; AMPATH website 2013.

Continued

Table 51-1   Selected Surgical Training Collaborations—cont'd

Collaborative Partners	Description of Method
Kamuzu Central Hospital (Lilongwe, Malawi)–University of North Carolina at Chapel Hill	UNC surgical and subspecialty surgical faculty visit KCH to instruct local surgeons in applicable specialty surgical skills Surgical residents from UNC spend their research year at KCH, supporting local surgical staff, providing continuity for visiting UNC faculty surgical instruction, and conducting research on global disease burden
College of Surgeons of East, Central, and Southern Africa (COSECSA)–Loma Linda University and Pan-African Academy of Christian Surgeons	Developed a rural-based surgical training program that has prepared graduates for formal regional accreditation exams (prepared by COSECSA or West African College of Surgeons) with a high pass rate Six training programs in four countries
University of Botswana–University of Toronto	Developed model for creating contextually relevant curriculum using surgical logs, local surgeons, and the Surgical Council on Resident Education (SCORE) curriculum
University of Guyana–Canadian Association of General Surgeons (CAGS)	CAGS assisted in needs assessment, proposed curriculum, and developed a module-based system for postgraduate surgical education alternating Guyanese and CAGS surgical faculty members Five residents have completed the 2-year course and are working in regional hospitals; another 9 residents are in the program
Moi University/Moi Teaching and Referral Hospital (Moi, Kenya)–AMPATH (Academic Model Providing Access to Healthcare) consortium	A consortium of North American academic health centers, led by Indiana University (IU), work with Moi University in Kenya to enhance medical education In general surgery, ENT (including facial plastics and reconstructive surgery) IU faculty rotate through Moi to treat patients and teach Kenyan medical students There are plans to establish a formal residency program in ENT

Today, global surgery fellowships abound in academic medical centers and offer residents the opportunity to obtain clinical and/or research exposure in developing countries—an experience thought to be well aligned with U.S. graduate medical education guidelines[23] (Table 51-2)—and further degree-oriented training in population health. Online and live continuing medical education courses have been designed for surgeons who wish to work in global health.[39,40]

Partnerships between academic medical centers and teaching hospitals in underresourced regions have a great potential to address the disparity between surgical disease burden and access to surgical care (Fig. 51-2).

Table 51-2   How a Clinical Experience in a Resource-Constrained Environment Fits the Competencies Outlined by the Accreditation Council for Graduate Medical Education (ACGME)

ACGME Competency	Global Health Application
Medical knowledge	Exposure to new clinical features of surgical diseases
Patient care	Shift back to focus on importance of history taking and physical examination
Professionalism	Coping with the difficulties of providing care in an austere environment to an underserved population; advocating for patients and the professionals who work daily in such settings
Interpersonal and communication skills	Cross-cultural communication and development of an understanding of the perception of medicine and surgery in a new cultural context
Practice-based learning and improvement	Application of medical knowledge to practice in a different setting and sharing past experiences with new colleagues; new sources of information and learning
Systems practice	Exposure to a vastly different practice environment and an understanding of cost-conscious care

Adapted from Ozgediz D, Wang J, Jayaraman S, et al. Surgical training and global health: initial results of a 5-year partnership with a surgical training program in a low-income country. Arch Surg 143:860-865; discussion 865, 2008.

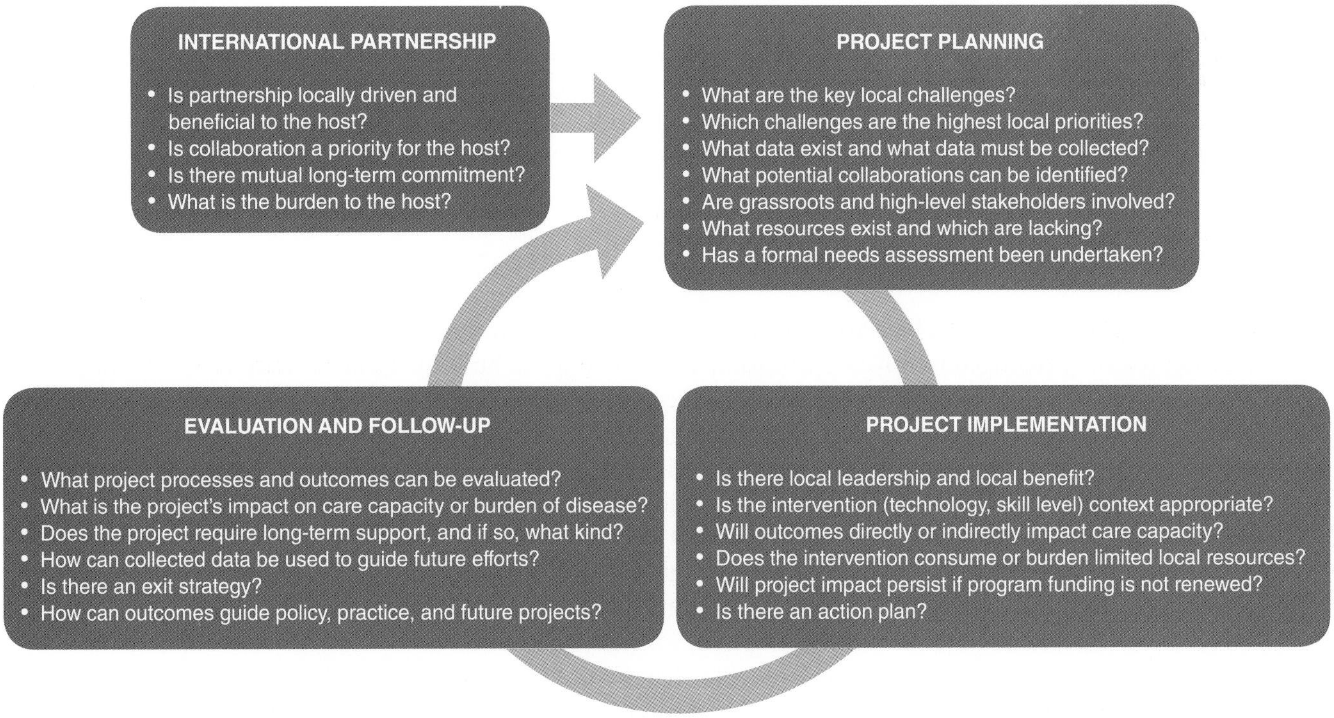

INTERNATIONAL PARTNERSHIP

• Is partnership locally driven and beneficial to the host?
• Is collaboration a priority for the host?
• Is there mutual long-term commitment?
• What is the burden to the host?

PROJECT PLANNING

• What are the key local challenges?
• Which challenges are the highest local priorities?
• What data exist and what data must be collected?
• What potential collaborations can be identified?
• Are grassroots and high-level stakeholders involved?
• What resources exist and which are lacking?
• Has a formal needs assessment been undertaken?

EVALUATION AND FOLLOW-UP

• What project processes and outcomes can be evaluated?
• What is the project's impact on care capacity or burden of disease?
• Does the project require long-term support, and if so, what kind?
• How can collected data be used to guide future efforts?
• Is there an exit strategy?
• How can outcomes guide policy, practice, and future projects?

PROJECT IMPLEMENTATION

• Is there local leadership and local benefit?
• Is the intervention (technology, skill level) context appropriate?
• Will outcomes directly or indirectly impact care capacity?
• Does the intervention consume or burden limited local resources?
• Will project impact persist if program funding is not renewed?
• Is there an action plan?

Fig. 51-2   Conceptual framework for capacity building through academic partnerships. (From Lipnick M, Mijumbi C, Dubowitz G, et al. Surgery and anesthesia capacity-building in resource-poor settings: description of an ongoing academic partnership in Uganda. World J Surg 37:488-497, 2013.)

Table 51-3   Selected University-Based Global Health Elective Opportunities
for Surgical Residents

Program	Resident Eligibility/Duration of Elective
Emory University Global Surgery Program (Ethiopia)	PGY-3 or PGY-4, 6 weeks
Stanford University General Surgery Residency International Elective (Zimbabwe)	PGY-3, 1 month
Vanderbilt University International Surgery Elective Rotation (Kenya)	PGY-4, 1 month
Loma Linda University International Surgery Rotation (Malawi)	PGY-4, 2 months
Alpert Medical School (Brown University) Rural Africa Surgical Elective (Kenya)	PGY-3, 2 months

Adapted from American College of Surgeons, 2013; Emory University Global Surgery Program website, 2013; Stanford University General Surgery Residency, 2013; Vanderbilt University Medical Center, General Surgery Residency, 2013; Loma Linda University Medical Center, General Surgery Residency, 2013; Alpert Medical School, Department of Surgery, 2013.

Critical components to the success of such collaborations include strong relationships, emphasis on mutual learning, and individual champions to ensure that local training needs supersede expatriate training needs.[41] These "twinning" programs provide greater opportunities to share much needed faculty, and contribute to the development of academic ecosystems that promote both acquisition of surgical skill and the development of future local faculty. There are successful examples of such collaborations across the globe[42-44] (see Tables 51-1 and 51-3). Encouraging academic productivity and teaching research skills both augments the quality of training and care provided and improves physician job satisfaction, thereby improving retention rates.[14] The founding and growth of societies such as the College of Surgeons of East, Central, and Southern Africa (COSECSA) and West African College of Surgeons (WACS) is evidence of global academic influence; these groups have begun to unify surgical training programs through formal accreditation mechanisms and develop educational resources for their members.

ONGOING CHALLENGES FOR GLOBAL SURGERY

Global surgical activities can be classified along a continuum, from short, weeks-long overseas surgical mission trips to prolonged multiyear institutional partnerships to build surgical capacity in developing countries. Investing in building long-term surgical capacity in developing countries offers the best solution.[43,45-47] Such capacity can only be built if the larger health ecosystems within which surgery is nested are both robust and supportive. In this regard, considerable and trenchant challenges remain. In many areas, government per capita spending on health care is tragically low (for example, in Eritrea, per capita annual government expenditures for health are USD $8),[30] and national strategies and financing schemes for surgical services are lacking. The lack of investment—or disinvestment—in health systems triggers physician exodus from many developing countries, further hindering access to quality surgical care. The World Health Organization's six building blocks of a functional health system illustrate the foundational work required (Box 51-3). Until key stakeholders (citizens, funders, and NGOs) mobilize and generate the political will to address health disparities in these countries, the task of reducing the global surgical disease burden will remain formidable.

Box 51-3   "Building Blocks" of Health Systems

- Good *health services* are those which deliver effective, safe, quality personal and non-personal health interventions to those that need them, when and where needed, with minimum waste of resources.
- A well-performing *health workforce* is one that works in ways that are responsive, fair and efficient to achieve the best health outcomes possible, given available resources and circumstances; that is, there are sufficient staff, fairly distributed, and they are competent, responsive, and productive.
- A well-functioning *health information* system is one that ensures the production, analysis, dissemination and use of reliable and timely information on health determinants, health system performance and health status.
- A well-functioning health system ensures equitable access to essential *medical products, vaccines, and technologies* of assured quality, safety, efficacy and cost-effectiveness, and their scientifically sound and cost-effective use.
- A good *health financing* system raises adequate funds for health, in ways that ensure people can use needed services, and are protected from financial catastrophe or impoverishment associated with having to pay for them. It provides incentives for providers and users to be efficient.
- *Leadership and governance* involves ensuring strategic policy frameworks exist and are combined with effective oversight, coalition building, regulation, attention to system design and accountability.

From World Health Organization, Western Pacific Region, 2013.

Preventing diseases that require surgical intervention is also important. Significant investments in injury prevention programs in developing countries (such as building safer roads for motor vehicles and campaigns to reduce interpersonal violence, and burn prevention through safer cooking methods) could dramatically reduce surgical burden in these countries.

The current challenge for facial plastic and reconstructive surgeons is to identify surgical training and/or intervention models that are sustainable and scalable in developing countries. Evaluation tools must be refined to address the following questions: "Do global facial plastic surgical programs effectively impact the health and well-being of the populations served?" "Are such programs making the most appropriate, culturally competent use of available financial, technical, and other resources to improve health outcomes in resource-poor areas?" Facial plastic surgeons have recently described an ambitious research agenda for global surgery as it relates to this field: "(1) collecting epidemiologic data to establish the met/unmet need, (2) measuring the effects of surgical services on the prevention of lifelong disability, (3) establishing benchmarks for quality of care, and evaluating cost-effectiveness."[46] These evaluation questions are designed to help identify programs with the ability to scale and transform successful global surgery programs in developing countries.

Many challenges for global surgery were summarized by the Bellagio Essential Surgery Group, an international consortium funded by both the Rockefeller and Bill and Melinda Gates Foundations. Its 2009 report on the future for surgery in sub-Saharan Africa laid out four principal recommendations for the field.[48] These remain relevant to facial plastic and reconstructive surgery in the global arena going forward:

- Strengthen surgical services at district hospitals
- Improve systems for the delivery of trauma care
- Expand the supply and quality of health workers with surgical skills
- Build evidence to inform interventions to improve access to surgery in sub-Saharan Africa

OPPORTUNITIES FOR GLOBAL FACIAL PLASTIC SURGERY

The potential contributions of facial plastic surgery to global health and surgical education are enormous and open ended. Surgeons from around the world are in a position to contribute to education in developing countries, and in the process improve and save lives. Surgeons whose main motivation is to forge a personal connection with individual patients may find medical mission trips to be a deeply satisfying experience, and a suitable initial foray into global health.

Validated and standardized assessment techniques need to be developed to better understand the root causes of deafness, facial anomalies, burns, and congenital defects. With a rigorous assessment approach, we will identify next generation, best evidence, and contextually appropriate solutions. Successful solutions will undoubtedly require innovative interventions in skills training (including training nonphysicians), policy creation, financing, quality assurance, equipment/supplies and supply lines, and community outreach; all of which are necessary for true systemic change.

Once these solutions are identified, collaboration with foreign governments to champion and scale these effective interventions on a national level will be required. As an example of a "next generation" approach, instead of operating on a small number of children with clefts or even training a few local surgeons in a given developing country, one could partner with a ministry of health and together declare a goal of national cleft lip eradication in all children age 2 or older, within a specified time frame. Delineating what it will take to achieve such ambitious population health goals will require deeper, more comprehensive approaches (such as public/private partnerships) than efforts to date.

Hospital and medical school departments need to establish clear academic career tracks for faculty members engaged in global health work, given the considerable field time they are likely to spend away from clinical practice[42]; and develop creative ways to finance global health programs (for example, set aside a percentage of clinical practice revenues to support departmental global health work). As evidenced by previous general surgery partnerships between North American and sub-Saharan African health institutions, such partnerships may yield fruitful scholarly contributions in the form of publications and joint conferences, and ultimately train the next generation of African surgeons.

Evaluation data on global facial plastic surgery collaborations could add to the body of scientific evidence regarding global surgery programs, which could inform policy decisions regarding the importance of funding surgical interventions as part of developing countries' health expenditures as a whole. Notably, a new scientific field known as implementation research is emerging. According to the Fogarty Institute at the National Institutes of Health, "the intent of implementation science and related research is to investigate and address major bottlenecks (social, behavioral, economic, and management) that impede effective implementation, test new approaches to improve health programming, as well as determine a causal relationship between the intervention and its impact."[49] Longitudinal implementation research on global facial plastic surgery collaborations is a promising new area of faculty research.

Collaborations with colleagues in the developing world facilitate "south to north" innovations in facial plastic surgery, in which medical innovations designed for application in developing countries could inform new applications in the developed world. Such innovations have occurred in other medical specialties; a low-cost Chlamydia Rapid Test that was designed for use in the context of a developing country proved so effective that it found a second commercial life in developed country markets, where it is now a market leader. The profits on the test from developed-country sales help the manufacturer offer the test at cost to governments of developing countries.[50] New communication technologies may help reduce the financial expense of intercontinental collaboration and offer better opportunity for longitudinal engagement. Telemedicine and telesurgery offer the ability to share clinical knowledge, provide mentorship, and introduce clinical simulation tools to local partners.

The research agenda for global facial plastic surgery must be expanded beyond evaluation of discrete surgical collaborations, in particular as related to the effectiveness and true impact of interventions (that is, including all collateral effects). For example, a training program that trains five surgeons from developing countries on basic facial plastic surgery techniques may stake a claim that they collectively repaired 500 clefts in the following year. Although this may sound like a large health impact, there are many questions that need to be asked to understand the true impact of the intervention. It is surprisingly easy to do more harm than good if impact assessment is limited to such vertical claims. For this example, a comprehensive health impact assessment must address the following:

- Is there a reimbursement structure that will provide incentive and sustain the surgeon's practice? Is there a reliance on philanthropy that is likely limited and time bound?
- Is the surgeon taken away from other vital activities (for example, appendectomies and other nonreconstructive surgeries)?
- Is a vehicle for training the next generation also being established?
- Is there a quality assurance system and accountability structure?
- Would the skills be better scaled for impact with focus on midlevel providers rather than physicians?
- Are safe anesthesia practices in place and/or do new models need to be developed?
- What are the postoperative care issues, such as travel?
- Are we training local research skills to gain local competency in asking the right questions for solution development?

Academic institutions and hospitals can further professionalize the field by developing a global facial plastic surgery ecosystem. Such an ecosystem might consist of the initiation of a peer-reviewed journal, a named subspecialty focus, a research forum or meeting, and the establishment of funded fellowships with a focus on global facial plastic and reconstructive surgery. Many of these field-building activities are already underway, although global facial plastic surgery is no exception to the rule that time and significant personal and institutional commitments are required to develop a field of practice. Given the recent interest in global surgery as a public health topic, the opportunity to engage in long-term field building now appears to be a viable and promising prospect that could significantly reduce disability in the developing world.

KEY POINTS

- There is a significant need for facial plastic and reconstructive surgical procedures in the developing world.
- Many opportunities exist for facial plastic surgeons and trainees to contribute to global health.
- Global surgical initiatives must be designed to improve local surgical health care in a sustainable manner.
- There is enormous emerging academic promise in the development of partnerships with hospitals and medical schools in the developing world.
- Next-generation global facial plastic surgery initiatives must align with population health goals of ministries of health from developing countries.
- Expanding the research agenda for global facial plastic surgery to include objective measures of impact and outcomes is critical to the advancement and maturation of the field.

REFERENCES

1. Koplan JP, Bond TC, Merson MH, et al. Towards a common definition of global health. Lancet 373:1993-1995, 2009.
2. Brown TM, Cueto M, Fee E. The World Health Organization and the transition from "international" to "global" public health. Am J Public Health 96:62-72, 2006.
3. Brandt AM. How AIDS invented global health. N Engl J Med 368:2149-2152, 2013.
4. Chu K, Stokes C, Trelles M, et al. Improving effective surgical delivery in humanitarian disasters: lessons from Haiti. PLoS Med 8:e1001025, 2011.
5. Weiser TG, Regenbogen SE, Thompson KD, et al. An estimation of the global volume of surgery: a modelling strategy based on available data. Lancet 372(9633):139-144, 2008.
6. Hughes CD, Babigian A, McCormack S, et al. The clinical and economic impact of a sustained program in global plastic surgery: valuing cleft care in resource-poor settings. Plast Reconstr Surg 130:87e-94e, 2012.
7. Corlew S, Fan VY. A model for building capacity in international plastic surgery: ReSurge International. Ann Plast Surg 67:568-570, 2011.
8. Bermudez L, Trost K, Ayala R. Investing in a surgical outcomes auditing system. Plast Surg Int. [Epub 2013 Jan 16]
9. Magee WP, Vander Burg R, Hatcher KW. Cleft lip and palate as a cost-effective health care treatment in the developing world. World J Surg 34:420-427, 2010.
10. Bickler S, Ozgediz D, Gosselin R, et al. Key concepts for estimating the burden of surgical conditions and the unmet need for surgical care. World J Surg 34:374-380, 2010.
11. Semer NB, Sullivan SR, Meara JG. Plastic surgery and global health: how plastic surgery impacts the global burden of surgical disease. J Plast Reconstr Aesthet Surg 63:1244-1248, 2010.
12. Grimes CE, Henry JA, Maraka J, et al. Cost-effectivness in low- and middle-income countries: a systematic review. World J Surg 38:252-263, 2014.
13. Moon W, Perry H, Baek RM. Is international volunteer surgery for cleft lip and palate a cost-effective and justifiable intervention? A case study from East Asia. World J Surg 36:2819-2830, 2012.
14. Corlew DS. Estimation of impact of surgical disease through economic modeling of cleft lip and palate care. World J Surg. 34:391-396, 2010.
15. Hsia RY, Mbembati NA, Macfarlane S, et al. Access to emergency and surgical care in sub-Saharan Africa: the infrastructure gap. Health Policy Plan 27:234-244, 2012.
16. Bickler SW, Rode H. Surgical services for children in developing countries. Bull World Health Organ 80:829-835, 2002.
17. Farmer P, Kim J. Surgery and global health: a view from beyond the OR. World J Surg 32:533-536, 2008.
18. Mishra B, Koirala R, Tripathi N, et al. Plastic surgery-myths and realities in developing countries: experience from eastern Nepal. Plast Surg Int 2011:870902, 2011.
19. Jovic G, Corlew DS, Bowman KG. Plastic and reconstructive surgery in Zambia: epidemiology of 16 years of practice. World J Surg 36:241-246, 2012.
20. Ozgediz D, Galukande M, Mabweijano J, et al. The neglect of the global surgical workforce: experience and evidence from Uganda. World J Surg 32:1208-1215, 2008.
21. Frenk J, Chen L, Bhutta ZA, et al. Health professionals for a new century: transforming education to strengthen health systems in an interdependent world. Lancet 376:1923-1958, 2010.
22. Mullan F. The metrics of the physician brain drain. N Engl J Med 353:1810-1818, 2005.
23. Ozgediz D, Wang J, Jayaraman S, et al. Surgical training and global health: initial results of a 5-year partnership with a surgical training program in a low-income country. Arch Surg 143:860-865; discussion 865, 2008.
24. Kasper J, Bajunirwe F. Brain drain in sub-Saharan Africa: contributing factors, potential remedies and the role of academic medical centres. Arch Dis Child 97:973-979, 2012.
25. Tyson AF, Boschini LP, Kiser MM, et al. Survival after burn in a sub-Saharan burn unit: challenges and opportunities. Burns 39:1619-1625, 2013.
26. World Health Organization. WH. Campaigns against acid violence spur change. 2011.
27. Murray C, Lopez A, Jamison D. The global burden of disease in 1990: summary results, sensitivity analysis and future directions. Bull World Health Organ 72:495-509, 1994.

28. Alkire B, Hughes CD, Nash K, et al. Potential economic benefit of cleft lip and palate repair in sub-Saharan Africa. World J Surg 35:1194-1201, 2011.

29. WHO Global Initiative for Emergency and Essential Surgical Care, 2013. Available at *http://www.who.int/surgery/globalinitiative/en/*.

30. WHO Global Health Expenditure Atlas, 2012. Available at *http://www.who.int/nha/atlas.pdf*.

31. Integrated Management for Emergency and Essential Surgical Care (IMEESC) Tool Kit. Available at *http://www.who.int/surgery/publications/imeesc/en/index.html*.

32. Interesting facts about Smile Train. Available at *http://www.smiletrain.org/assets/pdfs/smile-train-media-kit.pdf*.

33. 2011 Operation Smile annual impact report. Available at *http://www.operationsmile.org/news_events/publications/2011-annual-report/8.html*.

34. FACE to FACE International, 2013. Available at *http://www.facetofacesurgery.org/international/index.html*.

35. Martiniuk AL, Manouchehrian M, Negin JA, et al. Brain gains: a literature review of medical missions to low and middle-income countries. BMC Health Serv Res 12:134, 2012.

36. Nthumba PM. "Blitz surgery": redefining surgical needs, training, and practice in sub-Saharan Africa. World J Surg 34:433-437, 2010.

36a. Shrime MG, Sleemi A, Ravilla TD. Charitable platforms in global surgery: a systematic review of their effectiveness, cost-effectiveness, sustainability, and role training. World J Surg. [Epub 2014 March 29]

37. Patel PB, Hoyler M, Maine R, et al. An opportunity for diagonal development in global surgery: cleft lip and palate care in resource-limited settings. Plast Surg Int 2012:892437, 2012.

38. Magee WP, Raimondi HM, Beers M, et al. Effectiveness of international surgical program model to build local sustainability. Plast Surg Int 2012:185725, 2012.

39. International Humanitarian Surgery Skills Course. Feb 2-3, 2013. In Medicine SUSo, 2013.

40. University of British Columbia overview of courses, 2013. Available at *http://www.internationalsurgery.ubc.ca*.

41. Riviello R, Ozgediz D, Hsia RY, et al. Role of collaborative academic partnerships in surgical training, education, and provision. World J Surg 34:459-465, 2010.

42. Ozgediz D, Wang J, Jayaraman S, et al. Surgical training and global health. Arch Surg 143:860-865, 2008.

43. Pollock JD, Love TP, Steffes BC, et al. Is it possible to train surgeons for rural Africa? A report of a successful international program. World J Surg 35:493-499, 2011.

44. Mutabdzic D, Bedada AG, Bakanisi B, et al. Designing a contextually appropriate surgical training program in low-resource settings: the Botswana experience. World J Surg 37:1486-1491, 2013.

45. Lipnick M, Mijumbi C, Dubowitz G, et al. Surgery and anesthesia capacity-building in resource-poor settings: description of an ongoing academic partnership in Uganda. World J Surg 37:488-497, 2013.

46. Tollefson TT, Larrabee WF Jr. Global surgical initiatives to reduce the surgical burden of disease. JAMA 307:667-668, 2012.

47. Ozgediz D, Chu K, Ford N, et al. Surgery in global health delivery. Mt Sinai J Med 78:327-341, 2011.

48. Luboga S, Macfarlane SB, von Schreeb J, et al. Increasing access to surgical services in sub-Saharan Africa: priorities for national and international agencies recommended by the Bellagio Essential Surgery Group. PLoS Med 6:e1000200, 2009.

49. Frequently asked questions about implementation science. Available at *http://www.fic.nih.gov/News/Events/implementation-science/Pages/faqs.aspx*.

50. Health innovation transfer from south to north. Available at *http://www.rand.org/content/dam/rand/pubs/documented_briefings/2011/RAND_DB616.pds*.

Index